EPILEPSY AND SUDDEN DEATH
(Neurological Disease and Therapy Series/7)

Edited by: Claire M. Lathers and
           Paul L. Schraeder

Published: 1990
552 pages, bound, illustrated

$135.00 (U.S. and Canada)
$162.00 (All other countries)
(Prices subject to change without notice.)

marcel dekker, inc.
270 MADISON AVENUE • NEW YORK, NY 10016 • 212-696-9000

Epilepsy and Sudden Death

Neurological Disease and Therapy

Series Editor
William C. Koller
Department of Neurology
University of Kansas Medical Center
Kansas City, Kansas

Additional Volumes in Preparation

Epilepsy and Sudden Death

edited by

Claire M. Lathers

*Food and Drug Administration
Rockville, Maryland*

Paul L. Schraeder

*University of Medicine and Dentistry of New Jersey
Robert Wood Johnson Medical School
Camden, New Jersey*

Marcel Dekker, Inc.   New York and Basel

Library of Congress Catologing-in-Publication Data

Epilepsy and sudden death / edited by Claire M. Lathers, Paul L.
Schraeder.
    p. cm. -- (Neurological disease and therapy; v. 7)
    Includes bibliographical references.
    Includes index.
    ISBN 0-8247-8308-5 (alk. paper)
    1. Epilepsy--Risk factors. 2. Sudden death. 3. Epilepsy-
-Complications and sequelae. I. Lathers, Claire M. II. Schraeder,
Paul L. III. Series.
    [DNLM: 1. Death. Sudden--etiology. 2. Epilepsy--physiopath-
ology. W1 NE33LD v. 7 / WL 385 E64108]
    RC372.5.E624 1990
    616.8'53--dc20
    DNLM/DLC
    for Library of Congress   90-3424
                                                CIP

This book is printed on acid-free paper.

MARCEL DEKKER, INC.
270 Madison Avenue, New York, New York 10016

Current printing (last digit):
10 9 8 7 6 5 4 3 2 1

PRINTED IN THE UNITED STATES OF AMERICA

*To Bernie Robinson, for his love and words of wisdom
and to Carol, Schuyler, and Richard Lathers,
for their love, support, and encouragement in the completion
of this endeavor (CML)*

*To my wife Barbara
and to my daughters Maria and Ellen
for their patience, support and love (PLS)*

Series Introduction

Sudden and unexplained death is a mysterious and deadly complication of epilepsy. Doctors Lathers and Schraeder and their contributors discuss in detail the many central and autonomic nervous system changes in epilepsy as well as possible alterations in the cardiovascular and pulmonary system. This important topic has not received much attention in the past. This book provides a thorough discussion of all facets of epilepsy as it relates to the phenomena of sudden death. Both clinical data and basic science information are blended together to increase our understanding of this topic. This book provides valuable information for both the clinician who takes care of patients with seizures and the basic scientist who works in the laboratory studying the basic mechanism of the epilepsies.

William C. Koller, M.D., Ph.D.

Foreword

Lathers and Schraeder have assembled in this volume the experimental and clinical information available about sudden death and epilepsy. The contributors all struggle for insight into this problem, which, to my eye, resembles the field of sudden cardiac death 20 years ago. The epidemiologists identify the high risk group among epileptics as male, aged 20 to 40, and not compliant with anticonvulsant medications. The pathologist confirms these characteristics and notes that there usually is no gross cardiac or pulmonary pathology, but brain pathology is present in excess in those epileptics who die suddenly. In addition, the heart, lung, and liver weights tend to be high. Perhaps the heart is heavy due to repeated bouts of tachycardia and hypertension caused by seizure-related discharges of the sympathetic nervous system. The lungs and liver may be congested because of cardiac dysfunction. Studies using 24-hour simultaneous ambulatory recordings of the electroencephalogram and electrocardiogram show that most seizure activity is accompanied by marked sinus tachycardia caused by increased sympathetic nervous system activity. Bradycardia and ventricular arrhythmias are distinctly uncommon. These preliminary studies with ambulatory recordings have been fruitful and should be pursued.

Experimentally, electrical stimulation of certain areas in the brain can evoke ventricular tachyarrhythmias, even ventricular fibrillation. Other experimental work suggests that anticonvulsant medication (e.g., phenobarbital or phenytoin) can decrease the likelihood of arrhythmias substantially during electrically or chemically induced experimental seizures, primarily by reducing traffic on sympathetic nerves. The neural effects of these anticonvulsants decrease the heart rate and blood pressure during seizures.

Although many pieces of the epilepsy–sudden death puzzle are in place, the total picture is not clear. Death must ultimately come from serious compromise of cardiac or respiratory function in the form of ventricular fibrillation, asystole, or apnea. A recurrent theme in the speculations about sudden death in epileptics is the key role played by the autonomic nervous system. Knowledge about the causes of sudden death in coronary heart disease is more advanced and may provide some insight into sudden death in epileptics. In coronary heart disease, the number one cause of sudden death, the key element in the development of ventricular fibrillation is an arrhythmogenic myocardial substrate (e.g., large scars or substantial areas of ischemia), although the autonomic nervous system may trigger ischemia or arrhythmias. Holter recordings at the moment of sudden death in coronary heart disease usually show ventricular tachycardia that degenerates into ventricular fibrillation. Most patients who have been resuscitated from ventricular fibrillation can have ventricular tachyarrhythmias induced with programmed ventricular stimulation at any time. It is not difficult to imagine how changes in heart rate, blood pressure, and intrinsic electrophysiologic properties caused by sympathetic nervous system activity could evoke ischemic or scar-related ventricular tachyarrhythmias.

The case is quite different in epilepsy. The victims of sudden death are young and, at autopsy, are relatively free of coronary atherosclerosis. Their hearts are only slightly hypertrophied and free of the large myocardial scars that are present in victims of sudden death in coronary heart disease. For sudden death in epileptics, an arrhythmogenic myocardial substrate has not been identified. It is possible, but not likely, that intense sympathetic nervous system activity could cause ventricular fibrillation without a myocardial substrate. The sympathetic nervous system could cause ventricular fibrillation without a permanent myocardial substrate if combined with regional or global myocardial hypoxia engendered by apnea or neurogenic pulmonary edema. It should be recalled that there are other conditions in which the heart can fibrillate even though structurally normal. A striking example is the congenital long QT syndrome. In the congenital form of the long QT syndrome, there is an inequity in the distribution of cardiac sympathetic nerve terminals and in the flow of sympathetic nerve traffic to the heart. Increased sympathetic nerve traffic can cause heterogeneous electrophysiologic properties, torsade de pointes ventricular tachyarrhythmias, and ventricular fibrillation in the absence of myocardial hypertrophy or scarring. Malignant ventricular arrhythmias in the congenital long QT syndrome can be controlled with β-adrenergic blocking drugs or removal of the left stellate ganglion. It could be that the subset of epileptics most susceptible to sudden death have anatomic or functional maldistribution of the sympathetic nerve terminals in their hearts. If so, these patients would be in great danger during the autonomic storms related to seizures.

We seem a long way from understanding and controlling the problem of sudden death in epilepsy. How shall we proceed toward those goals? Additional epidemiologic inquiry should sharpen the focus on the high risk groups and we should study them intensely. Studies with ambulatory recordings will capture the events before and during sudden death. To understand this problem, we need recordings not only of the electroencephalogram and electrocardiogram, but also of respiration. Simultaneous recordings of these variables, and perhaps others (e.g., arterial oxygen saturation), during sudden death would permit us to evaluate the role of apnea or hypoxia. The role of the sympathetic nervous system could be explored more intensively with functional and biochemical evaluation of cardiac sympathetic nervous activity. Also, the anatomic distribution of cardiac sympathetic nerves in epileptics versus normals could be clarified by imaging with substances taken up by sympathetic nerve terminals in the heart. When we know the most common cause of sudden death in epileptics, we will be in a position to judge which animal models are relevant to human disease processes and select the appropriate models for study. Studies in relevant animal models will permit a quantum leap forward in our capability for generating relevant new knowledge and greatly accelerate the rate of progress. Once the experimental and clinical studies have clarified the pathophysiology of sudden death in epileptics, hypotheses about effective treatments will naturally follow and can be pursued in animal models, small pilot studies in epileptic patients, and, finally, large-scale clinical trials. Studies of the factors that govern compliance in epileptic patients should proceed now because the results can be put to immediate use controlling seizure disorders and will be important in planning effective means of controlling sudden death in this group in the future.

We are on the threshold of major advances in the problem of sudden death in epilepsy. The tools to advance our knowledge are at hand and we should energetically put them to use for the future benefit of patients with epilepsy. Knowledge gained from studies of sudden death in epileptics will very likely be useful for understanding sudden death in other situations as well.

J. Thomas Bigger, Jr., M.D.
Professor of Medicine and Pharmacology
College of Physicians and Surgeons
Columbia University
New York, New York

Foreword

Sudden death in persons with epilepsy continues to be an enigma despite its relatively common occurrence, accounting for approximately 15 percent of all deaths in persons with epilepsy. The most frequent causes of death in persons with epilepsy include: (1) a concomitant disease, (2) a brain disorder that also causes seizures, (3) status epilepticus, (4) accidental death as a result of a seizure, (5) suicide, and (6) sudden unexplained death due to an unknown cause. Overall, persons with epilepsy have a twofold increase in mortality from all causes. Past studies have failed to reveal any specific pathological findings. What has been found is that these patients die at an earlier age than the general population. The majority do not die from status epilepticus but many have low serum antiepileptic drug levels in the postmortem blood.

There are no specific pathological features although neurogenic pulmonary edema has, in the past, been suspected as one culprit. Cardiac arrhythmias accompanying epilepsy have been implicated in some cases, and in others cardiac arrhythmias have been suspected of mimicking epilepsy.

The authors of this book examine pathophysiology of sudden unexplained epileptic death. They examine apnea and bradycardia which can result from relatively minor and localized seizures on the basis of vegetative changes in the form of paroxysmal autonomic dysfunction. This frequently occurs during sleep. Past studies have implicated a hereditary prolonged QT syndrome, fatal syncope, and myocardial dysfunction. Like sudden infant death syndrome, the etiology has remained speculative.

Attention to this condition is one of the major unsolved problems in the management of the epilepsies. It remains a major cause of excess mortality, which, apart from other considerations, is reflected in unfavorable attention by the insurance industry with a major economic impact on all persons with epilepsy.

This book is a careful and painstaking compilation of basic scientific data relating events in the brain with those in the autonomic nervous system and relating events in the autonomic nervous system to effects in one of its main end organs, the heart. The book discusses the lockstep phenomenon and its relationship to autonomic dysfunction in the possible genesis of cardiac arrhythmias and epilepsy-related sudden unexplained death. Pathological changes are consistent with high catecholamine levels, which may be the final effector, possibly by excessive calcium ion influx, of the terminal event. Epilepsy-induced changes in GABA neurotransmission, possibly via intercellular second messengers such as cyclic nucleotide or via alterations in neuropeptide activity, may be implicated.

The association of cerebral lesions, particularly those of frontal lobe and neurogenic cardiographic changes associated with autonomic nervous system abnormalities, has long been reported. Over 80 years ago it was shown that catecholamine infusions might cause cardiac necrosis. This was mimicked by the condition of pheochromocytoma leading to myofibrillar degeneration with prominent contraction bands. Similar cardiac changes can be induced by stress.

There seems to be a relationship between various causes of excess catecholamine activity. These include cocaine, a compound that is associated with hypertension, ventricular tachycardia, seizures and sudden death, presumably by amplifying catecholamine effects. Pathological myocardial contraction bands are seen, as is the case in ischemia and as occurs after catecholamine infusion and in a stress-plus-steroid situation, which leads to myofibrillar degeneration where the cells die in an hypercontracted state with prominent contraction bands. This condition is considered to be similar to what is seen in postischemic reperfusion in which there appears to be an excess influx of calcium ions resulting in irreversible contracture. Similarly, the opening of the receptor-operated calcium channels by excessive amounts of norepinephrine may be a sort of final common path for these various sudden-death-inducing modalities.

The preceding considerations bring the subject of sudden unexplained epileptic death into line with what is already known about neurogenic changes in the cardiovascular system, as seen in subarachnoid hemorrhage and other stroke syndromes. As such they represent the physiological and pharmacological state-of-the-art and open new research vistas, bringing closer a sufficient understanding of this enigma, ultimately leading to its prevention.

The information presented in this book and the ideas generated by their analysis will be of major help to neuroscientists and to epileptologists in the development of more effective therapy of one of the remaining major unsolved problems in the epileptology.

Fritz E. Dreifuss, M.B., F.R.C.P., F.R.A.C.P.
Professor of Neurology
Director, Comprehensive Epilepsy Program
University of Virginia Health Sciences Center
Past-President, International League Against Epilepsy
Charlottesville, Virginia

Preface

Our collaboration in investigating possible neurogenic mechanisms of autonomic dysfunction in epilepsy started in 1979, after the sudden unexplained death of two patients of Paul Schraeder. At about that time, Claire Lathers presented a conference for the neurology residents at the Medical College of Pennsylvania in which she discussed human and experimental data on cardiovascular changes associated with seizures. The resultant collaboration developed an animal model to investigate cardiovascular autonomic dysfunction in association with epileptiform discharges. Subsequently, Dr. Harold Booker organized a symposium on sudden unexplained death for the American Epilepsy Society at the Epilepsy International meeting in Washington, D.C., in 1983. At that time it was evident that many people had concerns about introducing and highlighting the problem of sudden unexplained death in epilepsy to such a large public forum, as this concept contradicted the information given to patients by various self-help organizations, namely, that having epilepsy did not increase the risk of dying.

As a result of the symposium, Dr. Fritz Dreifuss encouraged the development of a book on sudden unexplained death in epilepsy. In the summer of 1987 the editors published a review of autonomic dysfunction, cardiac arrhythmias, and epileptiform activity (*Journal of Clinical Pharmacology 27*: 346-356). Shortly after publication, representatives of Marcel Dekker, Inc., expressed an interest in developing such a book, but with an emphasis on experimental data. This was subsequently modified to a broader overview of the clinical, pathological, and experimental phenomena relative to sudden unexplained death.

The phenomenon of sudden unexplained or unexpected death is prevalent throughout the spectrum of medicine in the United States. In sudden death, the victim dies unexpectedly without any sign of immediate cause. It should be recognized that the victim may have been in apparent good health or suffering from a known disease that was heretofore stable. The important point is that an immediate cause of death is not readily apparent upon postmortem examination. For example, of 1 million deaths attributed to cardiac causes, half may be sudden death, making this phenomenon the subject of major cardiac research into risk factors (e.g., stress). In addition, psychiatrists are well aware of the occurrence of sudden unexplained deaths in hospitalized psychiatric patients. The possible role of major psychotropic drugs in these deaths is controversial. Finally, the tragically common, yet unexplained, occurrence of sudden infant death syndrome in previously normal infants may account for up to 40% of infant deaths.

This book summarizes the current knowledge of one of the most common risk factors facing young persons with epilepsy, that is, cardiac arrhythmias and other types of potentially life-threatening autonomic dysfunction. The magnitude of the problem is apparent when one considers that epilepsy is a common condition with a prevalence of about 0.7% or more. However, there are many more persons who have seizures that are not necessarily defined as epilepsy, so that the lifetime risk of having any type of seizure may be as high as 10%. Thus, the population at risk for sudden unexplained death in relationship to a seizure or a history of seizures is significant. The prospective data from the Cook County Coroner's office indicate that the risk of sudden death in epilepsy may approach 1 in 200 persons in the general epilepsy population. If the population is that of males between ages 20 and 40 years with symptomatic epilepsy—that is, with some type of structural brain disease—who are noncompliant with antiepileptic drug use, the risk of sudden death may exceed 1 in 50.

The pathological observations in victims of sudden unexplained death in epilepsy, by definition, are unrevealing as to an immediate cause. However, a couple of associated findings are noteworthy. First, over two-thirds of the victims have definable brain pathology of various categories, explaining the epilepsy but not the deaths. Second, hemorrhagic pulmonary edema is a common but not universal finding in the lungs of victims and suggests that a major adrenergic component may exist in these deaths.

The neurophysiological observations in persons with epilepsy offer few clues to why some persons are more at risk for sudden death than others. The premorbid electroencephalograms from victims of sudden death are reported as showing greater variability in the paroxysmal activity in any given individual from one record to the next than is seen in a comparison group of other persons with epilepsy, suggesting that the victims may have more electrophysiological instability. The relatively recent availability of long-term multichannel simultaneous EEG and ECG monitoring may eventually provide some clues to the clinical electrophysiological correlates between brain discharges and potentially fatal cardiac arrhythmias. Research into this important area has thus far provided little clinically useful data.

That epileptiform discharges can be associated with severe, albeit transient, blood pressure alterations and cardiac arrhythmias is a well-recognized observation. The severity of these changes in certain unpredictable and undefined circumstances might well predispose susceptible persons to fatal arrhythmias and sudden death. Most of the currently available research data correlating epileptiform activity with autonomic dysfunction has been obtained from animal laboratory work. There are many similarities in the autonomic dysfunction induced by various arrhythmia models, including digitalis toxicity, myocardial infarction, psychotropic drug toxicity, and epileptiform discharges.

Over the past several years, various animal models of epileptiform-induced autonomic dysfunctions have been developed. These include systemic and intracerebroventricular pentylenetetrazol, intrahippocampal penicillin injection, and kindled seizures. Although the results of these various models may differ quantitatively, there is little qualitative difference in the cardiovascular changes noted with each. The occurrence of cardiac arrhythmias and blood pressure alterations in association with all degrees of epileptiform discharge, but not in all individual animals, raises the possibility that some individuals may be more susceptible to life-threatening arrhythmias than others. It may be that a combination of changes, that is, pathological, neurophysiological, biochemical, pharmacological, and genetic, may interact in some unfortunate individuals to produce a fatal event. Even interictal discharges may, in some individuals, present a risk. The use of increasingly sophisticated quantitative analysis of heretofore subtle but clinically important autonomic cardiovascular changes in association with all degrees of epileptiform activity should help in determining individual susceptibility to serious disruptions of function. There is little investigation of neurochemical risk factors in the production of autonomic dysfunction associated with epileptiform activity.

Drugs such as alcohol, cocaine, and psychotropic agents are known to be associated with an increased risk of arrhythmia. Whether use of these agents in persons with epilepsy predisposes them to an increased chance of sudden death is unknown, although an a priori risk seems evident. The most intangible risk factor in sudden death is that of stress. Cardiologists are cognizant of this relationship as a major problem predisposing to sudden death in persons with coronary artery disease. It seems strange that there is so little research into the risk of stress as a predisposing factor to arrhythmias in persons with epilepsy.

The prevention of sudden death is impossible without knowledge of its mechanisms and risk factors. Of the currently available antiepileptic drugs, phenobarbital and phenytoin have antiarrhythmic effects. However, determining whether therapeutic blood levels of these drugs prevent sudden death is impossible to ascertain, especially since most victims of sudden death have subtherapeutic or no levels of antiepileptic drugs. The material in this book is but the beginning of the task of determining why some individuals with epilepsy are at risk for premature death of an unexplained nature. Prevention will come only after the first task is completed.

Claire M. Lathers
Paul L. Schraeder

Contents

Contributors

Isha Agarwal Department of Pharmacology, The Medical College of Pennsylvania, Eastern Pennsylvania Psychiatric Institute, Philadelphia, Pennsylvania

John F. Annegers, Ph.D. Health Services, University of Texas Health Science Center at Houston School of Public Health, Houston, Texas

J. Thomas Bigger, Jr., M.D. College of Physicians and Surgeons, Columbia University, New York, New York

Sally A. Blakley, Ph.D. Health Services, University of Texas Health Science Center at Houston, School of Public Health, Houston, Texas

Lance D. Blumhardt, M.D. Department of Neurological Science, University of Liverpool and Walton Hospital, Liverpool, England

Arthur W. K. Chan, Ph.D. Research Institute on Alcoholism, New York State Division of Alcoholism & Alcohol Abuse, and State University of New York, Buffalo, New York

Issac L. Crawford, Ph.D. Department of Neurology, University of Texas Southwestern Medical Center and the Southwestern Regional Epilepsy Center, Veterans Administration Medical Center, Dallas, Texas

Jeffrey M. Dodd-o*   The Medical College of Pennsylvania, Eastern Pennsylvania Psychiatric Institute, Philadelphia, Pennsylvania

Kathleen M. Dolce[†]   Department of Drug Metabolism, Smith Kline & French Laboratories, King of Prussia, Pennsylvania

Fritz E. Dreifuss, M.D.   University of Virginia Hospital, Charlottesville, Virginia

Judy Gerard-Ciminera, M.D.   Department of Family Practice, Warminster General Hospital, Warminster, and Department of Family Practice, Holy Redeemer Hospital, Meadowbrook, Pennsylvania

Jeffrey H. Goodman, Ph.D.[‡]   Department of Neurology, University of Texas Southwestern Medical Center and Southwestern Regional Epilepsy Center, Veterans Administration Medical Center, Dallas, Texas

Richard W. Homan, M.D.[§]   Department of Neurology, University of Texas Southwestern Medical Center and Southwestern Regional Epilepsy Center, Veterans Administration Medical Center, Dallas, Texas

Stephen J. Howell   Department of Neurological Science, University of Liverpool and Walton Hospital, Liverpool, England

John R. Hughes, M.D., Ph.D.   Department of Neurology, College of Medicine, University of Illinois Medical Center, Chicago, Illinois

Kam F. Jim, Ph.D.**   Medical College of Pennsylvania, Eastern Pennsylvania Psychiatric Institute, Philadelphia, Pennsylvania

Clare Kahn, Ph.D.[†]   Department of Drug Metabolism, Smith Kline & French Laboratories, Upper Merion, Pennsylvania

Current affiliation:
  *Department of Biological Science, University of North Texas, Fort Worth, Texas.
  †Smithkline Beecham Pharmaceuticals, Swedeland, Pennsylvania
  ‡Neurology Research Center, Helen Hayes Hospital, New York State Department of Health, West Haverstraw, New York.
  §Department of Neurology, Medical College of Ohio, Toledo, Ohio.
  **Wyeth-Ayerst Research, Philadelphia, Pennsylvania.

Claire M. Lathers, Ph.D.* Department of Pharmacology, The Medical College of Pennsylvania, Eastern Pennsylvania Psychiatric Institute, Philadelphia, Pennsylvania

Jan E. Leestma, M.D. Chicago Neurosurgical Center, Columbus Hospital, Chicago, Illinois

William D. Matthews, Ph.D.** Department of Investigative Toxicology, Smith Kline & French Laboratories, Swedeland, Pennsylvania

John A. Messenheimer, M.D. Department of Neurology, School of Medicine, University of North Carolina, Chapel Hill, North Carolina

Daniel K. O'Rourke, M.D. Department of Neurosurgery, The Medical College of Pennsylvania, Eastern Pennsylvania Psychiatric Institute, Philadelphia, Pennsylvania

Wallace B. Pickworth, Ph.D. Addiction Research Center, National Institute on Drug Abuse, Baltimore, Maryland

Stephen R. Quint, Ph.D. Department of Neurology, School of Medicine, University of North Carolina, Chapel Hill, North Carolina

Paul L. Schraeder, M.D. Division of Neurology, Department of Medicine, University of Medicine and Dentistry of New Jersey, Robert Wood Johnson Medical School, Camden, New Jersey

Rochelle D. Schwartz, Ph.D. Department of Pharmacology, Duke University Medical Center, Durham, North Carolina

Michele M. Spino Department of Pharmacology, The Medical College of Pennsylvania, Eastern Pennsylvania Psychiatric Institute, Philadelphia, Pennsylvania

William H. Spivey, M.D. Department of Emergency Medicine, The Medical College of Pennsylvania, Eastern Pennsylvania Psychiatric Institute, Philadelphia, Pennsylvania

Current affiliation:

*Food and Drug Administration, Rockville, Maryland; Universities Space Research Association Division of Space Biomedicine, Working in NASA's Cardiovascular Laboratory in the Space Biomedical Institute; and Department of Pharmacology, Uniformed Services, University of Health Sciences, Bethesda, Maryland.

**Smithkline Beecham Pharmaceuticals, Swedeland, Pennsylvania.

Amy Z. Stauffer, M.D.* Department of Pharmacology, The Medical College of Pennsylvania, Eastern Pennsylvania Psychiatric Institute, Philadelphia, Pennsylvania

Michael B. Tennison, M.D. Department of Neurology, School of Medicine, University of North Carolina, Chapel Hill, North Carolina

Christopher F. Terrence, M.D.† Veterans Administration Medical Center, Newington, and Department of Neurology, University of Connecticut School of Medicine, Farmington, Connecticut

Laurie S. Y. Tyau, M.D. Department of Pharmacology, The Medical College of Pennsylvania, Eastern Pennsylvania Psychiatric Institute, Philadelphia, Pennsylvania

Braxton B. Wannamaker, M.D. Epilepsy Services and Research, Inc., Charleston, South Carolina

*Department of Pediatrics, University of Connecticut, Farmington, Connecticut.
†Veterans Administration Medical Center, East Orange, New Jersey.

1

Natural History of Epilepsy

JAN E. LEESTMA *Chicago Neurosurgical Center, Columbus Hospital, Chicago, Illinois*

I. INTRODUCTION

The term *seizure* is firmly rooted in lay and medical usage and often is erroneously used interchangeably with the term epilepsy. Seizures can be epileptic in nature, but they can also be nonepileptic and take the form of a syncopal attack, a fit of rage, a reflection of some somatic dysfunction, movement disorder, or behavioral reaction not caused by abnormal electrical discharges in the brain.

Epilepsy is a medical condition which most physicians know very well in practice but often find difficult to precisely define in a manner universally acceptable to all. Gastaut's (1973) definition captures many of the seminal elements of epilepsy: "A chronic brain disorder of various etiologies characterized by recurrent seizures due to excessive discharge of cerebral neurons." An important aspect of this definition is chronicity; as Gastaut points out, a single or occasional seizure that occurs in connection with an acute illness (high fever, toxic states, trauma) should not necessarily be considered epilepsy. Others would add the qualification that seizures be demonstrable on EEG before being accepted as true epilepsy (Wolf, 1985).

The classification of epileptic seizures and epileptic syndromes has evolved from personally propounded schemes to a more widely agreed upon classification as a result of the work of the General Assembly of the International League against Epilepsy (ILAE), which in 1981 drafted the International Classification of Epileptic Seizures (ICES). It was the intent of this collaborative effort to develop a system of classification that would be capable of evolution and not hinder the advancement of understanding about epilepsy (Porter, 1986; Wolf, 1985).

The ICES recognizes three major categories of epileptic seizures: (1) focal (partial or local) seizures, (2) generalized (convulsive or nonconvulsive) seizures, and (3) unclassified epileptic seizures (Commission on Classification and Terminology of the International League Against Epilepsy, 1981).

Focal seizures are those caused by the abnormal electrical behavior of a limited population of neurons. They can be subdivided into those that are simple and focal, those that are complex but focal and may or may not involve loss of consciousness, and those that begin focally but evolve into generalized tonic-clonic convulsions.

Generalized seizures can be subdivided into the absence seizures (previously petit mal), myoclonic seizures, clonic seizures, tonic seizures, tonic-clonic seizures, and atonic seizures or combinations of these.

Unclassified epileptic seizures are those that do not comfortably fit into the preceding categories. Status epilepticus is a separate designation for any of the groups in which the seizures are repetitive or continuous. When motor seizures are focal but continuous, they are referred to as epilepsia partialis continua (Commission on Classification and Terminology of the International League Against Epilepsy, 1981; Wolf, 1985). Some clinicians still retain the old designations: generalized tonic-clonic (GTC; grand mal), absence seizures (petit mal), psychomotor (temporal lobe), Jacksonian (focal motor), or complex seizures. But all of these are included in the newer scheme described above.

Another dimension of classification utilized by some (Parsonage, 1982) is whether the epilepsy is primary (probably genetically determined) or secondary to some other known or suspected process. The essential qualities of this distinction are also expressed by the designation preferred by some workers, that of idiopathic (of unknown etiology) or symptomatic (secondary to some disease process) origin. Sometimes seizures may not be chronic (and thus nonepileptic by some workers' definitions) but are linked with an underlying medical condition such as hypoglycemia, electrolyte disturbances, use or withdrawal from certain drugs, or other toxic states (Messing and Simon, 1986).

One further consideration in classifying epileptic seizures has to do with the frequency of attacks or level of activity. Epilepsy may be described as active, periodic or episodic, quiescent or inactive, or, perhaps, cured. Here too confusion occurs in classification, since it is questionable in the minds of some (Lennox, 1960; Loiseau, 1972) whether epilepsy is ever cured or is only quiescent for any period of time. The whole issue of discontinuance of pharmacological treatment of an epileptic seizure disorder once it has been diagnosed is a subject of considerable discussion and concern by clinicians (Loiseau, 1972; Penry, 1977; Richens, 1982; Schmidt, 1985).

II. EPIDEMIOLOGY OF EPILEPSY

A. Incidence

No population is spared from epilepsy. Extensive studies on the distribution, occurrence rates, and other population data regarding epilepsy have been conducted on a large scale in many countries. The incidence of epilepsy, the rate of occurrence of *new* cases each year per unit of population, is quite variable. The incidence of epilepsy in the general population ranges from about 11/100,000 in Norway (Krohn, 1961), to 20-22/100,000 in Poland (Grudzinska, 1973; Zielinski, 1974a,b), 30-54/100,000 in the United States (Hauser and Kurland, 1975; Kurland, 1959; Schoenberg, 1985), 30-70/100,000 in Great Britain (Brewis

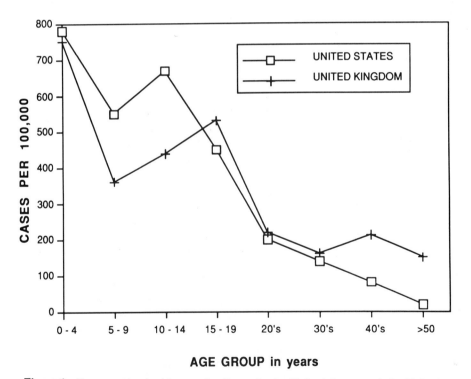

Figure 1 Comparative incidence of epilepsy in the United States and the United Kingdom in cases per 100,000 population by age groups. [Adapted from Epilepsy Foundation of America (1975) statistics; data from Great Britain (1969) and Lennox (1960).]

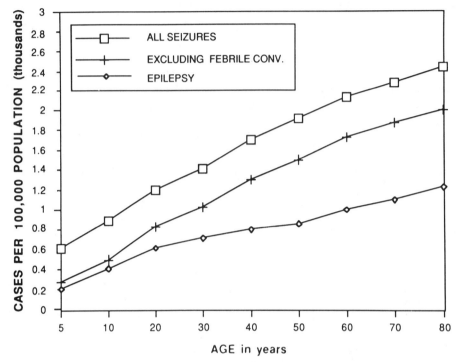

Figure 2 Cumulative incidence of seizures at various ages (by decades) in cases per 100,000 population. [Data derived from a study conducted in Denmark by Juul-Jensen and Foldspang (1983).]

et al., 1966; Pond et al., 1960), and intermediate rates in Denmark (Juul-Jensen and Ipsen, 1976), Japan, and other countries (Zielinski, 1982).

If the figures reported are realistic, at least 73,000–131,000 persons developed epilepsy in the United States in 1987 (Hoffman, 1988). But many feel that any statistics on incidence are always conservative owing to problems of definition, failure of sufferers to seek medical advice and diagnosis, and the failure of a central agency to collect or properly record data.

Most new cases of epilepsy arise in persons under the age of 20 years (see Figure 1) and there is a decreasing chance of developing epilepsy with each advancing decade. Males are more likely to develop epilepsy than females (Epilepsy Foundation of America, 1975; Zielinski, 1982).

B. Prevalence

The distribution of epilepsy within a given population at any one time is the prevalence of the disorder. Just as incidence figures are inaccurate, prevalence figures are even more so, dependent as they are on cumulative figures and population dynamics. Studies in various parts of the world show great diversity in prevalence figures. Important in analyzing these figures is an appreciation of how cases are selected or excluded. For example, based on a population study in Rochester, Minnesota (Hauser and Kurland, 1975), about 5.9% of the population will have at least one nonfebrile convulsion in their lifetime. It is highly questionable that this figure should be considered a measure of epilepsy prevalence, for if it were, it would mean that nearly 14 million persons in the United States would be affected. If prevalence rates for children are selected, 1–3% (10–30/1000) of children have had seizures, and, by some definitions, have epilepsy (Aicardi, 1985; Hauser, 1981; Lennox-Buchthal, 1982; Rose et al., 1973). If one considers the entire population, one arrives at a so-called lifetime prevalence rate. This figure also is subject to considerable variation. In Colombia the prevalence has been reported to be nearly 2% of the population (19.5/1000) but in Japan and Taiwan the rate may be as low as 0.13% (1.3–1.5/1000) (Rubio-Donnadieu, 1972; Zielinski, 1982). If cases are limited to those who have epilepsy that is clinically active, the reported prevalence rates in the general population of major industrialized nations of the Western hemisphere is probably between 0.57 and 0.78% (5.7–7.8/1000) (Hauser and Kurland, 1975; Zielinski, 1982). If a less strict definition of epilepsy is applied, the figure of about 1.2% of the population may be closer to reality (Juul-Jensen and Foldspang, 1983).

Just as the incidence of epilepsy is age related, prevalence figures reflect population demographics with a gradually increasing prevalence with age, until after age 50 when the number of affected persons begins to decline, and, for the general population, begins to plateau as illustrated in Figures 1 and 2 (Juul-Jensen and Foldspang, 1983; Zielinski, 1982).

C. Type of Disorder

The types of seizure disorders across the population are also nonuniform, as illustrated in Figure 3. Generalized tonic-clonic (grand mal) seizures are the most common in all age groups with absence (petit mal) attacks the next most common in childhood but comparatively rare in older age groups. So-called psychomotor (complex-partial) epilepsy is uncommon in young children but assumes a secondary position in adolescence and during the adult years (Epilepsy Foundation of America, 1975; Parke-Davis Co., 1958).

Implied by these trends is the phenomenon of change of seizure type in the same individual. It has been estimated that at least 50% of epileptic persons will

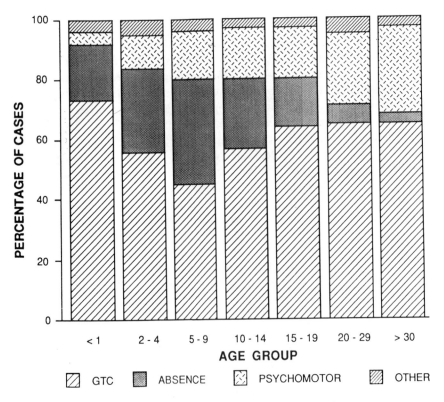

Figure 3 Types of seizure disorders by percentage incidence by age groups. Note the relative commonness of absence seizures in younger individuals and its relative rarity in older persons. [Data were derived from Parke-Davis (1958) and from Epilepsy Foundation of America (1975).]

display more than one type of seizure during their lifetime (Gibbs and Gibbs, 1952; Lennox, 1960). A not uncommon pattern is for an infant to suffer GTC convulsions in association with an acute illness, later to develop absence attacks, and as a young adult or adult to develop GTC or some other forms of seizure disorder.

III. ETIOLOGIES FOR EPILEPSY

A. Infants and Children

In the neonatal period the occurrence of seizures is a very serious event associated with a high mortality rate, due not to seizures per se but to the underlying conditions that give rise to seizure activity. In a recent prospective study (Holden et al., 1982) of 54,000 pregnancies, 277 infants (0.5%) developed seizures; about 35% of these infants did not survive. Most deaths occurred in the perinatal period, but some occurred up to seven years later. Of the 14 infants in the group who died at a year or more of age, most had severe "cerebral palsy" and continued seizure activity. The etiologies of the seizure disorders in the group of neonates included congenital CNS abnormalities (hydranencephaly, encephalocele, porencephaly, hydrocephaly), infectious diseases (cytomegalovirus, toxoplasmosis, herpes simplex, bacterial meningitis, or generalized sepsis), intracranial hemorrhages, respiratory and/or cardiac anomalies or insufficiency, fluid and electrolyte imbalance, or some other recognizable condition. It is interesting that about 70% of the 181 infants who survived had no subsequent development of epilepsy or other disability. Thirteen percent had "cerebral palsy," 19% had an IQ below 70, and 20% of the survivors suffered from epilepsy only. Other studies show similar results (Kurokawa et al., 1982; Matsumoto et al., 1983). Overall it appears that newborn infants suffer an incidence rate of seizures of about 0.6% (60/1000) (Brown, 1982). It is obvious that surviving newborns who experience seizures in the perinatal period do not make up a large percentage of the existing epileptic population.

The most heavily affected group of children who suffer seizures are the dler age group (1-5 years). The incidence of seizures in this group excee (50/1000). The most common etiology is the so-called febrile convuls' ally reported as being a generalized convulsion. On careful study en analysis, focality of onset can usually be demonstrated (Annegers Brown, 1982). At least 35% of all seizures observed in the unde group are due to fever and toxic states associated with infect' dation of America, 1975; Gesell and Amatruda, 1947). Ne ity is idiopathic or genetic epilepsy (about 24%), which r during febrile episodes, followed by seizures secondary brain malformation, or other CNS damage. Not to be which may account for about 15% of the cases, is child abuse. A long list of other possible causes. 20% of cases, includes infections, toxic or me' of metabolism, primary and metastatic brai cardi, 1985; Epilepsy Foundation of Am al., 1982).

The etiologic importance of infantile seizures (usually febrile convulsions) on the subsequent development of epilepsy is controversial. Rates of occurrence range from 10% to more than 20% (Annegers et al., 1979; Lennox-Buchtal, 1982; Lombroso, 1983). A complicating factor in febrile convulsions is the correlation with a positive family history for febrile convulsions, which doubles the risk of repeated seizures (Annegers et al., 1979, 1982; Lennox-Buchtal, 1972). Important also is the principle that the younger the age at which the individual develops seizures, the greater the chance that heredity plays a role in their etiology (Lennox-Buchthal, 1973; Schiottz-Christensen, 1972). Genetic interactions with epilepsy development are complex and may involve chromosomal abnormalities, subtle genetic defects, inherited metabolic diseases, and multigenetic inheritance (Jennings and Bird, 1981). There is considerable evidence that the tendency to develop epilepsy spontaneously may be inherited through an autosomal dominant gene (Metrakos and Metrakos, 1961).

Males appear more likely to develop continued seizures than are females (Millichap, 1968), and firstborn children are more likely to suffer a seizure disorder than are their siblings, a finding that Gowers noted more than 80 years ago (Orr and Risch, 1953). This may be related to a more prolonged labor period and hypoxic stress in the infant in primiparous women than in women who have born more than one child.

Children in the age group 5 years old and older who develop seizures will most likely have had them as infants, but they may occur for the first time in connection with some external event such as hypoxia or hyperventilation. Heredity, brain trauma, CNS infection, mental retardation syndromes, old birth injury or congenital brain lesions, migraine, and tumors are probably the most commonly implicated factors in the development of new seizures in this age group (Aicardi, 1985).

B. Adults

the adult years a number of important identifiable conditions are responsible
the development of seizures and epilepsy (Marsden and Reynolds, 1982).
most common predisposing condition is that the individual had seizures as
ld or has a strong family history of seizure disorder, i.e., in parents or
gs (Annegers et al., 1982; Porter, 1984).
ebral vascular diseases may account for 10-20% of unselected adult epi-
d for perhaps 50% of cases after the age of 50 years (Juul-Jensen, 1964;
son and Dodge, 1954), where cortical infarctions are probably the most
t lesion. Arteriovenous malformations are associated with a high per-
seizures in the younger adult, with as many as 40% of individuals
sion developing epilepsy (Wilson and Stein, 1984). Aneurysms, intra-
orrhages, subarachnoid hemorrhage, and intraventricular hemor-

rhages account for a lesser number of cases in younger adults. Brain trauma is probably the most frequently observed cause of adult seizures, occurring as a late complication of head injury in 20-50% of individuals who sustain an open or penetrating brain injury such as a gunshot wound (Caveness et al., 1979; Jennett, 1982; Salazar et al., 1985) and in about 10% of victims of blunt head trauma (Jennett and Teasdale, 1982; Walker and Erculei, 1969).

Tumors of the brain (primary or secondary) are also an important cause of epilepsy in the adult and may account for about 10% of cases of adult-onset epilepsy (Juul-Jensen, 1964). In partial or focal epilepsies, tumors may account for 30-40% of the etiologies (Currie et al., 1971; Raynor et al., 1959). Conversely, seizures are the presenting symptom in 60-80% of brain tumor cases (Meldrum and Corsellis, 1984).

Central nervous system infections, principally brain abscesses, are an important treatable cause of adult-onset seizures, with as many as 72% of surviving individuals continuing to suffer posttreatment seizures (Legg et al., 1973). Other infectious processes that may lead to the epileptic state include bacterial, fungal, and mycobacterial meningitis, viral encephalitis, and parasitic diseases. Degenerative and demyelinating diseases as well as various toxic and metabolic derangements including alcohol withdrawal (as discussed by Chan et al., Chapter 19, this book) and reactions to various illicit drugs or therapeutic agents account for the remaining cases.

IV. PATHOLOGICAL BASIS FOR EPILEPSY

The ultimate pathological basis for an epileptic state is always a matter of uncertainty since the techniques available to the neuropathologist are mostly measures of static phenomena and, for the most part, cannot display the dynamic processes involved in epilepsy. Nevertheless, empirical observations of postmortem material and the occasional surgical specimen when correlated with clinical observations, which may include intraoperative corticography or implanted electrode studies, provide inferential data regarding the types of lesions that may cause seizures. One common denominator of most epileptogenic lesions is that they may produce deafferentation of a population of neurons and/or alter the environment of a "trigger" population of neurons to enable or cause them to become a seizure focus (Goldensohn, 1985; Scheibel et al., 1974; Ward, 1969). The unfortunate fact is that as a group, when epileptic individuals come to autopsy, for whatever reason, a disappointing percentage (usually 10% or fewer) displays any lesion that could be construed as causative by ordinary techniques, yet if careful examination is done, microscopic mesial temporal lobe pathology is very common (Meldrum and Corsellis, 1984).

A. Lesions Observed in Epileptic Persons

The lesions expected and observed in epileptic persons at autopsy usually correlate with a known or suspected underlying and causal disease condition (so-called symptomatic epilepsy). In those individuals whose epilepsy is idiopathic or "hereditary," lesions are not usually found. In cases of symptomatic epilepsy lesions may be classified as follows (Mathieson, 1982):

Lesions acquired in utero: disorders of neuronal migration and maturation, in utero infections, miscellaneous malformations, phaecomatoses, vascular anomalies, inherited disorders

Lesions acquired in the perinatal period: hypoxic, toxic, and metabolic disorders, infection, circulatory disturbances, birth injury

Lesions acquired in childhood or adulthood: infection, neoplasia, vascular diseases, toxic and metabolic disorders, trauma, autoimmune and inflammatory disorders

An exhaustive review of these lesions is beyond the scope of this discussion and the interested reader is referred to several references for more information (Epilepsy Foundation of America, 1975; Laidlaw and Richens, 1982; Meldrum and Corsellis, 1984).

B. Ammon's Horn Sclerosis

Sclerosis of the mesial temporal lobe and hippocampal formation is probably the most consistently observed lesion in any epileptic person in whom no obvious cause for the seizure disorder can be observed. This was noted in 1880 by Sommer, after whom a portion of the mesial hippocampal region is named (Dam, 1982), but it had been noted earlier by Meynert (Dam, 1980). The prevalence of this lesion is highly variable, depending not only on the population under study but on the diligence of the neuropathological analysis. A number of early studies (Corsellis, 1957; Margerison and Corsellis, 1966; Sano and Malamud, 1953) on autopsy material indicate that about 50% of cases studied, which in many instances centered on persons with chronic active epilepsy, showed some degree of neuronal dropout and replacement gliosis in the hippocampus and/or the adjacent temporal lobe (Cavanagh et al., 1958). The lesion was grossly more often unilateral than bilateral, but microscopically bilaterality was the rule. Histological neuronal dropout associated with seizures may be confined to the Rose H3 (inner hippocampal) sector only, but dropout presumably due only to hypoxemia is typically placed in the Rose H1 (outer hippocampal) or Sommer's sector (Dam, 1980, 1982; Margerison and Corsellis, 1966). Mixtures and variability of neuronal loss as well as dropout outside the Ammon's horn complicate the interpretation of causality in human cases. A further discordant note comes from a comparative study of the hippocampus of epileptic and nonepileptic persons. In this study Morel and Wildi (1956) found mesial temporal lobe sclerosis in 20% of epileptics yet also found it in 40% of nonepileptic persons. In spite of this finding, most neuropathologists still regard Ammon's horn sclerosis in an epileptic individual as somehow related to his or her condition.

Sclerosis of the mesial temporal lobe(s) is considered both a cause and an effect of epilepsy. Numerous experimental studies have confirmed that induced seizure states in animals can bring about the lesion (Meldrum and Brierley, 1973), but there is considerable argument over whether it is the seizure state per se, the chemicals causing the seizures, or secondary phenomena such as hypoxia, cerebral edema, alterations in cerebral perfusion, or neurotransmitter milieu which causes death of neurons in the hippocampus (Meldrum, 1982; Meldrum and Brierley, 1973; Meldrum and Corsellis, 1984). With respect to a causal relationship of seizures to the hippocampus, many subscribe to the notion that a hippocampal lesion, however acquired, may act to "kindle" the seizure state or act as a primary epileptogenic focus (Dam, 1980; Wada, 1976). A good deal of the rationale for surgical removal of mesial temporal lobe structures in chronic active, and intractable, epileptics is rooted in this hypothesis (Penfield and Jasper, 1954; Ward, 1975, 1983).

C. Cerebellar Atrophy

A not uncommon finding in persons suffering from chronic intractable epilepsy is extensive cerebellar cortical atrophy. This atrophy may involve virtually the whole of the cerebellar cortex or may be somewhat circumscribed, though usually bilateral and symmetrical. The posterior-lateral portions of the cerebellum are most commonly affected and the vermis is usually spared. The microscopic appearance of the atrophy reveals extensive Purkinje and granular cell atrophy with replacement gliosis. Perhaps the etiology of cerebellar atrophy found in epileptics can be inferred by careful consideration of the topography of the atrophy, as suggested by Gessage and Urich (1985), who make the very important point that cerebral damage (as in hemiatrophy) may cause crossed cerebellar atrophy, which may be misinterpreted as due to some intrinsic aspect of epilepsy or its treatment.

Cerebellar atrophy in epileptic persons is often considered a toxic complication of phenytoin (Dilantin) therapy, but this contention is controversial. Experimental studies in animals has shown a specific effect of phenytoin on Purkinje cell axons that may lead to cerebellar atrophy, but phenytoin-caused cerebellar pathology in man remains inferential (Lindvall and Nilsson, 1984; Volk and Kirschgassner, 1985). Perhaps the greatest challenge to the phenytoin toxicity hypothesis is the fact that cerebellar atrophy was observed in chronic epileptics well before the availability of phenytoin as an anticonvulsant (Mathieson, 1982). In experimental seizure studies cerebellar neurons have been shown to be vulnerable, but as in the case of interpretation of causality of neuronal loss in the Ammon's horn in seizures, the same concerns have been raised for the cerebellum, e.g., direct effect by seizures vs. secondary hypoxia-ischemia alone or acting synergistically with phenytoin (Atillo et al., 1983; Dam, 1972; Dam et al., 1984; Siesjo and Wieloch, 1986). With regard to the relationship of cerebellar atrophy to intractability of seizure disorders, perhaps the cerebellum also has a dual cause and effect role: since the cerebellum exerts an inhibitory influence on the CNS, its degradation might remove an important inhibitory factor in some epileptic persons (Baier et al., 1984; Penry, 1977; Upton, 1982).

D. Other Neuropathological Changes Found in Epileptic Individuals

A host of neuropathological findings have been reported in the epileptic brain alone or in addition to lesions of the Ammon's horn and nearby temporal lobe structures and in the cerebellum. Prominent among these are congenital and presumably malformational-developmental phenomena such as neuronal-glial heterotopial, cerebral, and cerebellar cortical malformations, and dysgenetic lesions and other similar processes (Meencke and Janz, 1984; Meldrum and Corsellis, 1984). Traumatic lesions (contusions, hematomas, and "inner cerebral" traumatic leions), tumors, vascular malformations, and other acquired focal lesions of the cerebral hemispheres, such as lesions due to hypoxia, fever, or vascular insufficiency, as well as many toxic and metabolic conditions (known or unknown), have been reported as causes of the epileptic state and are commonly accepted as such by neuropathologists and clinicians.

More difficult to assess are the lesions that may be discovered only on microscopic examination of the chronically epileptic brain. These include the presumed effects of the seizures themselves or those that may follow status epilepticus. These changes occur according to many of the well-known patterns of selective vulnerability in hypoxia [which may attend the seizure episode(s)] (Schade and McMenemey, 1963), to microcirculatory deficiencies accompanying the seizure(s), or both (Meldrum and Corsellis, 1984). As mentioned earlier, it is often difficult to separate those lesions which are causal and those which are the effect of the seizure. One such change, about which little has been written in more than 20 years, is the pronounced subpial astrogliosis over the cerebral cortex observed in some chronic epileptic persons. Chaslin (1889) was apparently the first to note this lesion, but others such as Spielmeyer (1927), Scholz (1959), and Peiffer (1963) have reported it and hypothesized as to its etiology. Most regard this lesion as secondary to some aspect of the chronic epileptic process.

V. MORBIDITY AND MORTALITY IN EPILEPSY

A. Morbidity

Epileptic individuals suffer from many secondary effects of their seizure disorder which may be only annoying or may be life threatening. The behavioral, social, and lifestyle concomitants of seizure disorders have been extensively discussed elsewhere (Laidlaw and Laidlaw, 1982; Porter, 1984; Porter and Morselli, 1985), but may include severe behavioral disability including neurosis, psychosis, and suicidal behavior that may become life threatening. The epileptic state, especially if it is chronic and poorly controlled, may progressively affect intellectual function and learning. Sudden epileptic attacks may render the affected individual vulnerable to accident or injury that may be fatal. Examples are falls to hard surfaces or against protruding objects at dangerous or inopportune times (crossing streets, on stairs, in the bath). The injuries that may occur in connection with these events may include spinal, long bone, facial or cranial fractures, and brain injury, including epidural and subdural hematoma. Cortical brain contusions due to falls, most common in the poorly controlled epileptic person, may exacerbate the seizure disorder. When an epileptic person attempts to operate a vehicle such as a bicycle, motorcycle, or motor vehicle, there is always a risk of an attack occurring and resulting in a collision. Such accidents are not uncommon among teenagers who suffer from undiagnosed and untreated absence seizures and sometimes result in fatality (Leestma, 1988). Industrial and workplace accidents may involve amputations or more serious injuries to the epileptic person, especially if dangerous chemicals, heavy machinery, high voltages, high heat, or molten metals are part of the work environment. Accidental and fatal burns may result should a seizure occur when a person with epilepsy is smoking away from observers who may render assistance. Likewise, drowning may occur during bathing, swimming, or diving, should a seizure occur at that time. Such cases of accidental injury or death constitute a major form of morbidity and mortality for the epileptic individual (Epilepsy Foundation of America, 1975; Zielinski, 1974a,b, 1982).

Morbidity and disability due to epilepsy are significantly improved when anticonvulsant medication forms a part of the therapeutic regime. If case reports of clinical improvement are a realistic measure of therapeutic effectiveness, it appears that between 70 and 80% of individuals show important amelioration of their disease. However, clinical trials reveal a somewhat less dramatic response to drug therapy with those who experience major improvement, those with mild or moderate improvement, and those with no improvement or worsening of symptoms about equally represented (Coatsworth and Penry, 1972). There is no doubt that anticonvulsant drugs play a major role in the control of epilepsy, but the complications and side effects of therapy also constitute an important source

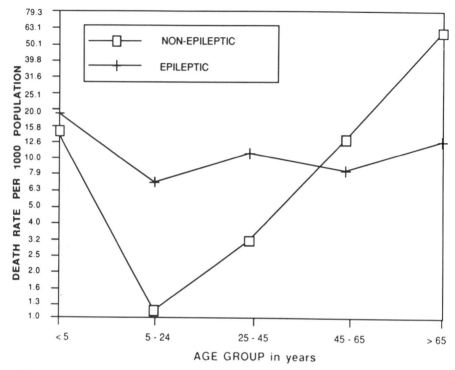

Figure 4 Comparative death rates in nonepileptic and epileptic persons by age groups and by death rates per 1000 population. [Data adapted from Lennox (1960) and Rodin (1968).]

of morbidity in the epileptic individual and possibly to the fetus in pregnant epileptic women (Porter, 1984; Woodbury et al., 1982).

B. Mortality

1. Life-Span Analysis

Accurate figures for mortality rates and life expectancy in epileptic persons and for deaths ascribable to epilepsy are acknowledged to be nearly impossible to obtain owing to the previously described problems in defining not only what constitutes epilepsy but also whether a given death was due to epilepsy or simply associated with it. Furthermore, methods of reporting vary so enormously that the method of case selection also influences the data. Nevertheless, considerable effort has been expended over many years to attempt an analysis of the question of mortality in the epileptic population.

The age-adjusted death rates for epilepsy worldwide vary significantly, with the locations showing the highest rates at about 3-4/100,000 population being Chile, Mexico, Portugal, Colombia, and Puerto Rico. Most other countries have epilepsy death rates of 1-2/100,000; Denmark and Iceland appear to have the lowest at about 0.4/100,000 persons (Zielinski, 1982).

Although it can be argued that the number of persons dying of epilepsy in the United States is relatively small (< 1/100,000 persons per year) (Zielinski, 1982), this figure does not do justice to the fact that the epileptic individual experiences double to triple the expected death rate of age-matched controls (Woodbury, 1978; Zielinski, 1974b). Furthermore, the median age at death for unselected persons with epilepsy may be between 32.5 and 43.5 years of age, compared to 68.3-69.5 years in nonepileptic persons, as reported for the years 1960-1966 by Rodin (1968). Similar statistics are reported by the Epilepsy Foundation of America (1975). At various ages the comparative death rates of epileptic and nonepileptic persons are often quite different, as seen in Figure 4, which is adapted from the data of Lennox (1960). Note that in the infant and toddler age group, the death rate in nonepileptic and epileptic individuals is not markedly different, but between age 5 and 24 years, the death rate for epileptic persons is nearly seven times that for nonepileptic persons and between 25 and 45 years it is about four times as high (Lennox, 1960). In those over 45 the nonepileptic population suffers a very significantly greater death rate than do persons with epilepsy of the same age, perhaps because persons with epilepsy tend to be more closely monitored by physicians and are probably more health conscious than other individuals. Within the population with epilepsy, men are more likely to die of some complication of epilepsy than are women, and nonwhites are more at risk than whites by a factor of more than 2:1 (Henriksen et al., 1967; Kurtzke, 1972; Kurtzke et al., 1973).

2. Causes of Death in Epilepsy

Reports regarding the causes of death in epileptic persons are heir to the same diversity and imprecision as any other population analysis of epilepsy. The method of case selection and definition (autopsy or death certificate data source), the population under study, the country in which the study was performed, and when it was performed all have a major effect on the data. All these factors should be born in mind when comparing data from various sources.

Table 1 is a compilation of data from several published series reporting causes of death in epileptic persons. These series span the 1900s and draw from highly variable populations ranging from series dominated by children, adults, or mixed

Table 1 Causes of Death in Epileptic Individuals

Cause of death	Range of occurrence	Average
Accidents	7-20%	> 10%
Suicide	3-22%	< 10%
Infections	1-58%	20%
Neoplasms	3-24%	< 10%
Stroke	1-3%	2%
Heart disease	3-16%	10%
Miscellaneous	9-27%	> 20%
Status epilepticus	3-6%	< 10%
Sudden unexpected death	6-41%	> 10%

Source: Freytag and Lindenberg (1964); Henriksen et al. (1967); Krohn (1963); Munson (1910); Neplokh (1965); Penning et al. (1969); Pond et al. (1960); Spratling (1902); Steinsiek (1950); Zielinski (1974b, 1982).

populations; institutionalized epileptics who may or may not have had psychiatric disability or may have been retarded. The definitions of what epilepsy represents are also variable, so ranges and estimates of an average in each category are given. In some series precise definitions of disease categories were not given and had to be interpreted. It is significant that in virtually every series, a category for sudden unexpected or unexplained death occurred.

In Table 1 accidental death includes drowning in the bath or while swimming (presumably in connection with a seizure), a not uncommon risk for the epileptic (Geertinger and Voigt, 1970). Other causes of accidental death are head injuries due to falls, industrial and occupational injuries, fire, traffic accidents, and unspecified accidents. Suicide is also a significant risk in the epileptic population (Camps, 1976). Infectious causes of death included tuberculosis (mainly in the older reports), pneumonia, generalized sepsis, meningitis, encephalitis, and other nonspecified conditions (Krohn, 1963; Rodin, 1968). Neoplasms causing death involved the brain more often than not but included both primary and secondary neoplasms, with many of these coming to light only at autopsy (Huntington et al., 1965). Most of the reports did not elaborate on and often did not specifically identify stroke as a cause of death and probably lumped these deaths under miscellaneous. Heart disease included myocardial infarctions and valvular disease as well as cardiac failure. Death due to pulmonary embolism may have been included in some reports with heart diseases but may also have been included in the miscellaneous category (Epilepsy Foundation of America, 1975; Henriksen et al., 1967; Kurtzke, 1972; Kurtzke et al., 1973; Zielinski, 1982).

Status epilepticus, when defined, usually conformed to the commonly accepted notion of this condition: a long series of successive, if not continuous seizures without remission until death or a moribund state occurred (Commission on Classification and Terminology of the International League Against Epilepsy, 1981). The sudden unexpected or unexplained death category undoubtedly encompassed many kinds of cases, mostly poorly defined, including individuals found dead and presumed to have recently suffered a seizure although showing no obvious anatomic pathological or clinical cause of death. Some of these series undoubtedly included cases of aspiration but probably most did not, and apparently these cases did not include those individuals dying in status epilepticus. Inferences of this sort can be made only by careful interpretation of the terminology employed by the individual authors of the various series summarized in Table 1.

The sudden unexpected death phenomenon is an important manner in which death occurs in the epileptic individual. It is the subject of much of this book and is dealt with epidemiologically and pathologically in Chapters 3 and 5 and in a number of articles in the medical literature (Freytag and Lindenberg, 1964; Hirsch and Martin, 1971; Jay and Leestma, 1981; Leestma et al., 1984, 1985, 1989; Terrence et al., 1975).

3. Comparison of Causes of Death in the Nonepileptic
   and Epileptic Populations

A great deal of information is available on the demographics and epidemiology of death in most industrialized nations. However, these data suffer from deficiencies not dissimilar from those encountered in any analysis of data on an epileptic population. Most large population data are derived from examination and tabulation of death certificates, which may not correctly identify the actual medical cause of death. Most individuals do not have autopsies and the death certificate represents a clinical diagnosis only (Kircher et al., 1985; Leestma and Magee, 1988; Nash, 1986; Schottenfeld et al., 1982). Furthermore, important underlying conditions that caused death often are not mentioned or are listed incorrectly. Comparisons, therefore, in reference to cause of death between a highly selected population such as persons with epilepsy and the general population are fraught with inherent errors. Nevertheless, some insight as to general trends and patterns can be gained from an examination of the data from the various series, regardless of the method of data collection.

From an examination of Table 2, several trends appear. An epileptic population is at risk for more deaths due to accident, suicide, and infection than would be expected within the general population. On the other hand, there appear to be fewer than expected deaths among persons with epilepsy due to neoplasms, stroke, and heart disease. However, if one examines statistics on causes of death in a medical examiner's service, additional important death rate information

Table 2 Comparisons in Causes of Death in Epileptic Persons and in the General Population[a]

Cause of death	Epileptics	General population
Accidents	> 10%	4%
Suicide	< 10%	1%
Infections	20%	7%
Neoplasms	< 10%	21%
Stroke	2%	7%
Heart disease	10%	35%
Miscellaneous	> 20%	23%

[a]Statistics for causes of deaths in epileptic persons are derived from the figures in Table 1; statistics for the general population, from the figures of the National Center for Health Statistics of the Department of Health and Human Services (Hoffman, 1988). The figures are probably not directly comparable since the U.S. vital statistics are obtained by examining causes of death listed in a sampling of 10% of all death certificates during an 11-month period in 1985–1986.

emerges. Using statistics from the Office of the Medical Examiner of Cook County, Illinois, which includes Chicago, about 17,000 of the expected 50,000 plus deaths (about one-third) come to the attention of the medical examiner (Office of the Medical Examiner, 1980). Of these, about 5500 are processed by the medical examiner in some detail. In an average year, about 3500 of these cases include an autopsy. The data in Table 3 come from reported statistics of

Table 3 Medical Examiner Death Statistics[a]

Causes of manner of death	Percentage of death certificates
Natural disease	64–66%
Homicide	10–11%
Suicide	4– 5%
Accident	20–22%
Undetermined	4– 5%

[a]Statistics extracted from Annual Report of the Office of the Medical Examiner, County of Cook, Chicago, Illinois (1980). These figures are based on investigation, inspection, and examination of the body and/or toxicological examination and autopsy analysis. Such results, from the selected population brought to the attention of the medical examiner, are inherently more accurate than statistics not based on such examinations.

death certificates generated by the Office of the Medical Examiner of Cook County and are generally comparable to similar statistics of other metropolitan medical examiner-coroner systems (Spitz and Fisher, 1973).

In interpreting these statistics it is important to realize that not every death is brought to the attention of the medical examiner or coroner; this is generally limited to those that occurred unobserved, outside the care of a physician, due to suspected or known foul play or criminal activity, during the first 24 hours of hospital admission, during surgery, anesthesia, or childbirth, while incarcerated or institutionalized, or under certain other special circumstances. The largest category of forensic case is the "natural" group which denotes deaths due to disease and other natural processes with no action on anyone's part; this includes nonaccidental and nonsuicide deaths in epileptic persons. Of these 64–66% of medical examiner's cases, about 7–12% (4–8% of all deaths under a medical examiner's purview regardless of manner) die suddenly and unexpectedly from a variety of causes. About 12–15% of this subgroup are sudden and unexpected deaths in epileptic persons (SUDEP) (Leestma et al., 1985; Office of the Medical Examiner, 1980). In Cook County, Illinois, this translates to between 60 and 80 deaths each year (at least one per week) of this type (Leestma et al., 1989). Special characteristics of this group of individuals set them apart from the other cases of sudden unexpected death in the general population. This very interesting and special group of individuals is specifically discussed in detail in Chapter 5.

VI. SUMMARY

Epilepsy is a complex though common condition, the precise definition of which is still controversial. All age groups are affected but the patterns and forms of epilepsy are somewhat age dependent. Epilepsy may result from injuries to the nervous system, toxic or metabolic disorders, or malformations and errors in development, or it may be inherited. The causes of epilepsy and the effects of epilepsy in the nervous system often result in very similar if not identical neuropathological changes. This is especially relevant in the hippocampal formation, where neuronal loss and gliosis are very common and have been interpreted as both cause and effect of epilepsy. The epileptogenic focus has been extensively studied in man and in experimental animals and much is known about the characteristics in a given population of neurons which make it electrophysiologically unstable. However, the means by which this instability is kindled, propagated, and ultimately inhibited is incompletely understood.

By all accounts, epilepsy is a condition that carries with it a significant morbidity and mortality reflected in a statistically shortened life expectancy. The epileptic state increases the chance for accidental injury and death and also carries with it a risk for sudden and unexpected death. Such epilepsy associated sudden deaths accounts for 12–15% of all sudden deaths in most medical examiner's caseloads. With about 1-2% of the general population suffering from epilepsy, the phenomenon of sudden death is greatly overrepresented in this population. This chapter sets the background for the remainder of this book, which is devoted to an analysis and investigation of this complex and challenging phenomenon and its related events and issues.

REFERENCES

Aicardi, J. (1985). The medical management of neonatal and infantile seizures and of febrile seizures. In *The Epilepsies*, R. J. Porter and P. L. Morselli (Eds.). Butterworths, London, pp. 206-226.

Annegers, J. F., Hauser, W. A., Elveback, L. R., and Kurland, L. T. (1979). The risk of epilepsy following febrile convulsions. *Neurology 29*:297-303.

Annegers, J. F., Hauser, W. A., Anderson, V. E., and Kurland, L. T. (1982). The risks of seizure disorders among relatives of patients with childhood onset epilepsy. *Neurology 32*:174-179.

Atillo, A., Soderfeldt, B., Kalimo, H., Olsson, Y., and Siesjo, B. K. (1983). Pathogenesis of brain lesions caused by experimental epilepsy. Light and electron-microscopic changes in the rat hippocampus following bicuculline-induced status epilepticus. *Acta Neuropathol. 59*:11-24.

Baier, W. K., Beck, U., Linge, H., and Hirsch, W. (1984). Cerebellar atrophy following diphenylhydantoin intoxication. *Neuropaediatrics 15*:76-81.

Brewis, M., Poskanzer, D. C., Rolland, C., and Miller, H. (1966). Neurological disease in an English city. *Acta Neurol. Scand. 42*:1-89.

Brown, J. K. (1982). Fits in children. In *A Textbook of Epilepsy*, J. Laidlaw and A. Richens (Eds.). Churchill-Livingstone, Edinburgh, pp. 34-67.

Camps, F. E. (Ed.) (1976). *Gradwohl's Legal Medicine*, 3rd ed. Year Book Medical, Chicago.

Cavanaugh, J. B., Falconer, M. A., and Meyer, A. (1958). Some pathogenic problems of temporal lobe epilepsy. In *Temporal Lobe Epilepsy*, M. Baldwin and P. Bailey (Eds.). Thomas, Springfield, Ill., pp. 140-148.

Caveness, W. F., Meirowsky, A. M., Rish, B. L., Mohr, J. P., Kistler, J. P., Dillon, J. D., and Weiss, G. H. (1979). The nature of posttraumatic epilepsy. *J. Neurosurg. 50*:545-553.

Chaslin, P. (1889). Note sur l'anatomie pathologique de l'épilepsie dite essentielle—las sclerose névrologique. *C. R. Séances Soc. Biolog. 1*:169-171.

Coatsworth, J. J., and Penry, K. (1972). Clinical efficacy and use. In *Antiepileptic Drugs*, D. M. Woodbury, J. K. Penry, R. P. Schmidt (Eds.). Raven Press, New York, pp. 87-101.

Commission on Classification and Terminology of the International League Against Epilepsy (1981). Proposal for revised clinical and electroencephalographic classification of epileptic seizures. *Epilepsia 22*:489-501.

Corsellis, J. A. N. (1957). The incidence of Ammon's horn sclerosis. *Brain 80*: 193-208.

Currie, S., Heathfield, K. W. G., Henson, R. A., and Scott, D. F. (1971). Clinical course and prognosis of temporal lobe epilepsy. A survey of 666 patients. *Brain* 94:173-190.

Dam, A. M. (1980). Epilepsy and neuron loss in the hippocampus. *Epilepsia 21*: 617-629.

Dam, A. M. (1982). Hippocampal neuron loss in epilepsy and after experimental seizures. *Acta Neurol. Scand. 66*:601-642.

Dam, M. (1972). The density and ultrastructure of the Purkinje cells following diphenylhydantoin treatment in animals and man. *Acta Neurol. Scand. (Suppl. 49) 48*:1-65.

Dam, M., Bolwig, T., Hertz, M., Bajorec, T., Lomax, P., and Dam, A. M. (1984). Does seizure activity produce Purkinje cell loss? *Epilepsia 25*:747-751.

Epilepsy Foundation of America (1975). *Basic Statistics on the Epilepsies.* F. A. Davis, Philadelphia.

Freytag, E., and Lindenberg, R. (1964). 294 medicolegal autopsies in epileptics. *Arch. Path. 78*:274-286.

Gastaut, H. (1973). *Dictionary of Epilepsy.* World Health Organization, Geneva.

Geertinger, P., and Voigt, J. (1970). Death in the bath. A survey of bathtub deaths in Copenhagen, Denmark, and Gothenberg, Sweden from 1961 to 1969. *J. Forensic Med. 17*:135-147.

Gesell, A., and Amatruda, C. (1947). *Developmental Diagnosis: Normal and Abnormal Child Development.* Harper and Row, New York.

Gessaga, E. C., and Urich, H. (1985). The cerebellum in epileptics. *Clin. Neuropathol. 4*:238-245.

Gibbs, E. L., and Gibbs, F. A. (1952). *Atlas of Electroencephalography*, Vol. 2. Addion Press, Cambridge.

Goldensohn, E. S. (1985). Neurophysiological approaches to basic mechanisms of seizures. In *The Epilepsies*, R. J. Porter and P. L. Morselli (Eds.). Butterworths, London, pp. 20-39.

Great Britain (1969). *People with Epilepsy.* Department of Health and Social Security. Central Health Services Council Advisory Committee on Health and Welfare of Handicapped Persons. London.

Grudzinska, B. (1974). Epidemiology of epilepsy in the population of a large industrial city. Coincidence and prevalence. *Neurol. Neurochir. Pol. 24*:175-180. (in Polish)

Hauser, W. A. (1981). The natural history of febrile seizures. In *Febrile Seizures*, K. B. Nelson and J. H. Ellenberg (Eds.). Raven Press, New York, pp. 5-17.

Hauser, W. A., and Kurland, L. T. (1975). The epidemiology of epilepsy in Rochester, Minnesota, 1935 through 1967. *Epilepsia 16*:1-66.

Henriksen, P. B., Juul-Jensen, P., and Lund, M. (1967). The mortality of epileptics. *Acta Neurol. Scand. 43*:164-167.

Hirsch, C. S., and Martin, D. L. (1971). Unexpected death in young epileptics. *Neurology 21*:682-690.

Hoffman, M. S. (Ed.). (1988). *The World Almanac and Book of Facts.* Ballantine, New York, p. 576.

Holden, K. R., Mellits, E. D., and Freeman, J. M. (1982). Neonatal seizures. I. Correlation of prenatal and perinatal events with outcomes. *Pediatrics 70*: 165-176.

Huntington, H. W., Cummings, K. L., Moe, T. I., O'Connell, H. V., and Wybel, R. (1965). Discovery of fatal primary intracranial neoplasms at medicolegal autopsies. *Cancer 18*:117-127.

Jay, G. W., and Leestma, J. E. (1981). Sudden death in epilepsy. *Acta Neurol. Scand. (Suppl. 82)63*:1-66.

Jennett, B. (1982). Post-traumatic epilepsy. In *A Textbook of Epilepsy*, J. Laidlaw and A. Richens (Eds.). Churchill-Livingstone, Edinburgh, pp. 146-154.

Jennett, B., and Teasdale, G. (1982). *Management of Head Injuries*. F. A. Davis, Philadelphia.

Jennings, M. T., and Bird, T. D. (1981). Genetic influences in the epilepsies. Review of the literature with practical implications. *Am. J. Dis. Child. 135*: 450-457.

Juul-Jensen, P. (1964). Epilepsy. A clinical and social analysis of 1020 adult patients with epileptic seizures. *Acta Neurol. Scand. (Suppl. 5) 40*:1-148

Juul-Jensen, P., and Foldspang, A. (1983). Natural history of epileptic seizures. *Epilepsia 24*:297-312.

Juul-Jensen, P., and Ipsen, J. (1976). Prevalence and incidence of epilepsy in greater Aarhus. In *Epileptology. Proceedings of the Seventh International Symposium on Epilepsy*, D. Janz (Ed.). Thieme, Stuttgard, p. 10.

Kircher, T., Nelson, J., and Burdo, H. (1985). The autopsy as a measure of accuracy of the death certificate. *New Engl. J. Med. 313*:1263-1269.

Krohn, W. (1961). A study of epilepsy in northern Norway, its frequency and character. *Acta Psychiatr. Scand. (Suppl. 150) 36*:215-225.

Krohn, W. (1963). Causes of death among epileptics. *Epilepsia 4*:315-321.

Kurland, L. T. (1959). The incidence and prevalence of convulsive disorders in a small, urban community. *Epilepsia 1*:143-161.

Kurokawa, T., Hanai, T., Kuroki, K., and Goya, N. (1982). Remission rate of epilepsy in children. In *Advances in Epileptology, 13th Epilepsy International Symposium*, H. Akimoto, H. Kazamatsuri, M. Seino, and A. Ward (Eds.). Raven Press, New York, pp. 121-123.

Kurtzke, J. F. (1972). Mortality and morbidity data on epilepsy. In *The Epidemiology of Epilepsy: A Workshop*, A. Milton and W. A. Hauser (Eds.). NINCDS Monograph 14, Department of Health, Education and Welfare, Washington, D.C.

Kurtzke, J. F., Kurland, L. T., Goldberg, I. D., Choi, N. W., and Reeder, F. A. (1973). Convulsive disorders. In *Epidemiology of Neurologic and Sense Organ Disorders*, APHA Monograph Series on Vital and Health Statistics, L. T. Kurland, J. F. Kurtzke, and I. D. Goldberg (Eds.). Harvard University Press, Cambridge, Mass., pp. 15-40.

Laidlaw, J., and Laidlaw, M. V. (1982). People with epilepsy—Living with epilepsy. In *A Textbook of Epilepsy*, J. Laidlaw and A. Richens (Eds.). Churchill-Livingstone, Edinburgh, pp. 513-544.

Laidlaw, J., and Richens, A. (Eds.). (1982). *A Textbook of Epilepsy*. Church-ill-Livingstone, Edinburgh.

Leestma, J. E. (1988). Forensic aspects of complex neural dysfunctions. In J. E. Leestma (Ed.), *Forensic Neuropathology*. New York, Raven, pp. 396–415.

Leestma, J. E., and Magee, D. J. (1988). Pathology and neuropathology in the forensic setting. In *Forensic Neuropathology*, J. E. Leestma (Ed.). Raven Press, New York, pp. 1–23.

Leestma, J. E., Kalelkar, M. B., Teas, S. S., Jay, G. W., and Hughes, J. R. (1984). Sudden unexpected death associated with seizures: Analysis of 66 cases. *Epilepsia 25*:84–88.

Leestma, J. E., Teas, S. S., Hughes, J. R., and Kalelkar, M. B. (1985). Sudden epilepsy deaths and the forensic pathologist. *Am. J. Forensic Med. Pathol. 6*:215–218.

Leestma, J. E., Walczak, T., Hughes, J. R., Kalelkar, M. B., and Teas, S. S. (1989). A prospective study on sudden unexpected death in epilepsy. *Ann. Neurol. 26*:195–203.

Legg, N. J., Gupta, P. C., and Scott, D. F. (1973). Epilepsy following cerebral abscess. A clinical and EEG study of 70 patients. *Brain 96*:259–268.

Lennox, W. G. (1960). *Epilepsy and Related Disorders*. Little, Brown, Boston.

Lennox-Buchthal, M. A. (1973). *Febrile Convulsions*. Little, Brown, Boston.

Lennox-Buchthal, M. A. (1982). Febrile convulsions. In *A Textbook of Epilepsy*, J. Laidlaw and A. Richens (Eds.). Churchill-Livingstone, Edinburgh, pp. 68–96.

Lindvall, O., and Nilsson, B. (1984). Cerebellar atrophy following phenytoin intoxication. *Ann. Neurol. 16*:258–260.

Loiseau, P. (1972). Quand faut-il arrêter un traitement antiépileptic? *Nouv. Presse Med. 1*:47–49.

Lombroso, C. T. (1983). A prospective study of infantile spasms: Clinical and therapeutic correlations. *Epilepsia 24*:135–158.

Margerison, J. H., and Corsellis, J. A. N. (1966). Epilepsy and the temporal lobes. A clinical, electroencephalographic and neuropathological study of the brain in epilepsy with particular reference to the temporal lobes. *Brain 89*:499–530.

Marsden, C. D., and Reynolds, E. H. (1982). Neurology. In *A Textbook of Epilepsy*, J. Laidlaw and A. Richens (Eds.). Churchill-Livingstone, Edinburgh, pp. 97–130.

Mathieson, G. (1982). Pathology and pathophysiology. In *A Textbook of Epilepsy*, J. Laidlaw and A. Richens (Eds.). Churchill-Livingstone, Edinburgh, pp. 437–487.

Matsumoto, A., Watanabe, K., Suiura, M., Negoro, T., Takaesu, E., and Iwase, K. (1983). Long-term prognosis of convulsive disorders in the first year of life: Mental and physical development and seizure persistence. *Epilepsia 24*: 321–329.

Meencke, H. J., and Janz, D. (1984). Neuropathological findings in primary generalized epilepsy: A study of eight cases. *Epilepsia 25*:8–21.

Meldrum, B. S. (1982). Pathophysiology. In *A Textbook of Epilepsy*, J. Laidlaw and A. Richens (Eds.). Churchill-Livingstone, Edinburgh, pp. 456–487.

Meldrum, B. S., and Brierley, J. B. (1973). Prolonged epileptic seizures in the primates: Ischemic cell change and its relation to ictal physiological events. *Arch. Neurol. 28*:10–17.

Meldrum, B. S., and Corsellis, J. A. N. (1984). Epilepsy. In *Greenfield's Neuropathology*, 4th ed., J. Hume Adams, J. A. N. Corsellis, and L. W. Duchen (Eds.). Wiley, New York, pp. 920–950.

Messing, R. O., and Simon, R. P. (1986). Seizures as a manifestation of systemic disease. In *Neurologic Clinics—Epilepsy*, Vol. 3, R. J. Porter and W. H. Theodore (Eds.). Saunders, Philadelphia, pp. 563–584.

Metrakos, K., and Metrakos, J. D. (1961). Genetics of convulsive disorders: II. Genetic and electroencephalographic studies in centrencephalic epilepsy. *Neurology 11*:474–483.

Millichap, J. G. (1968). *Febrile Convulsions*. Macmillan, New York.

Morel, F., and Wildi, E. (1956). Sclérose ammonienne et épilepsies (Etude anatomopathologique et statistique). *Acta Neurol. Belg. 2*:61–74.

Munson, J. F. (1910). Death in epilepsy. *Med. Rec. 77*:58–62.

Nash, I. (1986). The autopsy as a measure of accuracy of the death certificate. *New Engl. J. Med. 314*:1259.

Neplokh, I. (1965). Causes of death in epilepsy. *Zh. Neuropatol. Psikhiatr. 65*: 1382–1387. (in Russian)

Office of the Medical Examiner, County of Cook, Chicago, Illinois (1980). *Annual Report 1977-79*. Chicago, Cook County, Illinois.

Orr, J. K., and Risch, F. (1953). Is the order of birth a factor in epilepsy? *Neurology 3*:679–683.

Parke-Davis C. (1958). *Epilepsy: Patterns of Disease; Special Report*. Chicago.

Parsonage, M. (1982). Introduction. In *A Textbook of Epilepsy*, J. Laidlaw and A. Richens (Eds.). Churchill-Livingstone, Edinburgh, pp. xiv–xxv.

Peiffer, J. (1963). *Morphologische Aspekte der Epilepsien*. Springer, Berlin.

Penfield, W., and Jasper, H. (1954). *Epilepsy and the Functional Anatomy of the Human Brain*. Little, Brown, Boston.

Penning, R., Muller, C., and Ciompi, L. (1969). Mortality and cause of death in epileptics. *Psychiatr. Clin. 2*:85–92. (in French)

Penry, J. K. (Ed.). (1977). *Epilepsy: The Eighth International Symposium*. Raven Press, New York.

Pond, D. A., Bidwell, B. H., and Stein, L. (1960). A survey of epilepsy in fourteen general practices. I. Demographic and medical data. *Psychiatr. Neurol. Neurochir. 63*:217–236.

Porter, R. J. (1984). *Epilepsy. 100 Elementary Principles*. In *Major Problems in Neurology*, Vol. 12, John Walton (Ed.). Saunders, Philadelphia.

Porter, R. J. (1986). Recognizing and classifying epileptic seizures and epileptic syndromes. In *Neurologic Clinics—Epilepsy*, Vol. 3, R. J. Porter and W. H. Theodore (Eds.). Saunders, Philadelphia, pp. 495–508.

Porter, R. J., and Morselli, P. L. (Eds.) (1985). *The Epilepsies*. Butterworths, London.

Raynor, R. B., Payne, R. S., and Carmichael, E. A. (1959). Epilepsy of late onset. *Neurology 9*:111–117.

Richardson, E. P., and Dodge, P. R. (1954). Epilepsy in cerebral vascular disease: A study of the incidence and nature of seizures in 104 consecutive autopsy-proven cases of cerebral infarction and hemorrhage. *Epilepsia 3*: 49–74.

Richens, A. (1982). Clinical pharmacology and medical treatment. In *A Textbook of Epilepsy*, J. Laidlaw and A. Richens (Eds.). Churchill-Livingstone, Edinburgh, pp. 292–348.

Rodin, E. A. (1968). *The Prognosis of Patients with Epilepsy*. Thomas, Springfield, Ill.

Rose, S. W., Penry, J. K., Markush, R. E., Radloff, L. A., and Putnam, P. L. (1973). Prevalence of epilepsy in children. *Epilepsia 14*:133–152.

Rubio-Donnadieu, R. (1972). Epilepsy at the National Institute of Neurology in Mexico. In *The Epidemiology of Epilepsy: A Workshop*, A. Milton and W. A. Hauser (Eds.). NINCDS Monograph 14. Department of Health, Education and Welfare, Washington, D.C.

Salazar, A. M., Jabbari, B., Vance, S. C., Grafman, J., Amin, D., and Dillon, J. D. (1985). Epilepsy after penetrating head injury. I. Clinical correlates: A report of the Vietnam Head Injury Study. *Neurology 35*:1406–1414.

Sano, K., and Malamud, N. (1953). Clinical significance of sclerosis of the cornu ammonis. *Arch. Neurol. Psychiatr. 70*:40–53.

Schade, J. P., and McMenemey, W. H. (1963). *Selective Vulnerability of the Brain in Hypoxaemia*. F. A. Davis, Philadelphia.

Scheibel, M. E., Crandall, P. H., and Scheibel, A. B. (1974). The hippocampal-dentate complex in temporal lobe epilepsy. *Epilepsia 15*:55–80.

Schiottz-Christensen, E. (1972). Genetic factors in febrile convulsions. *Acta Neurol. Scand. 48*:538–546.

Schmidt, D. (1985). Discontinuation of antiepileptic drugs. In *The Epilepsies*, R. J. Porter and P. L. Morselli (Eds.). Butterworths, London, pp. 227–241.

Schoenberg, B. S. (1985). Epidemiology of epilepsy. In *The Epilepsies*, R. J. Porter and P. L. Morselli (Eds.). Butterworths, London, pp. 94–105.

Scholz, W. (1959). The contribution of patho-anatomical research to the problem of epilepsy. *Epilepsia 1*:36–55.

Schottenfeld, D., Eaton, M., Sommers, S. C., Alonso, D. R., and Wilkinson, C. (1982). The autopsy as a measure of accuracy of the death certificates. *Bull. N.Y. Acad. Med. 58*:778–794.

Siesjo, B. K., and Wieloch, T. (1986). Epileptic brain damage: Pathophysiology and neurochemical pathology. *Adv. Neurol. 44*:813–847.

Sommer, W. (1880). Erkrankung des Ammonshornes als ätiologishes Moment der Epilepsie. *Arch. F. Psychiatr. Nervenkrank 10*:631–675.

Spielmeyer, W. (1927). Die Pathogenese des eipleptischen Krampfes. *Z. ges. Neurol. Psychiatr. 109*:501–520.

Spitz, W. U., and Fisher, R. S. (Eds.) (1973). *Medicolegal Investigation of Death. Guidelines for the Application of Pathology to Crime Investigation*. Thomas, Springfield, Ill.

Spratling, W. P. (1902). The cause and manner of death in epilepsy. *Med. News* *80*:1225-1227.

Steinsiek, H. D. (1950). Uber Todesursachen und Lebensdauer bei genuiner Eplipsie. *Arch. Psychiatr. Z. Neurol. 183*:469-480.

Terrence, C. F., Wistoskey, H. M., and Perper, J. A. (1975). Unexpected unexplained death in epileptic patients. *Neurology 25*:594-598.

Upton, A. R. M. (1982). Cerebellar stimulation. In *A Textbook of Epilepsy*. J. Laidlaw and A. Richens (Eds.). Churchill-Livingstone, Edinburgh, pp. 430-436.

Volk, B., and Kirschgassner, N. (1985). Damage of Purkinje cell axons following chronic phenytoin administration: An animal model of distal axonopathy. *Acta Neuropathol. 67*:67-74.

Wada, J. A. (Ed.) (1976). *Kindling*. Raven Press, New York.

Walker, A. E., and Erculei, F. (1969). *Head Injured Men*. Thomas, Springfield, Ill.

Ward, A. A. (1969). The epileptic neuron: Chronic foci in animals and man. In *Basic Mechanisms of the Epilepsies*, H. H. Jasper, A. A. Ward, and A. Pope (Eds.). Little, Brown, Boston, pp. 263-268.

Ward, A. A. (1975). Theoretical basis for surgical therapy of epilepsy. In *Neurosurgical Management of the Epilepsies. Advances in Neurology*, Vol. 8, D. P. Purpura, J. K. Penry, and R. D. Walter (Eds.). Raven Press, New York, pp. 25-35.

Ward, A. A. (1983). Perspectives for surgical therapy of epilepsy. In *Epilepsy*, A. A. Ward, J. K. Penry, and D. Purpura (Eds.). Raven Press, New York, pp. 371-375.

Wilson, C. B., and Stein, B. M. (Eds.) (1984). Intracranial arteriovenous malformations. In *Current Neurosurgical Practice*, Charles B. Wilson (Ed.). Williams and Wilkins, Baltimore.

Wolf, P. (1985). The classification of seizures and the epilepsies. In *The Epilepsies*, R. J. Porter and P. L. Morselli (Eds.). Butterworths, London, pp. 106-124.

Woodbury, D. M., Penry, J. K., and Pippenger, C. E. (Eds.) (1982). *Antiepileptic Drugs*. Raven Press, New York.

Woodbury, L. A. (1978). Shortening of the life span and mortality of patients with epilepsy. *Plan for Nationwide Action on Epilepsy*, Vol. 4. Publication Number (NIH) 78:276. Department of Health, Education and Welfare, U.S. Public Health Service, Washington, D.C., pp. 107-114.

Zielinski, J. J. (1974a). *Epidemiology and medical-school problems of epilepsy in Warsaw*. Psychoneurological Institute, Warsaw.

Zielinski, J. J. (1974b). Epilepsy and mortality rate and cause of death. *Epilepsia 15*:191-201.

Zielinksi, J. J. (1982). Epidemiology. In *A Textbook of Epilepsy*, J. Laidlaw and A. Richens (Eds.). Churchill-Livingstone, Edinburgh, pp. 16-13.

2

A Perspective on Death of Persons with Epilepsy

BRAXTON B. WANNAMAKER *Epilepsy Services and Research, Inc.,*
Charleston, South Carolina

I. INTRODUCTION

Death among persons with epilepsy is more than a random event coincident with the usual causes of death among the nonepileptic population. Life ends earlier in general for the patient with epilepsy (Rodin, 1968). The mortality ratio is two to three times that of the general population (Hauser et al., 1980; Kurtzke, 1972). Identification of the causes of death or other factors that underlie these epidemiological features of epilepsy will undoubtedly lead us to methods of prevention.

Obviously, death can be the result of any number of natural or unnatural causes (accidents, homicide, suicide) that have no relationship to epilepsy. In those instances when death is attributable to the underlying disorder, death may be related as a direct or indirect consequence. Direct causes include status epilepticus; indirect causes can be head trauma or drowning subsequent to a seizure. Death may occur suddenly and without explanation. The term sudden unexpected unexplained death in epileptic persons is applied. Sudden means death occurring within one hour. Less rigorous temporal definitions, such as within 24 hours (as proposed by the World Health Organization), would lead to the inclusion of numerous heterogeneous etiologies. Unexpected refers to the fact that death is not imminent. There is no antecedent illness or symptom that would forecast the ensuing event. Unexplained is a term that will, I hope, be obviated in the future; it reflects our failure to demonstrate any anatomical pathological basis for the death. Death is the permanent ending of all life. "In epileptic persons" is the qualifying phrase to reflect our patients, who apparently have an etiology of the phenomenon which is possibly quite distinct.

Table 1   Causes of Sudden Death

Arteriosclerotic heart disease	Pulmonary embolism
Hypertensive heart disease	Asthma
Rheumatic heart disease	Racial/ethnic
Cerebrovascular disease	Epilepsy
Alcoholic liver disease	Epiglottiditis
Untreated infections	Myocarditis
Dissecting aneurysm of the aorta	Congenital heart disease

Sudden death is not unique to the epileptic population. Indeed, it may be a more common mode of death in other groups. In looking at some of the phenomena and/or diseases that lead to sudden death (Table 1), the most common is arteriosclerotic heart disease (coronary artery disease). In the United States, there are more than 300,000 sudden coronary deaths each year, representing half of the annual toll of coronary mortality (Kannel and Thomas, 1982). There are also unusual occurrences of sudden death. Healthy Filipino men may experience rapid unexpected death during sleep, a phenomenon termed "Bangungut." A similar series of enigmatic deaths was recently described in Southeast Asian refugees in the United States (Furst, 1982). Pokkuri is the term used for sudden cardiac deaths among apparently healthy Japanese soldiers during World War II (Sugai, 1959). In reading the literature on sudden death, one is struck that epilepsy frequently receives a mention, if only in passing. The congenital heart disorders include valvular lesions such as bicuspid aortic stenosis and the difficult differential diagnostic problem of the familial prolonged QT syndrome (De-Silvey and Moss, 1980).

The most common natural cause of sudden death for adults (44 years and older) is arteriosclerotic heart disease (Kuller et al., 1967); for young adults (20–39 years), in the Baltimore series of Kuller et al. (1966), alcoholism and fatty liver; for young adults in the New York series of Luke and Helpern (1968), asymptomatic coronary artery disease. Molander (1982) reported that in childhood and adolescence, common infectious diseases were the most frequent. Incidentally, in his series of 31 deaths in a 1- to 20-year age group, there were 2 deaths in children with epilepsy. Both were due to seizures.

Sudden death is not unique to humans. Sudden death in cattle, especially calves, is a common problem in farm practice (Bradley et al., 1981). "Flipover disease" is described as a sudden death syndrome in broiler chickens (Proudfoot et al., 1982; Steele et al., 1982). Horses and foals which die suddenly for the most part do so from cardiovascular disorders (Platt, 1982).

Table 2 Causes of Death—Epilepsy

Reference	Age group	Institutionalized/ noninstitutionalized	Total deaths	Death attributed to epilepsy
Munson, 1910	C, A	+/0	582	30.0%
Pigott et al., 1940	I, C	+/0	602	25.9%
Bridge, 1949	C	0/+	45	62.2%
Steinsiek, 1950	C, A	+/0	502	53.0%
Lennox, 1960	C, A	0/+	118	25.0%
Henriksen et al., 1970	A	0/+	104	26.0%
Sillanpää, 1973	I, C	+/+	18	44.4%
Zielinski, 1974	I, C, A	+/+	120	24.0%

Key: I = infants; C = children; A = adults.

One may gain better insight into the causes of death among persons with epilepsy by first considering the proportion of all deaths that can be attributed to epilepsy. A review of the literature (Bridge, 1949; Henriksen et al., 1970; Lennox, 1960; Munson, 1910; Pigott et al., 1940; Sillanpää, 1973; Steinsiek, 1950; Zielinski, 1974) indicates that an average of 42.7% of all deaths of persons with epilepsy can be attributed to the epilepsy (Table 2). Woodbury (1977), in his report to the National Commission for the Control of Epilepsy and Its Consequences based on the data from five of the above studies and from one other (Krohn, 1963), concluded that at least 50% of deaths could be attributed directly or indirectly to epilepsy. The most common specific causes of death among persons with epilepsy are natural events such as epileptic seizures and sudden death.

II. SPECIFIC CAUSES OF DEATH

A. Epileptic Seizures

A large number of studies provide detailed information about epileptic seizures as a cause of death. Table 3 includes only those instances of death directly due to a seizure. When an author ascribed a fatal accident to a seizure, the death was not attributed to the seizure. There is a broad range for death related to status epilepticus. A low of 1.2% (Pigott et al., 1940) originated in a 40-year experience with institutional patients from the New Jersey State Village for Epileptics. This is compared to the high of 46.7% (Bridge, 1949) in outpatients followed

Table 3 Causes of Death—Epileptic Seizures

Reference	Age group	Institutionalized/ noninstitutionalized	Total deaths	Status epilepticus	Seizure
Munson, 1910	C, A	+/0	582	10.1%	2.2%
Pigott et al., 1940	I, C	+/0	602	1.2%	5.3%
Bridge, 1949	C	0/+	45	46.7%	
Steinsiek, 1950	C, A	+/0	502	8.2%	
Lennox, 1960	C, A	0/+	118	8.4%	16.1%
Krohn, 1963	C, A	+/+	107	5.6%	
Penning et al., 1969	C, A	0/+	123		15.4%*
Sillanpää, 1973	I, C	+/+	18	5.6%	
Zielinski, 1974	I, C, A	+/+	120	5.8%	11.2%
Iivanainen and Lehtinen, 1979	C, A	+/0	179	8.9%	10.1%
Kurokawa et al., 1982	I, C	0/+	33		30.3%*

Key: I = infants, C = children; A = adults; * = combined in report.

Table 4 Causes of Death—Accidents

Reference	Age group	Institutionalized/ noninstitutionalized	Total deaths	Accidents
Bridge, 1949	C	0/+	45	17.8%
Steinsiek, 1950	C, A	+/0	502	4.6%
Krohn, 1963	C, A	+/+	107	13.1%
Penning et al., 1969	C, A	0/+	123	4.9%
Henriksen et al., 1970	C, A	0/+	104	11.0%
Zielinski, 1974	I, C, A	+/+	120	12.5%
Iivanainen and Lehtinen, 1979	C, A	+/0	179	16.1%
Hauser et al., 1980	C, A	0/+	187	6.4%

Key: I = infants; C = children; A = adults.

Table 5 Causes of Death—Suicide

Reference	Age group	Institutionalized/ noninstitutionalized	Total deaths	Suicides
Bridge, 1949	C	0/+	45	2.2%
Lennox, 1960	C, A	0/+	118	9.3%
Krohn, 1963	C, A	+/+	107	2.8%
Penning et al., 1969	A	0/+	123	3.3%
Henriksen et al., 1970	A	0/+	104	20.8%
Sillanpää, 1973	I, C	+/+	18	5.6%
Zielinski, 1974	I, C, A	+/+	120	11.7%
Iivanainen and Lehtinen, 1979	C, A	+/0	179	1.1%
Hauser et al., 1980	C, A	0/+	187	1.6%

Key: I = infants; C = children; A = adults.

Table 6 Causes of Death—Sudden Death

Reference	Age group	Institutionalized/ noninstitutionalized	Total deaths	Sudden deaths
Munson, 1910	C, A	+/0	582	17.0%
Krohn, 1963	C, A	+/+	107	13.1%
Sillanpää, 1973	I, C	+/+	18	11.2%
Zielinski, 1974	I, C, A	+/+	120	7.5%
Kurokawa et al., 1982	I, C	0/+	33	"a few"

Key: I = infants; C = children; A = adults.

in the clinics at Johns Hopkins University. However, other prevalence figures appear to be fairly consistent. If one considers all patients in these series, status epilepticus is the cause of death in 6.9% of patients, whereas an isolated seizure is the cause of death for 5.6% of patients. These studies suggest an average of 11.6% of all deaths among patients with epilepsy can be directly attributed to epileptic seizures in one form or another.

B. Accidents

Specific information published about accidental deaths (Table 4) includes all deaths by accident regardless of whether the seizure led to that accident. Drowning accidents are included if the authors specifically described that group. Indeed, when singled out, drowning was the most common cause of accidental death (Iivanainen and Lehtinen, 1979; Krohn, 1963). Orlowski, Rothner, and Lueders (1982) reported that the risk of submersion accidents in epileptic children is four times greater than in other children. Although an average of 8.6% of all deaths are caused by fatal accidents in the studies listed in Table 2, it is often difficult to determine clearly in any given patient what role a seizure may have had in the cause of death whether by drowning or by other accident.

C. Suicide

Another cause of death said to be relevant when considering deaths in persons with epilepsy is suicide. The accepted comparative figure for the proportion of deaths by suicide in the general population is 1.5% (Vital Statistics of the U.S., 1978). As seen in Table 5, Henriksen et al. (1970) report that the prevalence of suicide in Denmark is twice that of the next highest prevalence, which is Poland (Zielinski, 1974). More recent studies by Iivanainen and Lehtinen (1979) and by

Table 7 Studies Reporting Sudden Deaths with Other Specific Causes

| | Sudden death | Sudden death and | | |
Reference	Sudden death	Status epilepticus	Suicide	Accidents
Munson, 1910	17.0%	10.1%		
Krohn, 1963	13.0%	5.6%	2.8%	13.1%
Sillanpää, 1970	11.2%	5.6%	5.6%	
Zielinski, 1974	7.5%	5.8%	11.7%	12.5%

Hauser et al. (1980) did not reveal an excess of mortality by suicide in persons with epilepsy.

Penning et al. (1969) found no deaths attributed to suicide in patients between age 19 and 44; 10% of deaths were attributed to suicide in patients between 69 and 80 years of age. In contrast, Zielinski found most suicides in younger patients. Zielinski analyzed 97 deaths of epileptic patients who were confined to mental institutions and only 3.1% of these deaths were by suicide, whereas the proportion for his overall study population (120 deaths) was much greater. Krohn (1963) and Iivanainen and Lehtinen (1979) support the idea that fewer deaths by suicide are found in institutionalized patients as compared to outpatients. For all of the series in Table 5 the average proportion of deaths by suicide is 7.2%, a figure which is five times that of the general population. This signals a great nead for understanding and prevention of suicide in persons with epilepsy.

D. Sudden Unexpected Unexplained Death

Sudden death is reported as a distinct entity in five series (Table 6). Munson (1910) claimed sudden death as the cause of 17% of deaths in the Craig Colony in New York state. His value seems inflated in that some deaths were explained as suffocation and fatal accidents; however, the majority did not have assigned causes. As with recent studies (Leestma et al., 1984; Schwender and Troncoso, 1986), many patients were merely found dead in bed, an occurrence reported in some studies as "death due to a seizure."

The inclination to ascribe otherwise unexplained death in epileptic patients to a seizure whether or not it was witnessed is not appropriate. Borel (1966) refers to sudden death when attributing death to seizures during sleep in the belief that sudden death occurred only at night and had to be the result of a seizure. Iivanainen and Lehtinen (1979) also indicated that deaths due to a seizure per se had occurred due to a seizure during sleep. Certainly the various references to sudden death when a body is found in bed could by synonymous with those references to death due to an epileptic seizure. However, when reviewing the details of Henriksen et al. (1970), one finds a nearly normal mortality ratio for those patients who have seizures during sleep only.

Hirsch and Martin (1971) detailed clinical and laboratory studies of 19 victims of sudden death. Only six were in bed at the time of their demise. Of eight witnessed deaths, four persons died incident to generalized tonic-clonic seizures, two others had a very brief tonic phase, and two patients had no observed seizure activity. An 11-year-old girl just seated at school and a 13-year-old boy walking home after a snowball fight had brief tonic events. The other two persons without apparent seizure activity were a 13-year-old boy and a 15-year-old girl, each of whom dropped dead after emerging from a swimming pool. No gross or microscopic findings that would account for these events were discovered at autopsy on any of the cases in this study.

The series of Kurokawa et al. (1982) points to the lack of recognition or consideration of sudden deaths in persons with epilepsy. The phenomenon is often mentioned only in passing. In this study of 33 patients the causes of demise in 6 were unknown. Only one instance of sudden death was described and the other cases were not elaborated. These findings could be interpreted as indicating that sudden death explained 3 to 18 of the deaths. Thus it is clear that we need a wider recognition of the entity and inclusion of a definition in all future studies on causes of death in epilepsy.

The exact rate of sudden death among persons with epilepsy is not known. However, one can estimate confidently the prevalence of sudden death compared with the other causes of death when there is good concordance across studies for those other causes. The concordance is shown in Table 7. Three of the four studies are very close in their percentage of status epilepticus despite certain limitations. Munson (1910) reported the highest rate of death by status epilepticus, but his study was reported before the introduction of phenobarbital. Although some studies have fewer categories of causes of death (Munson, 1910; Sillanpää, 1970) than others (Krohn, 1963; Zielinski, 1974), the concordance of results for status, accidents, and suicide is quite good. A reasonable estimate of the proportion of sudden deaths in epilepsy based on these studies is 10–15%.

III. SUMMARY

The distribution of deaths among persons with epilepsy is difficult to know precisely. The four causes cited here are frequently listed as causes of death; as a group, they constitute the bulk of the 50% of deaths which are directly or indirectly attributable to epilepsy. Since the therapeutics, administration, and monitoring of antiepileptic drugs have continued to improve, the causes of death attributable directly to seizures should diminish. The complex of behavioral and psychological phenomena facing the person with epilepsy are not clearly understood, but their recognition and delineation should present some empirical guidelines from which we can alter the occurrences of death by accidents and suicide. The intriguing phenomenon of sudden and unexplained death in persons with epilepsy will therefore account for a higher proportion of deaths due to epilepsy.

The death of a young person with epilepsy, whatever the cause, can have an enormous impact, but death which occurs suddenly and without explanation is even more difficult for family and friends. Families who have long cared for the chronically afflicted person are not only bereft, but also questioning. Considering the unusual emotional bonds that have been established in the long-term care of a special person, many questions arise and lead to guilt and subsequent despondency surrounding these deaths. For the physicians who have lost patients in this fashion unnecessary concerns about negligence may surface. There are no standard responses to these situations. However, one of the repeated comments should be eliminated: "We know why he died . . . he had epilepsy." More satisfactory conclusions about death among persons with epilepsy may be routine in the foreseeable future.

REFERENCES

Borel, J. (1966). Sudden death in epilepsy. *Ann. Med. Psychol. 124*:729-730.

Bradley, R., Markson, L. M., and Bailey, J. (1982). Sudden death and myocardial necrosis in cattle. *J. Pathol. 13*:19-38.

Bridge, E. M. (1949). *Epilepsy and Convulsive Disorders in Children.* McGraw-Hill, New York, pp. 491-495.

DeSilvey, D. L., and Moss, A. J. (1980). Primidone in the treatment of long QT syndrome: QT shortening and ventricular arrhythmia suppression. *Ann. Intern. Med. 93 (Part 1)*:53-54.

Furst, G. (1982). Sudden, unexpected, nocturnal deaths among Southeast Asian refugees. *Am. J. Foresic Med. Pathol. 3*(3):177-279.

Hauser, W. A., Annegers, J. F., and Elveback, L. R. (1980). Mortality in patients with epilepsy. *Epilepsia 21*:399-412.

Henriksen, B., Juul-Jensen, P., and Lund, M. (1970). The mortality of epileptics. In *Proceedings of the International Congress of Life Assurance Medicine*, R. D. C. Brackenridge (Ed.). Pitman, London, pp. 139-148.

Hirsch, C. S., and Martin, D. L. (1971). Unexpected death in young epileptics. *Neurology 21*(7):682-690.

Iivanainen, M., and Lehtinen, J. (1979). Causes of death in institutionalized epileptics. *Epilepsia 20*:485-492.

Kannel, W. B., and Thomas, H. E., Jr. (1982). Sudden coronary death: The Framingham study. Part I: Epidemiology and pathology of sudden coronary death. *Ann. N.Y. Acad Sci. 382*:3–21.

Krohn, W. (1963). Causes of death among epileptics. *Epilepsia 4*:315–321.

Kuller, L., Lilienfeld, A., and Fisher, R. (1966). Sudden and unexpected deaths in young adults. *J. Am. Med. Assoc. 198*(3):158–162.

Kuller, L., Lilienfeld, A., and Fisher, R. (1967). An epidemiological study of sudden and unexpected deaths in adults. *Medicine 46*(4):341–361.

Kurokawa, T., Fung, K. C., Hanai, T., and Goya, N. (1982). Mortality and clinical features in cases of death among epileptic children. *Brain Dev. 4*:321–325.

Kurtzke, J. F. (1972). Mortality and morbidity data on epilepsy. In *NINDS Monograph No. 14*, M. Alter and W. A. Hauser (Eds.). Publication No. (NIH) 73-390. Department of Health, Education and Welfare, Washington, D.C.

Leestma, J. E., Kalelkar, M. B., Teas, S. S., Jay, G. W., and Hughes, J. R. (1984). Sudden unexpected death associated with seizures: Analysis of 66 cases. *Epilepsia 25*(1):84–88.

Lennox, W. G. (1960). *Epilepsy and Related Disorders*. Little, Brown, and Co., Boston, pp. 1000–1028.

Luke, J. L., and Helpern, M. (1968). Sudden unexpected death from natural causes in young adults. *Arch. Pathol. 85*:10–17.

Molander, N. (1982). Sudden natural death in later childhood and adolescence. *Arch. Dis. Child. 57*:572–576.

Munson, J. F. (1910). Death in epilepsy. *Med. Rec. 77*:58–62.

Orlowski, J. P., Rothner, A. D., and Lueders, H. (1982). Submersion accidents in children with epilepsy. *Am. J. Dis. Child. 136*:777–780.

Penning, R., Muller, C., and Ciompi, L. (1969). Mortality rate and causes of death in epileptics. *Psychiatr. Clin. (Basel) 2*:85–94.

Piggot, A. W., Weingrow, S. M., and Fitch, T. S. P. (1940). Convulsions in the chronic nervous diseases of infancy and childhood. A review of 1,660 cases. *Arch. Pediatr. 57*:92–111.

Platt, H. (1982). Sudden and unexpected deaths in horses. A review of 69 cases. *Br. Vet. J. 138*:417–429.

Proudfoot, F. G., Hulan, H. W., and McRae, K. B. (1982). The effect of crumbled and pelleted feed on the incidence of sudden death syndrome among male chicken broilers. *Poult. Sci. 61*:1766–1768.

Rodin, E. A. (1968). *The Prognosis of Patients with Epilepsy*. Thomas, Springfield, Ill., pp. 326–329.

Schwender, L. A., and Troncoso, J. D. (1986). Evaluation of sudden death in epilepsy. *Am. J. Forensic Med. Pathol. 7*(4):283–287.

Sillanpää, M. (1973). Medico-social prognosis of children with epilepsy. *Acta Paediatr. Scand. (Suppl.) 237*:77–80.

Steele, P., Edgar, J., and Doncon, G. (1982). Effect of biotin supplementation on incidence of acute death syndrome in broiler chickens. *Poult. Sci. 61*(5):909–913.

Steinsiek, H. D. (1950). Uber todesursachen und lebensdauer bei genuiner epilepsie. *Arch. Psych. Ztschr. Neurol. 183*:469–480.

Sugai, M. (1959). A pathological study on sudden and unexpected death, especially on the cardiac deaths autopsied by the medical examiners in Tokyo. *Acta Pathol. Jpn.* 9:723–752.

Vital Statistics of the U.S., Vol. 2 (1978). Mortality Publication No. 82-1101. National Center for Health Statistics, U.S. Department of Health and Human Services, Washington, D.C.

Woodbury, L. A. (1977). *Shortening of the Life Span and Mortality of Patients with Epilepsy. Plan for Nationwide Action on Epilepsy*, Vol. 4. Publication No. (NIH) 78-279. Department of Health, Education and Welfare, Washington, D.C., pp. 107–114.

Zielinski, J. J. (1974). Epilepsy and mortality rate and cause of death. *Epilepsia* 15:191–201.

3

Patterns of Overall and Unexplained Death Mortality Among Persons with Epilepsy

JOHN F. ANNEGERS and SALLY A. BLAKLEY *University of Texas Health Science Center at Houston School of Public Health, Houston, Texas*

I. INTRODUCTION

The purpose of this chapter is to review the patterns of mortality in persons with epilepsy. The following issues will be addressed: Do individuals with epilepsy have increased death rates? If elevated, is the increase in mortality associated with duration of epilepsy, use of or noncompliance with anticonvulsant drugs, etiology of epilepsy, age, or specific causes of death? Finally, are death rates from unexplained death increased? If so, are they associated with the factors listed here?

To accomplish this review it is necessary first to discuss the measures of the frequency of death and of association which are used in epidemiologic studies to examine patterns of mortality, the types of epidemiologic studies that have been conducted on mortality in patients with epilepsy and the strength and limitations of such studies, and the definition and classification of epilepsy.

A. Measures of the Frequency of Death and Association

The central measure of the frequency of death is the death rate, which is the number of deaths that occur in a defined population divided by the person-years at risk in that population. Person-years at risk are often estimated by the average or midyear population, and the rates are usually expressed as the number of deaths per 1000 person-years. Cause-specific death rates represent the number of deaths due to a specific cause, e.g., sudden death, divided by the person-years at risk; they are usually expressed per 100,000 person-years. Rates are also calculated for subgroups of the population defined by characteristics such as age, sex, race, time, and place; they are compared to evaluate the influence of these factors.

A completely different measure, but one often confused and erroneously used interchangeably with death rate, is proportional mortality. Proportional mortality represents the proportion of a series of deaths that is due to a specific cause, e.g., epilepsy.

Ratio measures of association are used to compare death rates in two populations. The ratio of the death rates between two groups is called a rate ratio. A rate ratio of 1.0 indicates no difference in the death rates between groups, rate ratios of > 1 indicate a high-risk group, and those of < 1 indicate a protected group. In many studies the number of deaths during follow-up of a cohort of people with epilepsy is compared to that expected if the cohort had had the same death rates as the general population, i.e., a standardized mortality ratio (SMR). A SMR is a close approximation of the rate ratio and can be adjusted for the age and sex composition of the study cohort. When possible in this review SMRs will be presented with 95% confidence intervals to indicate the precision of the point estimates.

B. Types of Epidemiological Studies

The nature and quality of information which an individual study provides on the patterns of mortality in people with epilepsy are dictated by the design and conduct of the study. Information on patterns of mortality in persons with epilepsy has generally come from four types of studies: case reports; autopsy series; proportional mortality studies; and cohort studies. It is important to review the strengths and limitations of these four types of studies.

Case reports and descriptions of autopsy series of patients with epilepsy provide important anecdotal information on causes of death and possible associations. However, they do not measure the relative association between specific causes of death and epilepsy or characteristics of patients with epilepsy. This is because such series do not provide the necessary information, person-years at risk, to determine death rates or to contrast death rates among people with epilepsy with rates among nonaffected populations. In addition, autopsy series are restricted to a selected and likely unrepresentative sample of all deaths among patients with epilepsy.

Proportional mortality studies give the proportions of deaths among individuals with epilepsy due to specific causes. The cause-specific proportions of deaths among persons with epilepsy are often compared with the proportional mortality in the general population to determine if the distribution of specific causes differs among patients with epilepsy, i.e., proportional mortality ratio. While these studies can be useful for suggesting specific causes of death that might be overrepresented among persons with epilepsy, a major limitation of proportional mortality studies is that they provide a measure of the relative proportions of deaths only and not a direct measure of the ratio of the rates of death. Consequently, an increased or decreased proportion of deaths from a specific cause among people with epilepsy relative to that in another population may be due to higher death rates from the cause of interest in patients with epilepsy or due to differences in their death rates from other causes. For example, even if the death rate from a specific cause were the same in people with epilepsy as the general population, but death rates from other causes were higher in people with epilepsy, the proportional mortality among the patients with epilepsy would show a deficit of deaths from the specific cause. This could be erroneously interpreted as a protective effect of epilepsy or of anticonvulsant medications. On the other hand if people with epilepsy had a twofold increase in mortality rates from a specific cause of death but also had a twofold increased death rate from all other causes of death, the proportional mortality ratio for the specific cause would be 1.0 and an important difference in death rates would not be detected.

In contrast, in cohort studies a series of patients with epilepsy is followed for known periods of time and deaths during follow-up are ascertained. From this information overall death rates and cause-specific death rates can be determined as both the numbers of deaths and person-years at risk are known. Then, to determine if overall death rates or those from specific causes are unusually high or low in people with epilepsy, the death rates in the epilepsy cohort are compared to those in the general population. To adjust for differences in death rates which may only reflect differences in the age and sex composition of the epilepsy cohort compared to the general population, SMRs can be computed. An SMR is the ratio of the numbers of deaths observed in the cohort to the number of deaths that would be expected to have occurred during follow-up if the epilepsy cohort had experienced the age- and sex-specific death rates in the general population.

C. Definition and Classification of Epilepsy

Epilepsy is defined as recurrent (two or more) unprovoked seizures, i.e., seizures not attributable to a known acute cause (Hauser and Kurland, 1975). By this definition, seizures in conjunction with acute insults to the central nervous system, e.g., head trauma, cerebrovascular disease, encephalitis, and ethanol withdrawal, are considered acute symptomatic seizures rather than epilepsy. However, subsequent recurrent unprovoked seizures in patients who have recovered from a central nervous system insult are classified as epilepsy due to a presumed etiology, i.e., remote symptomatic epilepsy. Patients with only one unprovoked seizure are classified as having isolated seizures rather than epilepsy.

Although febrile convulsions are related to epilepsy in that children with febrile convulsions are at an increased risk to epilepsy and the two conditions aggregate together in families, febrile convulsions usually have a benign course and are not associated with increased mortality (Hauser et al., 1980). Consequently, patterns of mortality among persons with febrile seizures only will not be included in this review.

Epilepsy is a common condition: the prevalence of active cases is about 0.7% and a person's risk of developing epilepsy to age 75 is about 3.5%. However, there are many seizure disorders that are not epilepsy and the lifetime risk for any type of seizure disorder is about 10%.

In cohort studies of mortality of patients with epilepsy it is possible to adhere to a strict definition of epilepsy by including only patients meeting the foregoing criteria. In contrast, studies that rely solely on death certificates to identify deaths in persons with epilepsy are subject to serious limitations. Most deaths among persons with epilepsy are not identified because epilepsy is rarely the underlying cause of death or even noted on the death certificate. On the other hand, some individuals will be erroneously classified as having epilepsy because they experienced acute symptomatic seizures near the time of death, as a result of which epilepsy was noted on the death certificate.

II. PATTERNS OF ALL-CAUSE MORTALITY

Studies in which the total death rates of a cohort of patients with epilepsy were compared to death rates in the general population or in which persons with epilepsy among insurance company policyholders were compared to other policyholders are presented in Table 1. Although the studies have various sources of patients with epilepsy and are from different time periods and countries, they are rather consistent in reporting a twofold to threefold increased mortality rate in people with epilepsy.

In this chapter updated mortality data from the Rochester cohort study of persons with epilepsy (Hauser et al., 1980) will be presented. In the Rochester study newly diagnosed cases of epilepsy among residents of Rochester, Minnesota, were identified through the medical records linkage system of the Rochester Project of the Mayo Clinic (Kurland et al., 1973). The present updated study includes 730 cases of epilepsy, meeting diagnostic and residency criteria, identified between 1935 and 1979 and who have now been followed through 1983 for a total of nearly 10,000 person-years after the diagnosis of epilepsy. In the present follow-up of the Rochester cohort the SMR for all-cause mortality is 2.2, representing the ratio of 237 deaths in the cohort to an expected number of 108 deaths if the epilepsy cohort had had the same death rates as the white population of the United States (Table 1).

Table 1 Standardized Mortality Ratios in Cohort Studies of Persons with Epilepsy

Reference	Country	Source of cohort	SMR	95% C.I.
	All patients with epilepsy			
Svensson and Astrand, 1969	Sweden	Insured	2.2	1.5–3.1
Singer, 1976	United States	Insured	1.3	0.8–1.8
Hutchinson and Sibigtroth, 1976	United States	Insured	3.1	2.4–4.0
Preston and Clark, 1966	United Kingdom	Insured	2.6	1.8–3.6
Penning et al., 1969	France	Series of patients	2.2	1.8–2.6
Alstrom, 1950	Sweden	Series of patients	2.4	2.0–2.8
Zielinski, 1974	Poland	Prevalence cases	1.8	1.6–2.1
Annegers et al., 1984	United States	Incidence cases	2.2	1.9–2.5
	Idiopathic epilepsy only			
Henriksen, 1970	Denmark	Insured	2.8	2.4–3.2
Alstrom, 1950	Sweden	Prevalence cases	1.5	1.1–1.9
Annegers et al., 1984	United States	Incidence cases	1.6	1.4–2.3

A. Etiology of Epilepsy

Most of the studies listed in Table 1 present SMRs for all patients with epilepsy. The SMRs reflect not only the effects of epilepsy and/or its treatment but also any effects attributable to the remote cause of damage to the central nervous system such as brain tumors, cerebrovascular disease, and head trauma, which are the presumed cause of about 25% of all epilepsy. The studies that present SMRs for all patients and separately for patients with idiopathic epilepsy (i.e., epilepsy without a presumed cause) show considerably lower SMRs for idiopathic epilepsy than for all patients with epilepsy (Table 1). Nevertheless, the SMRs for idiopathic epilepsy from Sweden and Rochester, Minnesota, still show a 50-60% increase in the death rates among persons with idiopathic epilepsy compared to the general population. The higher SMR for idiopathic epilepsy in the Danish insurance cohort is probably due to the fact that those in the comparison population, other insured persons, are healthier than the general popula-

Table 2 Standardized Mortality Ratios by Age Group in Persons with Epilepsy

Age group	Rochester	Warsaw	Denmark (Insurance)	New York Life (Insurance)
0–24	9.5 (6.3–13.6)			
0–29		3.5		4.7 (3.0–6.0)
10–29			3.3 (2.1–4.9)	
30–39				2.3 (1.1–4.4)
25–44	6.1 (4.2–8.5)			
30–49		3.4	5.6 (4.3–7.2)	
40+				1.8 (0.8–3.2)
50–59		2.5	1.5 (1.0–2.2)	
45–64	2.9 (2.1–3.9)			
60–69		1.8		
65+	1.6 (1.3–1.9)			
70+		1.5	0.7 (0.1–2.0)	

Source: Annegers et al., 1984, Zielinski (1974); Henriksen (1970); Hutchinson (1976).

tion and to the younger age distribution of the people with epilepsy in the Danish study.

Mortality differs as well among subgroups of patients with epilepsy with a presumed cause. In the Rochester study, persons with epilepsy as a result of a postnatal injury to the central nervous system had an SMR of 2.8 (2.3–3.4). Patients with epilepsy in association with a neurodeficit from birth, including cerebral palsy or mental retardation (defined as an I.Q. under 70), had a considerably higher SMR of 7.0 (4.6–10.2). The extremely high SMR in the neurodeficit group reflects the large number of observed deaths at relatively young ages where few deaths are expected. It is important to note that in these subgroups the increased mortality is almost entirely the result of the predisposing causes of the seizures rather than the seizures per se or their treatment.

B. Age

Mortality, as shown in Table 2, is increased at all ages among persons with epilepsy; however, the increase is not uniform across age groups. There is a sharp decline in the SMRs with age in all study populations. The higher SMRs in persons under age 25 are due to the extremely high relative death rates for patients with epilepsy in association with neurologic deficits. The increased death rates in

Table 3 Standardized Mortality Ratios by Etiology of Epilepsy and Duration
from Diagnosis: Rochester, Minnesota, Incidence Cases, 1935–1979

Years after diagnosis	All deaths		SMR	95% C.I.
	Observed	Expected		
Idiopathic Epilepsy				
0–9	61	32.3	1.9	1.6–2.4
10–19	24	19.7	1.2	0.8–1.8
20+	17	13.0	1.3	0.8–2.1
Total	102	65.1	1.6	1.3–1.9
Remote Symptomatic Epilepsy				
0–9	90	29.2	3.1	2.6–3.8
10–19	13	7.5	1.7	0.0–3.0
20+	5	1.9	2.6	0.9–6.1
Total	108	38.6	2.8	2.3–3.4
Epilepsy with Congenital Neurodeficits				
0–9	19	2.1	9.2	5.6–14.4
10–19	6	1.3	4.8	1.8–10.5
20+	2	0.5	3.9	0.5–14.2
Total	27	3.8	7.1	4.7–10.3

young adult life are consistent with the reports of autopsy series, suggesting that
mortality rates for people with epilepsy in this age group may be unusually high.
Although the SMRs decrease with age, in the Rochester and Warsaw cohorts the
death rates among the elderly with epilepsy (over 65 years) are still increased,
50–60%, above the rates in the general population of persons over 65.

C. Duration of Epilepsy

Standardized mortality ratios by duration after diagnosis for patients classified
by etiology of epilepsy in the Rochester study are shown in Table 3. For persons with idiopathic epilepsy, mortality was significantly increased (SMR = 1.9)
during the first 10 years after the diagnosis of epilepsy and was only slightly
increased thereafter. Persons with epilepsy due to a postnatal neurologic insult
have a threefold increased death rate during the first decade after diagnosis and

Table 4 Standardized Mortality Ratios by Duration from Diagnosis and Anticonvulsant Medication Status: Rochester, Minnesota, Incidence Cases, 1935–1979

Years after diagnosis	All deaths		SMR	95% C.I.
	Observed	Expected		
		On Medications		
0–9	117	41.2	2.8	2.4–3.4
10–19	23	18.4	1.3	0.8–1.9
20+	12	6.2	1.9	1.0–3.4
Total	152	65.5	2.3	2.0–2.7
		Off Medications		
0–9	53	22.1	2.4	1.8–3.2
10–19	20	10.1	2.0	1.2–3.1
20+	12	9.2	1.3	0.7–2.3
Total	85	41.5	2.1	1.7–2.6

a twofold increase after 10 years. Those with epilepsy in association with a congenital neurologic deficit had high mortality rates throughout follow-up.

Hutchinson and Sibigtroth (1976) also reported a decrease in the SMRs among males with grand mal seizures with time from the date of issue of the insurance policy. The SMR was 4.0 during the first 2 years, 3.2 from 2 to 5 years, and 2.6 from 5 to 10 years after issuance.

D. Medication Status

To evaluate the possible role of anticonvulsant medication in mortality among patients with epilepsy, the follow-up of the Rochester cohort was partitioned by medication status and duration-specific SMRs were computed (Table 4). The duration-specific SMRs show little effect of current or long-term anticonvulsant use on overall mortality rates among patients with epilepsy. Thus the increase in death rates in this population of persons with epilepsy appears to be unrelated to the use of anticonvulsant medications.

III. CAUSE-SPECIFIC MORTALITY IN PERSONS WITH EPILEPSY

A. Proportional Mortality

Over the last century numerous reports have described the proportions of deaths due to specific causes in persons with epilepsy (Munson, 1910; Steinsiek, 1950; Krohn, 1963; Loiseau and Henry, 1972; Iivanainen and Lehtinen, 1979). In these series, 6-19% of deaths have been directly attributed to seizures, 20-30% to pneumonia, and 10-20% to accidents, particularly drowning.

In our study of deaths during follow-up of newly diagnosed cases of epilepsy in Rochester, Minnesota, the major causes of death were cancer (20%), heart disease (19%), cerebrovascular disease (14%), accidents and suicide (6%), and epilepsy (5.5%) (Annegers et al., 1984). The difference in proportional mortality in the Rochester series compared to the earlier series reflects differences in the nature of the populations under study. In the Rochester study, causes of death were determined in a population-based cohort, whereas the series described above were predominantly comprised of institutionalized individuals. The proportions of deaths due to heart disease among the Rochester cohort, 19.0% for the total cohort and 22.5% for those with idiopathic epilepsy, are lower than expected in the total U.S. population, where about half of all deaths are due to heart disease. However, the lower relative proportion of heart disease deaths in the epilepsy cohort is due to the higher rates of deaths from other causes, as will be discussed below.

B. Cause-Specific Death Rates

Unfortunately, most cohort studies of persons with epilepsy do not provide details on cause-specific mortality rates or rates of sudden death. Death certificates were obtained for the 237 patients who were known to have died during follow-up of incidence cases of epilepsy in the Rochester study, and the underlying causes of death on the certificates were classified according to the International Classification of Disease, Ninth Revision. The SMRs for major causes of death for persons with idiopathic and remote symptomatic epilepsy in the Rochester cohort are presented in Table 5.

For persons with remote symptomatic epilepsy the SMR for cancer mortality was greatly increased, whereas for persons with idiopathic epilepsy there was only a slight overall increase in cancer mortality (SMR = 1.7), which was attributable to a few patients who had a malignant neoplasia at the time of the diagnosis of epilepsy. However, if the incidence of cancer is considered rather than cancer mortality, no significant increase in site-specific cancer rates was observed in the Rochester cohort, with the exception of brain tumors (Shirts et al., 1986). Similar findings in other cohorts of patients with epilepsy of little or no in-

Table 5 Cause-Specific Standardized Mortality Ratios by Cause of Epilepsy:
Rochester, Minnesota, Incidence Cases, 1935-1979

Cause of death	Deaths		SMR	95% C.I.
	Observed	Expected		
Idiopathic Epilepsy				
Heart disease[a]	28	27.8	1.0	0.7-1.5
Cancer	19	11.3	1.7	0.8-1.8
Cerebrovascular disease	17	13.0	1.3	0.8-2.1
Accidents and suicide	9	4.5	2.0	0.9-3.8
Remote Symptomatic Epilepsy				
Heart disease	28	17.4	1.5	0.97-2.2
Cancer	25	5.3	4.7	3.1-7.0
Cerebrovascular disease	25	5.5	4.6	2.9-6.7
Accidents and suicide	4	1.7	2.4	0.6-6.0

[a]International Classification of Disease codes 394, 410-414, 427, 429.

creased incidence of cancer of sites exclusive of the brain have been reported by
White et al. (1979) and Clemmensen and Hjalgrim-Jensen (1978).

The death rate from accidents and suicides was increased twofold in the
Rochester cohort and the increase was observed among persons with both idiopathic and acquired epilepsy. Penning et al. (1969), Henriksen et al. (1971),
and Zielinski (1974) also reported an excess of accidental deaths among epileptic patients.

The SMR for the broad category of heart disease was not significantly increased in either etiologic subgroup of persons with epilepsy (Table 5). However, there were marked age-specific differences in death rates from heart disease: the SMR for heart disease in the total cohort of persons under age 45 was
6.2 (2.3-13.5); in those aged 45-64 it was 2.5 (1.4-4.1). A significant increase
was observed even when the analysis was restricted to persons who had survived
10 or more years after the diagnosis of epilepsy. In the latter subgroup, the SMR
was 6.5 (1.3-19.4) among those under age 45 and was 3.1 (1.5-5.6) among
those aged 45-64.

C. Sudden Death

There are many reports of the causes of death found among autopsy series of
patients with epilepsy (Dasheiff and Dickenson, 1986; Falconer and Rajs, 1976;

Freytag and Lindenberg, 1964; Hirsch and Martin, 1971; Jay and Leestma, 1981; Leestma et al., 1984; Schwender and Troncoso, 1986; Terrence et al., 1975). In these studies the proportion of sudden deaths among patients with epilepsy, particularly at younger ages, appeared to be excessive. Freytag and Lindenberg (1964) reported that sudden death accounted for 63% of deaths among patients whose epilepsy was due to head trauma, brain tumors, or cerebrovascular lesions. Other autopsy series have reported that sudden deaths account for a high proportion of deaths among patients with idiopathic epilepsy. Because selection for postmortem examination is influenced by the circumstances of death and postmortems are more likely to be conducted when the cause of death is uncertain, these autopsy series would be expected to report a higher proportion of sudden unexplained deaths than would be found among all deaths of patients with epilepsy. The pathological findings from postmortem examinations of patients with epilepsy provide important information with respect to mechanisms underlying sudden death and these studies are discussed in detail in Chapters 1 and 5.

In the Rochester study, deaths in individuals who had no previous clinical diagnosis of ischemic heart disease and who died within 24 hours after the onset of symptoms suggestive of acute coronary insufficiency were classified separately as sudden cardiac deaths (Annegers et al., 1984). These were individuals suffering from no known lethal disease and for whom no other explanation of death was available, although postmortem findings were not included in determining the cause of death. Hence this classification is not strictly comparable to that of sudden death in studies where postmortem examinations have ruled out acute infarction or advanced coronary atherosclerosis as the cause of death.

Thirteen sudden cardiac deaths occurred during follow-up of the total cohort while only 5.7 were expected, based on rates in the general population of Rochester for an SMR of 2.3 (1.2-3.9). However, the increase appeared to be limited to those patients with remote symptomatic epilepsy, whose SMR for sudden cardiac death was 3.9 (1.7-7.7), compared to 1.2 (0.3-3.0) among patients with idiopathic epilepsy. The increased incidence in patients with remote symptomatic epilepsy was limited to those patients with cerebrovascular disease as the predisposing cause of the epilepsy; consequently, there appears to be no general increase in sudden cardiac death. However, the small numbers of deaths do not permit ruling out a threefold or smaller increase of sudden cardiac deaths in persons with idiopathic epilepsy.

There is evidence from autopsy series that many patients with epilepsy who die suddenly have subtherapeutic or absent serum levels of anticonvulsant drugs (Falconer and Rajs, 1976; Leestma et al., 1984; Terrence et al., 1975). Schwender and Troncoso (1986), however, found that most had detectable levels of anticonvulsants in postmortem blood and that more than half had therapeutic levels. In the Rochester study, the incidence of sudden cardiac death was not associated with anticonvulsant medication status. The SMR for patients on anti-convulsant medications of 2.7 (0.98–5.8) was similar to that for those not taking anticonvulsants, 2.0 (0.8–4.2). However, the level of compliance at the time of death for these patients was not determined.

Jay and Leestma (1981) suggested that the annual incidence of sudden death among individuals with epilepsy is at least 1/500–1000 and perhaps higher. In our study the annual risk of sudden cardiac death in the total cohort was 1/738, which is within the range estimated by Jay and Leestma. However, the annual risk for those over age 30 was 1/371 and the risk varied by etiology of epilepsy: for persons over age 30, the annual risk was only 1/1000 for those with idio-pathic epilepsy compared to almost 1/100 for those with remote symptomatic epilepsy.

IV. SUMMARY

Comparisons of death rates for people with epilepsy and those in the general population show that overall persons with epilepsy have a twofold increase in all-cause mortality. The increase is nearly three-fold in persons with epilepsy with a presumed cause; much of this excess is likely to be related to the under-lying brain injury that caused the epilepsy. Nevertheless, there is still a 50% in-crease in mortality among individuals with idiopathic epilepsy.

The increased death rate from all causes among persons with epilepsy is lim-ited to the first decade after diagnosis. Persons who have had epilepsy 10 years or more have a mortality rate similar to the general population.

Information on cause-specific death rates in persons with epilepsy is limited. In the Rochester study death rates for heart disease are not increased overall for persons with epilepsy, although there is a significant increase in persons under age 65. This increase in the younger age group persists 10 or more years after diagnosis.

The incidence of sudden cardiac death in the Rochester cohort is increased only in the subgroup of patients with remote symptomatic epilepsy, which was attributable to cerebrovascular disease as the predisposing cause. The incidence of sudden cardiac death does not appear to be increased in patients with idio-pathic epilepsy.

All-cause mortality and sudden cardiac death in persons with epilepsy in the Rochester study are not related to the prescribed use of anticonvulsant medica-tion.

REFERENCES

Alstrom, C. H. (1950). A study of epilepsy in its clinical, social and genetic aspects. *Acta Psychiatr. Neurol. Scand. (Suppl.)* 53:1–284.

Annegers, J. F., Hauser, W. A., and Shirts, S. B. (1984). Heart disease mortality and morbidity in patients with epilepsy. *Epilepsia 25*:699–704.

Clemmensen, J., and Hjalgrim-Jensen, S. (1978). Is phenobarbital carcinogenic? A follow-up study of 8078 epileptics. *Ecotox. Environ. Safety 1*:457–470.

Dashieff, R. M., and Dickinson, L. J. (1986). Sudden unexpected death of epileptic patients due to cardiac arrhythmia after seizure. *Arch. Neurol.*, 194–196.

Falconer, B., and Rajs, J. (1976). Post-mortem findings of cardiac lesions in epileptics: A preliminary report. *Forensic Sci. 8*:63–71.

Freytag, E., and Lindenberg, R. (1964). 294 medicolegal autopsies on epileptics. *Arch. Pathol. 78*:274–286.

Hauser, W. A., and Kurland, L. T. (1975). The epidemiology of epilepsy in Rochester, Minnesota. *Epilepsia 16*:1–66.

Hauser, W. A., Annegers, J. F., and Elveback, L. R. (1980). Mortality in patients with epilepsy. *Epilepsia 21*:399–412.

Henriksen, P. B., Juul-Jensen, P., and Lund, M. (1971). The mortality of epileptics. In *Epilepsy and Insurance*. Social Studies in Epilepsy, No. 5. International Bureau for Epilepsy, London, pp. 5–12.

Hirsch, C. S., and Martin, D. L. (1971). Unexpected death in young epileptics. *Neurology 21*:682–690.

Hutchinson, J. J., and Sibigtroth, J. C. (1976). Epilepsy in insured. In *Medical Risks: Patterns of Mortality and Survival*, R. D. Singer and L. Levinson (Eds.). Levington, Mass., pp. 2.34–2.35.

Iivanainen, M., and Lehtinen, J. (1979). Causes of death in institutionalized epileptics. *Epilepsia 20*:485–492.

Jay, G. W., and Leestma, J. E. (1981). Sudden death in epilepsy. *Acta Neurol. Scand. (Suppl.). 63*:1–66.

Krohn, W. (1963). Causes of death among epileptics. *Epilepsia 4*:315–321.

Kurland, L. T., Elveback, L. R., and Nobrega, F. T. (1973). Mayo Clinic records-linkage system in the Rochester-Olmsted Epidemiology Program Project. *Proceedings of the International Epidemiological Association*, August 1971, Primosten, Yugoslavia. Savremena Admiistracija, Belgrade, Yugoslavia.

Leestma, J. E., Kalelkar, M. B., Teas, S. S., Jay, G. W., and Hughes, J. R. (1984). Sudden unexpected death associated with seizures: Analysis of 66 cases. *Epilepsia 25*:84–88.

Loiseau, M. P., and Henry, P. (1972). Les causes de la mort chez les épileptiques. *Bordeaux Med. 5*:2643–2648.

Munson, J. F. (1910). Death in epilepsy. *Med. Rec. 77*:58–62.

Penning, R., Muller, C., and Ciompi, L. (1969). Mortalité et causes de décès des épileptiques. *Psychiatr. Clin. 2*:85–94.

Preston, T. W., and Clarke, R. D. (1966). An investigation into the mortality of impaired lives during the period 1947–1963. *J. Inst. Act. 92*:27–74.

Schwender, L. A., and Troncoso, J. C. (1986). Evaluation of sudden death in epilepsy. *Am. J. Forensic Med. Pathol. 7*:283–287.

Shirts, S. B., Annegers, J. F., Hauser, W. A., and Kurland, L. T. (1986). Cancer incidence in a cohort of patients with seizure disorders. *JNCI 77*:83–87.

Singer, R. A. (1976). Neurological and psychiatric disease. In *Medical Risks: Patterns of Mortality and Survival*, R. D. Singer and L. Levinson (Eds.). Levington Books, Levington, Mass., pp. 2.48–2.49.

Steinsiek, H. D. (1950). Uber Todesursachen und Lebensdauer bei genuiner Epilepsie. *Arch. Psychiatr. Z. Neurol. 183*:469–480.

Svensson, A., and Astrand, S. (1976). Substandard risks: Mortality in Sweden 1955–1965. Cooperation International pour les Assurances des Risque Aggraves. In *Medical Risks: Patterns of Mortality and Survival*, R. D. Singer and L. Levinson (Eds.). Levington Books, Levington, Mass., pp. 2.34–2.35.

Terrence, C. F., Wisotzkey, H. M., and Perper, J. A. (1975). Unexpected unexplained death in epileptic patients. *Neurology 25*:594–598.

White, S. J., McClean, A. E. M., and Howland, C. (1979). Anticonvulsants and cancer: A cohort study in patients with severe epilepsy. *Lancet 2*:458–460.

Zielinski, J. J. (1974). Epilepsy and mortality rate and cause of death. *Epilepsia 15*:191–201.

4

A Survey of EEG Changes Obtained in Epileptic Persons Prior to Sudden Unexplained Death

JOHN R. HUGHES *University of Illinois Medical Center, Chicago, Illinois*

I. INTRODUCTION

The phenomenon of sudden unexplained death in epilepsy (SUDEP) has now become established and relatively well known among epileptologists (Hirsch and Martin, 1971; Jay and Leestma, 1981; Leestma et al., 1984; Terrence et al., 1975). However, very little has been published regarding the EEGs of these patients before their death. Only one short account published by Hirsch and Martin (1971) could be found; they reported on 19 patients from an original series of 58. Two patients were said to have had a borderline normal record and definite EEG abnormalities were found in 17 (89%). In 14 of the 19 (74%) some type of paroxysmal epileptiform discharge was found and the authors commented that more than 50% had diffuse abnormalities with spikes or slow waves or both. No other details were provided. In a review of SUDEP, Jay and Leestma (1981) did not mention characteristics of EEGs obtained prior to death, although they did comment on the need to perform a careful cardiac work-up using simultaneous EEG–ECG recordings on patients with epilepsy. In a later report by Leestma et al. (1984) no comment was made about EEG, except to point out that cardiac changes have been associated not only with clinical seizures but also with electrographic ictal events. The goal of the present project was to survey in a more detailed way the EEG changes in patients with epilepsy who later had a sudden unexplained death, in the hope that these electrographic findings may shed some light on this important phenomenon.

II. METHODS

This investigation was part of a prospective study of SUDEP from cases referred to the Medical Examiner's Office of Cook County, Illinois, during 1983. The study included 60 known epileptic patients whose death was sudden and unexpected and also without obvious explanation. Medical investigators routinely performed scene investigations and also obtained medical records; they were specially trained to detect signs of foul play, suicide, and other circumstances that might assist the forensic pathologist in determining a cause of death. In all cases, a history of epilepsy was obtained from the family or witnesses and also was corroborated by medical records; however, details regarding different types of seizures, medication, and compliance could not be obtained in some instances. Scene investigation and interview of witnesses ruled out foul play, suicide, accident, or status epilepticus as the cause of death. A complete autopsy, performed by a forensic pathologist, confirmed that no anatomic cause of death could be demonstrated.

The EEGs that could be found were performed mainly (70%) in two laboratories (A and B) with electrodes placed in all laboratories according to the International System of Electrode Placement. Waking records were obtained on all patients; sleep records were done in lab A (10 patients, 29 records), but not in lab B (7 patients, 7 records). Also, in lab A hyperventilation and photic stimulation were included. Serial records were run on 8 patients on the average of one every 1.2 years. The time between the last EEG and death varied between 3 and 94 months with a mean of 43 months (median 46 months).

III. RESULTS

Table 1 shows that this study is based on 20 patients (16 males, 4 females) and 43 EEG records that could be found. The age range of the patients was from 10 to 54 years with a mean age of 36 years; the majority of patients were in the third and fourth decades. In 70% of the patients EEG abnormalities were found; 30% had normal tracings. However, only in half of the patients and two-thirds of the records were sleep tracings included; when only these more complete records were analyzed, 80% of the patients and 66% of the EEG tracings were found to be abnormal. Paroxysmal sharp waves or spikes were noted in 70% of patients and 52% of wake-sleep EEGs, and slow waves were seen in 60% of patients and 35% or records. As also seen in Table 1, the slow waves were mainly diffuse or temporal in location and the sharp waves or spikes were primarily temporal, accounting for 86% of the patients and 80% of the EEG records that showed some type of discharge. Only one patient showed bilaterally synchronous and symmetrical spike and wave complexes of a corticoreticular or generalized type.

Table 1 EEG Findings Prior to SUDEP

Findings	Patients	EEGs
All patients	20	43
Abnormal EEG	14 (70%)	28 (65%)
Slow only	6 (30%)	13 (30%)
Slow and sharp	5 (25%)	5 (12%)
Sharp only	3 (15%)	10 (23%)
Normal EEG	6 (30%)	15 (35%)
With wake and sleep	10	29
Abnormal EEG	8 (80%)	19 (66%)
Slow only	1 (10%)	4 (14%)
Slow and sharp	5 (50%)	6 (21%)
Sharp only	2 (20%)	9 (31%)
Normal EEG	2 (20%)	10 (34%)
With abnormal EEG	14	28
Slow	11 (79%)	18 (64%)
Diffuse	7 (64%)	12 (67%)
Temporal	6 (55%)	8 (44%)
Frontal	4 (36%)	3 (17%)
Sharp, spike	7 (50%)	15 (54%)
Temporal	6 (86%)	12 (80%)
Frontal	2 (29%)	3 (20%)
Bilateral spike and wave	1 (14%)	2 (13%)

Perhaps the most important finding in these patients was the variability of serial records. In 23 instances serial tracings (all with sleep) were run on 8 patients; the number of times that a different finding (in degree or type) appeared, compared to the previous record, was 17, or 74%. A comparison group of 20 patients was chosen from the Epilepsy Clinic and the files of the EEG Department, all with epilepsy of similar age (mean of 29 years), mean time of repeat record (1.0 year), and same-sex distribution (male 4:1), but otherwise picked randomly. The incidence of serial EEG records (all with sleep) that were different (in degree or type) from the previous EEG was 47%. The difference between the 74% of the SUDEP cases and 47% of the control group of typical patients with epilepsy was very significant ($t = 2.47; p = 0.007$).

Examples of the variability in EEG results can be found with L.C., a 37-year-old female, whose first record (September 1977) showed paroxysmal discharges on the right anterior and midtemporal area. The second record (April 1978) was normal, the third (May 1978) showed only a mild slow-wave abnormality on the left temporal area, and the fourth (June 1978) had a diffuse or generalized slow-wave abnormality, moderate in degree. In addition to the diffuse disorder, the fourth record also showed discharges on the right anterior temporal area and a focal slow-wave abnormality, moderate in degree, on the left posterior temporal and parietal areas. Thus in these four tracings obtained on L. C., EEG findings ranged from normal to abnormal, focal to diffuse, slow abnormalities, focal and diffuse together, paroxysmal discharges in two records, and none in two others.

A second example that demonstrates the variability of an epileptogenic focus was seen in A. V., a 26-year-old male. The first record (March 1977) showed only a moderate degree of diffuse slow wave abnormality, the next one (October 1978) also showed the diffuse abnormality but additionally contained only rare paroxysmal discharges on the right anterior temporal area, and the third (January 1979) again demonstrated the same diffuse finding but with such an active focus on the right anterior area that three ictal events with clinical manifestations were recorded. The last record (March 1979), taken two months later, failed to show any discharges but again manifested a diffuse slow-wave disorder, mild to moderate in degree. Hospitalization occurred twice for phenytoin (Dilantin) toxicity, once at the time of the second record, which showed only a few discharges, and also at the time of the fourth record, which included no discharges.

A third example of a changing record with regard to a spike focus was H. J., a 39-year-old male. His first record (October 1961) showed an active paroxysmal discharge on both frontal areas, the next (May 1972) was a normal record, and the third (April 1974) was also normal, before an active focus again appeared on the right frontal and temporal areas. A fourth example of variability is seen in R. J., a 25-year-old female, who showed bilaterally synchronous and symmetrical spike and wave complexes (13 seconds in duration) of a corticoreticular or generalized type in December 1981. Just four months later no such complexes appeared, even in a sleep tracing, but only 12 days after that time, the complexes appeared again. The last two records were taken without medication and with only sporadic compliance around the time of the first record.

Data obtained on a fifth patient demonstrates additional points on the question of variability. Seven records were done on B. W., a 45-year-old male. The first (March 1959) showed paroxysmal discharges and a slow-wave abnormality on the left anterior and midtemporal area. Ten years later a normal record was found (complete with a sleep tracing), but four years after that, discharges were seen on both frontal and midtemporal areas. Even though medication (phenytoin 100 mg TID, phenobarbital 30 mg TID) was taken on schedule by the patient and no clinical seizures had occurred for seven years, four generalized tonic-clonic (GTC) seizures suddenly appeared, one after the other, and were verified by witnesses. As a further emphasis on variability, the next record taken the day after the four breakthrough seizures had occurred was then perfectly normal, as was the record five years later. By the next full year (after the latter normal record) spike foci again appeared on both anterior temporal areas, even though no clinical attacks had occurred. In another year and a half a similar record was seen, but a clinical GTC attack had occurred the day before the record. The data from this patient demonstrate that even with compliance of medication the EEGs alternated back and forth between normal and abnormal with paroxysmal discharges, and the clinical picture changed from no attacks in seven years to four in one day. The variable character of the EEG and also the clinical events must be emphasized here. In the three other patients with repeat records two of them showed similar variability to those described above.

IV. DISCUSSION

The most important point that these data demonstrate in the SUDEP patients is the variability in their EEGs, significantly different from those of "typical" patients with epilepsy, whose EEGs usually show in adulthood foci that remain relatively constant in location in each tracing. At times, the variability appears even with compliance with the anticonvulsant regimen (B. W.). In other instances the patient was responsible for dramatic changes in the anticonvulsant levels by becoming toxic from overdosing (A. V.) and still in other cases medication was removed and then reinstituted (R. J.). Other patients, like L. J., had their seizure disorder complicated by alcoholism and noncompliance. Both of the latter factors would be expected to change the threshold for seizures to a significant degree, especially the sudden withdrawal from alcohol. If significant EEG, and therefore central nervous system, variability characterizes these patients, their status may suddenly change from a relatively benign to a severe condition. Thus R. W. experienced a benign seizure state without having had any attacks for seven years but then suddenly on one day had four GTC seizures, as an example of the change from a benign to severe condition that abruptly occurred. Wide swings of neuronal excitability or of threshold change to seizure, either self-induced or idiopathic, likely account for the uneven history of most of these patients. Thus evidence is seen for an unstable, changing environment of the central nervous system in SUDEP patients.

Other than a significant variability of central nervous system excitability, there are other likely reasons why some of these patients may have been at risk for death associated with their seizures. In the last two patients in this author's practice who were victims of SUDEP, both weighed over 350 pounds. Not only the cardiac load associated with such obesity, but also the additional load from a generalized tonic-clonic seizure that occurred in each, likely imposed a significant stress on cardiac function and may have been more than what could have been tolerated. Thus a cardiac arrest during the seizure may well have occurred in these two patients.

Table 1 shows that 86% of SUDEP patients with some paroxysmal pattern had a discharging focus within the temporal lobe. This localization is not surprising since nearly all of our patients were adults (one exception), and a temporal lobe focus is the most common focus in adulthood (Gibbs, 1952; Hughes, 1985). In the complex partial seizures that arise from the temporal lobe and those that generalize to a tonic-clonic type, the involvement of the autonomic nervous system has been clearly documented (Van Buren and Ajmone-Marsan, 1960) and significant changes within this system are also clear to any astute observer of these seizures. The storm of autonomic activity may take the form of sympathetic or parasympathetic impulses and many different types of cardiac changes, including ventricular arrhythmias and even cardiac arrest, have been associated with either electrographic seizures or clinically observed attacks (Mathew et al., 1970; Phizackerley et al., 1951; Sulg, 1967; Walsh et al., 1972). The close relationship between interictal discharges and cardiac autonomic neural discharge and arrhythmias has also been carefully investigated (Lathers and Schraeder, 1982) and more recently a lockstep phenomenon has been described in cats; cardiac sympathetic and vagal neural discharges have been reported as intermittently synchronized 1:1 with epileptiform activity (Lathers et al., 1987). Thus a possible mechanism has been delineated to explain the way in which not only ictal episodes but also interictal epileptiform activity may be related to cardiac changes that could result in death.

The prevalence of epileptiform activity at 40% (Table 1) in the 20 patients of this study would seem to be relatively low in any group of seizure patients, but sleep records are absolutely necessary to demonstrate the majority of foci and thus to confirm epilepsy by EEG. Therefore, when only sleep (and waking) records are considered, then the prevalence of paroxysmal discharges was 70%, a value that is similar to the 74% of SUDEP patients of Hirsch and Martin (1971) and the 77% found in a large population of patients with many different types of definite epilepsy (Hughes and Gruener, 1985). Thus our SUDEP patients were similar to other groups with seizures with regard to discharges in sleep records. The rate of 70% refers to the prevalence of discharges for a given patient in at least one record in contrast to the lower value of 52% (see Table 1) for all of the wake and sleep records done. The difference is a reflection of the variability from one record to another that was previously discussed. Also, a normal EEG was found at some time in 20% of the patients, but the same finding was seen in 34% of their records; these values are a further reflection of the wide swings of variable findings in the SUDEP group. The 20% normal rate is significantly different from the 5% found in a large group of patients with different types of epilepsy (Hughes and Gruener, 1985). The higher rate of normal EEGs in SUDEP patients may also be a reflection of variability in these same patients, especially since the majority of those with a normal record did not have serial tracings that may have then shown an abnormality on a second or third record.

V. SUMMARY

The 43 EEGs of 20 patients who had a sudden and unexplained death in epilepsy (SUDEP) were analyzed. In 70% of patients an abnormal EEG was found, but when wake and sleep records together were considered, 80% of patients showed an EEG abnormality. Paroxysmal sharp waves or spikes, mainly temporal, were seen in 70% of these patients and slow waves, mainly diffuse or temporal, were seen in an overlapping 60%. In 23 instances serial EEG records were run, showing a definite difference from the previous record in 74%; this incidence was significantly different from the 47% found in a comparison group of "typical" patients with epilepsy. Thus the major finding in this study was the variability of the EEG results in a given patient from one record to the next, likely reflecting an unstable and changing environment of the central nervous system. This instability within the brain, either idiopathic or self-induced, is likely an important factor in understanding the phenomenon of sudden unexplained death in epilepsy.

ACKNOWLEDGMENT

The author wishes to thank J. Leestma, T. Walczak, M. B. Kalelkar, and S. S. Teas for their contribution to the prospective study on SUDEP, of which the present EEG investigation was a part.

REFERENCES

Gibbs, F. A. (1952). Differentiation of mid-temporal, anterior temporal and diencephalic epilepsy. In *Temporal Lobe Epilepsy*, M. Baldwin and P. Bailey (Eds.). Thomas, Springfield, Ill., pp. 109–117.

Hirsch, C. S., and Martin, D. L. (1971). Unexpected death in young epileptics. *Neurology 21*:682–690.

Hughes, J. R. (1985). Long-term clinical and EEG changes in patients with epilepsy. *Arch. Neurol. 42*:213–223.

Hughes, J. R., and Gruener, G. (1985). The success of EEG in confirming epilepsy revisited. *Clin. EEG 16*(2):48–103.

Jay, G. W., and Leestma, J. E. (1981). Sudden death in epilepsy. *Acta Neurol. Scand. (Suppl. 82) 63*:1–66.

Lathers, C. M., and Schraeder, P. L. (1982). Autonomic dysfunction in epilepsy: Characterization of autonomic cardiac neural discharge associated with pentylenetetrazol-induced epileptogenic activity. *Epilepsia 23*:633–647.

Lathers, C. M., Schraeder, P. L., and Weiner, F. L. (1987). Synchronization of cardiac autonomic neural discharge with epileptogenic activity: The lockstep phenomenon. *Electroenceph. Clin. Neurophysiol. 67*:247–259.

Leestma, J. E., Kalelkar, M. B., Teas, S. S., Jay, G. W., and Hughes, J. R. (1984). Sudden unexpected death associated with seizures: Analysis of 66 cases. *Epilepsia 25*(1):84–88.

Mathew, N. J., Taori, G. W., Mathai, M. S., and Chandy, J. (1970). Atrial fibrillation associated with seizures in a case of frontal meningioma. *Neurology 20*: 725–728.

Phizackerley, P. J. R., Poole, W. E., and Whitty, C. W. M. (1951). Sinoauricular heart block as an epileptic manifestation (a case report). *Epilepsia 3*:89–91.

Sulg, I. A. (1967). Polygraph in differential diagnosis of paroxysmal loss of consciousness. *Electroenceph. Clin. Neurophysiol. 23*:389.

Terrence, D. F., Jr., Wisotskey, H. M., and Perper, J. A. (1975). Unexpected, unexplained death in epileptic patients. *Neurology 25*:594–598.

Van Buren, J. M., and Ajmone-Marsan, C. (1960). A correlation of autonomic and EEG components in temporal lobe epilepsy. *Arch. Neurol. Psychiatr. 3*: 683–703.

Walsh, G. O., Masland, W., and Goldensohn, E. S. (1972). Relationship between paroxysmal atrial tachycardia and paroxysmal cerebral discharge. *Bull. Los Angeles Neurol. Soc. 37*:28–35.

5

Sudden Unexpected Death Associated with Seizures: A Pathological Review

JAN E. LEESTMA *Chicago Neurosurgical Center, Columbus Hospital, Chicago, Illinois*

I. INTRODUCTION

Although there is no widely accepted and understood definition of sudden death, the term is used extensively in practice by pathologists and clinicians, lawyers, journalists, and the lay public. A pragmatic resolution of this definitional dilemma lies, perhaps, in developing the boundaries of the phenomenon, however fuzzy, and enumerating the general characteristics of cases to be included while recognizing a vital element of uncertainty. Without a doubt a vital element in the definition of sudden death is the element of the unexpected. The victim, in apparent good health or possibly suffering from a known disease that may in time be expected to be fatal, unexpectedly "drops dead" or is found dead without any obvious external sign of distress or a rapid decline in health. Another key element implies some dismay or uncertainty, perhaps only at first, of the cause for the sudden demise. These two components typify the "mysterious" quality that surrounds any such case.

The next level of definition, which is harder, involves the time frame for the phenomenon. What is *sudden*? As expected, there is wide variation in response to such a question. Without any further qualification, the time interval between which the victim is last seen alive and in no apparent distress and when found dead is commonly accepted to lie between 1 and 24 hours (Kuller, 1966; Kuller and Lilienfeld, 1966; Kuller et al., 1967). Many forensic pathologists, however, prefer more precise limits: less than 1 hour, less than 2 hours, less than 12 hours, etc. (Adelson and Hoffman, 1961; Atkins, 1977; Spain, 1964; Spain et al., 1969). Some (Davis and Wright, 1980) would prefer to identify those cases in which death occurred in minutes as having suffered very sudden death. Still others would designate as instant deaths those which occur within a few seconds, and as *rapid* those occurring in a few seconds up to about 10 minutes (Haerem, 1978). The time interval is dismissed as of little importance by still other forensic experts who prefer to regard the unexpected quality of the death as the more vital quality of distinction (Simpson, 1953).

Some discussions of the phenomenon of sudden and unexpected death add another descriptive to the term: unexplained death (Terrence et al., 1975). The usual objections to this designation are that not all sudden and unexpected deaths are unexplained and that there are varying degrees of certainty of causality from case to case, and not an inevitable, pervading, and overriding aura of the mysterious. Even in the most difficult cases in which causality is not precisely demonstrable, supportable hypotheses on the mechanism(s) of death are possible, based on the knowledge of the basic principles of human biology and pathology.

II. REVIEW OF THE PATHOLOGY OF SUDDEN UNEXPECTED DEATH

A. Prevalence

Sudden death is common and within the experience of every physician. At least 20% of all deaths in most urban centers and probably between 450,000 and 500,000 each year in the United States occur suddenly (Leestma et al., 1985; Luke and Helpern, 1968; Office of the Medical Examiner, Cook County, Illinois, 1980). It is not known how many of these deaths are truly unexpected, but this characteristic is probably present in most cases (DeSilva, 1982; DeSilva and Lown, 1978; Thiene et al., 1983). Suddenness of death is the most common characteristic in persons dying between ages 20 and 64 years. In large metropolitan areas in the United States, and probably other Western nations, sudden deaths, especially when they occur outside hospitals, are reported to the medical examiner or coroner's office, which maintains statistics on the causes and manner of death in all cases reported to them by legal statute. As a general rule, somewhat less than 1% of the population dies in any given year and in Cook County, Illinois, about half of all deaths (15,000–17,000 per year) are reported to the Medical Examiner's Office because (1) there was no physician in attendance who could or would execute a death certificate; (2) foul play or criminal activity might have been involved; (3) the individual died within 24 hours after admission to a hospital or during childbirth, surgery, or some other treatment; (4) the individual died in an institution or while incarcerated; or (5) the individual died in an accident. Ultimately, about 15–20% of all deaths in the county will be certified by the Medical Examiner (Office of the Medical Examiner, Cook

County, Illinois, 1980). This is similar to the practice in other large cities (Kuller, 1966; Kuller et al., 1967; Luke and Helpern, 1968). Upon review of the reported statistics of the Office of the Medical Examiner of Cook County, Illinois, and upon comparison of these figures with others from the medical examiners of other large cities (Spitz and Fisher, 1973), about 65% of all reported cases are judged to have died of "natural" causes, about 10% due to homicide, 4-5% of suicide, about 20% from accidents, and in about 5% no "manner" of death could be determined (Office of the Medical Examiner, Cook County, Illinois, 1980).

Although many individuals die suddenly by accident, homicide, or suicide, they could hardly be regarded as having died suddenly and unexpectedly or without obvious explanation. Most of the unexpected nontraumatic death cases fall into the death-by-natural-cause category. No precise figures are known regarding the percentage of all natural deaths that are sudden and unexpected, but it is fair to assume that a large percentage of reported cases are, since they would not have ended up at the medical examiner if they had not been sudden, unexpected, or immediately explained. Of this group of cases, between 7 and 10% of natural deaths are not only sudden and unexpected (4-8% of all medical examiner cases) but may be lacking in obvious anatomic pathological causes. In Cook County this amounts to about 600 cases each year. Evidence gathered from careful analysis of circumstances, medical inference, and special laboratory studies, which may include toxicological analysis or detailed analysis of the heart, brain, or other organs by subspecialty pathologists, may eventually lead to a determination of the medical cause of death or may not. Within this group of cases lie those who are presumed to have died of some complication of epilepsy including SUDEP cases (in Cook County there are at least 100 such cases each year).

B. Pathology of Sudden Unexpected Nontraumatic Deaths

In perhaps the largest compilation of autopsy series' statistics on sudden and unexpected deaths, Kuller and coworkers (1966, 1967) classified the anatomic causes of death from 20,981 autopsies from various series into the broad disease categories seen in Table 1. If other large series of cases are examined (e.g., those of Luke and Helpern, 1968; Moritz and Zamchek, 1946), very similar distributions of cases by etiology are observed (Schwartz and Walsh, 1971).

1. Cardiovascular Deaths

From a statistical perspective alone, given no other information, the assumption that most sudden unexpected nontraumatic deaths are likely due to sudden stoppage or malfunction of the heart would be justified. A further presumption is that the more rapid the death, the more likely it is to be due to failure of the heart. These conclusions are justified by an extensive literature which provides

Table 1 Autopsy-Proven Causes of Death in Cases
of Sudden and Unexpected Death in a General
Forensic Autopsy Population

Disease process of	Percentage of cases
Heart and/or aorta	56.1% (± 7.4%)
Respiratory	14.5% (± 6.4%)
Brain and meninges	15.8% (± 2.4%)
Digestive/urogenital	8% (± 1.7%)
Miscellaneous	9.5% (± 8.9%)

Source: Adapted from data of Kuller (1966) and
Kuller and Lilienfeld (1967).

information about other dimensions of the sudden coronary death syndrome
(Atkins, 1977; DeSilva, 1982; DeSilva and Lown, 1978; Greenberg and Dwyer,
1982; Haerem, 1978; Hinkle, 1982; Phillips et al., 1986).

When prospective data from large-scale controlled population studies are examined, between 20 and 25% of "new coronary events" manifest themselves as
sudden unexpected death (Greenberg and Dwyer, 1982; Haerem, 1978; Kuller,
1966; Kuller and Lilienfeld, 1967). Furthermore, in 45–80% of cases of sudden
coronary death, death occurred in less than 15 minutes, and in about 50%, death
occurred in a minute or less (Haerem, 1978).

Retrospective autopsy analysis (Kuller, 1966) of deaths due to cardiovascular
disease revealed that of witnessed deaths occurring within one hour of an acute
episode, 91% of deaths in men and 52% in women were due to coronary artery
disease. In cases in which witnessed death took over an hour, 55% of deaths were
due to coronary artery disease; in unwitnessed deaths in which the duration of
the final ictus was unknown, 60% of men and 35% of women were thought to
have died from coronary artery disease.

When the mechanism of cardiac death is sought, a great deal of difficulty is
encountered in precisely determining this (Johnson et al., 1984). The whole
problem of sudden coronary death has been referred to by Lovegrove and
Thompson (1978) as a "statistician's nightmare." To the pathologist, it is a constant source of professional frustration that in only 20–30% of acute "heart attack" deaths are thromboses of a coronary vessel found. Furthermore, 80% of
cases at autopsy have no evidence of recent myocardial necrosis or fibrosis and
nearly two-thirds have no evidence of any previous cardiac pathology (Baroldi
et al., 1979; Haerem, 1978; Lovegrove and Thompson, 1978). Other studies
sometimes indicate a higher frequency of older myocardial lesions and evidence

of some coronary artery pathology or myocardiopathy (Newman et al., 1982; Phillips et al., 1986). When a large group of "heart attack" victims were studied with respect to prior symptoms, about 25% had a history of coronary artery disease, about 33% had prior cardiac symptoms, yet more than 40% had no symptoms or history of heart disease before death (Myerburg and Davis, 1964).

Many hypotheses have been proposed to explain the distressing lack of pathological confirmation of an immutable clinical fact. These include lysis of an occluding thrombus or embolus, poor pathological technique, functional occlusion of a coronary vessel by an evanescent process (platelet aggregates, lipid droplets, vasospasm), and/or cardiac arrhythmia. The difficulty here is that many of these conditions have physiological consequences that may not be reflected in recognizable pathological alterations (Baroldi et al., 1979; Haerem, 1978).

From a clinical perspective, certainly the very sudden death cases (dying in minutes) are most probably due to a fatal cardiac arrhythmia, usually ventricular fibrillation since from 72 to 87% of such individuals, if monitored, show this arrhythmia, while up to 37% will show some form of bradyarrhythmia or cardiac standstill (Greenberg and Dwyer, 1982; Haerem, 1978). While coronary artery disease and/or sudden fatal arrhythmia is the most common cardiovascular cause of sudden unexpected death, other catastrophic conditions may kill as quickly (Topaz and Edwards, 1985). These include rupture of the heart and ventricular aneurysm, sudden valvular prolapse or incompetence including rheumatic valve disease (Jeresaty, 1985), idiopathic hypertrophic subaortic stenosis (IHSS; Powell et al., 1973), myocarditis (Wentworth et al., 1979), fatty infiltration of the heart (Parker, 1974), cardiac myopathy (Phillips et al., 1986), and rupture of an aortic aneurysm. Even though these conditions may be chronic, they may also be clinically unappreciated and may produce death suddenly. If pulmonary thromboembolism, gas embolism, amniotic fluid embolism, and fat and foreign body embolism are considered cardiovascular rather than pulmonary conditions, they too should be recognized as "vascular" causes of sudden death (Kuller, 1966).

2. Respiratory System Deaths

Pulmonary embolism might be considered under this heading and as such is an important, though poorly enumerated cause. There is no question that in the hospitalized or bedridden patient, this may be preventable, and it is certainly a treatable cause of sudden and unexpected death (Clagett and Reisch, 1988). Acute and chronic infectious processes of the lungs may cause death suddenly. Bacterial pneumonia, lung abscess, tuberculosis, and viral pneumonia are probably the most common of these. Some forms of asphyxia or suffocation due to upper airway obstruction might include aspiration of food (so-called "cafe" coronary), gastric contents, or foreign bodies (false teeth and dental bridges; Camps, 1976; Kuller, 1966; Spitz and Fisher, 1973) and may involve loss of pharyngeal guarding reflexes and massive aspiration of gastric contents in psychotic individuals under phenothiazine tranquilizer medication (Leestma and Koenig, 1968). Acute asthma and anaphylaxis may also produce asphyxial death as can sudden massive pulmonary edema. Sudden loss of thoracic air seal, as in rupture of emphysematous bullae, may also kill rapidly. Neurogenic causes of respiratory failure include "neurogenic" pulmonary edema (Moss et al., 1973; Terrence et al., 1981), apnea syndromes (Bliwise et al., 1988), and other even less well-defined conditions. A troublesome type of death to analyze is sudden death in the bath. Drowning is always a possibility, alone or in connection with a seizure. Sometimes a victim found in the bath does not appear to have drowned, and pathological confirmation of drowning is anything but straightforward (Geertinger and Voigt, 1970). In many cases, when obvious pathological changes of drowning are absent, SUDEP and cardiac causes of death must be considered.

3. Nervous System Diseases

When physical injury to the nervous system has been excluded, some form of acute intracerebral hemorrhage (ruptured aneurysm, hypertensive hemorrhage, ruptured vascular malformation, in this order; Kuller, 1966; Leestma, 1988a) is the most common cause of sudden collapse. Death seldom occurs in minutes after one of these catastrophes but more often takes several hours or longer to occur, especially where emergency medical assistance is available. Such conditions, to be sure, occur suddenly and usually unexpectedly, but unless the victim is unobserved, an antemortem clinical diagnosis is usually made and thus the death, when it occurs, is rarely unexpected or unexplained. Nevertheless, some reports of acute subarachnoid hemorrhage use the term immediate death (Kuller, 1966; Luke and Helpern, 1968). The mechanism of death in acute intracranial hemorrhage is complex and includes both chemical and mechanical factors (Leestma, 1988a).

Intracranial infections may also be found to have caused unexpected and sometimes sudden death, though usually several or many hours are required. Examples of infectious conditions which are discovered at autopsy in SUD cases include bacterial meningitis and/or brain abscess, tuberculosis (meningitis and/or tuberculoma), mycotic aneurysms and complications of infections such as acute hemorrhagic encephalitis (Shwartzman reaction), acute cerebral edema or hydrocephalus, cerebral hemorrhage and/or infarction, and rupture of purulent material into the ventricles or subarachnoid space. Occasionally poliomyelitis or viral encephalitis will not be suspected and comes to light only at autopsy, but most such deaths are not unexpected, merely unexplained or not understood (Leestma, 1988a).

Brain tumors may occasionally cause unexpected and sometimes rather rapid death, mostly due to decompensating acute hydrocephalus, hemorrhage into the tumor, and/or cerebral edema. Examples include sudden deaths due to colloid cysts of the third ventricle (Leestma and Konakci, 1981), metastatic tumors to the brain, subependymomas, and gliomas (Huntington et al., 1965; Leestma, 1988a).

Degenerative and other diseases of the nervous system, with the exception of the Landry-GuillianBarré syndrome, only rarely cause sudden death.

Epilepsy is only infrequently mentioned as an important or common cause of SUD in most autopsy series, yet there is increasing evidence that it may be more common than almost any other CNS-mediated form of sudden death (Leestma et al., 1984, 1985, 1989). This specific issue is discussed in detail later.

4. Digestive and Urogenital System Sudden Deaths

Sudden exsanguination from esophageal varices, perforated gastric ulcer, or duodenal ulcer may cause death in minutes. Such hemorrhages are comparatively rare in the genitourinary tract. Infections with generalized sepsis may cause shock states and sudden decompensation and death in rupture and perforation of the gastrointestinal tract and in cryptic or unappreciated infections of the kidney, bladder, and genital organs. Occasionally in elderly individuals or otherwise very sensitive persons with underlying cardiovascular disease, acute distention of the stomach, bowel, or bladder may produce a "reflex" death, which may challenge explanation, but these are comparatively rare (DeSilva, 1982; Engel, 1978). During childbirth or pregnancy amniotic fluid embolism or air embolism may lead to prostration and rapid death (Camps, 1976; Spitz and Fisher, 1973).

5. Miscellaneous Conditions

Sudden death during surgery, obstetrical delivery, bronchoscopy, or radiological procedures may occur and may challenge the abilities of all concerned to uncover the cause or mechanism. Certain hormone-secreting tumors such as pheochromocytomas and carcinoids may occasionally produce such cardiovascular stress that death results suddenly and unexpectedly. Tumors in various organs may suddenly hemorrhage, cause vascular or luminal obstruction, or embolize and cause sudden death. Delayed death after trauma from fat or other embolism may also cause sudden and unexpected death, though certainly not frequently or without some warning or appreciation of the underlying condition (Camps, 1976; Kuller, 1966; Spitz and Fisher, 1973).

C. The Problem of Physiological or Reflex Sudden Deaths

The phenomenon of sudden death in apparently healthy young individuals has been the subject of medical curiosity and investigation for centuries. The advancement of the science of pathology and the autopsy has swept much of the mystery away from such cases, but there still remains a hard core of cases in which no obvious anatomically demonstrable cause of death can be found. One explanation for the lack of autopsy findings is that the process responsible occurred so rapidly that no evidence of its existence is detectable grossly, microscopically, or by ordinarily applicable technical methods (Moritz and Zamchek, 1946). Another is that the process which caused death was "physiological" and either related to an exaggerated neurally mediated reflex or involving a pathological electrical event such as cardiac arrhythmia, which cannot be represented structurally and can be appreciated only in the living patient (Weiss, 1940). Occasionally, after rigorous studies of the cardiac conduction system, for example, structural lesions or anatomic variants may be found which probably caused the fatal events, yet no absolute confirmation is possible even then (Thiene et al., 1983). Conclusions about the mechanisms of such physiological death are based on circumstantial evidence and chance observations of ECG or other physiological measurements prior to death.

Most "reflex" or "physiological" deaths probably involve some neurally mediated abnormality of cardiac or vascular function and have been referred to by Weiss (1940) as "fatal syncope." Such sudden fatal events may occur in connection with stress, fright, strong emotion, dreams and nightmares, shock, extreme pain, or sudden blows to the chest, abdomen, head, or even extremities (DeSilva, 1982; DeSilva and Lown, 1978; Dimsdale, 1977; Doyle, 1976; Engel, 1978; Kuller, 1966; Lown et al., 1977). In virtually every culture, emotion-triggered sudden deaths have been described and often take an important place in folklore. In the Philippines these cases are referred to as bangungut, in Japan, as pokkuri, and among the Hmong people of Indochina the condition is regarded as almost epidemic (Baron et al., 1983; Kirschner et al., 1986; Melles and Katz, 1988). Mysticism and magic surround many of these kinds of cases, and hexes or curses are often blamed for deaths in certain cultures, most notably in so-called voodoo deaths in Haiti (Cannon, 1957) and in other countries (Cohen, 1988). When such cases have been thoroughly studied, the emotional overlay to underlying abnormalities of the cardiac conduction system has been described (Baron et al., 1983; Kirschner et al., 1986; Okada and Kawai, 1983). Similarly, the connection among sleep, dreaming, and nightmares in such cases is also common (Melles and Katz, 1988).

Every physician encounters individuals who may have one or more chronic diseases, may be grieving over the loss of a loved one, or may be of advanced age and suffering from one element of depression and who announce or otherwise inform family members, friends, or personnel that they want to die or will soon die—and they do. Autopsy examinations reveal the underlying disease process that was known clinically, but no obvious cause of death. The same phenomenon has been observed in concentration camp victims and in the special case of infants and young children who may be victims of abuse and neglect who simply fade away, having lost the "will to live" (Leestma, 1988a,b). This problem has been unevenly studied but has empirical and some experimental support (Spitz, 1965).

D. Sudden Infant Death Syndrome

Sudden infant death syndrome (SIDS), or crib death, is a distressingly common phenomenon in most countries and may represent 40% of all deaths in infancy. The mean age of victims is about three months, and SIDS is generally uncommon past the age of one year (Leestma, 1988a; Valdes-Dapeña, 1967). The SIDS designation is applied to those infant deaths that occur suddenly and unexpectedly and in which no obvious cause of death is determined by autopsy, thus ruling out obvious infections, tumors, malformations, or other common conditions.

Apnea, most commonly during sleep, is felt to be the most suspected mechanism of death, but why this should occur is still poorly understood. Some infants suffer numerous apneic episodes, sometimes requiring resuscitation, before they either die or recover completely. There is probably no single cause for SIDS but rather a multifactorial matrix of underlying conditions which may combine with an external event to cause death. Some of the factors are recent infection, involving the upper respiratory tract, of bacterial or viral origin; history of respiratory distress or perinatal ischemia or prematurity; underlying damage to brain stem reticular formation or respiratory centers; and/or the recent use of aspirin. Not every infant dying of SIDS displays all of these, but enough of them occur commonly that thay are probably involved. A number of mechanisms have been theorized for SIDS but have not been proven (Leestma, 1988a; Naeye, 1974; Valdes-Dapeña, 1967; Werne and Garrow, 1953a,b).

III. REVIEW OF THE PHENOMENON AND PATHOLOGY OF SUDDEN UNEXPECTED DEATH IN EPILEPTIC PERSONS

A. Historical Background

As early as 1902, Spratling noted that in a large population of institutionalized epileptic individuals, about 4% of the deaths which occurred over a number of years appeared to occur suddenly, unexpectedly, and, according to postmortem examination, apparently without demonstrable cause. A later study reported by Munson in 1910 noted that about 17% of deaths in a large epileptic population were sudden and unexpected, but this included a number dying from suffocation, aspiration, accident, and other discovered causes in addition to those in whom no anatomic cause of death could be determined. Over the intervening years many reports of sudden, unexpected, and often unexplained deaths of epileptic persons appeared in the literature. Typical among them are the reports of

Steinsiek (1950), Krohn (1963), Neplokh (1965), Freytag and Lindenberg (1964), Penning et al. (1969), Zielinski (1974a,b, 1982), Ziegler and Kamecke (1976), Hirsch and Martin (1971), Terrence et al. (1975), Leestma et al. (1984, 1985, 1989), and Copeland (1984). The unifying features of all these reports is that apparently normal epileptic individuals can suddenly and unexpectedly die without apparently demonstrable pathological cause, once status epilepticus, accidents, drowning, drug overdoses, intercurrent disease, and other demonstrable causes are ruled out. This phenomenon is not rare.

B. Recent Pathological Studies of SUDEP

As discussed in Chapter 1, SUDEP probably accounts for more than 10% of deaths in epileptic persons (Jay and Leestma, 1981; Leestma et al., 1984, 1985, 1989). Only recently has a significant effort been made to explain SUDEP cases in depth in an attempt to understand the phenomenon and to identify characteristics and a possible risk profile.

My coworkers and I have attempted to study the phenomenon from the perspective of the medical examiner's forensic pathologist, since one is more likely to confront such cases in this setting than anywhere else. We have identified suspected SUDEP cases by the following method over the past 10 years at the Office of the Medical Examiner of Cook County, Illinois:

1. When the lay investigator for the Medical Examiner's Office becomes involved in a case that clearly does not involve homicide, suicide, or accident but does involve the sudden unexpected death of an individual, the investigator is encouraged to inquire of family members, friends, or witnesses if the deceased suffered from seizures. Any medications at the death scene are examined and recorded, especially anticonvulsants.

2. When a given case is suspected to involve a seizure disorder, a specially prepared checklist (Figure 1), is consulted for assistance in eliciting and recording information that will enable analysis of the case.

3. When the body of the victim is brought to the Office of the Medical Examiner, a thorough external, toxicological, and autopsy examination, including examination of the brain, is done.

4. If an anatomically or toxicologically demonstrable cause of death can be found, the case is not considered a possible SUDEP.

5. In all suspected SUDEP cases, the brain is examined by a neuropathologist.

6. The designation of SUDEP is applied to the case only when there is an adequate history of a seizure disorder which usually would qualify the individual as having suffered from epilepsy and when the death was sudden and unexpected and anatomically and toxicologically unexplained.

EPILEPSY DEATH CHECK-LIST

ME Case No._____   Name:_____

Investigator:_____   Date:_____

How long did victim have seizures?   _____
How often?   _____
When was the last one?   _____
Was a seizure observed before death?   _____
Did victim take medication for seizures?   _____
Was a Brain Wave test (EEG) ever done?   _____
Hospital/Clinic where treated for seizures?   _____

Doctor who had treated victim: Name:_____
        Address/Phone: _____
Did victim:
  ( ) Drink heavily?   ( ) Use drugs?   ( ) Use marijuana?
  ( ) Have prior head injury? ( ) Have a brain operation?
  ( ) Have a brain disease?   ( ) Have meningitis/encephalitis?
  ( ) Any chronic health problem? Give details   _____
  ( ) Take insulin (diabetes)?
Additional Information:

Did victim take any of the following medications? (all that apply)

  ( ) Dilantin   ( ) Phenobarbital ( ) Mysoline   ( ) Tegretol
  ( ) Depakene   ( ) Zarontin   ( ) Celontin   ( ) Other:_____
Additional Information:

Description of Seizures: (check YES or NO to all that apply)

( ) Stiffening ( ) Violent jerking ( ) Mild Twitching ( ) Collapse
( ) Loud cry   ( ) Unconsciousness ( ) Staring spells ( ) of one side
( ) Loss of Bladder/Bowel control   ( ) Biting of tongue/cheeks
( ) Repeated automatic or senseless movements of hands, arms, legs
( ) Facial movements-grimacing-chewing movements, etc.
( ) Grogginess-sleeping after attacks
( ) Did victim have any warning of attack?   _____
( ) Could anything bring on an attack?   _____
( ) Could anything prevent an attack?   _____
Additional Information:

Information on labels of any medication found at scene:
Pharmacy, Rx number, Doctor, etc:

Figure 1 Epilepsy death checklist used by the Office of the Medical Examiner, Cook County, Illinois, for several years in collecting data on possible SUDEP cases. [From Leestma et al. (1985), reproduced with permission.]

There are several inherent sources of bias and error in such an approach. Potential cases of SUDEP may not be identified at the outset either because they never come to the attention of the medical examiner or because the investigator does not obtain or record relevant information which alerts the forensic pathologist to the possibility of SUDEP. Cases that could be SUDEP cases are eliminated because of the suspicion that natural disease processes, most notably arteriosclerotic cardiovascular disease, played a role or caused death with or without benefit of an autopsy. There is no way that contributory disease processes can adequately be dealt with unless a very much larger scale study is undertaken using nonepileptic control groups for comparison.

The case-selection method introduces an inherent exclusionary bias against older individuals, most of whom will show some degree of cardiovascular disease. It will also discriminate against very young potential victims, since some will be thought to be SIDS cases. In accident cases, when an epileptic person is drowned

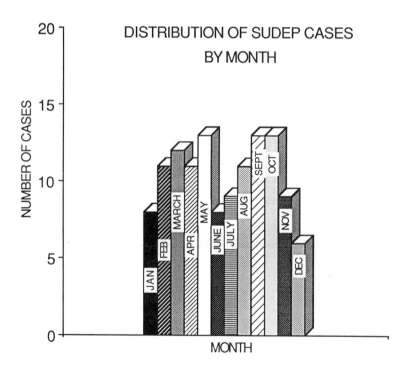

Figure 2 Occurrence of SUDEP by month. These data represent a collection of cases for a two-year time span (124 cases) at the Office of the Medical Examiner, Cook County, Illinois.

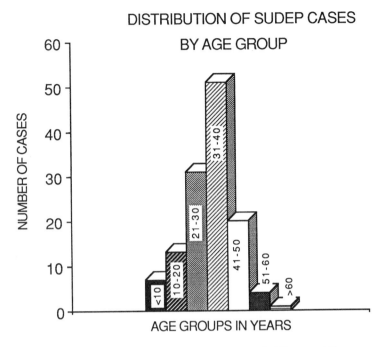

Figure 3 Age distribution by decade of 124 SUDEP cases. The mean and median age is 32 years, the mode is 33 years.

or traumatized, it may never be determined if the victim collapsed and would have died atraumatically were it not for special circumstances. Therefore, the figures derived by the methods employed are, if anything, conservative in terms of numbers.

Since the mid-1970s, with varying degrees of success, cases which have been identified as SUDEP have been collected at the Office of the Medical Examiner of Cook County, Illinois. In any given year between 60 and 80 cases are identified, amounting to at least one case per week among the nearly 100 cases subjected to autopsy each week at the Office. Thus in the course of about 10 years, over 500 cases were identified. Given the population base in Cook County of about 5.25 million persons, and the fact that about 10% of those dying in any year are autopsied by the Office of the Medical Examiner, it is possible to predict the number of SUDEP cases any other large metropolitan area is likely to experience. Informal contacts with the coronor or medical examiners in Denver, Miami, Los Angeles, and Baltimore have revealed remarkably similar incidence of the SUDEP phenonemon in those cities and in Chicago (Leestma et al., 1985; personal communication, 1985).

Table 2 Characteristics of the SUDEP Population Observed Over Nearly 10 Years in Cook County, Illinois, Office of the Medical Examiner

Age range	
4 months to 85 years	
Average age	
31.4 years	
Sex	
Male	74%
Female	26%
Race	
Black male	49%
White male	25%
Black female	11%
White female	15%
Seizure history duration	
More than 1 year	86%
More than 5 years	54%
Mean: 9.5 years Mode: 3 years	
Frequency of seizures	
< 1 seizure per year	9%
3–10 seizures per year	52%
> 1 seizure per week	39%
Type of seizure	
Generalized, usually GTC	96–98%
Circumstances of death	
Death in bed	37%
Dead in other room	25%
DOA in emergency room	22%
Other circumstances	12%

1. Population Characteristics of the SUDEP Group

Based on the most carefully studied 124 cases in our experience, which span 12 consecutive months bridging 1978–1979 and 12 consecutive months in 1983, we found representative characteristics of the SUDEP population as observed in Cook County (Chicago) (Leestma et al., 1984, 1985, 1989). The occurrence rate per month over the two-year span is depicted in Figure 2. It appears that the peak months for occurrence of SUDEP are February through May and August through October. There is no obvious explanation for this apparent seasonality. The age range is seen in Figure 3. Summary statistics on the 124 case series are given in Table 2.

Table 3 Drugs Taken by SUDEP Victims

Anticonvulsant medication	Percentage of cases
Phenytoin only	25%
Phenobarbital only	3%
Phenytoin and phenobarbital	33%
Phenytoin, phenobarbital, and other	10%
Phenytoin and carbamazepine	2%
Valproic acid and other	2%
Other combinations	2%
No known anticonvulsant	23%

Information regarding the SUDEP victims' seizures and their duration came from relatives, friends, witnesses, pharmacists, physicians, clinic records, and sometimes police records. Similar sources of information were used to ascertain the frequency of seizures. The types of seizures were deduced from descriptions taken down by the lay investigators at the scene (using the checklist shown in Figure 1), or information was obtained from medical records including EEGs. In only a few cases did death apparently occur after the first reported or observed seizure. Most SUDEP cases died in the course of normal everyday activities, usually at home, and most commonly in bed. When found in the home but not in bed, the victim was most often in an attitude of sleep (lying on a couch or sitting in a chair). None of these victims were entangled in bed clothing or died of asphyxia. Of these victims 3-5% were found in the bathroom, mostly in or near the tub or shower. All cases in which drowning was determined or suspected and those involving serious head injuries were eliminated from this study. Over 25% of SUDEP cases occurred in the presence of another individual, who either saw the fatal collapse or heard the victim call out or fall. These victims were almost always given medical assistance by the fire department rescue squad and were transported to a hospital emergency room where they died after varying intervals. Most, however, were admitted DOA, and the remainder were refractory to resuscitation and were declared dead later.

In about 23% of cases it was not possible to determine if the individual had ever taken or been prescribed anticonvulsant medication, but in the remaining 77% a number of combinations of medications were noted in pill bottles or found in pharmacy or other records. The pattern of medications that were being prescribed or taken by SUDEP victims is seen in Table 3.

Numerous other medications were found at the scene or were discovered to have been prescribed at one time or another for about half the SUDEP victims.

Table 4   Medical History Obtained from Family, Friends, or Other Witnesses of Deceased SUDEP Victims

Past medical/health history	Percentage of cases
In apparent good health	23%
Old head injury	27%
Gunshot wound to head	2%
History of hypertension	8%
Anemia/sickle cell disease	8%
Asthma	2%
Diabetes	2%
Miscellaneous	8%
Unknown	20%

The most common of these were tranquilizing medications [one of the benzodiazepines (21%), tricyclic antidepressants (7%), and phenothiazines (7%)]. Other drugs represented included diuretics, antihistaminics, disulfiram (Antabuse), and narcotic analgesics (2-5% each).

In at least half of SUDEP cases a history of substance abuse could be positively obtained. The most commonly abused substance was ethanol, reported in about at least 70% of victims whose history could be obtained. Intravenous drug use was reported in about 3-5% of cases, as was excessive (addictive) use of caffeine-containing beverages. About 5% of victims were known to use cannabis. About one-third of the victims used multiple substances at one time or another.

The past medical history of SUDEP victims, obtained from any available source, is displayed in Table 4.

2. Summary

It is apparent from a cursory examination of the population under study that they are young individuals, usually male and most likely black, who are in apparent good health, who probably abuse alcohol, have suffered some form of head injury in the past, and have most probably had anticonvulsant medication prescribed for their generalized seizures, which they have had for several years. If they are taking another medication, it is likely to be a tranquilizing medication. Their seizures are under moderate control. The SUDEP victim usually dies at home in the course of normal activities, usually sleep or preparing for or arising from sleep.

Table 5 Toxicological Results Obtained from Postmortem Blood Samples in 124 Victims of SUDEP

Phenytoin levels	Phenobarbital levels		
	None	Subtherapeutic	Therapeutic
None	50%	13%	7%
Subtherapeutic	8.7%	9.6%	0%
Therapeutic	7%	4.3%	0.9%

C. Toxicological Findings

In most suspected SUDEP cases heart blood, and probably other body fluids, such as urine and bile, as well as liver and other tissues, may be taken for toxicological examination. In the 124 SUDEP cases studied over two years by us (Leestma et al., 1984, 1985, 1989) 115 had such examinations. Blood samples were analyzed for phenytoin, phenobarbital, ethanol, opiates, tranquilizing drugs, and analgesics. In 50% of the cases, no detectable levels were found of either phenytoin or phenobarbital, or, for that matter, of any other anticonvulsant. The various combinations of drug levels are seen in Table 5.

In the very few cases in which primidone was detected, it was present alone in the therapeutic or greater range in three cases, in subtherapeutic concentrations with a subtherapeutic level of phenytoin in one case, and in only one further case were the levels of both drugs considered within therapeutic range. The therapeutic-range blood level for phenytoin was considered to be between 9 and 20 μg/ml and for phenobarbital between 9 and 25 μg/ml (Laidlaw and Richens, 1982). Reports by others of SUDEP cases confirm the pattern of noncompliance with anticonvulsant medication observed in our population (Copeland, 1984; Hirsch and Martin, 1971; Terrence et al., 1975).

D. Autopsy Findings

When cases that did not have a complete autopsy (7 cases which involved "head-only" autopsies) were reviewed, 117 cases yielded results for analysis. Some 38% of all cases were judged to show virtually no significant pathological abnormality that would merit inclusion in the diagnostic list of the autopsy. Incidental and other findings noted were not considered to be responsible for sudden death. These conditions included some degree of cerebral edema (32%), pulmonary emphysema (3%), some degree of cirrhosis or fatty liver (8.5%), chronic pancreatitis (3%), and other miscellaneous findings. Not specifically included for the com-

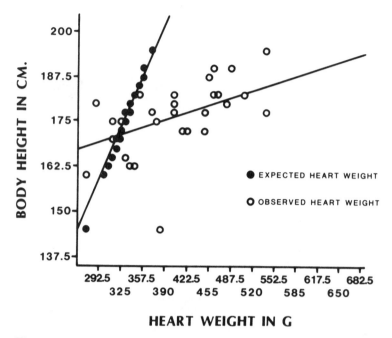

Figure 4 Scatter plot with linear regression lines illustrating the expected heart weight in 42 SUDEP males based on the formulation of Zeek (1942) (closed circles) compared with the observed heart weights in these men (open circles). The actual heart weights were about 150 g heavier than expected. The differences between expected and observed heart weights is statistically significant ($p < 0.0005$). [From Leestma et al. (1989), reproduced with permission.]

bined two-year series figures but specifically noted in the sixty 1983 cases were body height and weight and heart, lung, brain, and liver weights.

Of considerable interest was the finding that the hearts, lungs, and livers of male SUDEP victims were significantly ($p < 0.001$) heavier than the expected weights for these organs. Expected weight for the heart was derived from the regression equation based on body height and heart weight relationships in mature American males described by Zeek (1942). The comparison of these ideal and observed weights can be seen in Figure 4. The comparison between observed and ideal heart weights for women did not permit any statistical inference to be drawn from the data.

A similar scatter plot of expected and observed lung weights (Figure 5) showed a significant ($p < 0.001$) difference, as did the expected and observed liver weights. Here both male and female statistics were considered significantly different (heavier) from control organ weights. Histological examination of the

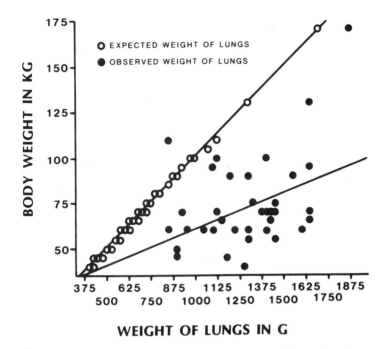

Figure 5   Scatter plot with linear regression lines illustrating the expected (open circles) and observed (closed circles) lung weights in 37 SUDEP cases of both sexes. Expected lung weights were estimated at 1% of body weight (Furbank, quoted by Simpson, 1953). Expected and observed weights are signficantly different ($p < 0.001$). [From Leestma et al. (1989), reproduced with permission.]

heart by routine screening sections did not reveal obvious pathology and in any case could not account for death. The histopathological appearances of the lungs and livers revealed passive congestion, and the lungs revealed both pulmonary edema and congestion (Leestma et al., 1989).

It was thought that there might be a statistical correlation between duration and/or frequency of epileptic attacks and the difference in expected (ideal) and observed weight of the heart in SUDEP cases, but no such correlation could be established.

The basis for cardiomegaly in SUDEP has not been determined and, to our knowledge, has not been specifically addressed in any prior report of SUDEP; however, it has been discussed in some detail in reports on SUD in Asian refugees in the United States (Baron et al., 1983). Kirschner et al. (1986) noted significant increase in heart weight (greater than 1 S.D. over expected weight) in 78% of their recent autopsied cases along with a general tendency for cardiac dilatation and abnormalities, probably congenital, in the cardiac conduction system and not in other SUD cases. The finding of cardiomegaly has also been reported in other types of SUD cases in Asians, Bangungut in the Philippines and in Pokkuri in Japan (Kirschner et al., 1986; Okada and Kawai, 1983). The significance of these observations is not known precisely, but surely they must have some bearing on the cause of death. Very little literature exists concerning possible pathology in the heart in SUDEP (Falconer and Rajs, 1976), but there are some reports that excessive sympathetic stimulation of the heart may cause subtle pathological changes (Savel'yeva and Posdnyakov, 1972). To overcome this difficulty, a thorough pathological analysis of the hearts of SUDEP victims could be undertaken, as was done in cooperation with the Centers for Disease Control in the Asian refugee deaths (Kirschner et al., 1986).

The degree of passive congestion in both liver and lung, as well as edema in the lungs, suggests some element of acute "backward" cardiac failure in the SUDEP cases. In some cases, the protein content of the pulmonary edema is high enough to appear in histological sections as a pink shadow in the alveoli. It is possible that the type and degree of pulmonary edema may be compatible with so-called neurogenic pulmonary edema of the type sometimes encountered in severe head injury (Moss et al., 1973; Terrence et al., 1981). The issue of cause and mechanism of such pulmonary edema is discussed in detail in Chapter 6 of this volume.

One issue of case selection which is inherent in any selection of special cases such as SUDEP victims is that true SUDEP cases are excluded because of underlying disease processes which either have nothing to do with the sudden death or are in some way contributory to the underlying mechanisms for SUDEP. Until and unless more is known about SUDEP it will not be possible to incude less clear-cut cases in any analysis.

E. Neuropathological Findings

It appears that SUDEP cases are much more likely to have obvious anatomic lesions of the brain than do epileptics who died under other circumstances. If one excludes microscopic alterations in the hippocampus, probably fewer than 10% of nonselected epileptics will show any grossly evident pathology in the brain (Corsellis, 1957; Margerison and Corsellis, 1966; Meldrum and Corsellis, 1984). Common lesions seen in these cases include gross Ammon's horn sclerosis, previously unsuspected vascular malformations, tumors, old traumatic contusions, cortical malformations in the brain, and a host of other conditions. These conditions appear much more common in the SUDEP group. The distribution of brain lesions in 124 SUDEP cases collected over two years is illustrated in Table 6.

If one takes into account the fact that more than one condition can be observed in a case and enumerates those cases with at least one of the foregoing

Table 6 Neuropathological Findings Observed in 124 Cases of SUDEP Examined by the Author

Pathological lesion	Percentage of cases
Old traumatic contusion(s)	26.1%
Hydrocephalus	8.4%
Old subdural hematoma(s)	7.6%
Leptomeningeal fibrosis	4.2%
Old penetrating injury or surgical site	10%
Vascular malformation	1.7%
Cortical or lacunar infarct(s)	7%
Cortical malformation/hamartoma	5.9%
Present or past brain tumor	4.2%
Other conditions	5%
Ammon's horn sclerosis	10%
Cerebellar atrophy	3.4%
Cerebral hemiatrophy	2.5%

neuropathological findings, about 70% of SUDEP cases have a grossly visible lesion in their brain. This lesion has been associated with, or blamed for, seizures in other individuals. The sites most likely to show a lesion are near the base of the brain in either the frontal or temporal lobes, regions which are said to have a lower seizure threshold than other locations (Laidlaw and Richens, 1982; Leestma, 1988b).

Of the tumors found in the cases of SUDEP, the distribution is similar to that found in other medical examiners' series (Huntington et al., 1965). Most were glial tumors, usually of low grade or in a period of relative control, various cysts at the base of the brain, and multiple lesions typically encountered in tuberous sclerosis (four cases included). Not all of these tumors were known clinically. The cortical malformations ranged from an anomaly which involved one hippocampal formation and blended into the adjacent basal ganglia to bilateral malformations, usually involving some portion of the temporal lobe including the hippocampus. Foreign bodies occasionally found in the brain incuded metallic fragments from old bullet wounds, stab wounds, or penetrating injuries. Bits of bone from old, usually unrecorded, traumatic events were also encountered, most frequently embedded in the frontal lobe. Ammon's horn sclerosis of varying degrees was found. There were six cases in which only one horn was affected (grossly) and an equal number with bilateral involvement. The contusions observed were most commonly at the frontal tip, orbital surface, or temporal tips or under surfaces and were thought to be mostly contrecoup and/or gliding contusions. Many of these cases also had chronic resolved subdural hematoma membranes.

F. Clinical Pathological Implications and Correlations

From the foregoing discussion regarding the experience with non-epilepsy-related sudden unexpected death, it is reasonable to expect that, in the absence of concrete causal findings at autopsy in a SUD victim, the death most probably involved failure by standstill or arrhythmia of the heart alone or combined with a circulatory embarrassment, possibly shock and/or an acute respiratory failure. It is therefore reasonable to extend this expectation to the SUDEP cases, since in most cases, no obvious anatomic cause of death can be found at autopsy. The connection of a sudden fatal cardiovascular collapse with some abnormality of brain function is compelling in the epileptic SUD victim. An examination of the SUDEP victims reveals a pattern of consistency in the findings in the general autopsy and in the brain, not to mention the circumstances and manner in which they die. Although there are many characteristics in these individuals which are not truly clinical symptoms, and thus might stretch the usual definition of a syndrome, a broader definition, like that of *Dorland's Medical Dictionary*—"The sum of signs of any morbid state"—would certainly qualify SUDEP as a syndrome, albeit a fatal one.

The careful study of 124 cases and the observation of perhaps 200 more such cases yield the following general bounds of definition for SUDEP. Usually the victim is a male, more commonly a black male, in his thirties, and who has suffered generalized (usually generalized tonic-clonic) epileptic seizures for two to three years or more, generally no more frequently than one seizure every month or two. He tends to abuse alcohol and to poorly comply with or never takes anticonvulsant medication. The SUDEP victim usually dies suddenly and unexpectedly; death may occur in the course of normal activities but is most commonly associated with retiring for bed, sleeping, or rising from bed at home. When the fatal attack is witnessed and assistance is available, resuscitative efforts are usually ineffective. When ECG data are available, ventricular fibrillation or standstill is commonly observed. Autopsy examination will most likely reveal no significant pathological findings to explain death, but the heart will be heavier than expected for the height and weight of the individual (men only), the lungs will be congested and edematous, and the liver will be congested. The brain will most probably show some structural, grossly evident lesion (most commonly posttraumatic) involving or impinging on the cerebral cortex, usually at the base of the brain. The brain will probably be somewhat under normal weight.

IV. SUMMARY

The description of the typical SUDEP victim suggests a number of conclusions regarding risk factors, pathogenesis, and mechanism. Risk of SUDEP in the general epileptic population is relatively small, having been estimated at between 1/525 and 1/2100 (Hirsch and Martin, 1971; Leestma, 1984, 1985; Terrence et al., 1975); however, when the general epileptic population is narrowed to more closely match the age and sex characteristics of the typical SUDEP case, the risk may approach 1/200. If the at-risk population is defined still more narrowly to select males between the ages of 20 and 40 years who have symptomatic epilepsy (posttraumatic, etc.) and may not comply with anticonvulsant medication, the risk of SUDEP may exceed 1/50 (Leestma et al., 1989).

If this risk estimate is even approximately correct, why is the SUDEP syndrome so poorly recognized by neurologists, neurosurgeons, and other medical practitioners? Perhaps the answer to this question can be appreciated from an examination of the lifestyle of the most commonly affected group, the norms of medical care practice, and the health-care "system" in the United States. In general, young individuals tend not to be especially concerned about their health, seeking medical care only when they are so seriously symptomatic that their vigorous lifestyle is affected. There may be a strong tendency to deny or belittle a potentially serious medical condition. Furthermore, a long-term relationship with a single physician is not common and becomes even less so as medical care is increasingly delivered via impersonal institutions such as HMOs, clinics, and emergency rooms. Care is often deferred since medical insurance is simply forgone by larger and larger proportions of the population, especially young individuals. Follow-up and tracking of patients is nearly impossible in the United States; therefore, a patient who does not return for treatment or follow-up disappears from medical observation and records. If such a patient were to die as a victim of SUDEP, he or she would be brought to the nearest emergency room of a hospital. Usually there is only the immediate concern of attempting to preserve life, and little attempt is made to obtain medical records or to contact past doctors once the patient has died. Furthermore, such deaths usually must be reported to the coroner or medical examiner, who will direct that the body be brought to that facility for examination or autopsy, thus bypassing the pathology department of the local hospital. The coroner or medical examiner is primarily charged with generating a death certificate and determining the cause and manner of death. Generally, little information is sought other than that required to perform this task, and feedback of information into the medical care system is limited by time and resources. Effectively, then, the case enters a separate track in the health-care system which compartmentalizes the SUDEP case insofar as the rest of the system is concerned.

As to pathogenesis and mechanism of death in SUDEP cases, much of this book is devoted to an exploration of this question. The role of centrally triggered or mediated cardiac electrical events acutely or chronically associated with the epileptic brain and the role of hemodynamic or neurogenic pulmonary vascular interaction in the process deserve further study.

With an understanding of the probable risk factors and at least some appreciation for the mechanism for SUDEP, some degree of prevention should be possible. This would logically involve education of physicians who manage epileptic persons, especially those with symptomatic epilepsy, as well as education of the most at-risk epileptic persons as to the dangers of poor medication compliance and hazards of lifestyle which render them vulnerable to sudden death.

REFERENCES

Adelson, L., and Hoffman, W. (1961). Sudden death from coronary disease: Related to a lethal mechanism arising independently of vascular occlusion or myocardial damage. *J. Am. Med. Assoc. 176*:129-135.

Atkins, J. M. (1977). Sudden death. In *Clinical Cardiology*. J. T. Willerson and C. A. Sanders (Eds.). Grune and Stratton, New York, pp. 623-628.

Baroldi, G., Falzi, G., and Mariani, F. (1979). Sudden coronary death. A postmortem study in 208 selected cases compared to 97 "control" subjects. *Am. Heart J. 98*:20-31.

Baron, R. C., Thacker, S. B., Gorelkin, L., Vernon, A. A., Taylor, W. R., and Choi, K. (1983). Sudden death among Southeast Asian refugees. An unexplained nocturnal phenomenon. *J. Am. Med. Assoc. 250*:2947-2951.

Bliwise, D. L., Bliwise, N. G., Partinen, M., and Dement, W. C. (1988). Sleep apnea and mortality in an aged cohort. *Am. J. Pub. Health 78*:544-547.

Camps, F. E. (Ed.) (1976). *Gradwohl's Legal Medicine*, 3rd ed. Year Book Medical, Chicago.

Cannon, W. B. (1957). "Voodoo" death. *Psychosomat. Med. 19*:182-190.

Clagett, G. P., and Reisch, J. S. (1988). Prevention of venous thromboembolism in general surgical patients. *Ann. Surg. 208*:227-240.

Cohen, S. I. (1988). Voodoo death, the stress response, and AIDS. *Adv. Biochem. Psychopharmacol. 44*:95-109.

Copeland, A. R. (1984). Seizure disorders. The Dade County experience from 1978 to 1982. *Am. J. Forensic Med. Pathol. 5*:211-215.

Corsellis, J. A. N. (1957). The incidence of Ammon's horn sclerosis. *Brain 80*: 193-208.

Davis, J. H., and Wright, R. K. (1980). The very sudden cardiac death syndrome: A conceptual model for pathologists. *Human Pathol. 11*:117-121.

DeSilva, R. A. (1982). Central nervous system risk factors for sudden cardiac death. In *Sudden Coronary Death*, H. M. Greenburg and E. M. Dwyer, Jr. (Eds.). New York Academy of Sciences, New York, pp. 143-161.

DeSilva, R. A., and Lown, B. (1978). Ventricular premature beats, stress and sudden death. *Psychosomatics 19*:649-661.

Dimsdale, J. E. (1977). Emotional causes of sudden death. *Am. J. Psychiatr.* *134*:1361-1366.

Doyle, J. T. (1976). Mechanisms and prevention of sudden death. *Mod. Concept. Cardiovasc. Dis. 45*:111-116.

Engel, G. L. (1978). Psychologic stress, vasodepressor (vasovagal) syncope and sudden death. *Ann. Intern. Med. 89*:403-412.

Falconer, B., and Rajs, J. (1976). Post-mortem findings of cardiac lesions in epileptics: A preliminary report. *Forensic Sci. 8*:63-71.

Freytag, E., and Lindenberg, R. (1964). 294 medicolegal autopsies in epileptics. *Arch. Pathol. 78*:274-286.

Geertinger, P., and Voigt, J. (1970). Death in the bath. A survey of bathtub deaths in Copenhagen, Denmark, and Gothenberg, Sweden from 1961 to 1969. *J. Forensic Med. 17*:135-147.

Greenberg, H. M., and Dwyer, E. M., Jr. (Eds.) (1982). *Annals of the New York Academy of Sciences*, Vol. 382, *Sudden Coronary Death*. New York Academy of Sciences, New York.

Haerem, J. W. (1978). Sudden unexpected coronary death. The occurrence of platelet aggregates in the epicardial and myocardial vessels of man. *Acta Pathol. Microbiol. Scand. 265 (Suppl)*:1-47.

Hinkle, L. E. (1982). Short-term risk factors for sudden death. In *Annals of the New York Academy of Sciences*, Vol. 382, *Sudden Coronary Death*, H. M. Greenberg and E. M. Dwyer, Jr. (Eds). New York Academy of Sciences, New York, pp. 22-38.

Hirsch, C. S., and Martin, D. L. (1971). Unexpected death in young epileptics. *Neurology 21*:682-690.

Huntington, H. W., Cummings, K. L., Moe, T. I., O'Connell, H. V., and Wybel, R. (1965). Discovery of fatal primary intracranial neoplasms at medicolegal autopsies. *Cancer 18*:117-127.

Jay, G. W., and Leestma, J. E. (1981). Sudden death in epilepsy. *Acta Neurol. Scand. (Suppl. 82) 63*:1-66.

Jeresaty, R. M. (1985). Mitral valve prolapse. An update. *J. Am. Med. Assoc. 254*:793-795.

Johnson, R. H., Lambie, D. G., and Spalding, J. M. K. (1984). Neurogenic abnormalities of the heart. In *Major Problems in Neurology*, Vol. 13, *Neurocardiology*, J. Walton (Ed). Saunders, London, pp. 59-111.

Kirschner, R. H., Eckner, F. A., and Baron, R. C. (1986). The cardiac pathology of sudden, unexplained nocturnal death in Southeast Asian refugees. *J. Am. Med. Assoc. 256*:2700-2705.

Krohn, W. (1963). Causes of death among epileptics. *Epilepsia 4*:315-321.

Kuller, L. (1966). Sudden and unexpected non-traumatic deaths in adults. *J. Chron. Dis. 19*:1165-1192.

Kuller, L., and Lilienfeld, A. (1966). Epidemiological study of sudden and unexpected deaths due to arteriosclerotic heart disease. *Circulation 36*:1056-1068.

Kuller, L., Lilienfeld, A., and Fisher, R. (1967). An epidemiological study of sudden and unexpected deaths in adults. *Medicine 46*:341-361.

Laidlaw, J., and Richens, A. (Eds.) (1982). *A Textbook of Epilepsy*, 2nd ed. Churchill-Livingstone, Edinburgh.

Leestma, J. E. (Ed.) (1988a). *Forensic Neuropathology*. Raven Press, New York.

Leestma, J. E. (1988b). Forensic aspects of complex neural dysfunctions. In J. E. Leestma (Ed.), *Forensic Neuropathology*. Raven Press, New York, pp. 396-415.

Leestma, J. E., and Koenig, K. L. (1968). Sudden death and phenothiazines. A current controversy. *Arch. Gen. Psychiatr. 18*:137-148.

Leestma, J. E., and Konakci, Y. (1981). Sudden unexpected death caused by neuroepithelial (colloid) cyst of the third ventricle. *J. Forensic Sci. 26*:486-491.

Leestma, J. E., Kalelkar, M. B., Teas, S. S., Jay, G. W., and Hughes, J. R. (1984). Sudden unexpected death associated with seizures: Analysis of 66 cases. *Epilepsia 25*:84-88.

Leestma, J. E., Teas, S. S., Hughes, J. R., and Kalelkar, M. B. (1985). Sudden epilepsy deaths and the forensic pathologist. *Am. J. Forensic Med. Pathol. 6*: 215-218.

Leestma, J. E., Walczak, T., Hughes, J. R., Kalelkar, M. B., and Teas, S. S. (1989). A prospective study on sudden unexpected death in epilepsy. *Ann. Neurol. 26*:195-203.

Lovegrove, J., and Thompson, P. (1978). The role of acute myocardial infarction in sudden cardiac death—A statistician's nightmare. *Am. Heart J. 96*: 711-713.

Lown, B., Verrier, R. C., and Rabinowitz, S. H. (1977). Neural and psychologic mechanisms and the problem of sudden cardiac death. *Am. J. Cardiol. 19*: 890-902.

Luke, J. L., and Helpern, M. (1968). Sudden unexpected death from natural causes in young adults. *Arch. Pathol. 85*:10-17.

Margerison, J. H., and Corsellis, J. A. N. (1966). Epilepsy and the temporal lobes. A clinical, electroencephalographic and neuropathological study of the brain in epilepsy with particular reference to the temporal lobes. *Brain 89*: 499-530.

Meldrum, B. S., and Corsellis, J. A. N. (1984). Epilepsy. In *Greenfield's Neuropathology*, 4th ed. J. Hume Adams, J. A. N. Corsellis, and L. W. Duchen (Eds.). Wiley, New York, pp. 920-950.

Melles, R. B., and Katz, B. (1988). Night terrors and sudden unexplained nocturnal death. *Med. Hypoth. 26*:149-154.

Moritz, A. R., and Zamchek, N. (1946). Sudden and unexpected deaths of young soldiers: Diseases responsible for such deaths during World War II. *Arch. Pathol. 42*:459-494.

Moss, G., Staunton, C., and Stein, A. A. (1973). The centoneurogenic etiology of the acute respiratory distress syndrome: Universal species independent phenomenon. *Am. J. Surg. 126*:137-141.

Munson, J. F. (1910). Death in epilepsy. *Med. Rec. 77*:58–62.

Myerburg, R. J., and Davis, J. H. (1964). The medical ecology of public safety. I. Sudden death due to coronary heart disease. *Am. Heart J. 68*:586–595.

Naeye, R. L. (1974). Hypoxemia and the sudden infant death syndrome. *Science 186*:837.

Neplokh, I. (1965). Causes of death in epilepsy. *Zh. Neuropatol. Psikhiatr. 65*: 1382–1387. (in Russian)

Newman, W. P., Tracy, R. E., Strong, J. P., Johnson, W. D., and Oalmann, M. C. (1982). Pathology of sudden coronary death. In *Annals of the New York Academy of Sciences*, Vol. 382, *Sudden Coronary Death*, H. M. Greenberg and E. M. Dwyer, Jr. (Eds). New York Academy of Sciences, New York, pp. 39–49.

Office of the Medical Examiner, County of Cook Chicago, Illinois (1980). *Annual Report 1977-79*. Chicago, Cook County, Illinois.

Okada, R., and Kawai, S. (1983). Histopathology of the conduction system in sudden cardiac death. *Jpn. Circ. J. 47*:573–580.

Parker, B. M. (1974). The effects of ethyl alcohol on the heart. *J. Am. Med. Assoc. 228*:741–742.

Penning, R., Muller, C., and Ciompi, L. (1969). Mortality and cause of death in epileptics. *Psychiatr. Clin. 2*:85–92. (in French)

Phillips, M., Robinowitz, M., Higgins, J. R., Boran, K. J., Reed, T., and Virmani, R. (1986). Sudden cardiac death in Air Force recruits. A 20-year review. *J. Am. Med. Assoc. 256*:2696–2699.

Powell, W. J., Whiting, R. B., Dinsmore, R. E., and Sanders, C. A. (1973). Symptomatic prognosis in patients with idiopathic hypertrophic subaortic stenosis (IHSS). *Am. J. Med. 55*:15–24.

Savel'yeva, I. A., and Posdnyakov, V. S. (1972). Pathological findings in the myocardium of epilepsy patients dying during convulsive crisis or status epilepticus. *Zh. Neuropatol. Psikhiatr. Korsakov 72*:1033–1037. (in Russian)

Schwartz, C. J., and Walsh, W. J. (1971). The pathologic basis of sudden death. *Prog. Cardiovasc. Dis. 13*:465–481.

Simpson, K. (ed.) (1953). *Modern Trends in Forensic Medicine*. Butterworths, London, pp. 54–65.

Spain, D. M. (1964). Anatomical basis of sudden cardiac death. In *Sudden Cardiac Death*, B. Surawicz and E. D. Pellegrino (Eds). Grune and Stratton, New York, pp. 6–15.

Spain, D. M., Bradess, V. A., Matero, A., and Tarter, R. (1969). Sudden death due to coronary atherosclerotic heart disease. Age, smoking habits, and recent thrombi. *J. Am. Heart Assoc. 207*:1347–1348.

Spitz, R. (1965). *The First Year of Life: A Psychoanalytic Study of Normal and Deviant Development of Object Relations*. International Universities Press, New York.

Spitz, W. U., and Fisher, R. S. (Eds.) (1973). *Medicolegal Investigation of Death. Guidelines for the Application of Pathology to Crime Investigation*. Thomas, Springfield, Ill.

Spratling, W. P. (1902). The cause and manner of death in epilepsy. *Med. News* *80*:1225–1227.

Steinsiek, H. D. (1950). Uber Todesursachen und Lebensdauer bei genuiner Epilepsie. *Arch. Psychiatr. Z. Neurol. 183*:469–480.

Terrence, C. F., Wistoskey, H. M., and Perper, J. A. (1975). Unexpected unexplained death in epileptic patients. *Neurology 25*:594–598.

Terrence, C. F., Rao, G. R., and Perper, J. A. (1981). Neurogenic pulmonary edema in unexpected unexplained death of epileptic patients. *Ann. Neurol. 9*:458–464.

Thiene, G., Pennelli, N., and Rossi, L. (1983). Cardiac conduction system abnormalities as a possible cause of sudden death in young adults. *Human Pathol. 14*:704–709.

Topaz, O., and Edwards, J. (1985). Pathologic features of sudden death in children, adolescents, and young adults. *Chest 87*:476–482.

Valdes-Dapeña, M. A. (1967). Sudden and unexpected death in infancy: A review of the world literature, 1954–1966. *Pediatrics 39*:123–138.

Weiss, S. (1940). Instantaneous "physiologic" death. *New Engl. J. Med. 223*: 793–797.

Wentworth, P., Jentz, L. A., and Croal, A. E. (1979). Analysis of sudden unexpected death in southern Ontario, with emphasis on myocarditis. *Can. Med. Assoc. J. 120*:676–680, 706.

Werne, J., and Garrow, I. (1953a). Sudden apparently unexpected death during infancy. I. Pathologic findings in infants found dead. *Am. J. Dis. Child. 29*: 633–676.

Werne, J., and Garrow, I. (1953b). Sudden apparently unexpected death during infancy. II. Pathologic findings in infants observed to die suddenly. *Am. J. Dis. Child. 29*:817–852.

Zeek, P. M. (1942). The weight of the normal human heart. *Arch. Pathol. 34*: 820–832.

Ziegler, H., and Kamecke, A. (1967). Uber unerwarteten Tod von Epileptkern. *Nervenarzt 38*:343–348.

Zielinski, J. J. (1974a). *Epidemiology and medical-social problems of epilepsy in Warsaw*. Psychoneurological Institute, Warsaw.

Zielinski, J. J. (1974b). Epilepsy and mortality rate and cause of death. *Epilepsia 15*:191–201.

Zielinski, J. J. (1982). Epidemiology. In *A Textbook of Epilepsy*, J. Laidlaw and A. Richens (Eds.). Churchill-Livingstone, Edinburgh, pp. 16–13.

6

Unexpected, Unexplained Death of Epileptic Persons: Clinical Correlation Including Pulmonary Changes

CHRISTOPHER F. TERRENCE* *Veterans Administration Medical Center, Newington, and University of Connecticut School of Medicine, Farmington, Connecticut*

I. INTRODUCTION

The sudden unexpected deaths of persons with epilepsy have been difficult for the clinical neurologist to deal with and have been almost uniformly disregarded by authors of neurological texts. This lack of appreciation by the neurologist of the possible outcome in a patient with epilepsy stems in part from the rarity of such an event but more likely from the common notion that a single seizure per se is not a potentially lethal event. Since people with epilepsy have so many seizures without lethal outcome, it is difficult for the neurologist to ascribe the unexplained death of a patient with epilepsy to a convulsion.

One of the first discourses on the causes of death in epilepsy was written by the medical superintendent of the Cambridge County Asylum in 1868. G. Mackenzie Bacon (1868) wrote:

The immediate cause of death in epilepsy is a matter which is not always easily solved, and one which is not often discussed in works of medicine, most probably from lack of information . . . the causes of death may be classed under the following categories: 1. Those arising from the long-continued effects of the disease on the body; 2. Deaths after a rapid succession of fits; 3. Sudden deaths in a fit; 4. Accidents due to fits.

Current affiliation: Veterans Administration Medical Center, East Orange, New Jersey

Bacon breaks the category of "sudden deaths in a fit" into three subsets: asphyxia from the spasms, mechanical suffocation, and last and most interesting "sudden loss of nervous power, due, probably to the state of the heart or its nerves."

The next review of epileptic deaths recorded in the literature was by Hector Geysen (1895) in his thesis entitled "De La Mort Inopinee Ou Rapide Chez Les Epileptiques." Geysen agrees with all of Bacon's proposed causes of death, and in addition stresses cardiac arrest as a cause of "mort subite pendant une crise." The importance of Geysen's work is that it was the first comprehensive clinical review of epileptic deaths.

In this century, Spratling's (1902) pioneering paper for the first time combined autopsy findings and clinical features as a methodology in studying epileptic deaths. He found that even after a complete autopsy, 4% of the deaths at the Craig Colony for Epileptics in Sonyea, New York, were the direct result of a seizure without any other pathological explanation. Based on an analysis of 220 deaths among residents of the epileptic colony, Spratling estimated the following percentages for every 100 epileptic deaths: 4% died as the direct result of a seizure; 24%, a result of status epilepticus; 12%, the result of an accident; 24%, the result of tuberculosis and other pulmonary afflictions; 26%, all other causes.

Ten years later in a clinical publication on death in epilepsy, Munson (1910) recounts the further experiences of physicians caring for epileptic patients at the Craig Colony for epileptics. Of the 2732 individuals admitted, 582 died while residents of the colony. There was a slight male excess death rate, with a mean age at the time of death of 30.8 years. Munson observed that about 12% of the resident epileptic population died either from a single seizure or without other obvious cause. Subsequent studies in both institutionalized and general epileptic populations after the advent of modern anticonvulsants reveal similar statistics for sudden death in epilepsy as a percentage of total epileptic deaths: Krohn (1963), 12%; Iivanainen and Lehtinen (1979), 10%; and Zielinski (1974), 13.8%. Munson (1910) described a typical case as follows:

F. C., No. 2258, a male was seen alive at midnight, and nothing unusual was noted. When the nurse made his next rounds at 1:30 A.M., he noted that the patient was not breathing in his usual manner, and on examination the patient was found to be dead. The physician's report states that the mouth and nose were clear, pillows wet with mucous, and urine had been voided. Face and neck were not cyanosed.

Munson made two invaluable contributions to those who were to study epileptic deaths in this century. First, he made the observations that death due to a seizure could occur from a brief seizure and that pulmonary "congestion" was a common accompaniment. And second, all cases of unexpected epileptic death should include as a minimum the following information: clinical history of patient, detailed examination of area at time of death, close external inspection of the body, and, most important, a detailed autopsy to exclude causes of death other than "conditions of purely epileptic character."

II. CASE CRITERIA

Before going on to discuss the clinical findings of death in epilepsy in the anticonvulsant era, this is an appropriate place to discuss the guidelines we have used in studying epileptic deaths (Terrence et al., 1975, 1980a,b). Although there has been some criticism of too much reliance on autopsy or medical examiners' series, because they represent deaths from a particular indigent population or are otherwise unrepresentative of the true epileptic population, this assertion is specious. As pointed out in the work of Jay and Leestma (1981),

> Examiners cases and those reported from hospitalized populations are difficult since they surely represent two different populations of persons . . . it should be pointed out that medical examiners' populations do not represent only those in lower socioeconomic groups, rather comprise all members of a society, the controlling factor being the nature of the death, its suddenness and unexpected quality in the absence of obvious serious illness in normal surroundings.

It is only through a detailed autopsy with toxicology that an investigator can exclude other cryptic causes of death. As we shall see, even some "modern" studies clearly lack enough pathological examination to make worthwhile conclusions as to the cause of death in an individual case.

In our work published in 1975 and 1980 (Terrence et al., 1980b), we used the following criteria for inclusion as case material in unexpected, unexplained death in epileptic patients:

1. A history of epilepsy was obtained from family or friends.
2. A complete autopsy was performed, with particular attention to the heart and respiratory system.
3. Cases of acute myocardial infarction, recent coronary occlusion, and heart disease of such severity that an arrhythmia might be a reasonable possibility were excluded. The mouth, pharynx, larynx, trachea, major bronchi, and lungs were examined for evidence of aspiration of food or other foreign material. If any of these findings were present, the case was excluded from the study. Patients who died of trauma were also excluded.
4. Tissue and blood samples taken at the time of autopsy failed to reveal any chemical or toxicological evidence likely to explain death.

5. Postmortem blood examination for anticonvulsants was available.
6. The patient did not die in a hospital.
7. There was reasonable certainty that status epilepticus was not part of the terminal episode, a premise based either on the report of a witness or on the description of the scene in the police report.
8. Blood specimens for drug analysis had to be drawn from the heart at the time of autopsy, and all autopsies had to be performed within 24 hours of death.
9. Past drug therapy and detailed medical history were obtained.

III.   CLINICAL CHARACTERISTICS

As pointed out by Massey and Schoenberg (1985), age-adjusted mortality rates for epilepsy have reportedly varied from such figures as 0.6 deaths/100,000/year in Denmark to 4.0 deaths/100,000/year in Portugal. The incidence of sudden epileptic death is difficult to calculate. All series must be reviewed with skepticism because of the small number of cases studied and the varying case inclusion criteria. Nevertheless, in our earlier work using figures from the Allegheny County Coroner's Office (Terrence et al., 1975), the risk for sudden death in the epileptic population was estimated to be about one death in a thousand patients at risk per year. In a later study done using the autopsy population from the Cook County Office of the Medical Examiner (Jay and Leestma, 1981), the authors reported an incidence of sudden death in epilepsy to be between 1/200 and 1/680 epileptic persons. Thus the best estimate to date is an incidence of 1/500-1000 patients at risk.

As mentioned previously, the median age of death is approximately 32 years. The reported range has been from a low median age at death of 26.0 years reported by Schwender and Troncoso (1986), to about 40 years reported by Rodin (1968). The history of epilepsy is usually longstanding. Hirsch and Martin (1971) reported a duration of epilepsy prior to death as 6 years. Krohn (1963) reported a figure of 16.7 years, which is similar to our earlier study (Terrence et al., 1975). Although not commented on in most reviews, there seems to be an excess representation of blacks as well as a slight preponderance of males. In our review from the Allegheny County Coroner's Office, blacks comprised almost 25% of the deaths in our series but made up only about 9% of the overall population of Allegheny County (Table 1). More recent studies (Leestma et al., 1985; Schwender and Troncoso, 1986) have reported a similar overrepresentation of blacks. At the present time the overrepresentation by blacks remains an enigma, but this excess black mortality in sudden epileptic death has also been reported in epileptic death rates in general. Kurland et al. (1973) reported a nonwhite excess of 240% for epileptic age-specific death rates in general for the United States.

Table 1 Unexpected, Unexplained Death in Epileptic Patients: Age, Race, and Sex

Race and sex	0–10	11–20	21–30	31–40	41–50	51–60	60+	Total
White male	1	1	3	4	5	1	1	16 (43%)
White female		4	3	1	2	1		12 (32%)
Black male		1		2	3			6 (16%)
Black female		3						3 (8%)
Total	2	9	6	7	10	2	1	37
Percentage of total cases	5%	24%	16%	19%	27%	5%	3%	100%
Percentage distribution of Allegheny County population	18%	18%	11%	12%	13%	12%	15%	100%

Source: Terrence et al., 1975, reproduced with permission of publisher.

Another striking feature of these patients is that they are ambulatory, noninstitutionalized individuals who are usually gainfully employed. In the Hirsch and Martin (1971) series, 13 cases had normal neurologic exams, and 6 had "mild to moderate retardation, but none was sufficiently impaired to require institutionalization." Consonant with their normal lifestyle, the frequency of premorbid seizure activity was in no way alarming. Hirsch and Martin (1971) did not quantify the seizure frequency in their cases but stated they were "infrequent or rare." Seizure frequency was reported in our later, larger series (Terrence et al., 1975) to be less than one seizure per month in all but 2 patients of the 37 reported. Youth and infrequency of seizures was also noted with uneasiness by Loiseau and Henry (1972). On the face of it, young patients with infrequent seizures should most logically be better risks, but this does not appear to be the case. The electroencephalographic abnormalities reported in most series show a preponderance of generalized rather than focal abnormalities (Hirsch and Martin, 1971; Terrence et al., 1975). Surprisingly, in no series is complex partial epilepsy the predominant electroencephalographic or clinical seizure type reported. The typical seizure pattern is tonic-clonic.

In the past, the circumstances of death were commonly and erroneously used to ascribe a cause of death in patients known to have epilepsy. Prior to the turn of the century, if an epileptic was found dead in bed, it was assumed the patient suffocated in bedclothes (Spratling, 1902). Spratling stressed the importance of pillows and bedclothes as one of the major causes of asphyxia leading to death during a seizure. Hirsch and Martin (1971) and numerous later studies (Lewis, 1978; Loiseau and Henry, 1972; Schwender and Troncoso, 1986; Terrence et al., 1975) demonstrated that there is no pathologic proof of asphyxia in almost all these cases. Although not proven in any particular study, there does seem to be an overrepresentation of deaths occurring during sleep, or just after arising from sleep. Some authors (Schwender and Troncoso, 1986) reported data indicating 79.3% of their cases died in bed or the bedroom, a figure almost double the incidence reported by our group (Terrence et al., 1975) and by Hirsch and Martin (1971). Borel (1966) was one of the first authors commenting on death in epilepsy to stress the inordinately high frequency with which unexpected unexplained death in epileptic persons is associated with sleep. At present this information is only anecdotal and warrants more investigation. Such overrepresentation may be related to the potential of sleep as an activation process of epileptiform activity (Pompeiano, 1968).

A second pitfall in deducing the cause of death in epilepsy occurs when the decedent is found in the tub or shower. It is important to perform an autopsy in all such cases, for most of the time drowning will not be the cause of death, as we have found on a number of occasions.

Although the most frequent circumstance of death is "found dead," probably the next most common circumstance is "death after a witnessed seizure." A bizzare such case would be the death of an epileptic "while the patient was talking on the phone" (Schwender and Troncoso, 1986). A more typical case would be the following, from our 1980 series (Terrence et al., 1980b, patient 7). A 19-year-old white man had had a grand mal seizure disorder since 5 years of age. Anticonvulsant medications prescribed before death included phenytoin, 100 mg, and phenobarbital, 30 mg, each three times daily. He had infrequent grand mal seizures and was known to go for days at a time without taking his anticonvulsant medications. On the night preceding death the patient drank two small glasses of beer and returned home at about 2:00 A.M. At 10:00 A.M. he was roused by a friend for work. After talking to him for a few minutes, the friend saw him get up and go to the bathroom to wash up for work. Fifteen minutes later the patient was found by his friend on the bathroom floor, deeply cyanotic and in the midst of a grand mal seizure. A paramedic team arrived within minutes and found the patient to be in cardiopulmonary arrest. Cardiopulmonary resuscitation was attempted but the patient was pronounced dead on arrival at the hospital. The general autopsy, including brain examination, was both grossly and microscopically unremarkable except for pulmonary edema. Plasma phenytoin and phenobarbital levels were both subtherapuetic at 5.8 and 3.2 μg/ml respectively, and blood alcohol was negative.

Such a case is quite routine in studies of death in epilepsy, but it is important that the autopsy be performed prior to final case disposition. A case in point is one which we studied in the late seventies. A 13-year-old girl with a long history of seizures well controlled on phenytoin and phenobarbital fell to the floor and stiffened up with a few "twitching" movements noted by her parents. She was taken to a hospital unconscious and was pronounced dead. It was felt by the treating physicians that she died as a result of a convulsion, but autopsy revealed not only the cause of her death but also the etiology of her convulsive disorder. She had a large subependymal glioma, which had caused marked hydrocephalus and central herniation. The rest of the autopsy revealed other pathological stigmata of tuberous sclerosis, including typical cardiac lesions. Without an autopsy this case would have been inappropriately labeled death due to a convulsion.

Another pitfall is to ascribe death without toxicological and anticonvulsant blood determinations. In the studies of Zielinski (1974), Krohn (1963), and others (Iivanainen and Lehtinen, 1979; Lund and Gormsen, 1985; Mackay, 1979), suicide or self-poisoning is always a small but significant percentage of all epileptic deaths. Only with the aid of postmortem blood levels can the investigator be sure that an inadvertent or willful overdosage was not the cause of death (Bruce and Smith, 1977).

IV. ANTICONVULSANTS

As described above we have a wealth of clinical information concerning the death of the epileptic patient, but we are still without an explanation. Hirsch and Martin (1971) put it succinctly: "We do not know why a seizure, apparently no different from those which the patient has survived in the past, should prove fatal at a particular time." Although not commented on by Hirsch and Martin (1971), drug levels for anticonvulsants drawn at the time of autopsy in their series were either negative or subtherapeutic in over 90% of cases studied. All 19 patients had been prescribed anticonvulsants; in 9 patients two or more anticonvulsants had been prescribed prior to death, but almost none had therapeutic levels at the time of death. It was not until four years later in a larger autopsy study of 37 cases that our group found and commented on a similar pattern of absent or subtherapeutic anticonvulsant levels (Terrence et al., 1975). Although 17 of the patients in our study had phenytoin prescribed, none had therapeutic levels of the drug. Similarly, only 3 of 24 patients prescribed phenobarbital had therapeutic levels of the drug. If one compares the frequency of subtherapeutic or absent anticonvulsant levels in our work and that of Hirsch and Martin with that reported by other authors studying an ambulant epileptic population, the difference is striking. In a group of 111 patients given phenytoin for epilepsy, Lascelles et al. (1970) found that about 45% had therapeutic blood levels. A comparison of our patients with those reported by Lund et al. (1964) and Lascelles et al. (1970) dramatically demonstrates that therapeutic blood levels of at least one anticonvulsant were much less frequent in our series than in their ambulatory epileptic populations.

Studies subsequent to our 1975 report have found similar low frequency of therapeutic anticonvulsants in this group of epileptic deaths (Bowerman et al., 1977; Copeland, 1984; Leestma et al., 1985; Lund and Gormsen, 1985). Leestma (1985) reported that "one feature of SUD-epilepsy cases is that either medications have not been prescribed, no history of prescription is known, or the victim neglected to take prescribed medications for his/her condition." In Hirsch and Martin's (1971) and our (Terrence et al., 1975) series, almost all the cases had information not only on anticonvulsants prescribed but on the prescribed dosages. Such information would not support the assertion that suboptimal dosages were consistently prescribed to account for the findings of subtherapeutic or absent blood levels of anticonvulsants in this group of patients. On the contrary, the most logical explanation of these subtherapeutic or absent levels is either recent discontinuation or noncompliance with the prescribed drug regimen (Bowerman et al., 1977; Terrence, 1983).

Does this information agree with the clinical information we have? I think the answer is yes. This is a group of young, ambulatory patients with seemingly well-controlled seizures who are prime candidates for either noncompliance or impulsive discontinuation because of undesired side effects.

As pointed out in our work (Terrence, 1983) and stressed by Lund and Gormsen (1985), some sudden deaths in epilepsy clearly occur with therapeutic levels of anticonvulsants; however, the high frequency of subtherapeutic and absent levels of anticonvulsants clearly imply this as a risk factor for such deaths.

V. NEUROGENIC PULMONARY EDEMA

A frequent but not universal finding in these cases is pulmonary edema. As a complication of tonic-clonic seizures, pulmonary edema was first reported by Shanahan (1908). He reported on 11 patients who developed pulmonary edema following a single convulsion or multiple convulsions. Four patients died, and both autopsied cases demonstrated pulmonary edema. Two years later, Ohlmacher (1910) published a paper entitled "Acute Pulmonary Edema as a Terminal Event in Certain Forms of Epilepsy." Forty-one deaths followed a single seizure or were nocturnal deaths. Only three deaths from a single seizure and associated pulmonary edema were described by Ohlmacher in detail, but in none was the pulmonary edema deemed to be the direct cause of death. That same year Munson (1910) stressed the importance of pulmonary edema in such cases. "The importance of this factor is . . . that it is a frequent and dangerous condition, following all forms of the epileptic attack, even single grand mal seizures."

Our group reported on eight cases of unexpected unexplained death in young ambulatory epileptics (Terrence et al., 1980b). These cases were studied with special attention to the heart and lungs at the time of postmortem examination. Lung weights uniformly exceeded the expected values (Furbank, 1967), with gross evidence of hemorrhagic pulmonary edema. Microsocpic examination revealed moderate to severe pulmonary edema with protein-rich fluid as well as alveolar hemorrhage. Although this is sometimes misconstrued, it is important to stress that "after autopsy . . . there was no anatomical or chemical evidence sufficient to explain the deaths" (Terrence et al., 1980b). The finding of pulmonary edema is common in this group of deaths (Leestma et al., 1985), but it is neither a universal finding nor the cause of death.

Interestingly, several recent reports implicate neurogenic pulmonary edema as a risk factor in discontinuation or noncompliance of anticonvulsants (Bloom, 1968; Bonbrest, 1965; Chang and Smith, 1967; Green et al., 1975; Sarkar and Munshi, 1977). Archibald and Armstrong (1978) reported a 32-year-old-patient who had a history of noncompliance in taking phenytoin and had three episodes of postictal pulmonary edema. In fact the demographics and clinical histories of postictal pulmonary edema patients and sudden epileptic deaths are all too similar: they are young with infrequent tonic-clonic seizures.

The frequent finding of pulmonary edema in these deaths does suggest an adrenergic component to these deaths (Theodore and Robin, 1976; Urabe et al., 1961). The exact interplay of the autonomic nervous system in these deaths is discussed by other authors of this volume. Suffice it to say that any explanation of the exact mechanism of death in these individuals must solve the tantalizing question posed by Hirsch and Martin in 1971. Youth, noncompliance, and autonomic disturbances all seem to be risk factors. The interrelation of these factors remains a mystery. I feel we have advanced from the pessimism of Krohn (1963) as to the cause of sudden death in epilepsy. "It happens now and again that an epileptic is found dead and no one knows what has happened . . . . Autopsy has been performed in seven of our thirteen cases, but has made us none the wiser." Clinical and autopsy studies have improved our knowledge of risk factors in these patients. Clearly, patients should be admonished from the self-withdrawal of anticonvulsants. Such an act seems to be a risk factor for a lethal convulsive episode, quite different from the seizures the patient survived in the past.

ACKNOWLEDGMENTS

I wish to thank Drs. Gutti Rao and Joshua Perper for their support in the study of sudden epileptic deaths. I would also like to pay fond tribute to the memory of Dr. Howard Wisotzkey, who challenged me to study sudden death in epilepsy while I was a neurology resident.

REFERENCES

Archibald, R. B., and Armstrong, J. D. (1978). Recurrent postictal pulmonary edema. *Postgrad. Med. 63*:210–213.
Bacon, G. M. (1868). On the modes of death in epilepsy. *Lancet 1*:555–556.
Bloom, S. (1968). Pulmonary edema following a grand mal seizure. *Am. Rev. Respir. Dis. 97*:292–294.
Bonbrest, H. C. (1965). Pulmonary edema following an epileptic seizure. *Am. Rev. Respir. Dis. 91*:97–100.
Borel, J. (1966). La mort subite dans l'èpilepsie. *Ann. Medico-Psychol. 124*: 729–730.
Bowerman, D. L., Levisky, J. A., Urich, R. W., and Wittenberg, P. H. (1977). Premature deaths in persons with seizure disorders—Subtherapeutic levels of anticonvulsant drugs in postmortem blood specimens. *J. Forensic Sci. 12*: 522–526.
Bruce, A. M., and Smith, H. (1977). The investigation of phenobartitone, phenytoin and primidone in the death of epileptics. *Med. Sci. Law 17*:195–199.
Chang, C. H., and Smith, C. A. (1967). Postictal pulmonary edema. *Radiology 89*:1087–1089.
Copeland, A. R. (1984). Seizure disorders. The Dade County experience from 1978 to 1982. *Am. J. Forensic Med. Pathol. 5*:211–215.

Furbank, R. A. (1967). Appendix of conversion data, normal values, nomograms and other standards. In *Modern Trends in Forensic Medicine*, Vol. 2. K. Simpson (Ed.). London, Butterworth, pp. 348–353.

Geysen, H. (1895). De la mort inopinée ou rapide chez les épileptiques. *Thesis.* Faculté de Médecine et de Pharmacie de Lyon.

Green, R., Platt, R., and Matz, R. (1975). Postictal pulmonary edema. *N.Y. State J. Med. 75*:1257–1261.

Hirsch, C. S., and Martin, D. L. (1971). Unexpected death in young epileptics. *Neurology* (Minneap) *21*:682–690.

Iivanainen, M., and Lehtinen, J. (1979). Causes of death in institutionalized epileptics. *Epilepsia 20*:485–492.

Jay, G. W., and Leestma, J. E. (1981). Sudden death in epilepsy. A comprehensive review of the literature and proposed mechanisms. *Acta Neurol. Scand. (Suppl. 82)63*:5–66.

Krohn, W. (1963). Causes of death among epileptics. *Epilepsia 4*:315–321.

Kurland, L. T., Kurtzke, J. F., and Goldberg, I. D. (1973). *Epidemiology of Neurologic and Sense Organ Disorders.* Harvard University Press, Cambridge, Mass, p. 29.

Lascelles, P., Kocen, R., and Reynolds, E. (1970). The distribution of plasma phenytoin levels in epileptic patients. *J. Neurol. Neurosurg. Psychiatr. 33*: 501–505.

Leestma, J. E., Teas, S. S., Hughes, J. R., and Kalelkar, M. B. (1985). Sudden epilepsy deaths and the forensic pathologist. *Am. J. Forensic Med. Pathol. 6*:215–218.

Lewis, J. A. (1978). Death and epilepsy. *Proc. Ann. Meet. Med. Sect. Am. Counc. Life Insur. 3*:121–131.

Loiseau, P., and Henry, P. (1972). Les causes de la mort chez les épileptiques. *Bordeaux Méd. 5*:2643–2648.

Lund, A., and Gormsen, H. (1985). The role of antiepileptics in sudden death in epilepsy. *Acta Neurol. Scand. 72*:444–446.

Lund, M., Jorgensen, R., and Kuhl, V. (1964). Serum diphenylhydantoin in ambulant patients with epilepsy. *Epilepsia 5*:51–58.

Mackay, A. (1979). Self-poisoning—A complication of epilepsy. *Br. J. Psychiatr. 134*:277–282.

Massey, E. W., and Schoenberg, B. S. (1985). Mortality from epilepsy. International patterns and changes over time. *Neurolepidemiology 4*:65–70.

Munson, J. F. (1910). Death in epilepsy. *Med. Rec. 77*:58–62.

Ohlmacher, A. P. (1910). Acute pulmonary edema as a terminal event in certain forms of epilepsy. *Am. J. Med. Sci. 139*:417–422.

Pompeiano, O. (1968). Sleep mechanisms. In *Basic Mechanisms of the Epilepsies*, H. H. Jasper, A. A. Ward, and A. Pope (Eds.). Little, Brown, Boston, pp. 453–473.

Rodin, E. A. (1968). *The Prognosis of Patients with Epilepsy.* Thomas, Springfield, Ill., p. 167.

Sarkar, T. K., and Munshi, A. T. (1977). Postictal pulmonary edema. *Postgrad. Med. 61*:281–286.

Schwender, L. A., and Troncoso, J. C. (1986). Evaluation of sudden death in epilepsy. *Am. J. Forensic Med. Pathol.* 7:283–287.

Shanahan, W. T. (1908). Acute pulmonary edema as a complication of epileptic seizures. *N.Y. Med. J.* 54:54–56.

Spratling, W. P. (1902). The causes and manner of death in epilepsy. *Med. News* 80:1225–1227.

Terrence, C. F. (1983). Unexpected, unexplained death of epileptic persons: Clinical correlation. *Epilepsia* 24:515–516.

Terrence, C. F., Rao, G., and Perper, J. (1980a). Neurogenic pulmonary edema in unexpected, unexplained death in epileptic patients. *Ann. Neurol.* 8:96.

Terrence, C. F., Rao, G. R., and Perper, J. A. (1980b). Neurogenic pulmonary edema in unexpected, unexplained death of epileptic patients. *Ann. Neurol.* 9:458–464.

Terrence, C. F., Wisotzkey, H. M., and Perper, J. A. (1975). Unexpected, unexplained death in epileptic patients. *Neurology* (Minneap) 25:594–598.

Theodore, J., and Robin, E. D. (1976). Speculations on neurogenic pulmonary edema (NPE). *Am. Rev. Respir. Dis.* 113:405–411.

Urabe, M., Segawa, Y. U., Tsubokawa, T., Yamamoto, K., Araki, K., and Izumi, K. (1961). Pathogenesis of the acute pulmonary edema occurring after brain operation and brain trauma. *Jpn. Heart J.* 2:147–169.

Zielinski, J. J. (1974). Epilepsy and mortality rate and cause of death. *Epilepsia* 15:191–201.

7

The Role of EEG Monitoring in the Diagnosis of Epilepsy-Related Cardiac Arrhythmias and of Cardiac Arrhythmias Mimicking Epilepsy

STEPHEN J. HOWELL and LANCE D. BLUMHARDT *University of Liverpool and Walton Hospital, Liverpool, England*

I. INTRODUCTION

That events within the central nervous system can affect heart rate and rhythm has been well established from studies of lesioned animals, from stimulation experiments in both animals and man, and from observations on patients with a variety of cerebral lesions including stroke, subarachnoid hemorrhage, and head injury. These topics have been well reviewed in recent articles (Lathers and Schraeder, 1982, 1987; Schraeder and Lathers, 1989; Talman, 1985).

The striking autonomic effects of epileptic seizures have long been known (Jackson, 1887; Temkin, 1971) but are perhaps less well recognized by clinicians than the alternative possibility that seizures may be precipitated by cardiac arrhythmias. However, during the last few years an increasing number of case reports of seizure-associated arrhythmias have been published. The recent introduction of simultaneous ambulatory monitoring of the ECG and electroencephalogram (SAMMEE) has improved our ability to record undiagnosed symptomatic attacks to determine whether a cerebral or cardiac dysrhythmia is the primary precipitating event.

SAMMEE is of importance for two main reasons. First, a seizure precipitated cardiac arrhythmia may lead to misdiagnosis if ambulatory ECG (AECG) or Holter monitoring alone is carried out in a patient with undiagnosed episodes of loss of consciousness. A cardiac arrhythmia during an unrecognized seizure may then be erroneously interpreted as the primary reason for symptoms. Examples of inappropriate pacemaker insertion (Gilchrist, 1985) and antiarrhythmic drug treatment (Pritchett et al., 1980) in this situation have been reported. Second, it has been suggested that cardiac arrhythmias may be the cause of some unexplained sudden deaths in young epileptics (Jay and Leestma, 1981; Leestma et al., 1984).

In this chapter we will review some of the evidence for seizure-induced cardiac arrhythmias and for seizures precipitated by cardiac arrhythmias, from case reports and experimental studies carried out prior to the availability of ambulatory EEG, and describe how recent developments which have facilitated the capture of symptomatic events on cassette tape may shed more light on this rather obscure area of clinical practice.

II. SEIZURE-ASSOCIATED CHANGES IN CARDIAC RATE AND RHYTHM

A. Induced Seizures in Man

Some of the best evidence that epilepsy is a potent cause of cardiac rate and rhythm changes comes from laboratory studies of induced seizures in which both EEG and ECG have been monitored.

1. Chemically Induced Seizures

In some laboratory studies seizures have been induced in paralyzed patients with intravenous pentylenetetrazol (Mosier et al., 1957; Van Buren, 1958; Van Buren and Ajmone-Marsan, 1960; White et al., 1961). In these studies the patients were usually paralyzed and ventilated and atropine was frequently used. Some patients in these studies developed generalized seizure activity from the start, whereas others had focal seizures which became secondarily generalized. Most authors tend to agree that EEG seizure activity must be bilateral before autonomic changes result.

In these studies the most frequently observed cardiac effect of a seizure appeared to be a tachycardia (95%); bradycardias were much less common (Van Buren, 1958). The cardiac rate changes were noted to be of abrupt onset and offset (Van Buren and Ajmone-Marsan, 1960). If a generalized seizure is induced, rapid heart rate increases of 50–150% may be observed in the tonic phase, but the pulse slows rapidly when seizure activity ceases (Mosier et al., 1957; White et al., 1961).

Ictal cardiac arrhythmias are less commonly described than sinus tachycardias. Mosier and colleagues (1957) observed arrhythmias in 9 of their 41 patients (22%). These were usually in the clonic phase and included supraventricular and ventricular ectopic beats and short runs of bigeminy and ventricular tachycardia (VT). Other studies have reported a higher incidence of cardiac irregularities (53%), including premature atrial or ventricular beats, conduction blocks, VT, and prolonged bradycardia with coupling, the arrhythmia usually occurring as the seizures subsided (White et al., 1961). Unfortunately, neither the arrhythmias nor their relationship to the EEG seizure activity is illustrated or described in detail in these reports.

2. Electrically-Induced Seizures

Many studies have been published on the cardiac effects of seizures induced by electric shock therapy (ECT) (see Perrin, 1961, for review). When ECT is unmodified by the use of antiarrhythmic drugs, there is an initial brief slowing in heart rate (which may be blocked by atropine) followed by a rapid rise to 130–190 bpm. Midway through the clonic phase the pulse rate begins to fall; by the end of the seizure it may reach levels below the preshock rate. It is at this time that arrhythmias may occur. A second less marked phase of tachycardia may follow. For example, Brown and coworkers (1953) found the heart rate had dropped to a mean of 51 bpm below the base rate within 3 seconds of the shock, rising to 61 bpm above base 30 seconds later. The rate then rapidly declined to preshock levels but fluctuated for the remaining five minutes of the recording period. This triphasic response is less commonly seen in the authors' own ambulatory recordings of spontaneous seizures (see below).

As in chemically induced seizures, a high prevalence of tachycardias and low frequency of bradycardias are reported. Green and Woods (1955) described a sinus bradycardia of two or three seconds preceding the ictal tachycardia and, in a few patients, a more marked sinus bradycardia was seen after the convulsion. Arrhythmias were seen in 79 (40%) of 200 recordings. All were due to premature beats, except in one patient who developed a nodal rhythm. Ventricular premature beats were often multifocal and bigeminy developed in 19 cases. A slight prolongation of the PR interval was observed in one record in one patient, but no other conduction disturbances were seen. Patients were pretreated with atropine, given intravenous thiopentone and suxamethonium, and ventilated with a face mask and bag. While the initial bradycardia in ECT-induced seizures can be blocked by atropine, the frequency of late arrhythmias is reduced by adequate oxygenation, suggesting that they may be largely secondary to hypoxia (McKenna et al., 1970).

The cardiovascular effects of seizures induced by direct stimulation of the brain have also been reported. Electrical afterdischarges are frequently mentioned (Delgado et al., 1960), but it is usually not clear whether the described autonomic effects were due to induced seizures, since stimulation of various areas of the brain may affect heart rate without seizure induction.

Other authors have described cardiac activity during spontaneous or induced seizures but the results are not separately described or discussed by seizure type (Erikson, 1939; Van Buren, 1958). However, in Erikson's study the majority of the seizures recorded appear to be Jacksonian in type. Acceleration of the heart rate was usual, occurring in each patient in at least one attack, whereas slowing of the heart rate occurred in only two attacks.

The studies of seizures during paralysis have demonstrated that ictal effects on heart rate and rhythm are common and not due to motor activity, but it is difficult to know what relevance these findings have to spontaneous seizures in epileptic patients. Bradycardias could be masked by pretreatment with atropine, and many of the patients did not have spontaneous generalized seizures (i.e., the induced seizure type was not their usual seizure). Furthermore, the apparatus, venepuncture, and the convulsant drug, pentylenetetrazol, produced an increase in the level of sympathetic activity prior to the seizures, as Van Buren (1958) acknowledged. It is therefore necessary to turn to reports of the autonomic effects of spontaneously occurring epileptic seizures.

B. Spontaneous Seizures

1. Circumstantial Evidence of Seizure-Associated Arrhythmias from Case Reports Without Monitored Ictal EEG

Bradycardia/Sinus Arrest.   One of the earliest observations of the cardiac effects of epilepsy was that of Russell (1906), who noted cessation of the pulse during an epileptic seizure. However, Erikson (1939) subsequently found no changes in the ECG during fits, despite fading or loss of the pulse. He concluded that earlier reports of transient ictal cardiac arrest were due to difficulty palpating the pulse.

In 1954 Phizackerley and colleagues reported a 71-year-old woman with attacks of epigastric discomfort and a feeling of great apprehension, sometimes going on to loss of consciousness. Witnesses reported that she became pale and limp with no convulsion or incontinence. The period of unconsciousness lasted for less than 30 seconds and was followed by headache. Attacks were not abolished by phenobarbital. An interictal routine laboratory EEG (REEG) showed right anterior temporal spikes. In some attacks the pulse was normal at onset, but in others the pulse ceased abruptly and loss of consciousness occurred when asystole continued for more than five seconds. When the pulse could not be felt the ECG showed complete sinoauricular block. She was treated with tincture of belladonna and had no further episodes of loss of consciousness, although the attacks of epigastric discomfort and apprehension continued. If, as the authors suggest, we assume that the arrhythmia in this case was secondary to a complex partial seizure (CPS), the response to treatment suggests that loss of consciousness was due to the asystole and not the epileptic seizure per se.

In a similar case report, a 35-year-old man with undiagnosed blackouts was observed in a coronary care unit where an attack was noted to begin with déjà vu (Smaje et al., 1987). A progressive slowing of heart rate culminated in asystole for 20 seconds with loss of consciousness and twitching. Atropine was administered intravenously and the patient recovered. Five similar attacks followed over the next hour and a pacemaker was inserted. An REEG showed an excess of irregular slow waves over the left temporal region. The pacemaker was removed and phenytoin introduced, but further seizures occurred. Computed tomography and magnetic resonance imaging showed a suprasellar epidermoid. Although no simultaneous EEG was available, the sensation of déjà vu prior to loss of consciousness suggested that the asystole was secondary to a seizure and not to distortion of the hypothalamus by the tumor.

Erikson (1939) recorded the ECG during 54 seizures in 17 patients. Eighteen of these seizures were induced by stimulation of the cerebral cortex during neurosurgical procedures, 11 occurred during therapy with a hydration regimen, 2 were induced by hyperventilation, and 23 were spontaneous. Four of the 54 seizures were described as grand mal, eight petit mal, one psychomotor, and the remainder Jacksonian. Acceleration of the heart rate was usual and bradycardias occurred in only two seizures. The magnitude of these changes was not reported.

Supraventricular Arrhythmias. Here again the evidence is largely circumstantial. For example, Mathew and coworkers (1970) described a 36-year-old man who was found to be in atrial fibrillation after his first seizure. A further fit one month later was not associated with an arrhythmia. An REEG showed slow activity in the left frontal and anterior temporal regions and a parasagittal meningioma was removed. The cardiac rhythm prior to the seizure is not known, so in this case the evidence that the seizure caused the arrhythmia is suggestive but scarcely compelling.

Other authors have assumed that effective treatment with anticonvulsants (ACD) implies an epileptic etiology. Pritchett and colleagues (1980) described two cases with arrhythmias they considered were secondary to partial seizures. The first, a 21-year-old man, developed attacks of palpitation, dizziness, and dyspnea, some with loss of consciousness. AECG monitoring recorded two asymptomatic episodes of supraventricular tachycardia (SVT). Treatment with a variety of antiarrhythmics was ineffective. Cardiac electrophysiology was normal. REEG showed right temporal sharps and spikes. Introduction of carbamazepine was associated with cessation of the attacks. The second case was a 15-year-old with episodes of loss of consciousness associated either with SVT or with SVT and bradycardia. Several antiarrhythmics and phenobarbital were ineffective. A variety of asymptomatic arrhythmias were recorded on AECG, including sinus pauses, junctional rhythm, multifocal ventricular tachycardia, and atrioventricular (AV) block. Cardiac electrophysiology was normal. REEG showed left temporal slow activity and bilateral spike and wave bursts. A ventricular pacemaker was fitted and phenytoin prescribed. There were no further episodes of loss of consciousness, but episodes of SVT continued despite the use of antiarrhythmics. Two years later he was found dead in a swimming pool with a functioning pacemaker. The authors point out that paroxysmal SVT is rarely a cause of loss of consciousness and that 90% of patients with spontaneous SVT have abnormal cardiac electrophysiology.

Other reports have suggested links between temporally unrelated paroxysmal supraventricular arrhythmias and REEG abnormalities on the basis of arrhythmia resolution with ACD (Pogliali, 1971). Apart from the lack of evidence from simultaneous recordings in such reports, there is at least a theoretical objection to this conclusion, as these drugs also have an antiarrhythmic action (Rosen et al., 1967; Steiner et al., 1970).

Ventricular Arrhythmias. Again, although the circumstantial evidence in these reports may be highly suggestive, the exact sequence of events remains necessarily equivocal in view of the lack of EEG data. For example, Dasheiff and Dickinson (1986) reported the case of a 48-year-old man who had a long history of epilepsy and a previous myocardial infarction. REEG showed left temporal theta activity and spikes. He was admitted for consideration of epilepsy surgery. Depth electrodes were inserted and slow ACD withdrawal undertaken. After one CPS with secondary generalization he complained of pain in his chest and left arm. ECG showed areas of ST elevation and T wave inversion. After a further partial seizure he suffered a cardiorespiratory arrest. Resuscitation was immediately commenced. Ventricular fibrillation proceeded into asystole and resuscitation was unsuccessful. No anatomical cause of death was found at autopsy.

2. Seizure-Associated Arrhythmias Confirmed by Monitored Ictal EEG

A few case reports include data obtained with routine ECG and EEG techniques.

Bradycardia/Sinus Arrest. Katz and coworkers (1983) recorded the EEG and ECG during CPS in two patients. Seizure activity arising in the temporal regions became generalized with periods of sinoatrial arrest of 8–10 seconds starting shortly after seizure onset. Cardiological studies were normal, although details were not given in the report.

Coulter (1984) reported an infant with cyanotic attacks from the age of 3 months. Seizures were recorded with EEG telemetry and ECG. Paroxysmal low-amplitude 10- to 12-Hz activity was followed by high-amplitude slow waves in the left temporal region. Respiratory arrest occurred at this stage and was followed by generalized slow activity and a bradycardia. Attacks were controlled with phenobarbital and carbamazepine.

In another report, Kiok and colleagues (1986) described a 23-year-old man with a history of epilepsy who had two episodes of bradycardia (one followed by a transient tachycardia) associated with CPS. There were also periods of sinus arrest lasting up to nine seconds. EEG during seizures showed increases in amplitude and decreased frequency of rhythmic 7- to 9-Hz waves over the right midtemporal region.

In some cases the confusion is considerable and diagnosis may be delayed. For example, Gilchrist (1985) reported a young man with a history of generalized tonic-clonic seizures refractory to phenytoin. Pseudoseizures were suspected and ACDs were withdrawn. The attacks continued and AECG monitoring captured an unwitnessed attack with loss of consciousness. There was an abrupt change from sinus rhythm to a junctional escape rhythm of 20 bpm followed sequentially by 4.8 seconds of asystole, an SVT of 160 bpm, and, finally, reversion to sinus rhythm. A diagnosis of sick sinus syndrome was made and a demand ventricular pacemaker fitted. However, subsequent simultaneous EEG and ECG monitoring showed seizure activity in the left temporal region associated with SVT during an attack. Eventually, treatment with carbamazepine (and not the pacemaker) abolished the attacks.

Supraventricular Arrhythmias. Walsh and colleagues (1968) presented two cases of seizure-associated SVT. The first was a 14-year-old boy with a 2-year history of paroxysmal tachycardia. An ECG showed this to be an atrial tachycardia occasionally with a Wenkebach phenomenon. An REEG showed runs of 3.5- to 4.5-Hz slow waves in the posterior temporo-occipital region. A period of tachycardia occurred during a paroxysmal cerebral discharge, but it is not stated if the tachycardia also occurred at other times without accompanying cerebral discharges. The second case, reported in more detail in another report, was a 4-year-old boy with episodes of SVT often preceded by a feeling of fear (Walsh et al., 1972). Antiarrhythmic therapy was unsuccessful but attacks ceased on phenytoin. Phenytoin was subsequently withdrawn when a rash developed. An REEG showed bilateral spike and wave and sharp–slow wave complexes occurring in short bursts of less than two seconds duration, which were associated with changes in the RR interval on the ECG. A 2-second burst accompanied by swallowing preceded an irregular bradycardia of 6 seconds duration which was in turn followed by a paroxysmal atrial tachycardia of 200–240 bpm lasting 1.5 hours.

Seizure-associated SVTs also occurred in the case reported by Gilchrist (1985).

3. Series Reporting ECG During Epileptic Seizures

Petit Mal Epilepsy. Until recently, most available data on spontaneous seizure activity and the autonomic nervous system concerned 3/second spike and wave absences. The cardiac effects of this type of seizure appears to be relatively minor from most reports. For example, Mirsky and Van Buren (1965) recorded 1000 bursts of generalized spike and wave or polyspike and wave in 11 patients. Only four patients showed slight slowing of the heart rate. Similarly, Bogacz and Yanicelli (1962) recorded the ECG during 132 mostly 3/second discharges in 23 patients and found only minor changes in the RR interval, although these were associated with 64% of the bursts. The study of Johnson and Davidoff (1964) also included eight patients with typical petit mal EEG discharges. In seven of eight bursts with clinical accompaniments there were associated changes in heart rate, although the magnitude of the changes was not stated.

Fischgold and Arfel-Capdevielle's study (1955) showed the variable autonomic effects that different seizures can have in the same individual. During nine attacks of petit mal recorded in one patient, bradycardia occurred in four, tachycardia in one, tachycardia followed by bradycardia in another, with no changes in the remaining three.

Temporal Lobe Seizures. Van Buren (1958) included seven spontaneous temporal lobe seizures in his report of the autonomic features of temporal lobe epilepsy (TLE). The features of these 7 attacks were not separated from those of the induced seizures, but 19 of the 20 seizures recorded showed bursts of tachycardia, whereas bradycardia occurred in only 1. Marshall and colleagues (1983) reported ictal changes in heart rate in 12 consecutive patients with CPS. All were associated with a tachycardia of between 120 and 180 bpm.

Mixed Seizures or Seizures of Uncertain Type. Delgado and colleagues (1960) recorded asymptomatic spontaneous bursts of spike and wave (3/second) from scalp and temporal lobe depth electrodes in two epileptic patients and found no changes in the ECG. Johnson and Davidoff (1964) recorded spontaneous seizures in 48 patients with a history of epilepsy or episodic loss of consciousness and no focal neurological or REEG abnormalities. Of 10 patients with clinical seizure manifestations during atypical spike and slow-wave bursts, 8 showed changes in heart rate (3 patients had seizure-associated bradycardias but most had tachycardias). Only 1 of 21 patients who had bursts without obvious clinical effect had an associated change in heart rate. Forty-eight slow wave discharges in eight patients were not accompanied by any changes. White and coworkers (1961) described the cardiac effects of three spontaneous seizures. Two were very brief and associated with little cardiovascular change, but one lasted 65 seconds and was associated with an increase in heart rate from 85 to 196 bpm.

III. CARDIAC ARRHYTHMIAS MIMICKING EPILEPSY

In the cardiological literature there are many clinical reports in which the descriptions of attacks ascribed to cardiac arrhythmias have features suggestive of epilepsy, particularly temporal lobe epilepsy. The diagnostic possibilities include anoxia-induced seizures secondary to the cardiac arrhythmia or perhaps an overlap in the symptoms of hindbrain ischemia and temporal lobe seizures. Without ictal EEG recordings, it is difficult to separate these two mechanisms.

A. Case Reports Without Simultaneous EEG

Typical symptoms of a cardiac episode in one man were described by Storstein (1949): episodes of loss of consciousness coupled with an imperceptible pulse, facial pallor, fixed and dilated pupils, followed by cyanosis and "clonic convulsions of the head and arms." When heart sounds and pulse recommenced the patient flushed. He was amnesic for the attacks. The ECG showed episodes of ventricular fibrillation (although it is not clear whether these were recorded during attacks). Interestingly, the attacks of one of the original two cases reported by Stokes (1846) began with something very like an epigastric aura ("a lump . . . in the stomach, which passes up through the right side of the neck into the head, where it seems to pass away with a loud noise resembling thunder, by which he is stupified").

Major convulsions have been described in association with arrythmias, although in many reports the evidence for the sequence of events remains circumstantial and some cases may have been examples of reflex anoxic seizures or vagal nonepileptic attacks (Stephenson, 1978). For example, Duvernoy and coworkers (1980) reported two patients with arrhythmias associated with major convulsions. The first had a long history of fainting spells. She lost consciousness during a venepuncture and convulsed. Holter monitoring showed sinus arrest lasting 16.2 seconds. Treatment with atropine reduced the number of attacks, but they did not cease until a pacemaker was implanted. The second patient also had a convulsion associated with venepuncture and AECG showed asystole of 11.6 seconds. A pacemaker was implanted and the attacks ceased, although the duration of follow-up and response to further venepuncture are not reported.

Convulsions may also occur in patients with long QT syndromes (Romano-Ward and Jervell–Lange-Nielsen). For example, Singer and coworkers (1974) reported a 22-year-old woman who had an episode of loss of consciousness with rigidity followed by clonic movements of all extremities and urinary incontinence. An interictal ECG showed a long QT interval. A month later, the patient again lost consciousness and was converted from ventricular fibrillation (VF) to sinus rhythm by DC countershock. She regained consciousness but then had a series of multifocal seizures which were controlled with intravenous barbiturate. One week later she lost consciousness and had a left-sided focal motor seizure. An ECG again showed VF, and DC countershock once more converted this to sinus rhythm. Despite treatment with antiarrhythmics and ACD she had a further episode of loss of consciousness with major motor seizures associated with VF. Control was apparently finally achieved with bretylium tosylate. In a similar case, Chaudron and colleagues (1976) reported a girl who, from the age of 5, had attacks of loss of consciousness which were diagnosed as epilepsy. At age 14 she had two convulsions preceded by a sensation of cardiac arrest. Later in the same year she was admitted apparently in status epilepticus. ECG showed bursts of ventricular flutter and multifocal ventricular tachycardia. She was successfully treated with intravenous lidocaine. An ECG showed a long QT interval.

Other examples are reviewed by Lambert and Fairfax (1980) but in all these cases it is, of course, impossible to be certain that the arrhythmias were the primary event and not secondary to possible epileptic seizures (although circumstantial evidence that the convulsions were secondary to arrhythmias is strong).

Ambulatory ECG monitoring without EEG has also been carried out in a number of studies of patients with undiagnosed episodic symptoms who are attending neurological clinics (DeBono et al., 1982; Schott et al., 1977). However, the diagnostic significance of the detected arrhythmias remains doubtful in many of these cases because recordings were seldom obtained during symptomatic episodes and the long-term results of treating the arrhythmias have not been reported.

B. Case Reports with Simultaneous EEG

There are surprisingly few clinical descriptions of symptoms ascribed to cardiac arrhythmias which contain EEG data obtained during the attacks. Pearson (1944) reported a 52-year-old woman with episodes of dizziness or loss of consciousness. After preliminary pallor she would develop a fearful expression, turning her head and eyes to the right with clenching and sometimes grinding of the teeth and swallowing movements. Sometimes her respiration would be sighing while her arms were flexed at the elbows and the hands raised "in a series of jactitating contractions of the forearms and clutching movements of the hands." Although this description might to the neurologist seem alarmingly reminiscent of CPS, simultaneous recording of the ECG and EEG during her attacks showed asystole on the ECG and only "minimal change in rhythm due to cerebral anoxemia" on the EEG. Unfortunately, the records are not shown in the published article. It should be noted that some CPS can be accompanied merely by flattening or attenuation of the EEG or even by normal EEG activity in scalp recordings (Lieb et al., 1976).

Regis and coworkers (1961) also recorded slowing and flattening on the EEG during Stokes–Adams attacks. Their patient either became confused with anxiety and intense sweating or would lose consciousness with "some tonic and clonic jerks." Tucker and Yoe (1956) described a 58-year-old woman with complete heart block and frequent episodes of loss of consciousness, sometimes with convulsions. Typical episodes began with a "rising feeling" then a pounding in the chest, a feeling of heat, pallor, and loss of consciousness, sometimes followed by a tonic convulsion with incontinence. Simultaneous EEG and ECG recording showed bouts of VT. When the VT lasted more than 10 seconds the EEG would slow and the patient was described as staring, pale, and confused. Short tonic convulsions occurred if VT lasted 18 seconds or more. After long runs of VT the EEG became flat.

The attacks of patients with the long QT syndrome have occasionally been recorded on ECG and EEG. For example, Driver and Selby (1977) described a 17-year-old who had attacks of facial pallor with a cry, dizziness, extension of the arms, and head turning. She also had drop attacks, episodes involving only a brief loss of attention, and nocturnal attacks in which she was incontinent of urine. ACDs were ineffective and an ECG showed frequent torsade de pointe VT. Simultaneous ECG and EEG demonstrated that clinical attacks occurred only when VT lasted five seconds or more. The EEG showed high-voltage frontal slow waves during attacks. There was some response to mexiletine. No QT data were included in the report.

Braham and colleagues (1981) reported a patient with episodes of loss of consciousness precipitated by minor surgery and injections which had been diagnosed as epilepsy at the age of 12 and treated with ACDs. The initial attacks were accompanied by myoclonic jerks. An ECG showed bradycardia then asystole associated with brief loss of consciousness and slow activity in the frontal regions on the EEG. A sinus arrest of 58 seconds was recorded on one occasion, and this attack terminated "with a few convulsive movements." Diagnosis and treatment with atropine at the age of 21 was followed by one year free of attacks, suggesting that this may have been yet another example of reflex vagal nonepileptic seizures (Stephenson, 1978).

C. Series with Simultaneous EEG

Gastaut (1985) and Gastaut and Fischer-Williams (1957) in response to the case report of Lloyd-Smith and Tatlow (1958), reported the EEG and ECG findings during 100 syncopal attacks in 71 subjects. All but seven of these episodes were provoked by firm ocular pressure for 10 seconds. With cardiac asystole lasting 8–12 seconds, consciousness and tone were lost. The EEG showed slow activity of about 3/second. With longer periods of asystole, the EEG became "silent" and the record showed only artifact during a tonic, opisthotonic spasm with clenched fists and a few jerks. Pupil dilatation and urinary or fecal incontinence also occurred. Gastaut states that he did not observe EEG seizure activity during these syncopal episodes. He suggested that the EEG in the case of Lloyd-Smith and Tatlow shows only slow activity with superimposed movement artifact and not spike and wave complexes as the authors had claimed.

Stephenson (1978) reported the effects of ocular compression in children diagnosed clinically as having reflex anoxic seizures. Asystole of more than two seconds was produced in the majority, and seizures provoked in some. Of 29 cases, 19 had tonic seizures with or without clonic jerks while the other 10 had atonic seizures without convulsion. Somewhat similar attacks were reported by Aminoff and colleagues (1988), who recorded ECG and EEG during ventricular arrhythmias induced to test implanted automatic defibrillators. In 15 episodes of induced ventricular arrhythmia in 11 patients, consciousness was lost. During unconsciousness motor activity occurred in 10 of the 15 episodes, with generalized tonic contractions of axial muscles accompanied or followed by irregular jerking of all extremities in 7 episodes, generalized rigidity without clonic activity in 1, and irregular facial movements or eyelid flutter without any tonic activity in the remaining 2. As circulation was restored, tonic flexion of the trunk or drawing up of the limbs was seen in 3 patients. Subjects were dazed and confused or slow to respond for up to 30 seconds after recovering consciousness. The EEG showed slowing of the background activity in 13 of the 15 episodes in which consciousness was lost, beginning 10–15 seconds after the induction of the ventricular arrhythmia. This was followed by flattening of the trace in 9 episodes. In the 2 remaining episodes, the record became attenuated without the development of slow activity. After the circulation was restored there was a gradual return to normal rhythms. The ictal EEG in syncope, therefore, is usually different from that in epilepsy, with the possible exception of electrodecremental seizures and partial seizures with a negative ictal EEG.

IV. SAMMEE IN EPILEPSY AND "POSSIBLE EPILEPSY"

Graf and colleagues (1982) recorded simultaneous ECG and EEG during symptomatic syncopal attacks in three patients, one of whom had a bilateral burst of spikes in the ictal AEEG record and simultaneously developed ventricular bigeminy. They were unable to explain this finding, which suggests that the occurrence of arrhythmias secondary to epileptic seizures is not widely recognized, even among those working in the ambulatory monitoring field.

Only two groups have reported the results of recording seizures in substantial numbers of epileptic patients. Blumhardt and coworkers (1986) reported 74 spontaneous seizures recorded by SAMMEE in 26 patients with a clinical diagnosis of CPS. Of these, 71 were typical or minor versions of the patients' usual seizures and 3 were asymptomatic nocturnal seizures. There was an abrupt acceleration in 67, rising to a maximum of over 120 bpm in 67%. The highest rate recorded was 201 bpm. There was no significant heart rate change during 7 seizures. In a minority of attacks there was a brief initial bradycardia. Unequivocal seizure activity was recorded on the AEEG in 66 seizures (42 unilateral and 24 bilateral). The increase in heart rate was greatest in young, untreated patients. Changes in cardiac rhythm occurred in 22 seizures in 11 patients and consisted mainly of abrupt accelerations and decelerations toward the end of the EEG seizure. One patient had several short episodes of SVT during and immediately after the EEG seizure.

By contrast, Keilson and colleagues (1987) found no significant cardiac arrhythmias during 56 AEEG seizures in 17 patients, although some were associated with a sinus tachycardia. Some seizures were apparently focal, but it is not clear what type they were or whether they were symptomatic. More recently the same group reported 82 seizures in 30 patients (Kielson et al., 1988). Of these, 95% were associated with a tachycardia of more than 100 bpm and 56% with a tachycardia of more than 150 bpm. Again, no ictal arrhythmias were observed.

SAMMEE has also been undertaken in patients with undiagnosed episodes of impaired consciousness where epilepsy or cardiac arrhythmias are more likely to be confused. Callaghan and McCarthy (1981) recorded patients with episodes of loss of consciousness and a normal interictal REEG. Monitoring revealed "epileptic features" in six patients with a provisional diagnosis of syncope and cardiac arrhythmias as a cause for attacks in three. It is not clear in exactly how many patients attacks were recorded, or in how many cases the diagnoses were based on interictal recordings only. The same authors (Callaghan and McCarthy, 1982) reported similar results in patients with episodes of loss of consciousness and normal routine and sleep EEG: 32 had attacks that were clinically diagnosed as epileptic and 16 as syncopal. Of the 32 diagnosed as epileptic, none was found on monitoring to have a cardiac origin. Of the 16 diagnosed clinically as syncopal, 5 were thought to have a cardiac basis (a paroxysmal tachycardia in 2 and heart block in 3). How often these episodes were associated with symptoms is not clear, and the results of treatment and follow-up are not given.

Blumhardt (1985) reported the results of a study of 145 patients with episodes of disturbed consciousness which remained unexplained after review by a neurologist. A typical event was recorded during SAMMEE in 29. Four had epileptic attacks on AEEG and another three had cardiac arrhythmias during attacks. The remainder showed no definite abnormality during typical attacks. At follow-up on average 26.7 months after monitoring, 14 of the 41 patients with equivocal or normal SAMMEE during attacks were now asymptomatic, 7 had psychiatric diagnoses, 3 had been diagnosed as epileptic, and in 2, symptoms had been attributed to cardiac arrhythmias and successfully treated. Five patients were lost to follow-up and 13 continued to have symptoms and remained undiagnosed. Of the remaining 97 in whom no symptoms had been recorded, 15 had been diagnosed epileptic and in 2 symptoms had been attributed to cardiac arrhythmias. Symptoms had resolved spontaneously in a majority of the remaining cases.

V. SUMMARY

There seems little doubt that most generalized convulsive seizures and symptomatic temporal lobe seizures are associated with autonomic cardiovascular changes, usually an abrupt tachycardia that may be preceded or followed by brief periods of bradycardia. The heart rate changes that occur during petit mal absences appear to be relatively minor. Data from both induced (Brown et al., 1953; White et al., 1961) and spontaneous seizures (Blumhardt et al., 1986) show that the end of the seizure and return of the heart rate toward preseizure levels may be associated with some irregularity of rate and minor arrhythmias. Serious arrhythmias appear uncommon but are reported following ECT-induced seizures. Case reports also provide evidence that significant arrhythmias (particularly asystole) do occasionally occur during spontaneous seizures.

Although the potential for the misdiagnosis of epileptic seizures as cardiac dysrhythmias certainly exists (Gilchrist, 1985), it is difficult to know from present series how commonly this may occur. When a cardiac arrhythmia has been recorded by AECG in association with dizziness or a blackout and appropriate antiarrhythmics or a pacemaker fails to stop the attacks, we do not know how often these patients will turn out to have epilepsy. The results of investigating a series of such patients for epilepsy have yet to be reported.

The clinical picture is further obscured by those patients whose symptoms are due to a secondary arrhythmia triggered by a minor focal seizure, rather than to the seizure itself. Such patients may be partially responsive to therapy for their arrhythmia (e.g., Phizackerley et al., 1954). On the other hand, some arrhythmias that may seem alarming and relevant, such as prolonged asystole at the onset of a seizure, may actually be secondary, despite their timing in relation to the scalp-recorded EEG seizure (see Figure 1) and their treatment may have no effect on the seizure disorder. A further complication is the possibility of cardiac rate and rhythm changes triggered by seizures which do not show up on simultaneous AEEG traces (Smith et al., 1989). Scalp EEG negative seizures are well recognized (Lieb et al., 1976) and may occur in as many as 20% of CPS patients during AEEG (Blumhardt et al., 1986). To date, the cardiac accompaniments of only a small number of spontaneous seizures have been reported and much larger studies of epileptics and patients with attacks not responding to cardiological treatments are required.

Convulsive movements during episodes of loss of consciousness secondary to cardiac arrhythmias are probably common if the arrhythmia reduces cardiac output and is sufficiently prolonged. Convulsive movements and other epileptiform features which occur in a minority of syncopal attacks or reflex anoxic seizures may result in the misdiagnosis of a cardiac dysrhythmia as epilepsy. Therefore, in cases of diagnostic doubt, or when "epilepsy" proves refractory to ACDs, an attempt to record an attack using SAMMEE should be considered.

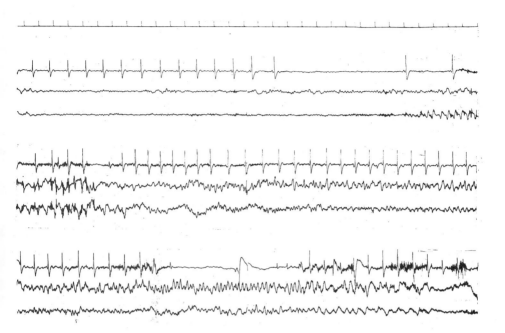

Figure 1   SAMMEE recording (Oxford Medilog four-channel recorder) of seizure in adult epileptic patient whose CPS and tonic-clonic seizures were poorly controlled by ACDs. Onset of rhythmic EEG seizure activity is preceded by asystole, although attenuation of the EEG in the left scalp trace appears even earlier. All seizures were associated either with similar periods of asystole or bradycardias. Pacemaker insertion resulted in correction of the ictal arrhythmias but had no effect on the characteristics of the seizures or their frequency or severity. The three sections of traces are continuous. ECG modified lead II. EEG leads are T4-P4 above and T3-P3 below. Time markers one second.

The investigation of arrhythmias associated with epileptiform and other attacks of disturbed consciousness (using SAMMEE) has just begun and much is still to be discovered. For the present, one can say that arrhythmias caused by epileptic seizures and arrhythmias producing attacks that mimic epilepsy both occur. The EEG features of syncope, even when the attacks involve convulsive movements, are usually different from those of epilepsy (Aminoff et al., 1988; Gastaut, 1958). Simultaneous recording of EEG and ECG should therefore distinguish most arrhythmias causing syncope from those which are secondary to epileptic seizures. How often this is of practical importance is as yet unknown.

REFERENCES

Aminoff, M. J., Scheinman, M. M., Griffin, J. C., and Herre, J. M. (1988). Electrocerebral accompaniments of syncope associated with malignant ventricular arrhythmias. *Ann. Intern. Med.* 108:791–796.

Blumhardt, L. D. (1985). The diagnostic value of ambulatory ECG/EEG recording: A follow-up study of 145 patients with unexplained transient non-focal neurological symptoms. In *Proceedings of the Fifth International Symposium on Ambulatory Monitoring.* C. Dal Palu and A. C. Pessina (Eds.). Cleup, Padua, pp. 675–683.

Blumhardt, L. D., Smith, P. E. M., and Owen, L. (1986). Electrocardiographic accompaniments of temporal lobe epileptic seizures. *Lancet 1*:1051–1056.

Bogacz, J., and Yanicelli, E. (1962). Vegetative phenomena in petit mal epilepsy. *World Neurol. 3*:195–208.

Braham, J., Hertzeanu, H., Yahini, J. H., and Neufeld, H. N. (1981). Reflex cardiac arrest presenting as epilepsy. *Ann. Neurol. 10*:277–278.

Brown, M. L., Huston, P. E., Hines, E. M., and Brown, G. M. (1953). Cardiovascular changes associated with electroconvulsive therapy in man. *Arch. Neurol. Psychiatr. 69*:601–608.

Callaghan, N., and McCarthy, N. (1981). Twenty-four hour EEG monitoring in patients with normal routine EEG findings. In *Advances in Epileptology. XIIth International Symposium*, M. Dam, and J. K. Penry (Eds.). Raven Press, New York, pp. 357–379.

Callaghan, N., and McCarthy, N. (1982). Ambulatory EEG monitoring in fainting attacks with normal routine and sleep EEG records. In *Mobile Long-Term EEG Monitoring*, H. Stefan and W. Burr (Eds.). Fischer, Stuttgart, pp. 61–65.

Chaudron, J. M., Heller, F., Van Den Berghe, H. B., and Le Bacq, E. G. (1976). Attacks of ventricular fibrillation and unconsciousness in a patient with prolonged QT interval. A family study. *Am. Heart J. 91*:783–791.

Coulter, D. L. (1984). Partial seizures with apnea and bradycardia. *Arch. Neurol. 41*:173–174.

Dasheiff, R. M., and Dickinson, L. J. (1986). Sudden unexpected death of epileptic patient due to cardiac arrhythmia after seizure. *Arch. Neurol. 43*:194–196.

DeBono, D. P., Warlow, C. P., and Hyman, N. M. (1982). Cardiac rhythm abnormalities in patients presenting with transient non-focal neurological symptoms: A diagnostic grey area? *Br. Med. J. 284*:1437–1439.

Delgado, M. R., Mihailovic, L., and Sevillano, M. (1960). Cardiovascular phenomena during seizure activity. *J. Nerv. Ment. Dis. 130*:477–487.

Driver, M. V., and Selby, P. J. (1977). Apparent epilepsy due to intermittent ventricular tachyarrhythmia (Romano–Ward syndrome). *Electroenceph. Clin. Neurophysiol. 43*:289.

Duvernoy, W. F. C., Nair, M. R. S., and Zobl, E. G. (1980). Convulsive disorder mimicked by prolonged asystole and cured by permanent pacing. *Heart Lung 9*:711–714.

Erikson, T. C. (1939). Cardiac activity during epileptic seizures. *Arch. Neurol. Psychiatr. 41*:511–518.

Fischgold, H., and Arfel-Capdevielle (1955). Modifications respiratoires dans les paroxysmes épileptiques. *Electroenceph. Clin. Neurophysiol. 7*:165–168.

Gastaut, H. (1958). Syncope and seizure. *Electroenceph. Clin. Neurophysiol. 10*: 571–572.

Gastaut, H., and Fischer-Williams, M. (1957). Electroencephalographic study of syncope, its differentiation from epilepsy. *Lancet 2*:1018–1025.

Gilchrist, J. M. (1985). Arrhythmogenic seizures: Diagnosis by simultaneous EEG/ECG recording. *Neurology 35*:1503–1506.

Graf, M., Brunner, G., Weber, H., Auinger, C., and Joskowicz, G. (1982). Simultaneous long-term recording of EEG and ECG in "syncope" patients. In *Mobile Long-Term EEG Monitoring*, H. Stefan and W. Burr (Eds.). Fischer, Stuttgart, pp. 67–75.

Green, R., and Woods, A. (1955). Effects of modified ECT on the electrocardiogram. *Br. Med. J. 1*:1503–1505.

Jackson, H. (1887). Remarks on evolution and dissolution of the nervous system. In *Selected Writings of Hughlings Jackson*, J. Taylor (Ed.). Hodder and Stoughton, London, pp. 106–108.

Jay, G. W., and Leestma, J. E. (1981). Sudden death in epilepsy. *Acta Neurol. Scand (Suppl. 82)63*:1–66.

Johnson, L. C., and Davidoff, R. A. (1964). Autonomic changes during paroxysmal EEG activity. *Electroenceph. Clin. Neurophysiol. 17*:25–35.

Katz, R. I., Tiger, M., and Harner, R. N. (1983). Epileptic cardiac arrhythmia: Sinoatrial arrest in two patients. A potential cause of sudden death in epilepsy? *Epilepsia 24*:248.

Keilson, M. J., Hauser, W. A., Magrill, J. P., and Goldman, M. (1987). ECG abnormalities in patients with epilepsy. *Neurology 37*:1624–1626.

Keilson, M. J., Hauser, W. A., and Magrill, J. (1988). ECG changes during electrographic seizures. *Neurology (Suppl. 1)38*:302.

Kiok, M. C., Terrence, C. F., Fromm, G. H., and Lavine, S. (1986). Sinus arrest in epilepsy. *Neurology 36*:115–116.

Lambert, C. D., and Fairfax, A. J. (1980). Cerebral effects of cardiac arrhythmias. In *Handbook of Clinical Neurology*, Vol. 39, *Neurological Manifestations of Systemic Diseases*, Part II, P. J. Vinken and G. W. Bruyn (Eds.). Elsevier, Amsterdam, pp. 259–271.

Lathers, C. M., and Schraeder, P. L. (1982). Autonomic dysfunction in epilepsy: Characterisation of autonomic discharge associated with pentylenetetrazol-induced epileptogenic activity. *Epilepsia 23*:633–647.

Lathers, C. M., and Schraeder, P. L. (1987). Review of autonomic dysfunction, cardiac arrhythmias, and epileptogenic activity. *J. Clin. Pharmacol. 27*:346–356.

Leestma, J. E., Kalelkar, M. B., Teas, S. S., Jay, G. W., and Hughes, J. R. (1984). Sudden unexpected death associated with seizures: Analysis of 66 cases. *Epilepsia 25*:84–88.

Lieb, J. P., Walsh, G. O., Babb, T. L., Walter, R. D., and Crandall, P. H. (1976). A comparison of EEG seizure patterns recorded with surface and depth electrodes in patients with temporal lobe epilepsy. *Epilepsia 17*:137–160.

Lloyd-Smith, D. L., and Tatlow, W. F. T. (1958). Syncope and seizure. *Electroenceph. Clin. Neurophysiol. 10*:153–157.

Mameli, P., Mameli, O., Tolu, E., Padua, G., Giraudi, D., Caria, M. A., and Melis, F. (1988). Neurogenic myocardial arrhythmias in experimental focal epilepsy. *Epilepsia 29*:74–82.

Marshall, D. W., Westmoreland, B. F., and Sharbrough, F. W. (1983). Ictal tachycardia during temporal lobe seizures. *Mayo Clin. Proc. 58*:443–446.

Mathew, N. T., Taoti, G. M., Mathai, K. V., and Chandy, J. (1970). Atrial fibrillation associated with seizure in a case of frontal meningioma. *Neurology 20*: 725–728.

McKenna, G., Engle, R., Brooks, H., and Dalen, J. (1970). Cardiac arrhythmias during electroshock therapy: Significance, prevention and treatment. *Am. J. Psychiatr. 127*:530–533.

Mosier, J. M., White, P., Grant, P., Fisher, J. E., and Taylor, R. (1957). Cerebroautonomic and myographic changes accompanying induced seizures. *Neurology 7*:204–210.

Mirsky, A. F., and Van Buren, J. M. (1965). On the nature of the "absence" in centrencephalic epilepsy: A study of some behavioural, electroencephalographic and autonomic factors. *Electroenceph. Clin. Neurophysiol. 18*:334–348.

Pearson, R. S. B. (1944). Sinus bradycardia with cardiac asystole. *Br. Heart J. 7*:85–90.

Perrin, G. (1961). Cardiovascular and other physiologic changes accompanying EST. *Acta Psychiatr. Neurol. Scand. (Suppl. 152)36*:1–45.

Phizackerley, P. J. R., Poole, E. W., and Whitty, C. M. W. (1954). Sino-auricular heart block as an epileptic manifestation. *Epilepsia 3*:89–96.

Poggiali, I. (1971). Considerazioni su di un caso di tachycardia parossistica sopraventricolare e giunzionale con alterazioni elettroencefalografiche. *Clin. Pediatr. 53*:260–270.

Pritchett, E. L. C., McNamara, J. O., and Gallagher, J. J. (1980). Arrhythmogenic epilepsy: An hypothesis. *Am. Heart J. 100*:683–688.

Regis, H., Toga, M., and Righini, C. (1961). Clinical, electroencephalographic and pathological study of a case of Adams–Stokes syndrome. In *Cerebral Anoxia and the Electroencephalogram*, H. Gastaut and J. S. Meyer (Eds.). Thomas, Springfield, Ill., pp. 295–303.

Rosen, M., Lisak, R., and Rubin, I. L. (1967). Diphenylhydantoin in cardiac arrhythmias. *Am. J. Cardiol. 20*:674–678.

Russell, A. E. (1906). Cessation of the pulse duing the onset of epileptic fits. *Lancet 2*:152–154.

Schott, G. D., McLeod, A. A., and Jewitt, D. E. (1977). Cardiac arrhythmias that masquerade as epilepsy. *Br. Med. J. 1*:1454–1457.

Schraeder, P. L., and Lathers, C. M. (1989). Paroxysmal cardiovascular dysfunction and epileptogenic activity. *Epilepsy Res. 3*:55–62.

Singer, P. A., Crampton, R. S., and Bass, N. H. (1974). Familial QT prolongation syndrome. Convulsive seizures and paroxysmal ventricular fibrillation. *Arch. Neurol. 31*:64–66.

Smaje, J. C., Davidson, C., and Teasdale, G. M. (1987). Sino-atrial arrest due to temporal lobe epilepsy. *J. Neurol. Neurosurg. Psychiatr. 50*:112–113.

Smith, P. E. M., Howell, S. J. L., Owen, L., and Blumhardt, L. D. (1989). Profiles of instant heart rate during partial seizures. *Electroenceph. Clin. Neurophysiol. 72*:207–217.

Steiner, C., Wit, A. L., Weiss, H. B., and Damatoa, A. H. (1970). The antiarrhythmic actions of carbamazepine. *J. Pharm. Exp. Therap. 173*:323.

Stephenson, J. P. B. (1978). Reflex anoxic seizures ("white breath holding"): Nonepileptic vagal attacks. *Arch. Dis. Child. 53*:193–200.

Stokes, W. (1846). Observations on some cases of permanently slow pulse. *Dublin Q. J. Med. Sci. 2*:73–85.

Storstein, O. (1949). Adams–Stokes attacks caused by ventricular fibrillation in a man with an otherwise normal heart. *Acta Med. Scand. 133*:437–441.

Talman, W. T. (1985). Cardiovascular regulation and lesions of the central nervous system. *Ann. Neurol. 18*:1–12.

Temkin, O. (1971). *The Falling Sickness*, 2nd ed. Johns Hopkins Press, Baltimore, pp. 40–42.

Tucker, J. S., and Yoe, R. H. (1956). Simultaneous EEG–ECG recording: Study of a case with complete heart block and paroxysmal ventricular tachycardia. *Electroenceph. Clin. Neurophysiol. 8*:129–132.

Van Buren, J. M. (1958). Some autonomic concomitants of ictal automatism. *Brain 81*:505–528.

Van Buren, J. M., and Ajmone-Marsan, C. (1960). A correlation of autonomic and EEG components in temporal lobe epilepsy. *Arch. Neurol. 3*:683–703.

Walsh, G., Masland, W., and Goldensohn, E. (1968). Paroxysmal cerebral discharge associated with paroxysmal atrial tachycardia. *Electroenceph. Clin. Neurophysiol. 24*:187.

Walsh, G. O., Masland, W., and Goldensohn, E. (1972). Relationship between paroxysmal atrial tachycardia and paroxysmal cerebral discharges. *Bull. L.A. Neurol. Assoc. 37*:28–35.

White, P. T., Grant, P., Mosier, J., and Craig, A. (1961). Changes in cerebral dynamics associated with seizures. *Neurology 11*:354–361.

8

The Relation of Paroxysmal Autonomic Dysfunction and Epileptogenic Activity

PAUL L. SCHRAEDER *University of Medicine and Dentistry of New Jersey, Robert Wood Johnson Medical School, Camden, New Jersey*

CLAIRE M. LATHERS* *The Medical College of Pennsylvania, Eastern Pennsylvania Psychiatric Institute, Philadelphia, Pennsylvania*

I. INTRODUCTION

Almost every patient having a generalized tonic-clonic seizure manifests autonomic abnormalities. These include diaphoresis, cardiac arrhythmias, hypertension, hypotension, pupillary abnormalities, loss of sphincter control, apnea, neurogenic pulmonary edema, and hyperpyrexia. The wonder of it all is that the patient recovers from the event, which reflects the effectiveness of autonomic homeostasis. In recent years, autonomic dysfunction also has been reported in patients with focal epileptiform discharges in the temporal lobes in association with complex partial seizures. Data from various animal models are beginning to show that even interictal discharges can be associated with a variety of disturbances of cardiovascular function. The accumulation of clinical and experimental evidence showing that epileptiform discharges of generalized and focal distribution can be accompanied by potentially serious disruptions of autonomic control of cardiovascular and pulmonary function suggests that the syndrome of unexplained sudden death in epilepsy may be the result of sudden failure of autonomic homeostatic safeguards. The risk factors leading to such failure are unknown. This chapter will review the spectrum of clinical autonomic changes associated with varying degrees of epileptiform discharges.

II. GENERALIZED SEIZURES

Quantitative data on the disruption of autonomic nervous system function in association with generalized tonic-clonic seizures in controlled circumstances

---

Current affiliation: FDA, Rockville, Maryland.

have been reported primarily with the use of electroconvulsive therapy (ECT) in psychiatric patients. The effects of convulsions attenuated by subparalyzing doses of curare offer the best model for study. Brown et al. (1953) evaluated 24 patients under such conditions, subjected to a fully convulsive ECT dose, resulting in 31 convulsions. At the beginning of the ECT, the average systolic blood pressure (BP) decreased 20 mm Hg below control and the mean diastolic BP decreased 50 mm Hg. Additional evidence that autonomic dysfunction occurred at this early stage in ECT was manifested by the presence of concurrent bradycardia. The expected response to a fall in BP should be tachycardia mediated by the carotid sinus reflex (Milnor, 1974). As the convulsions continued the BP and heart rate (HR) increased above control, only to fall below control levels at the end of the convulsion. The latter decrease in BP was again followed by another elevation, which gradually returned to control levels. Bradycardia continued throughout the postictal period. Although respiratory arrest lasted for an average of 52 seconds from the onset of ECT, several patients experienced several minutes of apnea.

In a second group of experiments, these same investigators found that subconvulsive ECT shocks in 15 partially curarized patients failed to induce clinical seizures or apnea. Nonetheless, the same pattern of BP and HR variation occurred as was seen in the partially curarized patients subjected to a fully convulsive ECT shock. The fact that the BP and HR changes were similar in both patient groups indicated that the cardiovascular changes resulted from the cerebral discharges rather than the physiological consequences of the clinical seizure.

McKenna et al. (1970) emphasized that cardiac arrhythmias commonly occur during routine ECT even with use of adequate muscle paralysis. Of patients undergoing ECT, 28–43% were observed to have various cardiac arrhythmias such as premature ventricular contractions, often with bigeminy or trigeminy. This high percentage of observed cardiac arrhythmias observed during routine ECT led this author to suggest that the risk of death from fatal cardiac arrhythmias may be increased in persons with coronary artery disease who undergo ECT. The possibility of multiple risk factors, in this case ECT-induced seizures plus coronary artery disease, increasing the risk of sudden death is introduced in this same article. This concept of multiple risk factors in sudden death needs to be considered in the discussion of any population at risk for sudden unexplained death.

Seizures induced by pentylenetetrazol (PTZ) provide another model of generalized tonic-clonic seizures. Cleckley et al. (1942) documented the marked elevation in BP in unparalyzed patients with seizures induced by intravenous PTZ. These investigators attributed the BP elevation to the increased intrathoracic and intra-abdominal pressure resulting from the clinical convulsions. Mosier et al. (1957) and White et al. (1961) studied the effects of PTZ-induced seizures in patients with epilepsy. The subjects were paralyzed with intravenous succinylcholine with the exception of one distal lower limb, which had a tourniquet inflated to just above the systolic BP. This latter technique allowed monitoring of localized tonic-clonic seizure activity without production of a generalized clinical convulsion, which would disrupt the EEG recordings. The subjects were continuously ventilated and the electrocardiogram (ECG) and BP were monitored. In some patients, focal seizures preceded the generalized event with no concurrent BP or ECG changes. All patients had generalized tonic-clonic seizure discharges induced by PTZ during which a variety of associated autonomic changes were observed. Varying degrees of hypertension and tachycardia occurred during seizure discharges in all patients. A variety of significant ECG changes and arrhythmias were observed during PTZ-induced seizures (Mosier et al., 1957; White et al., 1961), including premature ventricular contractions, bigeminy, premature atrial contractions, ventricular tachycardias, elevated or depressed ST segments and T waves, conduction blocks, and bradycardia. One patient (Mosier et al., 1957) suffered an acute myocardial infarction. These studies in human subjects indicate that major cardiovascular changes are correlated with generalized electrographic seizure discharges even when the clinical tonic-clonic events are prevented with neuromuscular blockade.

Thus, as evidenced by common clinical observation and the clinical studies just described, a generalized seizure, even if only electrographic, is a major physiological stress to the body. Whether abnormalities of autonomic function are attributable to adrenal medullary and/or neurogenic effects is an important unanswered question. Neurogenic effects on cardiovascular function produce a very rapid change in BP, HR, and cardiac rhythm. The lag time can be measured in terms of seconds or even a fraction thereof. This question of lag time is important when trying to determine whether cardiac arrhythmias and BP changes are due to neurogenic effects and/or adrenal medullary secretions. Published evidence suggests that neurogenic factors produce rapid, major changes in BP and cardiac rhythm, whereas the humorally mediated response occurs at a much slower rate. Adrenal catecholamines most certainly are liberated in response to seizures produced by PTZ (Hahn, 1960). However, Doba et al. (1975) found that with an intact sympathetic nervous system the pressor response associated with seizure activity was not abolished by adrenalectomy. This latter observation indicates that the adrenal gland has but a minor role in mediating the pressor response to a seizure. Ceremyzynski et al. (1969) reported that even though adrenal medullary secretions were involved in the production of cardiac arrhythmias, the catecholamines did not reach significant levels until 2–25 minutes after coronary occlusion. Since ectopic cardiac beats are observed to occur within 15–30 seconds after coronary occlusion, it would seem unlikely that the rapid, acute onset of a cardiovascular response to a stress such as coronary artery occlusion or a seizure is humorally mediated. Instead, this rapid responsiveness would argue strongly in favor of a neurogenic mechanism for the commonly observed rapid onset of seizure-related cardiovascular changes.

Although PTZ-induced seizures provide a standard model of primary generalized epilepsy, one must also consider whether the autonomic effects are secondary to the ictal discharges alone, or whether PTZ exerts a direct action on peripheral organs (e.g., the heart and blood vessels). Stone (1972) stated that PTZ has no direct activating effect on muscle or nerve fibers but does stimulate autonomic ganglia even when all preganglionic impulses have been eliminated by preganglionic nerve section. Toman and Davis (1949) indicated that the major peripheral actions of PTZ were mediated via the central rather than the peripheral nervous system. Also in support of the primary central action of PTZ are the observations of Hildebrandt (1937), as translated and quoted by Hahn (1960), that PTZ did not exert any positive inotropic action on the heart. Therefore, it would appear unlikely that the cardiovascular changes observed in these human studies are due to any direct action of PTZ on the heart and peripheral vascular system, but rather are the result of centrally mediated autonomic dysfunction associated with the generalized PTZ-induced epileptiform discharges with or without accompanying clinical convulsions.

III. FOCAL SEIZURES

When autonomic dysfunction is found in association with seizures, it is commonly assumed that the precipitating event is a generalized tonic-clonic seizure resulting from generalized epileptiform cerebral discharges. However, neither generalized clinical seizures nor generalized epileptiform discharges which are unaccompanied by clinical seizures are the sine qua non for production of autonomic dysfunction. Van Buren (1958) observed the effects of temporal lobe seizure automatisms resulting either from hyperventilation or subthreshold doses of PTZ. He found that paroxysmal tachycardia occurred in association with clinical automatisms in 12 of his 13 patients. Only one individual experienced bradycardia. Blood pressure elevation occurred in over half of the subjects. A rapid fall in the galvanic skin response and inhibition of gastric motility were commonly observed at the onset of the seizure. Expiratory apnea or hypoventilation occurred during all automatisms. In general, the disturbances of vegetative function varied widely and unpredictably at different times in the same patient and between patients from one seizure to another. There did not appear to be any predictable pattern of autonomic dysfunction for any given individual.

Van Buren and Ajmone-Marsan (1960) subsequently correlated autonomic phenomena (e.g. apnea, BP changes, HR, esophageal peristalsis) with varying degrees of epileptiform activity. They found great variability in the correlations between acute autonomic changes and bilaterally synchronous cerebral discharges in any one patient experiencing recurrence of the same type of electrographic discharges at different times. Autonomic disturbances also occurred in association with the patients' acknowledged clinical auras, even when unaccompanied by epileptiform discharges on the scalp EEG. This lack of clinical EEG correlation suggested that the auras were the result of discharges occurring in brain regions not accessible to the scalp EEG. They found that bilaterally synchronous frontal discharges were most likely to be associated with autonomic changes. However, at other times, despite the occurrence of the same type of EEG discharges even in the same patient, no autonomic manifestations were observed. This variability of the autonomic response to morphologically similar EEG bursts in the same and different patients led the authors to conclude that these epileptiform discharges were neither massive nor indiscriminate in engulfing every available neuronal circuit. They hypothesized that within regions of the brain representing autonomic nervous system function, epileptiform discharges follow as yet undefined anatomical pathways within the diencephalon or brain stem.

Also of more than passing interest was the conclusion by Van Buren and Ajmone-Marsan (1960) that focal epileptiform discharges limited to one temporal region were not accompanied by any changes in autonomic function. This conlusion is not supported by more recent work. Patients with unilateral temporal lobe discharges indeed can have significant associated autonomic abnormalities. Katz et al. (1983) described a 63-year-old man with no known history of epilepsy who had documented periods of asystole thought to be cardiac in origin. Because he complained of a rising sensation in his stomach prior to some of his syncopal episodes, an EEG utilizing nasopharyngeal electrodes was recorded. This patient was found to have isolated right mesiotemporal spikes immediately prior to and during 15 seconds of asystole, documenting that focal epileptiform discharges limited to one temporal region can cause potentially life-threatening disruption of myocardial rhythm. Presumably, excessive vagal tone, consequent to epileptiform discharges, resulted in asystole. Bonvallet and Gary Bobo (1972) found that stimulation of various topographical areas of the amygdala could result in bradycardia and respiratory deactivation or tachycardia and respiratory activation. These studies confirmed, at least in the cat, that major sympathetically or vagally mediated cardiac rhythm changes can occur consequent to discharges limited to very specific regions of the temporal lobe.

That focal temporal discharges can cause major cardiac arrhythmias is further documented by the clinical studies of Marshall et al. (1983). The patients in this study, ranging in age from 15 to 78 years, had focal ictal discharges limited to one temporal lobe, with accompanying complex partial seizures. In each instance, within a few seconds after onset of the isolated, unilateral ictal discharges, the patients experienced runs of tachycardia, including runs of premature ventricular beats. The maximal HR ranged from 120 to 180 bpm with the tachycardia lasting an average of 45 seconds after the termination of the seizure. The author suggested that the autonomic phenomena responsible for such seemingly inconsequential tachycardia may have more serious consequences in persons with a history of underlying cardiac disease. This latter caveat is similar to that expressed by McKenna et al. (1970) in discussing the risks of ECT-induced arrhythmias.

Cardiologists have long recognized the importance of the correlation of tachyarrhythmias with the risk of sudden death in persons with a history of cardiac disease (DeSilva, 1982). It is widely accepted that episodic tachycardia may be of little consequence in persons with a healthy myocardium but may be a risk factor for sudden death in an elderly population with coronary artery disease or in younger patients with clinically silent abnormalities of cardiac conduction. The subtle nature of the relationship between a history of seizures and occurrence of tachycardia is supported by the findings of Blumhardt et al. (1986) using 24-hour EEG/ECG monitoring. These investigators found that some individuals with a history of temporal lobe epilepsy experienced cardiac acceleration before the onset of any recognizable surface EEG disturbance. Based on these observations, they suggested that discharges in deep limbic circuits may produce autonomic effects with no visible surface EEG manifestations, a conclusion supported by the experimental work of Bonvallet and Gary Bobo (1972).

The variety of autonomic changes accompanying focal epileptogenic discharges is rather diverse and a function of the region of the brain which is stimulated. Penfield and Jasper (1954) observed the autonomic responses to cortical stimulation in humans subjected to epilepsy surgery under local anesthesia. Suprasylvian stimulation resulted in uncontrolled salivation, and stimulation of the insula resulted in a variety of gastrointestinal symptoms. Anterior and inferior cingulate gyrus stimulation produced apnea; however, this apnea was unusual in that it was easily overcome by the patient consciously willing himself to breathe. In contrast, stimulation of rolandic and uncal regions produced apnea that could not be overcome by voluntary effort on the part of the awake patient. Supplemental motor area cortical stimulation produced abdominal sensations, acceleration of the heart rate, the sensation of flushing, and various pupillary changes. These clinical neurophysiological observations demonstrate that localized discharges in the temporal lobe and medial frontal cortex are often associated with major respiratory and cardiovascular changes and that a major dramatic and electrophysiological event in the form of a generalized tonic-clonic seizure is not necessary to produce clinically obvious autonomic dysfunction.

IV. INTERICTAL DISCHARGES

The next logical step in considering the minimal degree of epileptiform activity necessary to produce autonomic dysfunction involves the interictal discharge.

Although there is no clinical literature on this subject, there are data from animal studies concerning the effects of interictal spikes on autonomic function. The studies of Lathers and Schraeder (1982, 1987), Lathers et al. (1987), and Schraeder and Lathers (1983) monitoring the intrathoracic cardiac sympathetic and vagal branch discharges demonstrated that the discharge patterns in these nerves varied widely in association with the different degrees of epileptiform discharges. These researchers observed a most intriguing phenomenon, consisting of cardiac sympathetic nerve discharges which were time-locked to the bilateral cortical interictal spikes induced by PTZ (Lathers et al., 1987; Stauffer et al., 1989). During the interictal discharges, this time-locked event, termed the lockstep phenomenon, waxed and waned among all of the monitored cardiac sympathetic branches. The latency between the spike on the electrocorticogram and the discharges in the cardiac sympathetic branches ranged from 30 to 100 milliseconds, indicating that the cortical discharges preceded the cardiac neural discharges and probably were conducted through a multisynaptic pathway within the central nervous system. Only one of the five cats in which the vagal branches were recorded manifested this lockstep phenomenon in association with interictal spikes. In all cats manifesting the lockstep phenomenon, the ECG exhibited peaking, inversion, and biphasic T waves as well as P wave changes consisting of peaking, flattening, and biphasic configuration; variable Q wave changes and widened QRS intervals suggested neurogenically mediated interference in myocardial conduction time. Premature ventricular contractions occurred in one cat in association with interictal spikes. The lockstep phenomenon has also been significantly correlated with variability in the mean arterial BP.

Mameli et al. (1988) recently confirmed the disruptive effect of interictal spikes on cardiac rhythm and blood pressure with a model utilizing microinjection of aqueous penicillin into the hypothalamus of the rat. These investigators found that interictal spikes triggered a short-latency cardiac arrhythmia with sinus bradycardia and junctional rhythm. They also noted lengthening of intervals between blood pressure waves with a significant drop in diastolic blood pressure. With cessation of the discharges, cardiac rhythm and diastolic blood pressure returned to baseline. Prolonged ictal discharges (1-1.5 minutes) seemed to trigger sinus and junctional bradyarrhythmias, which lasted longer than that associated with the interictal spikes. Supraventricular extrasystoles, sinus arrest and bigeminal ventricular extrasystoles, and a decrease in both systolic and diastolic BP also occurred during ictal discharges. Because of the short latency of these cardiac and hemodynamic responses relative to the spike discharges, the author concluded that paroxysmal disruptions of autonomic function were neurogenic rather than humoral or metabolic in origin.

Thus there is an increasing body of experimental evidence to suggest that even minimal epileptiform discharges in the form of interictal spikes are associated with measurable disruptions of neural control of cardiac rhythm and blood pressure. Although these findings have yet to be confirmed in patients with epilepsy, they tend to lend support to the clinical observation that autonomic dysfunction can occur even when only minimal epileptiform discharges are present. The observation that synchronized events in the cerebrum, even in the form of seemingly innocuous interictal spikes, can have an effect on cardiovascular autonomic regulation may well be explained by the evolving concept of chaos (Pool, 1989). This concept of biological rhythms holds that healthy physiological systems have innate variability. Loss of variability, that is, a transition to a more ordered state (e.g., ictal and interictal discharges) signals an impaired system. The applicability of this interesting and only recently recognized concept of chaos in both neural and cardiac function warrants more investigation as it applies to the risk factors of sudden death.

V. NEUROGENIC PULMONARY EDEMA

A common seizure-related phenomenon is the occurrence of bilateral pulmonary infiltrates seen in patients during the postictal period. Although at one time thought to be a form of aspiration pneumonia, this phenomenon is more likely to be neurogenic pulmonary edema resulting from a massive centrally mediated adrenergal discharge induzed by seizures. Terrence et al. (1981) consider this phenomenon to be a factor in unexplained sudden death in epilepsy. However, these authors acknowledge that a likely mechanism of sudden death involves the combination of neurogenic pulmonary edema and ventricular arrhythmia. Although the observation of postmortem pulmonary edema only adds to speculations about the pathophysiological mechanisms of sudden death, it is clear that there is a relationship between epileptogenic activity and acute pulmonary changes. Simon et al. (1982) showed that seizures in sheep model can produce acute pulmonary edema. They found a neurogenically induced increase in pulmonary microvascular pressure with an accompanying prolonged change in endothelial conductance to protein.

The clinical relevance of acute neurogenic pulmonary edema is emphasized by the recent report of Koppel et al. (1987), which described three patients in whom unilateral pulmonary edema occurred secondary to generalized tonic-clonic seizures. The recent observation of adult respiratory distress syndrome (ARDS) induced by nonconvulsive electrographic status epilepticus also emphasized the profound effect epileptiform discharges may have on the lung (Schraeder, 1987). Although such clinical observations only add to speculations about the pathophysiological mechanisms, the relationship between epileptiform activity and acute pulmonary changes cannot be in question.

VI. ICTAL APNEA

Apnea is often observed in association with clinical seizures. The cortical stimulation studies of Penfield and Jasper (1954) clearly demonstrated that apnea can result from stimulation of rolandic and uncal cortex and the cingulate gyrus in humans. However, in recent years the question of ictal apnea and episodic apnea and bradycardia as seizure manifestations has become controversial. Fenichel et al. (1980) showed that episodic apnea usually occurs without HR changes. Nonetheless, there is a small group of infants in whom ictal events are manifested by apnea and bradycardia. Coulter (1984) demonstrated that a localized epileptogenic discharged limited to the temporal region can result in apnea and bradycardia. This clinical observation correlates well with the experimental work of Bonvallet and Gary Bobo (1972), which demonstrated topographically defined bradycardia and apnea centers in the amygdala of the rat. Therefore, it would seem logical to postulate that the potential risks involved in having repeated episodes of seizures, manifested by apnea and bradycardia, can put susceptible patients at risk for sudden death. The factors making a patient susceptible are unknown. These clinical and electrographic observations again provide evidence that even well-localized epileptogenic discharges without bilateral secondary spread can result in potentially life-threatening alterations of vegetative function.

VII. POSSIBLE PATHOPHYSIOLOGICAL MECHANISMS OF UNEXPLAINED SUDDEN DEATH

By definition there is no pathological cause for sudden unexplained death. It is known that males are more at risk than females by a three to two ratio. The mean age at the time of death is slightly more than 30 years and accounts for over 15% of mortality in epilepsy (Hirsch and Martin, 1971; Jay and Leestma, 1981; Krohn, 1963; Leestma et al., 1984). Hirsch and Martin (1971) also found that 6 of their 19 sudden death victims had a prior history of generalized tonic-clonic seizures, while 11 of the 19 had a mixed seizure disorder including generalized tonic-clonic seizures, which were apparently well controlled. Syncopal seizures were also mentioned, presumably in reference to the brief tonic events associated with cardiogenic cerebral hypoperfusion. Of the eight witnessed deaths, four victims had brief generalized tonic-clonic seizures, while two others had a minimal tonic seizure. Two victims had no observed seizure activity at the time of death. In no instance was there a history of frequent seizures prior to death, so that neither the severity of the disorder prior to death nor the severity of the ictal event at the time of death was a factor. There is, therefore, a question whether a seemingly physiologically benign epileptiform discharge could produce enough disruption of autnomic function to result in sudden death. The additive risk factors that might set up a life-threatening substrate are unknown.

Paroxysmal autonomic dysfunction associated with epileptogenic discharges may be a factor in these deaths, presumably by causing a disruption of cardiac and/or respiratory function. In the several published postmortem series, up to half of the patients died during sleep (Hirsch and Martin, 1971; Jay and Leestma, 1981; Krohn, 1963; Leestma et al., 1984). Since sleep is an activator of epileptogenic activity, it could be a contributing mechanism associated with death. However, half or more of the victims were awake just prior to their demise. Another factor may be low antiepileptic drug levels, since most of the victims had subtherapeutic or no detectable levels postmortem (Jay and Leestma, 1981; Leestma et al., 1984). The presence of low antiepileptic drug levels raise speculation that the patients were noncompliant, thus increasing the risk of drug withdrawal seizures. It seems unlikely that sudden apnea is the cause of death in patients who were alert just prior to the morbid event, but apnea may be a factor in the patients who died during sleep. A more plausible explanation for death, especially in the group dying during daytime, is a paroxysmal cardiac arrhythmia induced by epileptiform discharges, especially in association with simultaneous acute neurogenic pulmonary edema (Simon et al., 1982; Terrance et al., 1981).

The role of stress also must be considered in sudden death. Psychophysiologically induced arrhythmias in association with stress are well documented (DeSilva, 1982). Although the relationship of stress to the risk of sudden death in epilepsy is unclear, the occurrence of a seizure can cause release of catecholamines from the adrenal medulla (Doba et al., 1975), possibly predisposing the heart to the development of arrhythmias when confronted with a sudden sympathetic neural barrage induced by epileptogenic discharges. Another risk factor is the concurrent use of psychotropic drugs. Leestma and Koenig (1968) described sudden death associated with seizures in persons taking phenothiazines. Phenothiazine use can well lower seizure threshold (Lathers and Lipka, 1987; Lipka and Lathers, 1987). The risk of seizure induction increases to almost 9% with clinical use of high doses of these drugs (Logothetis, 1967). There are also experimental observations of increased epileptogenic activity in guinea pig hippocampal slices exposed to low doses of phenothiazines (Oliver et al., 1977). This latter observation is of interest since low doses of these agents are often used in the management of behavioral symptoms in persons with epilepsy.

VIII. SUMMARY

Although autonomic dysfunction commonly accompanies generalized tonic-clonic clinical seizures, it can also be associated with even minimal degrees of epileptiform activity. How the many variables discussed in this chapter apply to the mechanism of unexplained sudden death in persons with epilepsy is unclear. From a clinical standpoint, it seems prudent to undertake 24-hour ambulatory

EEG/ECG routinely on young persons with unexplained cardiac arrhythmias and in individuals with recent seizures of unexplained etiology who have normal routine EEGs. This brief review obviously raises more questions that it answers about the mechanism of autonomic dysfunction and seizures; it is intended to emphasize that this phenomenon may be multifactorial in origin, requiring coordinated research among the disciplines of cardiology, neuropharmacology, and clinical neurophysiology.

REFERENCES

Blumhardt, L. D., Smith, P. E. M., and Owen, L. Electrocardiographic accompaniments of temporal lobe epileptic seizures. *Lancet 1*:1051–1056.

Bonvallet, M., and Gary Bobo, E. (1972). Changes in phrenic activity and hearing elicited by localized stimulation of amygdala and adjacent structures. *Electroenceph. Clin. Neurophysiol. 32*:1–16.

Brown, M. I., Huston, P. E., Hines, H. M., and Brown, G. W. (1953). Cardiovascular changes associated with electroconvulsive therapy in man. *Arch. Neurol. Psychiatr. 69*:601–608.

Ceremyzynski, L., Staszewska-Barczak, J.,and Herbaczynska-Cedra, K. (1969). Cardiac rhythm disturbances and the release of catecholamines after coronary occlusion in dogs. *Cardiovasc. Res. 3*:190–197.

Cleckley, H., Hamilton, W. P., Woodbury, R. A., and Volpitto, P. P. (1942). Blood pressure studies in patients undergoing convulsive therapy. *South. Med. J. 35*:37

Coulter, D. L. (1984). Partial seizures with apnea and bradycardia. *Arch Neurol. 41*:173–174.

DeSilva, R. A. (1982). Central nervous sytem risk factors for sudden cardiac death. *Annals of New York Academy of Sciences*, Vol. 382, New York Academy of Sciences, New York, pp. 143–161.

Doba, N., Beresford, J. R., and Reis, J. (1975). Changes in regional blood flow and cardiodynamics associated with electrically and clinically induced epilepsy in the cat. *Brain Res. 90*:115–132.

Fenichel, G. M., Olson, B. J., and Fitzpatrick, J. E. (1980). Heart rate changes in convulsive and nonconvulsive neonatal apnea. *Ann. Neurol. 7*:577–582.

Hahn, F. (1960). Analeptics. *Pharmacol. Rev. 12*:447–530.

Hildebrandt, E. (1937). Pentamethylenetetrazol (Cardiazol). *Handb. exp. pharmacol. 5*:151–183.

Hirsch, C. S., and Martin, D. L. (1971). Unexpected death in young epileptics. *Neurology 21*:682–690.

Jay, G. W., and Leestma, J. E. (1981). Sudden death in epilepsy. A comprehensive review of the literature and proposed mechanisms. *Acta Neurol. Scand. (Suppl. 82) 63*:1–66.

Katz, R. I., Tiger, M., and Harner, R. N. (1983). Epileptic cardiac arrhythmia: Sinoatrial arrest in two patients. *Epilepsia 24*:248.

Koppel, B. S., Pearl, M., and Perla, E. (1987). Epileptic seizures as a cause of unilateral pulmonary edema. *Epilepsia 28*(1):41–44.

Krohn, W. (1963). Causes of death among epileptics. *Epilepsia 4*:315–321.

Lathers, C. M., and Lipka, L. J. (1987). Cardiac arrhythmia, sudden death and psychoactive agents. *J. Clin. Pharmacol. 27*:1–14.

Lathers, C. M., and Schraeder, P. L. (1982). Autonomic dysfunction in epilepsy: Characterization of cardiac neural discharge associated with pentylenetetrazol-induced seizures. *Epilepsia 23*:633–647.

Lathers, C. M., and Schraeder, P. L. (1987). Review of autonomic dysfunction, cardiac arrhythmias, and epileptogenic activity. *J. Clin. Pharmacol. 27*:346–356.

Lathers, C. M., Schraeder, P. L., and Weiner, F. L. (1987). Synchronization of cardiac autonomic neural discharge with epileptogenic activity: The lockstep phenomenon. *Electroenceph. Clin. Neurophysiol. 67*:247–259.

Leestma, J. E., and Koenig, K. L. (1968). Sudden death and phenothiazines: A current controversy. *Arch. Gen. Psychiatr. 18*:137–148.

Leestma, J. E., Kalelkar, M. B., Teas, S. S., Jay, G. W., and Hughes, J. R. (1984). Sudden unexpected death associated with seizures. Analysis of 66 cases. *Epilepsia 25*:84–88.

Lipka, L. J., and Lathers, C. M. (1987). Psychoactive agents, seizure production, and sudden death in epilepsy. *J. Clin. Pharmacol. 27*:169–183.

Logothetis, J. (1967). Spontaneous epileptic seizures and electroencephalographic changes in the course of phenothiazine therapy. *Neurology 17*:869–877.

Mameli, P., Mameli, O., Tolu, E., Padua, G., Giraudi, D., Caria, M. A., and Melis, F. (1988). Neurogenic myocardial arrhythmias in experimental focal epilepsy. *Epilepsia 29*:74–82.

Marshall, D. W., Westmoreland, B. F., and Sharbrough, F. W. (1983). Ictal tachycardia during temporal lobe seizures. *Mayo Clin. Proc. 58*:443–446.

McKenna, G., Engle, R. P., Brooks, H., Dalent, J. (1970). Cardiac arrhythmias during electroshock therapy: Significance, prevention and treatment. *Am. J. Psychiatr. 127*:530–533.

Milnor, W. R. (1974). The cardiovascular control system. In *Medical Phys*, V. B. Montcastle (Ed.). C. V. Mosby, St. Louis, pp. 958–983.

Mosier, J. W., White, P., Grant, P., Fisher, J. E., and Taylor, R. (1957). Cerebroautonomic and myographic changes accompanying induced seizures. *Neurology 7*:204–210.

Oliver, A. P., Hoffer, B. J., and Wyatt, R. J. (1977). The hippocampal slice: A system for studying the pharmacology of seizures and for screening anticonvulsive drugs. *Epilepsia 18*:543–548.

Penfield, W., and Jasper, H. (1954). Summary of clinical analysis and seizure patterns. In *Epilepsy and the Functional Anatomy of Human Brain*. Little, Brown, Boston, pp. 830–831.

Pool, R. (1989). Is it healthy to be chaotic? *Science 243*:604–607.

Schraeder, P. L. (1987). Adult respiratory distress syndrome (ARDS) associated with nonconvulsive status epilepticus. *Epilepsia 28*:605.

Schraeder, P. L., and Lathers, C. M. (1983). Cardiac neural discharge and epileptogenic activity in the cat: An animal model for unexplained sudden death. *LIFE Sciences 32*:1371-1382.

Simon, R. P., Bayne, L. L., Tranbaugh, R. F., and Lewis, F. R. (1982). Elevated pulmonary flow and protein content during status epilepticus in sheep. *J. Appl. Physiol. 52*:91-95.

Stone, W. E. (1972). In *Experimental Models of Epilepsy: A Manual for the Laboratory Worker*. D. P. Purpura, J. K. Penry, D. Tower, D. Woodbury, and R. Walters (Eds.). Raven Press, New York, pp. 407-422.

Stauffer, A. Z., Dodd-o, J., and Lathers, C. M. (1989). The relationship of the lockstep phenomenon and precipitous changes in mean arterial blood pressure. *Electroenceph. Clin. Neurophysiol. 72*:340-345.

Terrence, C. E., Rao, G. R., and Pepper, J. A. (1981). Neurogenic pulmonary edema in unexpected, unexplained death in epileptic patients. *Neurology 25*: 594-595.

Toman, J. E. P., and Davis, J. P. (1949). The effects of drugs upon the electrical activity of the brain. *Pharmacol. Rev. 1*:425-492.

Van Buren, J. M. (1958). Some autonomic concomitants of ictal automatism. *Brain 81*:505-528.

Van Buren, J. M., and Ajmone-Marsan, C. (1960). A correlation of autonomic and EEG components in temporal lobe epilepsy. *Arch. Neurol. 3*:683-703.

White, P. T., Grant, P., Mosier, J., and Craig, A. (1961). Changes in cerebral dynamics associated with seizures. *Neurology 11*:354-361.

9

Autonomic Dysfunction, Cardiac Arrhythmias, and Epileptogenic Activity

CLAIRE M. LATHERS* *The Medical College of Pennsylvania, Eastern Pennsylvania Psychiatric Institute, Philadelphia, Pennsylvania*

PAUL L. SCHRAEDER *University of Medicine and Dentistry of New Jersey, Robert Wood Johnson Medical School, Camden, New Jersey*

I. INTRODUCTION

Sudden unexplained death in epilepsy is a syndrome for which there is no single or usual explanation. Electrical instability of the heart may be the unifying mechanism for cardiac arrhythmia and sudden death. Contributing factors in the pathogenesis of cardiac sudden death include stress-related release of catecholamines (Lathers and Roberts, 1980); changes in platelet aggregation; arteriosclerotic coronary artery disease; cardiac pathology including rare myocardial tumors; embolism, rupture, or abnormalities in the structure of the AV junction; changes in the autonomic neural control of the heart; and cardiac arrhythmias (James, 1983). Potentially fatal changes in catecholamine release and the related consequence of alterations in the neural control of cardiac rhythm (Lathers et al., 1977, 1978) would not be detected at autopsy. The role of autonomic neural mechanisms in the development of cardiac arrhythmias in sudden death will be reviewed by comparing data obtained in four animal models: digitalis toxicity, coronary occlusion, experimental epilepsy, and the use of phenothiazines.

II. DIGITALIS TOXICITY AND CORONARY OCCLUSION

Ouabain was administered intravenously every 15 minutes until death in anesthetized cats with a right thoracotomy to record postganglionic cardiac sympathetic neural discharge (Lathers, 1980; Lathers et al., 1974, 1977). Neural discharge in the minute prior to the onset of arrhythmia was increased in one nerve,

---

Current affiliation: FDA, Rockville, Maryland.

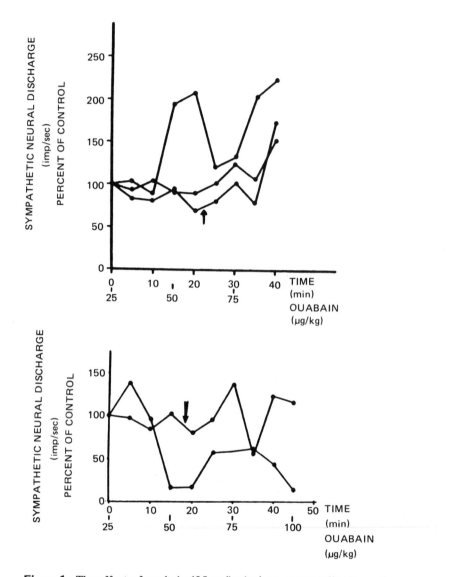

Figure 1   The effect of ouabain (25 μg/kg i.v.) on postganglionic cardiac sympathetic neural discharge (impulses/second). The data are graphed as a function of time in minutes. In the upper graph, two postganglionic cardiac nerves were monitored in one cat; in the lower graph, three nerves were monitored in another cat. [From Lathers (1980), reproduced with permission.]

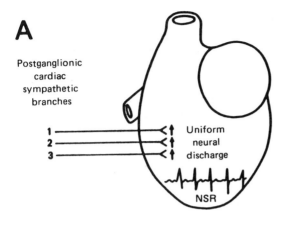

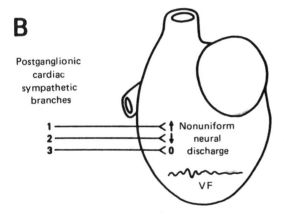

Figure 2 Postganglionic cardiac sympathetic neural discharge in three branches innervating the ventricle. (A) Nerve activity in all branches is enhanced (↑) above control and is designated a uniform neural discharge. (B) Never activity is increased in one branch (↑), decreased in a second (↓), and shows no change in a third (○); this trend is designated a nonuniform neural discharge. [From Lathers and Schraeder (1987), reproduced with permission.]

decreased in another, and decreased to a lesser extent in the third nerve (Figure 1, upper graph). Immediately prior to ouabain-induced arrhythmia, neural discharge was slightly increased in one postganglionic cardiac sympathetic nerve and depressed in the other when a second animal was examined (Figure 1, lower graph). This discharge pattern was designated nonuniform (Lathers, 1980; Lathers et al., 1974, 1977). When neural discharge in each of three postganglionic sympathetic branches was increased, this was a uniform neural discharge (Figure 2A). Discharge was also designated uniform when all neural activity was decreased or unchanged. The uniform postganglionic cardiac sympathetic neural discharge was hypothesized to be necessary at the cardiac myocardial junctions to maintain normal electrical excitability and automaticity, i.e., normal sinus rhythm. In contrast, a nonuniform neural discharge occurred when activity in one sympathetic branch was increased and that in a second was decreased, while discharge was not altered in a third (Figure 2B). Nonuniform neural discharge was hypothesized to be manifested in the heart as inhomogeneity of myocardial electrical excitability and conduction patterns, as demonstrated by Han and Moe (1964), who found that myocardial nonuniformity could cause ventricular arrhythmias, including ventricular fibrillation.

A second animal model used in our laboratory mimics the arrhythmias occurring in victims of sudden death due to acute myocardial infarction. An abrupt acute coronary occlusion of the left anterior descending coronary artery is done in anesthetized cats, resulting in nonuniform cardiac sympathetic neural discharge (Lathers, 1981; Lathers et al., 1978). The associated arrhythmia was suppressed by cardiac-selective beta-adrenergic blocking agents (Lathers and Spivey, 1987). These digitalis toxicity and coronary occlusion studies raised the question of whether the animal model of neural nonuniformity and arrhythmias could be developed to investigate experimental mechanisms of sudden unexplained death in persons with epilepsy.

III. EXPERIMENTAL EPILEPTOGENIC ACTIVITY

The model was designed to examine autonomic cardiac neural discharge and arrhythmias associated with epileptogenic activity since paroxysmal autonomic dysfunction is one possible explanation for sudden unexplained death in epilepsy (Terrence et al., 1975). To explore the possibility that altered autonomic function may be one factor, a study was designed using the anesthetized cat. Varying doses of pentylenetetrazol were used since this animal model of epilepsy is an established method to produce interictal and ictal epileptogenic activity (Hahn, 1960). The cardiovascular changes in blood pressure, heart rate, and ECG associated with interictal and ictal activity were examined to determine if alterations in interictal and ictal activity correlated with nonuniform cardiac autonomic neural discharge known to be associated with arrhythmia development. It was hypothesized that detection of arrhythmia with subconvulsant interictal activity would provide a possible explanation for the fact that some epileptic persons die unexpectedly during minimal clinical seizures or even without observed seizure activity; no pathological abnormalities are found on autopsy.

Pentylenetetrazol was administered every 10 minutes in doses which elicited one of three categories of epileptogenic activity. The first category was designated prolonged ictal activity and was characterized by polyspike discharges greater than 10 seconds in duration. The second was brief ictal activity, characterized by groups of polyspikes of less than 10 seconds duration. The third was designated interictal activity and characterized as spike or polyspike complexes occurring at a rate of about 1/second; the interictal activity was often interspersed between the prolonged and the brief ictal discharges. All types of epileptogenic activity were quantified. The interictal activity was counted as spikes per minute; both types of ictal activity were measured as duration of ictal discharges occurring each minute.

In eight of nine cats, the administration of 10 mg/kg pentylenetetrazol elicited only interictal activity. One of the nine cats exhibited prolonged ictal activity; another manifested no epileptogenic activity. The dose of 20 mg/kg pentylenetetrazol elicited ictal activity in most cats. With increasing doses of pentylenetetrazol, the amount of interictal activity decreased and the duration of ictal activity was increased, with maximum duration of ictal activity occurring after doses of 100 or 200 mg/kg pentylenetetrazol (PTZ).

Interictal activity elicited by 10 mg/kg PTZ was associated with a brief but significant decrease in the mean heart rate lasting for one minute; little or no change in heart rate was noted thereafter. Little change in heart rate occurred with the development of interictal and/or ictal activity developing after 20 mg/kg PTZ. However, as epileptogenic activity increased following higher doses of pentylenetetrazol, the heart rate was significantly increased. Likewise, the mean arterial blood pressure was significantly elevated with the occurrence of interictal discharge; this trend continued as epileptogenic activity increased. Although the initial injection of each dose of pentylenetetrazol caused a decrease in mean arterial blood pressure, the overall response was an increase.

Interictal activity elicited by 10 mg/kg PTZ was associated with a variety of changes in the electrocardiogram, including alterations in the P, T, and Q waves and in the QRS complexes; ventricular tachycardia; and, in one animal, a premature ventricular contraction. With increasing degrees of both interictal and ictal activity, the number of animals exhibiting the foregoing electrocardiogram changes increased, with some additional animals exhibiting premature atrial contractions. The total number of animals exhibiting premature ventricular contractions increased with increasing duration of epileptogenic activity.

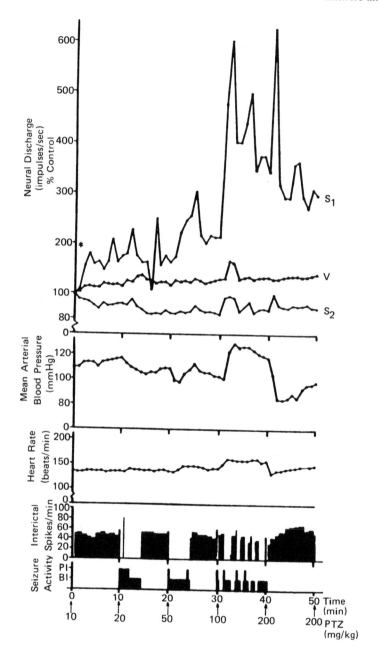

Data from one animal are illustrated in Figure 3. Interictal discharge elicited with the 10 mg/kg dose of PTZ was associated with an increase in the mean arterial blood pressure. However, the sympathetic response was atypical in that the neural discharge in one of the sympathetic nerves was decreased, while that in a second nerve was increased. The expected physiological response for all sympathetic neural discharge would be changed in the same direction. For contrast, a typical physiological sympathetic neural response is depicted in Figure 4. During the control period of each experiment, prior to the induction of epileptogenic activity and the associated changes in the electrocardiogram, a test dose of 5 μg/kg of histamine was administered intravenously. The injection of histamine caused the blood pressure in the cat to fall, with a concomitant increase in the sympathetic neural discharge in both branches. As the blood pressure returned to the prehistamine level, the sympathetic discharge in both branches was decreased. This response was always obtained in all postganglionic sympathetic branches during the control period. However, as depicted in Figure 3, when the blood pressure increased with the onset of interictal activity after the administration of 10 mg/kg PTZ, the neural discharge in only one sympathetic nerve decreased. Discharge in the second nerve increased. This is an example of autonomic dysfunction in the discharge of the cardiac sympathetic nerves. The asterisk in Figure 3 marks the occurrence of autonomic sympathetic neural dysfunction associated with an alteration in the T wave amplitude and the P–R interval in the electrocardiogram.

These experimental animal data provide a possible pathophysiological explanation for sudden autonomic dysfunction in individuals who had no observed clinical seizure and only seizures of minimal severity proceding their demise (Hirsch and Martin, 1971; Iivananien and Lehtinen, 1979; Jay and Leestma,

---

Figure 3 Autonomic cardiac neural discharge and epileptogenic activity as a function of time (minutes) for the data obtained in one cat. Neural discharge (impulses/second, percentage of control) is illustrated for two postganglionic cardiac sympathetic branches (S_1, S_2) and for the vagus nerve (V) in the first graph. Mean arterial blood (mm Hg) and heart rate (bpm) are illustrated as a function of time in the second and the third graphs from the top, respectively. Interictal activity in spikes/minute is illustrated in the fourth graph and the duration of ictal activity (prolonged ictal, solid boxes; brief ictal, crosshatched boxes) in seconds is seen in the bottom graph. The arrows along the abscissa indicate injections of PTZ 10, 20, 50, 100, 200, and 2000 mg/kg i.v., which were given every 10 minutes. The asterisk indicates the first occurrence of a change in the ECG. [From Lathers and Schraeder (1982), reproduced with permssion.]

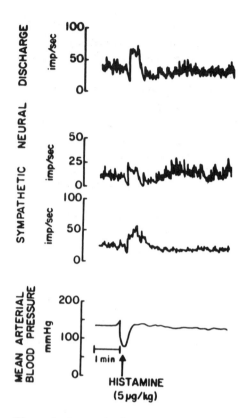

Figure 4 Sympathetic neural discharge (upper two panels) and the mean arterial blood pressure response monitored in one cat. The arrow indicates the injection of histamine (5 μg/kg i.v.). [From Lathers and Schraeder (1987), reproduced with permission.]

1981; Spratling, 1902; Terrence et al., 1975; Zielinski, 1974). Our data suggest that from time to time, interictal nonconvulsive activity may be associated with cardiac neural dysfunction with consequent abnormalities of conduction and rhythm, making certain persons with epilepsy susceptible to developing fatal arrhythmias. The cardiac neural and cardiovascular alterations were also observed, as might be expected, with ictal activity and at the time of death (Lathers and Schraeder, 1987).

Mean parasympathetic and sympathetic neural discharge for all animals were calculated. An increase in the standard deviation of mean parasympathetic neural discharge occurred with the onset of interictal discharge. The development of increasing degrees of epileptogenic activity was associated with a further increase in the standard deviation. By definition, a large standard deviation of the mean indicates that there is large range among the values included within the mean. Thus the neural discharge in some nerves was increased above control, whereas that in others was decreased or showed little or no change. These changes demonstrated autonomic dysfunction within the parasympathetic division. A very large standard deviation was also seen in the mean sympathetic neural discharge, although it did not occur until after the large standard deviation developed in the mean parasympathetic discharge. Thus there was autonomic dysfunction within both the parasympathetic and the sympathetic divisions of the autonomic nervous system and in an imbalance between the two divisions.

Two earlier studies (Onuma, 1957; Orihara, 1952) examined the effect of subconvulsive or convulsive doses of pentylenetetrazol on cervical sympathetic and parasympathetic autonomic discharge. Increases and/or decreases in the neural discharge within both divisions of the autonomic nervous system occurred, as observed for the autonomic cardiac nerves in our studies. Onuma (1957) emphasized that sympathetic neural activity was hyperexcited and that increased ictal activity was associated with an imbalance between the sympathetic and parasympathetic discharge. This evidence supports our findings for the cardiac autonomic nerves.

Schraeder and Celesia (1977) reported that even minimal subclinical interictal epileptogenic activity had a wide-ranging effect on cerebral function, as monitored from the auditory cortex of the cat. We theorized that if the recorded interictal activity found in our study were likewise to have an effect on regions of the cerebrum involved in autonomic regulation, an autonomic imbalance in cardiac neural discharge and arrhythmias might occur. These changes could be one factor contributing to sudden unexplained death in the epileptic patient.

The question of whether a pharmacologic agent could be found to eliminate the autonomic cardiac neural discharge dysfunction and the associated arrhythmia was raised. Phenytoin (Gillis et al., 1971; Roberts, 1970; Schlosser et al., 1975) and chlordiazepoxide (Schallek and Zabransky, 1966) both had been shown to depress cardiac sympathetic neural discharge and to abolish cardiac arrhythmias (Evans and Gillis, 1974, 1975; Gillis, 1969; Gillis et al., 1971, 1972, 1974; Pace and Gillis, 1976; Raines et al., 1970). We hypothesized that the pharmacologic agent which would provide the best protection against the autonomic dysfunction associated with the epileptogenic activity is one that exhibits anticonvulsant, antiarrhythmic, and cardiac neural depressant activity (Lathers and Schraeder, 1982). Since phenobarbital has both anticonvulsant and antiarrhythmic properties, it was decided to examine this agent in our experimental model. Phenobarbital caused a significant depression of sympathetic neural discharge and a fall in the mean arterial blood pressure prior to the administration of PTZ; this change in the sympathetic neural discharge was the opposite of the predicted response to a fall in blood pressure. Neural depression

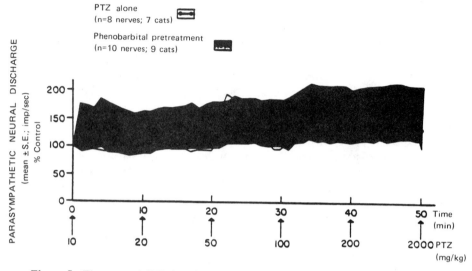

Figure 5 The mean ± S.E. for the parasympathetic neural discharge monitored in seven cats (8 nerves) receiving only pentylenetetrazol is depicted by a white area that became black when the values overlapped with those obtained in the phenobarbital group. The data obtained in only the nine cats (10 nerves) pretreated with phenobarbital prior to the administration of pentylenetetrazol are depicted by the gray area. [From Lathers and Schraeder (1987), reproduced with permission.]

continued for the next 70 minutes. In contrast, phenobarbital did not significantly alter the parasympathetic neural discharge from control. A comparison of the parasympathetic neural discharge monitored in those animals pretreated with phenobarbital and those receiving only pentylenetetrazol found no significant difference in the standard errors of the mean (Figure 5). The sympathetic neural discharge monitored after the administration of pentylenetetrazol in the animals pretreated with phenobarbitol did not differ from that monitored in cats receiving only pentylenetetrazol (Figure 6).

An anticonvulsant effect was obtained since phenobarbital prevented the interictal subconvulsant epileptogenic activity elicited by PTZ 10 mg/kg and shifted the dose response curve to the right. In general, the duration of ictal activity was decreased by phenobarbital. Phenobarbital did not exhibit an antiarrhythmic effect; the incidence of cardiac arrhythmias and the types of arrhythmias were the same in animals with and without phenobarbital pretreatment. Phenobarbital did not modify parasympathetic neural discharge, although it initially depressed the sympathetic discharge. As the pentylenetetrazol induced

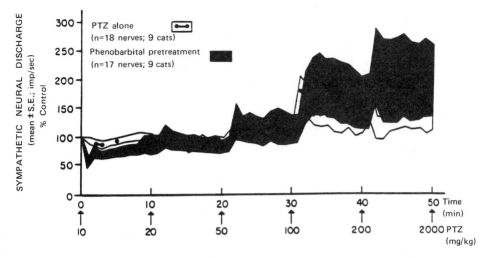

Figure 6 The mean ± S.E. for the sympathetic neural discharge monitored in nine cats (18 nerves) receiving only pentylenetetrazol is depicted by the white area; values in this group overlapping those obtained for the nine cats (17 nerves) pretreated with phenobarbital are designated by the black area. Areas depicting only values from the phenobarbital group are designated by the gray area. [From Lathers and Schraeder (1987), reproduced with permission.]

epileptogenic activity, there was no significant difference between the two groups. These data suggest that phenobarbital is not the ideal agent for the prevention of autonomic neural dysfunction and cardiac arrhythmias associated with epileptogenic activity.

IV. SOME POSSIBLE MECHANISMS FOR AUTONOMIC DYSFUNCTION AND SUDDEN DEATH IN EPILEPTIC PERSONS

A. The Lockstep Phenomenon

Lathers and colleagues first described the finding that cardiac sympathetic and vagal neural discharges were intermittently synchronized 1:1 with epileptogenic discharge, i.e., the lockstep phenomenon (LSP), in 1983. This relationship was designated as real when it was locked 1:1 and semilocked when the relationship was almost 1:1. The abnormal cardiac neural discharge and cardiac arrhythmias were associated with subconvulsant interictal activity and thus it was suggested that if sudden cardiac arrhythmias are a cause of sudden unexpected death, then the LSP may be a factor in the mechanism of unexplained death in persons with epilepsy who exhibited no overt seizure activity at the time of demise (Lathers et al., 1987). Stauffer et al. (1988) found that a higher mean proportion of time was spent in precipitous changes in blood pressure, i.e., < 23 mm Hg in a 10-second interval, in association with an unstable LSP pattern. An unstable LSP pattern was defined as all time intervals of 10 seconds or more during which the LSP existed but the interspike intervals were not constant. Dodd-o and Lathers (Chapter 13, this book) also noted that when stable LSP was lost, both precipitous mean arterial blood pressure changes and the incidence of ECG changes occurred more frequently. They suggested that development of the abnormal rhythmic activity of the unstable LSP may alter neurotransmitter release and initiate autonomic dysfunction, thereby having a possible contributory role in sudden unexplained death in epileptic persons.

In another study Lathers and Schraeder (Chapter 12, this book) found no direct correlation between the occurrence of LSP and the appearance of abnormalities in the ECG. They noted the importance of central neuronal outflow in altering the peripheral efferent discharge to the heart and that efferent sympathetic discharge can initiate abnormalities in the ECG (Lathers et al., 1977, 1978). It was suggested that the development of the LSP may precede the occurrence of changes in the ECG or vice versa. All of these LSP studies (Dodd-o and Lathers, Chapter 13, this book; Lathers et al., 1983, 1987; Lathers and Schraeder, Chapter 12, this book; Stauffer et al., 1988) suggest that at least four mechanisms can be postulated through which LSP may be related to arrhythmia and sudden death in persons with epilepsy:

1. Excessive stimulation of an electrically unstable heart previously damaged.
2. The occurrence of nonuniform postganglionic cardiac sympathetic discharge or an imbalance between the sympathetic and parasympathetic neural innervation of the heart.
3. Sinus arrest and bradycardia associated with seizures and induced by the parasympathetic nervous system.
4. The development of precipitous blood pressure changes. Definitive experiments will have to be done to verify these possibilities.

B. Simultaneous Electroencephalogram and Electrocardiogram in Humans

The clinical relevance of our data is emphasized by the findings of McLeod and Jewitt (1978). Through the use of 24-hour continuous electrocardiogram monitoring, 300 patients are not selected for suspected epilepsy were screened. Of these patients, 36% exhibited major arrhythmias, many of which were ominous. The observation that these arrhythmias were found in asymptomatic patients is important since it strengthens the hypothesis that neurally induced autonomic arrhythmias may be a contributory mechanism in the sudden unexplained deaths in persons with epilepsy. Schott et al. (1977) studied patients with suspected idiopathic epilepsy, four of whom had abnormalities on routine 12-lead electrocardiograms. None of the patients had any cardiac symptoms and only one had a transient focal abnormality in the EEG. However, after prolonged continuous electrocardiographic monitoring, these patients manifested cardiac arrhythmias. Treatment with antiarrhythmic agents or the installation of a pacemaker eliminated the seizures. It was concluded that treatable cardiac arrhythmias may underlie epilepsy more often than is generally recognized and it was suggested that physicians consider the possibility that cardiac arrhythmias occasionally mimic epilepsy.

Based on their experimental animal data, Schraeder and Lathers (1983) suggested that there may be interindividual variability in susceptibility to arrhythmias, so that a smaller, as yet unidentified group of persons at risk is more susceptible to autonomic dysfunction induced by epileptogenic activity. They suggested that the autonomic dysfunction observed in association with even minimal epileptogenic activity produced cardiac arrhythmias that could contribute to sudden unexplained death in the epileptic population. The suggestion that interindividual variability may be a factor in explaining susceptibility to arrhythmias was recently documented in two studies in humans (Blumhardt and Oozeer, 1982; Keilson et al., 1987). Blumhardt and Oozeer (1982) noted that simultaneous EEG and ECG recordings from patients with established epilepsy have demonstrated the occurrence of nonepileptic and epileptic events on the same tape. They emphasized that the negative findings obtained in some patients must be cautiously interpreted and the outcome established by long-term follow-up studies. Only a few patients had a clear ECG or EEG abnormality accounting for the symptoms of repeated episodes of disturbed consciousness for which no diagnosis had been established by routine methods. They concluded that simultaneous recordings of ECG and EEG are of initial value in the clinical workup of patients with unexplained attacks but emphasized that unequivocally positive diagnostic records will be obtained only in a minority of patients. This is true because attacks generally occur with such widely varying frequencies that a high detection rate cannot be expected, even if recordings are extended for periods of up to a week in duration. Nonetheless, their study did find some patients with ECG and EEG abnormalities.

Ambulatory monitoring of the ECG and the EEG in 338 consecutive patients with epilepsy for 20–24 hours, including an overnight sleep period, detected high-risk (based on historical potential for sudden death) cardiac arrhythmias in 18 (5.3%) patients (Keilson et al., 1987). It was concluded that the incidence of serious cardiac arrhythmias predisposing to sudden death is not increased in patients with epilepsy but is similar to the incidence reported for the nonepileptic population. The finding of 5.3% epileptic persons with high-risk arrhythmias in this study is very important since the study showed that some epileptic persons are more susceptible to autonomic dysfunction and the development of serious arrhythmias. The occurrence of these arrhythmias may place these particular epileptic persons at risk for sudden death. Furthermore, the identical incidence of cardiac arrhythmias in both groups suggests that adding epilepsy to benign arrhythmias may increase the risk of transformation to a mortal arrhythmia at some time.

C. Role of Stress in Sudden Death in Epileptic Persons

Another possible explanation for the development of arrhythmias and epileptogenic activity is the role of stress. Induced psychological stress in animals may lead to myocardial degeneration and sudden death. Monkeys subjected to electric shock developed bradyarrhythmia and death in asystole (Corley et al., 1975). Pigs, on the other hand, developed ventricular tachyarrhythmias rather than asystole (Johanssen et al., 1974). Stress induced in rats was found to be associated with microthrombic and myocardial necrosis (Haft, 1979). In other studies using experimental coronary arterial occlusion in dogs (Corbalon et al., 1974) and pigs (Skinner et al.,1975), it was found that tachyarrhythmias occurred more readily when the animals were also subjected to the stress of an unfamiliar adverse environment as compared to a familiar or comfortable environment. The importance of environmental stress in the person with epilepsy is obvious, since stress is an ongoing factor in the lives of these individuals. Stress may contribute both to the induction of seizures (Feldman and Paul, 1976; Friis and Lund, 1974) and to the induction of autonomic dysfunction centrally, which, in turn, may modify cardiac peripheral neural discharge and produce the cardiac arrhythmias that may be fatal.

When considering central mechanisms such as stress which may be involved in the production of arrhythmias, one must also realize that a patient taking nonepileptic drugs may also be predisposed to the development of arrhythmias. For example, phenothiazines are associated with the phenomenon of sudden unexplained death in psychiatric patients (Leestma and Koenig, 1968) and individuals with epilepsy often are treated with phenothiazines as part of the management of psychiatric symptoms. Several studies (Lathers and Lipka, 1986; Lathers et al., 1986) examined the effect of the infusion of chlorpromazine or thioridazine on the heart rate, blood pressure, and electrocardiogram in the cat. As the drugs were infused, the heart rate was depressed and the mean arterial blood pressure fell. Associated changes in the electrocardiogram included a loss of the P wave, the occurrence of premature ventricular contractions, and ventricular fibrillation. Thus these agents have the potential to modify the autonomic parameters of blood pressure, heart rate, and the electrocardiogram. The question of whether the potential for phenothiazines to induce cardiovascular autonomic dysfunction means that the use of phenothiazines in individuals is a factor in sudden unexplained death remains to be answered. The reader is referred to a recent review of this topic (Lipka and Lathers, 1987). The definitive answer to this question remains to be discerned.

D. Central Biochemical Changes Associated with Epileptogenic Activity

A number of central biochemical mechanisms may contribute to or explain, in part, the development of cardiac arrhythmias in association with the epileptogenic activity that may ultimately induce sudden unexplained death in some epileptic persons. In the recent study of Lathers et al. (1988) (D-Ala^2)methionine-enkephalinamide (DAME, 500 μg/kg) was given intracerebroventricularly (i.c.v.) to nine cats anesthetized with alpha-chloralose. Epileptogenic activity and hypotension occurred in all cats (maximum fall ranging from 6 to 46 mm Hg; duration of 6-35 minutes). In six cats the heart rate decreased, in two it increased, and in one it showed little or no change. The duration of heart rate changes varied from 18 to 76 minutes. Naloxone (100 μg/kg) was given intravenously (i.v.) to six cats after DAME. Naloxone suppressed or abolished the epileptogenic activity in all six cats, reversed the DAME-induced hypotension and increased the heart rate in three cats, decreased it in two, and produced no change in one. These results indicate that DAME may produce epileptogenic activity and cardiovascular changes through an action on central opiate receptors.

Possible mechanisms involved in the development of cardiac arrhythmias and/ or sudden unexplained death in some epileptic patients are summarized in Figure 7 (Kraras et al., 1987; Lathers et al., 1988). Enkephalins injected into the central nervous system elicit seizure activity (Frenk et al., 1978; Snead, 1983). Pentylenetetrazol increased enkephalin levels in the amygdala and the hippocampal, septal, and hypothalamic areas (Vindrola et al., 1983). It may be that the PTZ-induced increases in central enkephalin levels within the autonomic center of the hypothalamus inhibited the release of gamma aminobutyric acid (GABA) and thus led to the production of epileptogenic activity and autonomic dysfunction in the experiments of Lathers and Schraeder (1982). The central roles of GABA and neuropeptides are discussed in detail in Chapters 17 and 18 of this book.

That the cardiac neural dysfunction and arrhythmias occurring in association with epileptogenic activity is due, at least in part, to modification of centrally mediated neural control of cardiac rhythm was demonstrated by the study of Evans and Gillis (1975). The posterior region of the hypothalamus of the cat was stimulated every five minutes; cardioacceleration increased postganglionic sympathetic neural discharge, and an increase in blood pressure was elicited. In the control period, stimulation of the hypothalamus increased sympathetic discharge

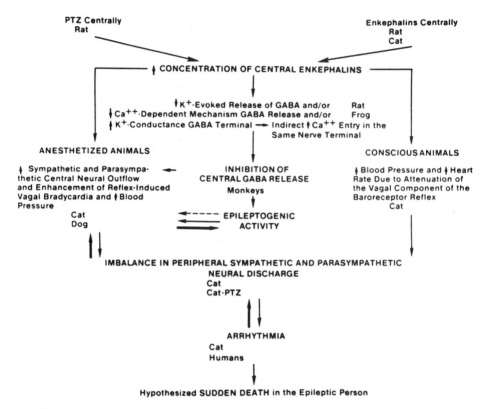

Figure 7 Hypothesized biochemical and autonomic mechanisms involved in the development of cardiac arrhythmias and/or sudden unexplained death in persons with epilepsy. [From Lathers et al. (1988), reproduced with permission.]

but did not elicit arrhythmia; i.e., this was a subarrhythmogenic stimulus. When stimulation was repeated in the presence of a low dose of ouabain, a neural depressant effect occurred but arrhythmia did not develop. When the hypothalamus was again stimulated in the presence of a higher dose of ouabain, there was an increase in sympathetic neural discharge and subsequent changes in the electrocardiogram. These data demonstrate that central autonomic centers within the hypothalamus can modify peripheral cardiac nerve impulses to the heart and produce arrhythmias.

V. SUMMARY

Similarities in autonomic dysfunction associated with arrhythmias and death in animal models for digitalis toxicity, myocardial infarction, psychotropic toxicity, and epileptogenic activity are reviewed. Pertinent points discussed in this chapter include the fact that central autonomic dysfunction may elicit or may be elicited by either interictal or ictal epileptogenic activity. That changes in peripheral cardiac sympathetic or parasympathetic neural discharge are associated with the epileptogenic activity and may produce arrhythmia were discussed (Carnel et al., 1985; Kraras et al., 1987; Lathers and Schraeder, 1982, 1987; Lathers et al., 1984, 1987; Schraeder and Lathers, 1983, 1988; Suter and Lathers, 1984). When pentylenetetrazol (i.v.) was given to anesthetized cats, autonomic dysfunction was associated with both interictal and ictal epileptogenic activity. The autonomic dysfunction was manifested by the fact that autonomic cardiac nerves did not always respond in a predictable manner to changes in blood pressure; the development of a marked increase in variability in mean autonomic cardiac nerve discharge; and the appearance of a very large increase in the variability of the discharge rate of parasympathetic nerves first and in sympathetic discharge second. The altered autonomic cardiac nerve discharge was associated with interictal epileptogenic activity and arrhythmias, which may contribute to sudden unexplained death in epileptics. It may well be that various changes—pathological, neurophysiological, biochemical, and pharmacological— at times interact in a manner that is unfortunate for the patients with epilepsy.

As summarized by James (1983), given the fact that the nerves to the heart have such an important function in both normal and abnormal cardiac activity, it is surprising that they have received so little attention in postmortem studies. James suggested that the condition of the intracardiac nerves and the autonomic ganglia should be investigated routinely during autopsy.

The animal model described may be used to screen for new anticonvulsant agents which also prevent the autonomic neural dysfunction and cardiac arrhythmias. Since phenobarbital (20 mg/kg i.v., 60 minutes prior to PTZ) exhibited anticonvulsant but not antiarrhythmic and neural depressant activity, the antiepileptic drug does not appear to be a useful agent to prevent the autonomic dysfunction associated with epileptogenic activity in this animal model.

ACKNOWLEDGMENT

The original research was funded by NIH Grant BRSGRR-4518, a grant from the Epilepsy Foundation of America, and NIH Grant HL13666.

REFERENCES

Blumhardt, L. D., and Oozeer, R. (1982). Simultaneous ambulatory monitoring of the EEG and ECG in patients with unexplained transient disturbances of consciousness. In *Proceedings of the 4th International Gent 1981 Symposium on Ambulatory Monitoring and the Second Gent Workshop on Blood Pres-*

sure Variability, F. D. Stott, E. B. Raferty, D. L. Clement, and S. L. Wright (Eds.). Academic Press, New York, pp. 171–182.

Carnel, S. B., Schraeder, P. L., and Lathers, C. M. (1985). Effect of phenobarbital pretreatment on cardiac neural discharge and pentylenetetrazol-induced epileptogenic activity in the cat. *Pharmacology 30*:225–240.

Corbalon, R., Verrier, R. L., and Lown, B. (1974). Psychological stress and ventricular arrhythmia during myocardial infarction in conscious dog. *Am. J. Cardiol. 34*:692–696.

Corley, K. C., Mauck, H. P., and Shiel, F. O. (1975). Cardiac responses associated with "yoked-chair" shock avoidance. *Psychophysiology 12*:439.

Evans, D. E., and Gillis, R. A. (1974). Effect of diphenylhydantoin and lidocaine on cardiac arrhythmias induced by hypothalamic stimulation. *J. Pharmacol. Exp. Ther. 191*:506–517.

Evans, D. E., and Gillis, R. A. (1975). Effect of ouabain and its interaction with diphenylhydantoin on cardiac arrhythmias induced by hypothalamic stimulation. *J. Pharmacol. Exp. Ther. 195*:577–586.

Feldman, R. G., and Paul, N. L. (1976). Identity of emotional triggers in epilepsy. *J. Nerv. Ment. Dis. 162*:345–353.

Frenck, H., Urca, G., and Liebeskind, J. C. (1978). Epileptic properties of leucine- and methionine-enkephalin: Comparison with morphine and reversibility by naloxone. *Brain Res. 147*:327–337.

Friis, M. L., and Lund, M. (1974). Stress convulsions. *Arch. Neurol. 31*:155–159.

Gillis, R. A. (1969). Cardiac sympathetic nerve activity: Changes induced by ouabain and propranolol. *Science 66*:508–510.

Gillis, R. A., McClellan, J. R., Sauer, T. S., and Standaert, F. G. (1971). Depression of cardiac nerve activity by diphenylhydantoin. *J. Pharmacol. Exp. Ther. 179*:599–610.

Gillis, R. A., Raines, A., Sohn, Y. J., Levitt, B., and Standaert, F. G. (1972). Neuroexcitatory effects of digitalis and their role in the development of cardiac arrhythmias. *J. Pharmacol. Exp. Ther. 183*:154–168.

Gillis, R. A., Thibodeaux, H., and Barr, L. (1974). Antiarrhythmic properties of chlordiazepoxide. *Circulation 49*:272–282.

Haft, J. I. (1979). Role of platelets on coronary artery disease. *Am. J. Cardiol. 4*:1197–1206.

Hahn, F. (1960). Analeptics. *Pharmacol. Rev. 12*:447–530.

Han, J., and Moe, G. K. (1964). Nonuniform recovery of excitability in ventricular muscle. *Circ. Res. 14*:44–60.

Hirsch, C. S., and Martin, D. L. (1971). Unexpected death in young epileptics. *Neurology 21*:682–690.

Iivanainen, M., and Lehtinen, J. (1979). Causes of death in institutionalized epileptics. *Epilepsia 20*:485–491.

James, T. N. (1983). Chance and sudden death. *J. Am. Coll. Cardiol. 1*:164–183.

Jay, G. W., and Leestma, J. E. (1981). Sudden death in epilepsy. A comprehensive review of the literature and proposed mechanisms. *Acta Neurol. Scand. (Suppl. 82):63*:1–66.

Johanssen, G., Jonsson, L., Lanneck, N., Blomgren, L., Lindberg, P., and Poupa, O. (1974). Severe stress-cardiopathy in pigs. *Am. Heart J. 87*:451–457.

Keilson, M. J., Hauser, W. A., Magrill, J. P., and Goldman, M. (1987). ECG abnormalities in patients with epilepsy. *Neurology 37*:1624–1626.

Kraras, C. M., Tumer, N., and Lathers, C. M. (1987). The role of enkephalins in the production of epileptogenic activity and autonomic dysfunction: Origin of arrhythmia and sudden death in the epileptic patient? *Med. Hypotheses 23*:19–31.

Lathers, C. M. (1980). Effect of timolol on postganglionic cardiac and preganglionic splanchnic sympathetic neural discharge associated with ouabain-induced arrhythmia. *Eur. J. Pharmacol. 64*:95–106.

Lathers, C. M. (1981). Models for studying sequelae to "Induced Myocardial Infarction." In *Mammalian Models for Research on Aging*, National Academy Press, Washington, D.C., pp. 224–228.

Lathers, C. M., and Lipka, L. J. (1986). Chlorpromazine: Cardiac arrhythmogenicity in the cat. *Life Sci. 38*:521–538.

Lathers, C., and Roberts, J. (1980). Minireview: Digitalis cardiotoxicity revisited. *Life Sci. 27*:1713–1733.

Lathers, C. M., and Schraeder, P. L. (1982). Autonomic dysfunction in epilepsy: Characterization of autonomic cardiac neural discharge associated with pentylenetetrazol-induced epileptogenic activity. *Epilepsia 23*:633–647.

Lathers, C. M., and Schraeder, P. L. (1987). Review of autonomic dysfunction, cardiac arrhythmias, and epileptogenic activity. *J. Clin. Pharmacol. 27*:346–356.

Lathers, C. M., and Spivey, W. H. (1987). The effect of timolol, metroprolol, and practolol on postganglionic cardiac neural discharge associated with acute coronary occlusion-induced arrhythmia. *J. Clin. Pharmacol. 27*:582–592.

Lathers, C. M., Roberts, J., and Kelliher, G. J. (1974). Relationship between the effect of ouabain on arrhythmia and interspike intervals (I.S.I.) of cardiac accelerator nerves. *Pharmacologist 16*:201.

Lathers, C. M., Roberts, J., and Kelliher, G. J. (1977). Correlation of ouabain-induced arrhythmia and nonuniformity in the histamine-evoked discharge of cardiac sympathetic nerves. *J. Pharmacol. Exp. Therap. 203*:467–479.

Lathers, C. M., Kelliher, G. J., Roberts, J., and Beasley, A. B. (1978). Nonuniform cardiac sympathetic nerve discharge. *Circulation 57*:1058–1064.

Lathers, C. M., Weiner, F. L., and Schraeder, P. L. (1983). Synchronization of cardiac autonomic neural discharge with epileptogenic activity: The locked-step phenomenon. *Circ. Res. 31*:630A.

Lathers, C. M., Schraeder, P. L., and Carnel, S. B. (1984). Neural mechanisms in cardiac arrhythmias associated with epileptogenic activity: The effect of phenobarbital in the cat. *Life Sci. 34*:1919–1936.

Lathers, C. M., Flax, R., and Lipka, L. J. (1986). The effect of C_1 spinal cord transection or bilateral adrenal vein ligation on thioridazine-induced arrhythmia in the cat. *J. Clin. Pharmacol. 26*:515–523.

Lathers, C. M., Schraeder, P. L., and Weiner, F. L. (1987). Synchronization of cardiac autonomic neural discharge with epileptogenic activity: The lockstep phenomenon. *Electroencephalogr. Clin. Neurophysiol. 67*:247–259.

Lathers, C. M., Tumer, N., and Kraras, C. M. (1988). The effect of intracerebroventricular D-Ala^2 methionine enkephalinamide and naloxone on cardiovascular parameters in the cat. *Life Sci. 43*:2287–2298.

Leestma, J., and Koenig, K. K. (1968). Sudden death and phenothiazines. *Arch. Gen. Psychiatr. 18*:137–148.

Lipka, L. J., and Lathers, C. M. (1987). Psychoactive agents, seizure production, and sudden death in epilepsy. *J. Clin. Pharmacol. 27*:169–183.

McLeod, A. A., and Jewitt, D. E. (1978). Role of 24-hour ambulatory electrocardiographic monitoring in a general hospital. *Br. Med. J. 1*:1197–1199.

Onuma, T. (1957). Relationships of the predisposition to convulsions with the action potentials of the autonomic nerves and the brain. II. Changes in action potential of the autonomic nerves and the brain under conditions for increasing the predisposition to convulsions. *Tohoku J. Exp. Med. 65*:121–129.

Orihara, O. (1952). Comparative observations of the action potential of autonomic nerve with EEG. *Tohoku J. Exp. Med. 57*:43–54.

Pace, D. G., and Gillis, R. A. (1976). Neuroexcitatory effects of digoxin in the cat. *J. Pharmacol. Exp. Ther. 199*:583–600.

Raines, A., Levitt, B., Standaert, F. G., and Sohn, Y. J. (1970). The influence of sympathetic nervous activity on the antiarrhythmic efficacy of diphenylhydantoin. *Eur. J. Pharmacol. 11*:293–297.

Roberts, J. (1970). The effect of diphenylhydantoin on the response to accelerator nerve stimulation. *Proc. Soc. Exp. Biol. Med. 134*:274–280.

Schallek, W., and Zabransky, F. (1966). Effects of psychotropic drugs on pressor responses to central and peripheral stimulation in the cat. *Arch. Int. Pharmacodyn. Ther. 161*:126–131.

Schlosser, W., Franco, S., and Sigg, E. B. (1975). Differential attenuation of somatovisceral and viscerosomatic reflexes by diazepam, phenobarbital, and diphylhydantoin. *Neuropharmacology 14*:525–531.

Schott, G. D., McLeod, A. A., and Jewitt, D. E. (1977). Cardiac arrhythmias that masquerade as epilepsy. *Br. Med. J. 1*:1454–1457.

Schraeder, P. L., and Celesia, G. G. (1977). The effects of epileptogenic activity upon auditory evoked responses in cats. *Arch. Neurol. 34*:677–682.

Schraeder, P. L., and Lathers, C. M. (1983). Cardiac neural discharge and epileptogenic activity in the cat: An animal model for unexplained death. *Life Sci. 32*:1371–1382.

Schraeder, P. L., and Lathers, C. M. (1989). Paroxysmal cardiovascular dysfunction and epileptogenic activity. *Epilepsy Res. 3*:55–62.

Skinner, J. E., Lie, J. T., and Entman, M. L. (1975). Modification of ventricular fibrillation latency following coronary artery occlusion in the conscious pig: The effects of psychological stress and beta-adrenergic blockade. *Circulation 51*:656–671.

Snead, O. C. (1983). Seizures induced by carbachol, morphine, leucine-enkephalin: A comparison. *Ann. Neurol. 13*:445–451.

Spratling, W. T. (1902). The causes and manner of death in epilepsy. *Med. News 80*:1225–1227.

Stauffer, A. Z., Dodd-o, J., and Lathers, C. M. (1989). The relationship of the lockstep phenomenon and precipitous changes in mean arterial blood pressure. *Electroencephalogr. Clin. Neurophysiol. 72*:340–345.

Suter, L., and Lathers, C. M. (1984). Modulation of presynaptic gamma aminobutyric acid release by prostaglandin E_2: Explanation for epileptogenic activity and dysfunction in autonomic cardiac neural discharge leading to arrhythmias. *Med. Hypotheses 15*:15–30.

Terrence, C. F., Wisotzkey, H. M., and Perper, J. A. (1975). Unexpected, unexplained death in epileptic patients. *Neurology 25*:594–598.

Vindrola, O., Asai, M., Zubieta, M., and Linares, G. (1983). Brain content of immunoreactive (leu_5) enkephalin and (met_5) enkephalin after pentylenetetrazol-induced convulsions. *Eur. J. Pharmacol. 90*:85–89.

Zielinski, J. J. (1974). Epilepsy and mortality rate and cause of death. *Epilepsia 15*:191–201.

10

Arrhythmias Associated with Epileptogenic Activity Elicited by Penicillin

CLAIRE M. LATHERS* *The Medical College of Pennsylvania, Eastern Pennsylvania Psychiatric Institute, Philadelphia, Pennsylvania*

PAUL L. SCHRAEDER *University of Medicine and Dentistry of New Jersey, Robert Wood Johnson Medical School, Camden, New Jersey*

I. INTRODUCTION

The association of autonomic dysfunction, clinical epilepsy, and sudden unexplained death has been the subject of many studies (Leestma et al., 1984; Terrence et al., 1975). Lathers and Schraeder (1982; Schraeder and Lathers, 1983) observed autonomic dysfunction in cats after epileptogenic activity induced by pentylenetetrazol (PTZ). A marked increase in variability in mean autonomic cardiac sympathetic and parasympathetic neural discharge was associated with the epileptogenic activity. It was hypothesized that if altered cardiac neural discharge also occurs in the patient with epilepsy, cardiac arrhythmias and sudden unexplained death may occur. The ideal agent to prevent these events should possess anticonvulsant, antiarrhythmic, and cardiac neural depressant properties.

This study developed a new small-animal model to study autonomic dysfunction in association with epileptogenic activity produced by injecting penicillin into the hippocampus of the cat. Epileptogenic activity was monitored as it spread to the left and right hippocampi and cerebral cortices. Data were analyzed to determine whether changes in the autonomic parameters of mean arterial blood pressure and heart rate were associated with both the interictal and the ictal epileptogenic activity. Phenobarbital was administered to determine whether it suppressed the epileptogenic and arrhythmic activity.

Current affiliation: FDA, Rockville, Maryland.

II. METHOD

The stereotaxic hippocampal injection of aqueous penicillin solution in 11 cats anesthetized with general anesthesia elicited both interictal and ictal activity. Cats were anesthetized intravenously (i.v.) with alpha-chloralose (80 mg/kg) and surgically prepared for monitoring the mean arterial blood pressure, lead II ECG, and for drug administration as described by Lathers and Schraeder (1982). A burr hole was made in the region of the posterior sylvian and posterior ectosylvian gyri bilaterally after the animal was placed into a stereotaxic head holder (David Kopf Instruments). A microcannula and a concentric bipolar recording electrode were inserted into the hippocampus using coordinates obtained from a stereotaxic atlas of the cat brain (Snider and Niemer, 1961).

Electrocorticographic recording electrodes were placed on the left and right (motor) cortices and the hippocampi. Penicillin was injected into the right hippocampus (coordinates A+7, HD-6.0, and RL+11.8). Motor cortex activity was recorded because of evidence that the frontal cortex is involved in cardiovascular regulation (Yingling and Skinner, 1976). Epileptogenic activity, interictal and ictal spikes, was elicited by the right hippocampal injection of penicillin as an aqueous solution of 400,000 U/ml colored with methylene blue in order to verify postmortem the injection recording site. A microsyringe in stereotaxic carrier was used to inject 0.0025 ml of penicillin (1000 U). The epileptogenic activity, quantified in spikes per minute, was correlated with changes in mean arterial blood pressure, heart rate, and ECG.

Either 20 or 40 mg/kg sodium phenobarbital (Elkins Sinn, Inc.), dissolved in 5 ml of physiologic (0.9%) saline, was infused into the femoral vein at a rate of 0.5 ml/min, followed by a 2-minute wash at the same rate with saline. Phenobarbital was administered after the injection of penicillin into the hippocampus.

One-factor repeated-measures analysis of variance (ANOVAs) were run where the independent variable was time (every four minutes) and the dependent measure was either heart rate or blood pressure. This was repeated for both penicillin and phenobarbital, creating four separate analyses. When a significant F-ratio (using the Huynh-Feldt correction to degrees of freedom) was obtained, the Newman–Keuls post-hoc procedure for determining which pairwise comparisons were significant was run at alpha = 0.05 (Winer, 1962). ANOVAs were done using biomedical programs (BMPD), subprogram P2V. Post-hoc tests were accomplished using the Statistical Package for the Social Sciences (SPSS), subprogram one way.

III. RESULTS

Changes in the electrocardiogram that were observed after the administration of 1000 U of penicillin in 11 cats included T wave inversion in 5, changes in the ST

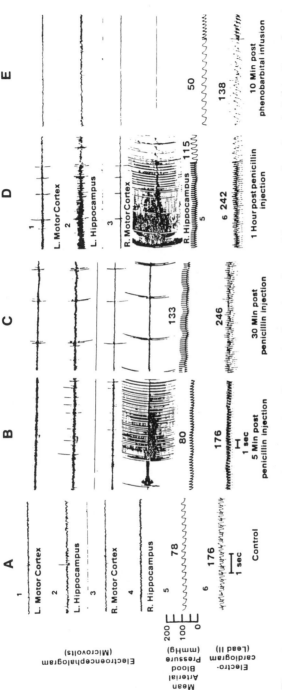

Figure 1 Changes in the electroencephalogram and cardiovascular function observed in one cat after the administration of penicillin (100 U/µl) into the right hippocampus. Phenobarbital (40 mg/kg i.v.) was administered two hours after the administration of penicillin. Panel A, left motor cortex; panel B, left hippocampus; panel C, right motor cortex; panel D, right hippocampus; panel E, blood pressure; and row 6, electrocardiogram. The numbers above the mean arterial blood pressure and electrocardiogram tracings indicate the blood pressure and heart rate values in mm Hg and bpm, respectively. The labels on the panels indicate data obtained in the control period and the times at which the data were obtained after the administration of penicillin and phenobarbital 40 mg/kg i.v.

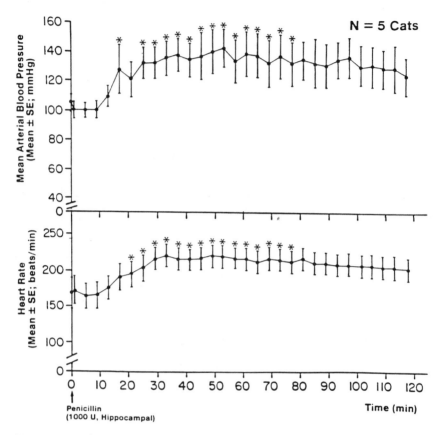

Figure 2 The effect of hippocampal injection of penicillin (1000 U/μl) on mean arterial blood pressure (mm Hg) and heart rate (bpm). Data are graphed as a function of time in minutes and are expressed as the mean ± S.E. for another group of five cats. The asterisks indicate values that are significantly different from control.

and PR intervals in 4 and 3, respectively, alterations in the QRS complex in 4, and ST depression in 2. The administration of phenobarbital 20 mg/kg i.v. to four additional cats or 40 mg/kg i.v. to nine additional cats abolished the penicillin-induced changes in the ECG. The ECG changes included alterations in the P and QRS waves, the appearance of a U wave, and premature ventricular contractions. At some experimental times, the premature ventricular contractions occurred prior to the appearance of the epileptogenic activity; at other times in the same cat the premature ventricular contractions appeared just after the ini-

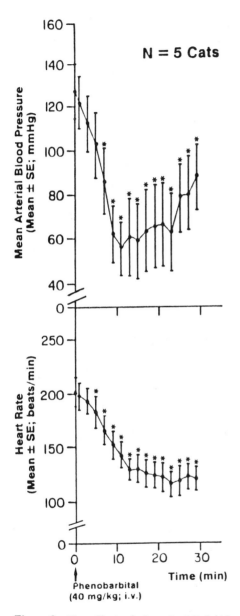

Figure 3 The effect of phenobarbital (40 mg/kg i.v.) on penicillin-induced changes in blood pressure (mm Hg) and heart rate (bpm). Data are graphed as a function of time in minutes and are expressed as the mean ± S.E. and were obtained in the same five cats depicted in Figure 2. Phenobarbital was given two hours after the administration of penicillin. The asterisks indicate values that are significantly different from control.

·tiation of the epileptogenic activity. The changes in the ECG were not caused by anesthesia or by surgical stress since they were not observed in the control period. In the rare event that anesthesia initiated arrhythmias, the cat was not included in the study.

Data from one cat are depicted in Figure 1. Penicillin 1000 U/μl induced interictal activity in the left motor cortex and in the left and right hippocampi one minute after administration (not shown). Ictal activity developed in the right hippocampus five minutes after the injection of penicillin and was associated with a 5-mm Hg increase in the mean arterial blood pressure (column B). Interictal activity was evident in all four electrocorticograms at minute 12 (not shown). Thirty minutes after the administration of penicillin (column C), the mean arterial blood pressure increased to 133 mm Hg and the heart rate to 246 bpm. Interictal spikes were observed in both motor cortices and ictal discharge in both hippocampi one hour (column D) and two hours (not shown) after penicillin administration. Mean arterial blood pressure and heart rate values were still increased from control. Penicillin-induced interictal and ictal activity was suppressed minute 5 of the infusion of phenobarbital (not shown) and was abolished minute 10 after 40 mg/kg iv phenobarbital (column E). Penicillin-induced increases in blood pressure and heart rate were also reversed to values lower than the control. Blood pressure and heart rate values were slightly higher than control 30 minutes after phenobarbital; no epileptogenic activity was apparent (not shown).

The hippocampal injection of penicillin (1000 U/μl) in six cats increased the mean arterial blood pressure from a control of 92 ± 12 to 106 ± 10 mm Hg at 30 minutes after penicillin. Heart rate was increased from the control of 179 ± 15 to 199 ± 13 bpm at this time. The change in heart rate was significant ($p < 0.05$) but the change in blood pressure was not. The administration of phenobarbital (20 mg/kg i.v.) decreased mean arterial blood pressure from the pre-phenobarbital control of 115 ± 14 to 79 ± 14 mm Hg ($p < 0.05$) 22 minutes after phenobarbital. Heart rate was decreased from 204 ± 19 to 162 ± 12 bpm ($p < 0.05$) at this time. To determine whether a higher dose of phenobarbital (40 mg/kg i.v.) would completely abolish the penicillin-induced epileptogenic activity, five additional cats received hippocampal injections of penicillin (1000 U/μl). The effect of penicillin on the mean arterial blood pressure and heart rate in these five additional cats is depicted in Figure 2. Mean arterial blood pressure increased from the control of 105 ± 5 to 143 ± 13 mm Hg 52 minutes after the administration of penicillin; heart rate increased from 170 ± 22 to 218 ± 16 bpm ($p < 0.05$) 34 minutes post penicillin. When phenobarbital (40 mg/kg i.v.) was administered to these five cats, it decreased mean arterial blood pressure from the pre-phenobarbital control of 128 ± 14 to 56 ± 28 mm Hg and heart rate from 201 ± 15 to 117 ± 14 bpm ($p < 0.05$) at 12 and 22 minutes, respectively (Figure 3). Comparison of the effect of 20 and 40 mg/kg i.v. phenobarbital revealed that the magnitude of the decrease in blood pressure and heart rate after the larger dose was twice that of the lower dose.

IV. DISCUSSION

This study showed that penicillin-induced hippocampal epileptogenic discharges were associated with increases in mean arterial blood pressure and heart rate and changes in the ECG. The dose of 20 mg/kg phenobarbital i.v. reversed the associated increases in blood pressure and heart rate and attenuated the epileptogenic activity; 40 mg/kg phenobarbital i.v. completely abolished epileptogenic activity and reversed the associated changes in the cardiovascular parameters.

This study demonstrated that the use of general anesthesia with hippocampal injections of aqueous penicillin elicited both interictal and ictal spike activity, in contrast to intracortical penicillin into the cerebral convexity, which does not usually progress to ictal activity in cats under general anesthesia (Prince, 1972). Several of our preliminary experiments (unpublished observations), utilizing alpha-chloralose anesthesia and cortical injection of penicillin, elicited only interictal spike activity in the primary focus and in the minor focus, i.e., the homologous contralateral cortical area, within 3 to 10 minutes. Afterdischarges did not develop for as long as seven hours after the intracortical injection of penicillin. In contrast, when ether was used for induction of anesthesia, followed by local anesthesia, afterdischarges within a mean time of 105 minutes after penicillin injection (Schraeder and Celesia, 1977). Thus the use of alpha-chloralose and cortical convexity injection of penicillin reliably elicits only interictal spikes and therefore is useful only to examine the effect of interictal discharge on autonomic cardiovascular function. In contrast, this study found that injection of penicillin into the hippocampus in animals anesthetized only with alpha-chloralose resulted in the progressive development of interictal to ictal discharges. Thus the use of general anesthesia in the model utilizing hippocampal injection of penicillin does not preclude investigation into the effects of ictal discharge.

The significance of the data reported in this study is that interneuronal pathways connect the hippocampal area to the autonomic cardiovascular areas within the hypothalamus. The hippocampal formation, the amygdaloid complex, the septal region, the gyrus fornicatus, the piriform lobe, and the caudal orbital frontal cortex constitute the limbic forebrain structures (Nauta and Haymaker, 1969). The fornix system forms the main efferent pathways from the hippocampus. Fiber systems originating in the limbic forebrain are among the most conspicuous afferents of the hypothalamus. Hippocampal afferents come from the medial septal nucleus and cingulate and the parahippocampal regions of the gyrus fornicatus. The amygdaloid complex is connected with the hypothalamus

by the stria terminalis and the ventral amygdalofugal pathway. The septoamyg-
dalar complex projects directly to the hippocampus (Swanson and Cowan,
1979). The hypothalamus is then, at least in part, under cerebral cortical control in its influence on the maintenance of homeostasis, by virtue of its neural
relationships with both divisions of the autonomic nervous system and with both
lobes of the pituitary gland. "When the connections of the septo-hippocampal
complex are considered as a whole, the conclusion emerges that it essentially
forms the gateway between the hypothalamus and the limbic cortical regions"
(Swanson, 1983). It is quite possible that with spread of interictal activity in
the hippocampus to the hypothalamus, the subclinical epileptogenic activity
alters the function of other areas of the brain, with resultant simultaneous
changes in the autonomic control of mean arterial blood pressure, heart rate and
rhythm, and cardiac neural discharge in the periphery.

Furthermore, cardiovascular regulation is a function of neuronal activity in
the cerebral cortex, the amygdala, and the medullary reticular formations. Car-
dioacceleratory and cardioinhibitory centers exist at these levels of the nervous
system, with selective activation producing either increased or decreased heart
rate. Vasopressor and vasodepressor centers also exist at these central sites and
produce their effects through reticulospinal connections to the preganglionic
sympathetic neurons of the intermediolateral cell column and through connections to preganglionic parasympathetic neurons. In addition to descending input
from higher centers, the cardiovascular centers also receive input from peripheral
receptors, the most important of which are the baroreceptors of the carotid
sinus and the aortic arch.

While peripheral autonomic dysfunction in cardiac autonomic nerves can precede the changes in the ECG associated with subconvulsant interictal discharge,
interictal activity alone can also be associated with premature ventricular contractions (Lathers and Schraeder, 1982). Thus minimal epileptogenic activity
(single spikes) can be associated with altered cardiac neural discharge and arrhythmias. Schraeder and Celesia (1977) reported that even minimal epileptogenic activity has a wide-ranging effect on cerebral functions monitored at the
auditory cortex of the cat. If, then, subclinical epileptogenic activity were to
likewise have an effect on other functions of the brain, i.e., autonomic regulation, producing autonomic imbalance in cardiac autonomic neural discharge with
subsequent arrhythmias, this type of activity could be a contributing factor to
the mechanism of unexpected death in epilepsy. That this sequence could occur
in the person with epilepsy is supported by the anatomical relationships among
the cerebral cortex, the hippocampi, and the hypothalamus.

The anatomical and physiological relationship of the frontal cortex with the
hypothalamus is complex; studies stimulating the dorsolateral surface of both
hemispheres have reported both a rise or a fall in blood pressure and increases or

decreases in heart rate (Hoff et al., 1963). Cortical stimulation evoked dilatation of pupils, retraction of the nictitating membrane, piloerection, salivation, sweating, and gastric motility and secretion. The autonomic localization in the motor and premotor cortex corresponds closely with the somatotopic representation (Brooks and Koizumi, 1974).

The focal model of epilepsy used in this study produced cardiovascular changes that were similar to those produced by pentylenetetrazol-induced epileptogenic activity (Lathers and Schraeder, 1982; Schraeder and Lathers, 1983). These data support the hypothesis that focal epileptogenic activity can produce alterations in cardiac electrical activity making the heart susceptible to arrhythmias that may cause sudden unexplained death in epileptic persons. The clinical significance of the data obtained in this type of epileptogenic model is emphasized by Blumhardt et al. (1986). They reported that in some patients with temporal lobe epilepsy, cardiac acceleration preceded the onset of recognizable rhythmic surface EEG seizure activity; this may reflect the onset of electrical discharge in deep limbic circuits and the connections of these structures with the autonomic nervous system. Arrhythmias were observed at times when there were no seizure discharges on the EEG in some patients. Blumhardt and colleagues also noted that the autonomic effects of temporal lobe epilepsy on heart rate and rhythm may be more severe in untreated younger patients. Their suggestion agrees with the observation that young epileptic patients are at high risk of sudden unexplained death.

The present study used an animal model that allowed testing of a pharmacologic agent which possesses antiepileptic, antiarrhythmic, and neural depressant activity. Future use of this model should help in the development of better therapeutic regimens designed to eliminate the autonomic dysfunction and arrhythmias associated with epileptogenic activity and ultimately contribute to our understanding of the risk factors for sudden unexplained death in epilepsy. If the data indicate that the autonomic changes are secondary to seizures, the primary clinical therapeutic goal would be to use a pharmacologic agent with maximum anticonvulsant potency. However, if interictal activity is associated with a risk of autonomic dysfunction, questions must be raised about the current therapeutic goal for epilepsy, which is to suppress seizures but not interictal discharges. In the latter case, a new type of drug may be required.

V. SUMMARY

Penicillin-induced epileptogenic activity (1000 U/ml) was recorded bilaterally from the hippocampi and the motor cortices of 11 anesthetized cats. The onset of epileptogenic activity ranged from 1 second to 16 minutes. Epileptiform activity, consisting of interictal discharges (n = 3) or ictal discharges (n = 3), first occurred at the injection site, the right hippocampus. Blood pressure increased from 92 ± 12 (control) to 106 ± 10 at 30 minutes and 115 ± 10 mm Hg 60 minutes after penicillin ($p > 0.05$). Heart rate increased from 179 ± 15 (control) to 194 ± 13 at 30 minutes and 216 ± 13 bpm 60 minutes after penicillin ($p > 0.05$). Maximum increases in blood pressure and heart rate were 55 ± 15 mm Hg and 59 ± 15 bpm, respectively ($p < 0.05$). ECG alterations included: P-R interval changes; increased P wave amplitude; QRS complex changes; T wave inverstion; ST elevation, and the appearance of premature ventricular contractions. Phenobarbital (20 mg/kg i.v.) diminished the epileptogenic activity and depressed the blood pressure to 79 ± 14 mm Hg at 23 minutes from 115 ± 14 mm Hg (10 minutes before phenobarbital; $p < 0.05$). Heart rate was decreased to 162 ± 12 from the pre-phenobarbital control of 204 ± 19 bpm ($p > 0.05$). To determine whether a higher dose of phenobarbital (40 mg/kg i.v.) would completely abolish the penicillin-induced epileptogenic activity, five additional cats received penicillin G sodium 1000 U/μl into the right hippocampus. In these cats the penicillin also produced epileptogenic activity and increased the blood pressure from 105 ± 5 to 143 ± 13 and the heart rate from the control 170 ± 22 to 218 ± 16 ($p < 0.05$). Phenobarbital (40 mg/kg i.v.) significantly reversed the effect of penicillin on the blood pressure and heart rate. Blood pressure fell from the pre-phenobarbital control of 128 ± 14 to 56 ± 18 mm Hg and heart rate fell from 201 ± 15 to 117 ± 14 bpm ($p < 0.05$). This dose of phenobarbital also prevented the penicillin-induced epileptogenic activity. Thus phenobarbital diminished the epileptogenic activity and autonomic dysfunction induced by penicillin. The autonomic dysfunction and epileptogenic activity induced by the peripheral intravenous administration of pentylenetetrazol (Lathers and Schraeder, 1982) are similar to those induced by the hippocampal injection of penicillin.

ACKNOWLEDGMENTS

This study was funded by the Epilepsy Foundation of America. The authors are indebted to Dr. Nihal Tumer, Valerie Farris, and Larry Pratt for technical help, Dr. Edward Gracely for statistical analyses, and Michele Spino for typing the manuscript.

REFERENCES

Blumhardt, L. D., Smith, P. E. M., and Owen, L. (1986). Electrocardiographic accompaniments of temporal lobe epileptic seizures. *Lancet 1*:1051-1056.
Brooks, C. M., and Koizumi, K. (1974). The hypothalamus and control of integrative processes. In *Medical Physiology*, 13th ed. V. B. Mountcastle (Ed.). C. V. Mosby, St. Louis, pp. 813-836.

Hoff, E. C., Kell, J. F., Jr., and Carrol, M. N., Jr. (1963). Effects of cortical stimulation and lesions on cardiovascular function. *Physiol. Rev. 43*:68–114.

Lathers, C. M., and Schraeder, P. L. (1982). Autonomic dysfunction in epilepsy: Characterization of autonomic cardiac neural discharge associated with pentylenetetrazol-induced epileptogenic activity. *Epilepsia 23*:633–647.

Leestma, J. E., Kalelkar, M. B., Teas, S. S., Jay, G. W., and Hughes, J. R. Sudden unexpected death associated with seizures: Analysis of 66 cases. *Epilepsia 25*:84–88.

Nauta, W. J. H., and Haymaker, W. (1969). Hypothalamic nuclei and fiber connections. In *The Hypothalamus*, W. Haymaker, E. Anderson, and W. J. H. Nauta (Eds.). Thomas, Springfield, Ill., pp. 136–209.

Prince, D. A. (1972). Topical convulsion drugs and metabolic antagonists. In *Experimental Models of Epilepsy. A Manual for the Laboratory Worker*, D. P. Purpura, J. K. Peney, D. Tower, D. M. Woodbury, and R. Walter (Eds.). Raven Press, New York, pp. 51–84.

Schraeder, P. L., and Celesia, G. G. (1977). The effects of epileptogenic activity on auditory evoked potentials in cats. *Arch. Neurol. 34*:677–682.

Schraeder, P. L., and Lathers, C. M. (1983). Cardiac neural discharge and epileptogenic activity in the cat: An animal model for unexplained death. *Life Sci. 32*:1371–1382.

Snider, R. S., and Niemer, W. T. (1961). *A Stereotaxic Atlas of the Cat Brain*. University of Chicago Press, Chicago.

Swanson, L. W. (1983). The hippocampus and the concept of the limbic system. In *Neurobiology of the Hippocampus*, W. Seifert (Ed.). Academic Press, London, pp. 3–20.

Swanson, L. W., and Cowan, W. M. (1979). The connections of the septal region in the rat. *J. Comp. Neurol. 186*:621–656.

Terrence, C. F., Wisotzkey, H. M., and Perper, J. A. (1975). Neurogenic pulmonary edema in unexpected, unexplained death in epileptic patients. *Neurology 25*:594–598.

Winer, B. (1962). *Statistical Principles in Experimental Design*, 2nd ed. McGraw-Hill, New York.

Yingling, C. D., and Skinner, J. E. (1976). Selective regulation of thalamic sensory relay nuclei by nucleus reticularis thalami. *Electroencephalogr. Clin. Neurophysiol. 41*:476–482.

11

Acute Cardiovascular Response During Kindled Seizures

JEFFREY H. GOODMAN*, RICHARD W. HOMAN†, and ISSAC L. CRAWFORD
*University of Texas Southwestern Medical Center and Southwestern Regional
Epilepsy Center, Veterans Administration Medical Center, Dallas, Texas*

I. INTRODUCTION

The high incidence of sudden unexplained death in the epileptic population not
only poses a serious problem for the epileptic patient but is also a challenge to
the clinician and an unsolved mystery for the basic scientist. A reasonable hypothesis is that if seizures disrupt autonomic regulation of the cardiovascular
system, then the consequent generation of cardiac arrhythmias may underlie
sudden unexplained death. Clearly, spontaneous seizures in man (Gilchrist,
1985; Marshall et al., 1983; Pritchett et al., 1980) and experimentally induced
seizures in animlas (Doba et al., 1975; Lathers and Schraeder, 1982) can be
accompanied by cardiac arrhythmias. There is also a case report of sudden cardiac death immediately following a complex partial seizure (Dashieff and Dickinson, 1986). However, no direct evidence has been provided that definitely
links sudden unexplained death to seizure occurrence. A recent report by Keilson et al. (1987) revealed that the incidence of serious cardiac arrhythmias is no
greater in epileptic patients than in the general population. Since there is no clinical marker that identifies those epileptic patients most at risk for sudden death,
a greater research emphasis placed on basic experimental models of epilepsy may
reveal new directions for clinical studies.

Current affiliation:
*New York State Department of Health, West Haverstraw, New York.
†Department of Neurology, Medical College of Ohio, Toledo, Ohio.
Portions of this chapter adapted from Goodman, J. H., Homan, R. W., and Crawford, I. L.,
(1990). Kindled Seizures Elevate Blood Pressure and Induce Cardiac Arrhythmias. *Epilepsia*
(in press).

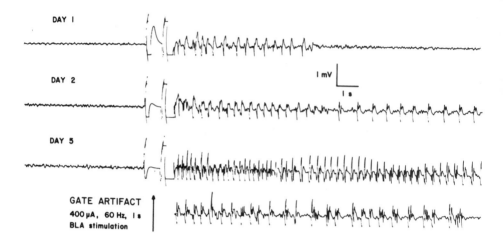

Figure 1 Growth of seizure afterdischarge during the kindling process. The lower electrograph for day 5 is a continuation of that shown before and after the fifth stimulus.

Cardiovascular changes occur during several types of experimentally induced seizures: electroconvulsive treatment (Petito et al., 1977; Plum et al., 1968; Wasterlain, 1974; Westergaard et al., 1978); pentylenetetrazol (Doba et al., 1975; Lathers and Schraeder, 1982; Plum et al., 1968); bicuculline (Meldrum and Horton, 1973); and penicillin (Lathers and Schraeder, Chapter 10, this book; Mameli et al., 1988). However, these models have inherent limitations due to the presence of anesthetics, paralytic agents with artificial ventilation, or widespread exposure of the CNS to chemical convulsants or electrical current.

In the kindling seizure model, repeated spaced presentations of an initially subconvulsive electrical stimulus eventually leads to a permanent change in brain function (Goddard et al., 1969; Homan and Goodman, 1988). This change is characterized by the occurrence of a generalized motor seizure each time the stimulus is presented. During the kindling process there is a progressive increase in electrical afterdischarge activity (Figure 1), with spread of the afterdischarge to remote brain regions. Eventually, clinically apparent seizures develop, progressing through five distinct behavioral stages (Racine, 1972; Figure 2). Early stages in the kindling process (stages 1 and 2) are equivalent to partial seizures. Spread of the seizure first occurs at stage 3, while a stage 5 seizure is equivalent to a generalized tonic-clonic convulsion. This is a key feature of kindling, since partial as well as generalized seizures can be examined in the same animal.

A stage 5 generalized seizure usually occurs after 9-10 days of amygdaloid stimulation. To elicit spontaneous interictal spiking or spontaneous seizures requires 100-300 days of daily stimulation (Pinel and Rovner, 1978). For this

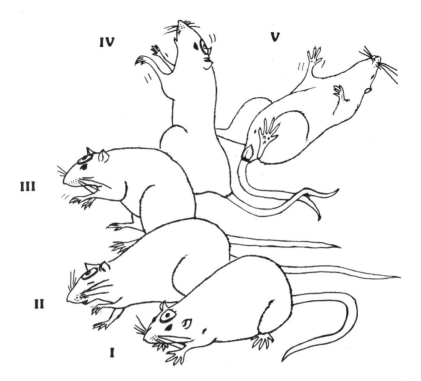

Figure 2 Behavioral stages of kindled seizures. The five stages are those identified by Racine (1972).

reason these types of epileptiform activity are difficult to investigate in the kindling model. However, in contrast to chemical models, no drug is injected, and therefore one does not have to distinguish the direct from the nondirect effects of nonexperimental drugs. Thus far few major morphological alterations have been found in the kindled focus, in contrast to injection of heavy metals or thermal injury to produce convulsions; both of the latter procedures result in neuronal loss and glial proliferation.

The kindling model is well suited for an examination of the relationship between seizures and the cardiovascular system without the presence of drugs. Kindled seizures can be initiated in a discrete region of the brain of unanesthetized, unrestrained animals (Racine, 1972, 1978). We have utilized this model to explore the acute cardiovascular changes that occur during amygdaloid-kindled seizures. We will review the results of our studies and also discuss the significance of these changes with respect to the potential value of kindling as a model of seizure-induced cardiac arrhythmias. Speculation on the relationship of our findings to the clinical phenomenon of sudden unexplained death will also be presented.

II. METHODS

To examine the effect of kindled seizures on the cardiovascular system of the rat, male Sprague-Dawley rats (275–325 g) were anesthetized with ketamine (90 mg/kg) and xylazine (15 mg/kg) by intramuscular injection. Teflon-coated stainless steel electrodes (100 μ) were stereotaxically implanted in the basolateral amygdalae or the olfactory bulbs according to previously reported methods used in our laboratory (Campbell and Crawford, 1980; Crawford, 1986; Walker et al., 1981). Each animal was allowed to recover a minimum of one week before the kindling process was initiated. During the kindling process each animal was stimulated once daily for 1 second (400 μA, 60 Hz, 1-msec square wave, bipolar pulse) until three consecutive stage 5 generalized seizures occurred. A chronic femoral artery catheter filled with heparinized saline was then surgically implanted to allow for the direct measurement of blood pressure in unanesthetized rats during the kindled seizure. Following recovery from catheterization (a minimum of 24 hours) ECG electrodes were placed across the chest, a kindled seizure was initiated, and changes in blood pressure, heart rate, and ECG were measured. Controls, with electrodes and catheter, were treated in a similar manner without undergoing the kindling process. In a separate group of rats, blood pressure and heart rate were measured during amygdaloid kindling acquisition. Amygdaloid electrodes and the arterial catheter were implanted as described above. These animals did not have ECG electrodes, so changes in the ECG were not measured. Since the arterial catheter remained patent for only five days, these animals were stimulated twice a day during the kindling process. The other stimulus parameters were the same as previously described. After each stimulus, changes in behavioral seizure score, afterdischarge duration, blood pressure, and heart rate were measured.

III. RESULTS

A. Effect on Blood Pressure and Heart Rate

Figure 3 shows the typical cardiovascular response during a stage 5 generalized amygdaloid-kindled seizure. The response was characterized by an abrupt increase in systolic and diastolic pressure, which lasted 20–30 seconds after initiation of the seizure. Superimposed on this change in pressure was a profound bradycardia occasionally accompanied by premature ventricular contractions. A summary of the effect of the seizure on mean arterial pressure (MAP) and heart

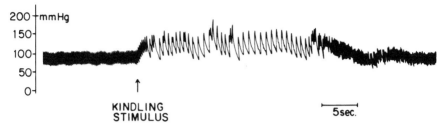

Figure 3 Typical blood pressure response during an amygdaloid-kindled seizure. Arrow indicates when stimulus was delivered.

rate is seen in Figure 4. MAP was significantly elevated for 20 seconds after initiation of the kindled seizure. During the first 10 seconds of the seizure MAP approximated 150 mm Hg while mean heart rate was decreased 50%. The increase in MAP was concomitant with increases in systolic, diastolic, and pulse pressure (Table 1). Changes in pressure and heart rate were greatest in the first 10-15 seconds of the seizure; however, both parameters returned to baseline before the end of the seizure afterdischarge.

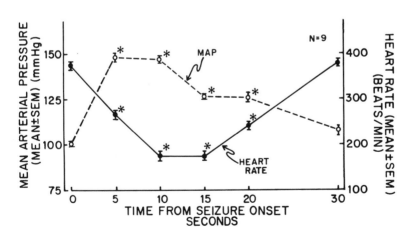

Figure 4 Graphic comparison of changes in mean arterial pressure (MAP) and heart rate during the first 30 sec. after initiation of stage 5 amygdaloid kindled seizures (* – $p < 0.01$). SEM equals standard error of the mean. Reprinted from Goodman et al., 1990, *Epilepsia* (in press).

Table 1 Effect of Amygdaloid-Kindled Seizures on Blood Pressure[a]

Mean ± SEM mmHg	N	Baseline	Time from seizure initiation (seconds)						
			5	10	15	20	30	60
Systolic pressure (mean ± SEM)	9	131.1 ±1.4	192.8** ±2.6	197.8** ±3.3	171.1** ±1.5	163.3** ±1.9	142.2 ±1.4	131.4 ±2.1
Diastolic pressure (mean ± SEM)	9	85.0 ±1.1	126.1** ±2.2	121.1** ±1.5	103.9* ±1.6	108.3** ±2.2	90.6 ±1.9	85.9 ±1.5
Pulse pressure (mean ± SEM)	9	46.1 ±1.0	66.7** ±2.3	76.7** ±2.2	67.2** ±1.6	55.0 ±1.3	51.7 ±1.0	45.6 ±1.6

[a]One repeated-measure ANOVA followed by Neuman-Keuls, compared to baseline value.
*$p < 0.05$; **$p < 0.01$
SEM = standard error of the mean.
Reprinted from Goodman et al., 1990, Epilepsia (in press), Raven Press.

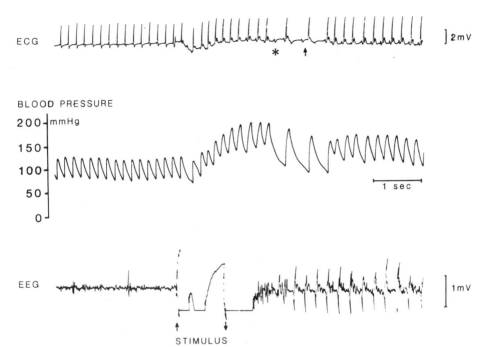

Figure 5 Electrograph of the effect of Stage 5 amygdaloid kindled seizure on the electrocardiogram (ECG) and blood pressure. Notice the isolated P wave (*) and increased P–R interval (small arrow) that correspond with irregular changes in the blood pressure recording and the afterdischarge in the EEG. The up and down arrows under the EEG indicate the beginning and end of the kindling stimulus. This is followed by a period of amplifier block. Reprinted from Goodman et al., *Epilepsia* (in press).

B. Effect of the Seizure on the Electrocardiogram

The effect of the kindled seizure on the heart was determined by making simultaneous recordings of blood pressure and the ECG from animals during kindled seizures. During the seizure the bradycardia present in the pressure recording was consistently present in the ECG of each animal. In most of the animals, additional irregularities were detected in the ECG during the bradycardia. Occasionally, premature ventricular contractions were also observed. These changes, as illustrated in Figure 5, included nonconducted P waves and increases in the P–R interval, which are indicative of conduction heart block (Berne and Levy, 1981).

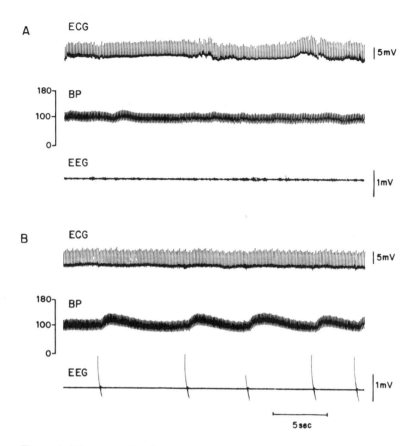

Figure 6 Electrograph of blood pressure. EEG-electroencephalogram, ECG-electrocardiogram in a kindled rat before (A) and three minutes after a kindling stimulus (B). Note the transient rise in pressure after each interictal, epileptiform spike-wave complex.

C. Seizure Dependency

The possibility existed that the cardiovascular response observed during the kindled seizure was simply the result of electrical stimulation of the amygdala, a known cardiovascular control center. To test this hypothesis, rats not previously kindled were stimulated with a single kindling train. In each instance the stimulus elicited a small seizure afterdischarge; however, no change in blood pressure or heart rate was detected. This suggests the cardiovascular changes that occurred in kindled animals in response to the same stimulus were seizure dependent.

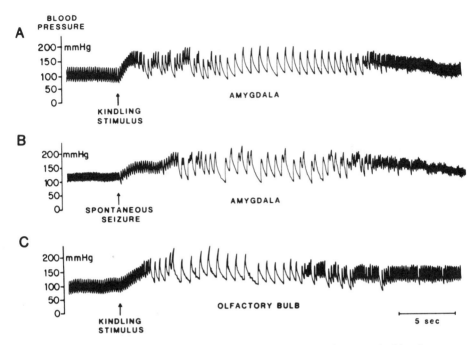

Figure 7   Effect of kindled seizures on blood pressure: (A) change in blood pressure during an amygdaloid kindled Stage 5 generalized seizure. (B) Change in blood pressure during a spontaneous generalized seizure that occurred 3 min after a stimulus-induced amygdaloid kindled seizure. (C) Blood pressure response during a Stage 5 generalized seizure initiated in the olfactory bulb.

Electrically kindled seizures can be followed by postictal spiking. When this occurred in several animals, postictal spikes were accompanied by increases in blood pressure (Figure 6). These postictal spikes often develop into spontaneous seizures two or three minutes after the stimulus-induced seizure. These seizures, electrographically and behaviorally, mimicked stimulus-induced seizures. The cardiovascular responses during the secondary spontaneous seizures (Figure 7B) were qualitatively the same as those recorded during amygdaloid-kindled seizures (Figure 7A).

D. Autonomic Changes in Non-Amygdaloid-Initiated Seizures

To determine whether kindled seizure–induced autonomic changes were restricted to seizure initiation in the amygdala, we kindled animals in the olfactory bulb. Figure 7C shows the cardiovascular changes that occurred during an

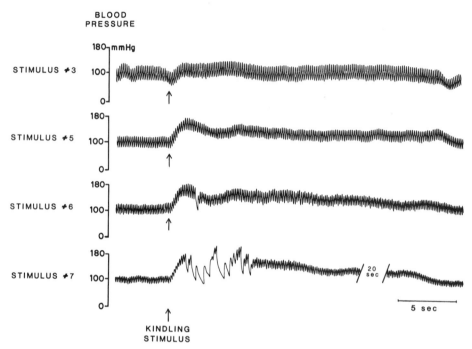

Figure 8 Changes in blood pressure during kindling acquisition. Notice the delayed appearance of the arrhythmic response after the sixth and seventh stimulation. Arrows indicate when stimulus was delivered. Reprinted from Goodman et al., *Epilepsia* (in press).

olfactory bulb–kindled seizure. These changes were qualitatively the same as those recorded during amygdaloid-kindled seizures.

E. Cardiovascular Changes During Kindling Acquisition

The initial stimulus in the kindling process did not elicit a pressor response or a change in heart rate. However, as kindling was continued, several changes were observed. Figure 8 shows the progressive changes in the pressure and arrhythmic responses during the kindling process. The first cardiovascular change was a small rise in pressure with no change in heart rate. With subsequent stimulations the pressor response continued to increase. In contrast, the arrhythmic response developed at a different rate. The arrhythmia did not occur until after the sixth stimulation. Continued stimulation resulted in an increase in the duration and the severity of the arrhythmia while the magnitude of the pressor response remained the same. The cardiovascular response present after the seventh stimulation occurred during a stage 2 seizure, before seizure generalization had developed.

IV. DISCUSSION

The results from the foregoing experiments identify an experimental seizure model that simultaneously evaluates altered cardiovascular function. The cardiovascular response during amygdaloid-kindled seizures was characterized by a large increase in blood pressure accompanied by a profound bradycardia. These changes were present during partial (Figure 8) as well as generalized seizures. It is important to recognize that these results were obtained from unanesthetized animals, thereby eliminating one of the confounding variables associated with other experimental seizure models.

A. Role of the Amygdala

The amygdala is an important cardiovascular control center with numerous connections to brain stem (Hopkins and Holstege, 1978; Schwaber et al., 1980; Takeuchi et al., 1982) and limbic (De Olmos, 1972) structures that regulate the autonomic nervous system. The connections to the hypothalamus through the stria terminals (De Olmos and Ingram, 1972) and ventral amygdalofugal pathways (Millhouse, 1969) are particularly relevant since these pathways mediate amygdala-induced changes in cardiovascular function (Faiers et al., 1975; Galosy et al., 1982; Hilton and Zbrozyna, 1963). Stimulation of the amygdala in the rat (Faiers et al., 1975; Le Doux et al., 1982; Mogenson and Calaresu, 1973), cat (Heinemann et al., 1973; Stock et al., 1978), and monkey (Reis and Oliphant, 1964) has been shown to affect blood pressure and heart rate. Specific changes with basal amygdaloid stimulation in unanesthetized animals include a decrease in blood pressure with no change or an increase in heart rate (Heinemann et al., 1973; Stock et al., 1978) or a bradycardia followed by an increase in blood pressure (Reis and Oliphant, 1964).

With these observations in mind, a predictable response to an electrical stimulus in the amygdala of kindled rats would be an alteration of cardiovascular function. However, a single stimulus train in the amygdala of implanted control animals had no effect on blood pressure or heart rate. The difference between this result and those of past studies may be due to the use of different stimulus parameters, specifically stimulus frequency and duration. The observation that a single stimulus train (1 second, 400 μA, 60 Hz) did not elicit cardiovascular changes in control animals suggests that the cardiovascular changes in kindled animals are seizure dependent. This is supported by the observations that postictal spikes are accompanied by an increase in pressure and that secondary spontaneous seizures, in the absence of a kindling stimulus, result in the same abnormal cardiovascular changes that occur during stimulus-induced seizures. Similar changes observed during olfactory bulb–kindled seizures suggests that this response is not limited to seizures initiated in the amygdala.

B. The Pressor Response

The hypertension observed during generalized kindled seizures was similar to pressor changes reported to occur in several other experimental seizure models: ECT (Petito et al., 1977; Plum et al., 1968; Wasterlain, 1974; Westergaard et al., 1978); PTZ (Doba et al., 1975; Lathers and Schraeder, 1982; Plum et al., 1968); and bicuculline (Johansson and Nilsson, 1977; Meldrum and Horton, 1973). The pressor response during the kindled seizure was characterized by a rapid elevation in MAP to approximately 150 mm Hg. The normal response to an increase in MAP is an increase in vascular resistance, minimizing the increase in cerebral blood flow. However, increases in MAP of this magnitude were observed by Plum et al. (1968) during ECT- and PTZ-induced seizures to interrupt cerebral autoregulation, thereby causing cerebral blood flow to become pressure dependent. Such major MAP elevations can also compromise the blood–brain barrier (Johansson and Nilsson, 1977; Suzuki et al., 1984; Westergaard et al., 1978).

The sudden rise in blood pressure during the kindled seizure may be due to activation of sympathetic pathways. Plum et al. (1968) demonstrated that severing the spinal cord in dogs eliminated the increase in blood pressure and cerebral blood flow that occurred during seizures initiated with ECT or PTZ. A massive autonomic discharge has been reported to accompany generalized seizures (Meldrum et al., 1979) and in other seizure models the seizure-induced rise in pressure can be prevented with ganglionic blockers (Meldrum, 1976), alpha-adrenergic blockers, or chemical sympathectomy (Doba et al., 1975).

C. The Arrhythmogenic Response

It is not surprising that kindled seizures are accompanied by cardiac arrhythmias. There are several reports of arrhythmias associated with other types of experimentally induced seizures in animals (Delgado et al., 1960; Doba et al., 1975; Lathers and Schraeder, 1982; Wasterlain, 1974). These arrhythmias were probably due to abnormal autonomic activity induced by interictal or ictal seizure activity.

The bradycardic response that occurred during the kindled seizure was probably mediated by the parasympathetic system. The irregularities observed in the ECG during the seizure indicate the bradycardia was due to a conduction heart block (Berne and Levy, 1981). The parasympathetic system could be activated by two different mechanisms. The most obvious would be the activation of baroreceptor reflexes by the large pressor response (Frysinger et al., 1984). However, the parasympathetic system could also be activated centrally by the seizure. Lathers et al. (1987) demonstrated that cardiac arrhythmias associated with PTZ-induced interictal or ictal seizure activity result from autonomic dysfunction, i.e., an imbalance in neural activity within and between sympathetic and parasympathetic nerves to the heart. Seizure-induced coactivation of the sympathetic and parasympathetic systems is another possibility (Doba et al., 1975).

D. The Cerebral Ischemic Response

The hypertension and bradycardia that occurred during the kindled seizure resemble cardiovascular changes that occur in response to an increase in intracranial pressure, the Cushing response (Cushing, 1902; Doba and Reis, 1972; Hoff and Reis, 1970), or to cerebral ischemia (Dampney et al., 1979; Guyton, 1948). The rapid onset of the seizure-induced cardiovascular response makes it unlikely that these changes were the result of an increase in intracranial pressure or cerebral ischemia. However, the kindled changes may be mediated through the same central pathways. The cardiovascular changes during cerebral ischemia are mediated by coactivation of sympathetic and parasympathetic systems at the level of the lower brain stem (Kumada et al., 1979). The kindled seizure may activate the same pathways to induce changes in cardiovascular function.

E. Clinical Relevance

The etiology of sudden death in epileptic patients remains undefined and may not be the same in all patients. Evidence suggests that it may be associated with events occurring at the time of a seizure and perhaps is precipitated by a seizure. The finding that many patients who are found dead have subsequently been shown to have subtherapeutic anticonvulsant levels supports this hypothesis (Dasheiff and Dickinson, 1986). Of particular importance is the possibility that the interaction between seizures and the cardiovascular system underlies the sudden unexplained death that has been estimated to occur in 5-17% of epileptic patients (Leestma et al., 1984). Our observations obtained during kindled seizures may be relevant to similar cardiovascular changes seen during seizures in epileptic patients. Hypertension has been observed during spontaneous seizures (Meyer et al., 1966; Van Buren, 1958; Van Buren and Ajmone-Marsan, 1960; White et al., 1961) and ECT (Elliot et al., 1982). There are also case reports of ictal tachycardia (Marshall et al., 1983; Metz et al., 1978; Pritchett et al., 1980) and bradycardia (Devinsky et al., 1986; Coulter, 1984; Gilchrist, 1985; Kiok et al., 1986).

F. Kindling as a Model of Seizure-Induced Arrhythmias and Sudden Unexplained Death

In the past a good experimental model to study this relationship was lacking. Experimental seizure models such as ECT, PTZ, and bicuculline have inherent limitations due to the presence of anesthetics, paralytic agents, or widespread exposure of the CNS to chemical convulsants. In addition, these are models of generalized seizures, which precludes the examination of the effect of partial seizures on the cardiovascular system. The kindling model does not have these limitations. However, it is difficult to study the effect of interictal seizure activity on cardiovascular function in kindled animals. To study these changes the PTZ model in anesthetized cats has been useful (Carnel et al., 1985; Lathers and Schraeder, 1982; Lathers et al., 1984, 1987).

Kindled seizures are initiated in a discrete region of the brain of unanesthetized, unrestrained animals. Kindling also progresses through a series of distinct stages that allows for the examination of the effect of partial as well as generlized seizures on the cardiovascular system. In light of our results, the kindling seizure model appears to be well suited for studies that examine the relationship between seizures and the cardiovascular system.

Several questions remain to be answered. Do seizures have a progressive effect on the cardiovascular system? Is the severity of the seizure related to the degree of cardiac involvement? Is the quality of the arrhythmic response dependent on the site of origin of the seizure? Can repeated kindled seizures increase the susceptibility of kindled animals to cardiovascular changes associated with minimal discharges, i.e., interictal spikes? All of these questions have yet to be addressed in the kindling seizure model.

V. SUMMARY

The effect of seizures on cardiovascular function was evaluated during kindled seizures in conscious rats. This relationship was also examined during kindling acquisition. The typical cardiovascular response during a generalized kindled seizure consisted of a large increase in blood pressure accompanied by a profound bradycardia during the first 20-30 seconds of the seizure. Similar changes in heart rate and blood pressure were observed during amygdaloid- and olfactory bulb-kindled seizures as well as secondary spontaneous siezures, suggesting these changes were seizure dependent but not limited to seizures initiated in the amygdala. These cardiovascular changes were also present during partial seizures early in the kindling process.

These results suggest that kindling is a useful seizure model in which to study the underlying mechanism of seizure-induced arrhythmias and possibly the clinical phenomenon of sudden unexplained death.

REFERENCES

Berne, R. M., and Levy, M. N. (1981). *Cardiovascular Physiology*. C. V. Mosby, St. Louis, p. 46.

Campbell, G. A., and Crawford, I. L. (1980). A gated electronic switch for stimulation and recording with a single electrode. *Brain Res. Bull.* 5:485–486.

Carnel, S. B., Schraeder, P. L., and Lathers, C. M. (1985). The effect of phenobarbital pretreatment on cardiac neural discharge and pentylenetetrazol-induced epileptogenic activity. *Pharmacology 20*:225–240.

Coulter, D. (1984). Partial seizures with apnea and bradycardia. *Arch. Neurol. 41*:173–174.

Crawford, I. L. (1986). Relationship of glutamic acid and zinc to kindling of the rat amygdala: Afferent transmitter systems and excitability in a model of epilepsy. In *Excitatory Amino Acids and Epilepsy*, R. Schwarcz and Y. Ben-Ari (Eds.). Plenum, New York, pp. 611–623.

Cushing, H. (1902). Some experimental and clinical observations concerning states of increased intracranial tension. *Am. J. Med. Sci. 124*:375–400.

Dampney, R. A. L., Kumada, M., and Reis, D. J. (1979). Central neural mechanisms of the cerebral ischemic response. *Circ. Res. 45*:48–62.

Dasheiff, R. M., and Dickinson, L. J. (1986). Sudden unexpected death of epileptic patient due to cardiac arrhythmia after seizure. *Arch. Neurol. 43*:194–196.

Delgado, J. M., Mihailovic, L., and Sevillano, M. (1960). Cardiovascular phenomena during seizure activity. *J. Nerv. Ment. Dis. 130*:477–487.

De Olmos, J. S. (1972). The amygdaloid projection field in the rat as studied with the cupric-silver method. In *The Neurobiology of the Amygdala*, B. Eleftheriou (Ed.). Plenum, New York, pp. 145–204.

De Olmos, J. S., and Ingram, W. R. (1972). The projection field of the stria terminalis in the rat brain: An experimental study. *J. Comp. Neurol. 146*:303–334.

Devinsky, O., Price, B. H., and Cohen, S. I. (1986). Cardiac manifestations of complex partial seizures. *Am. J. Med. 80*:195–202.

Doba, N., and Reis, D. J. (1972). Localization within the lower brainstem of a receptive area mediating the pressure response to increased intracranial pressure (the Cushing response). *Brain Res. 47*:487–491.

Doba, N., Beresford, H. R., and Reis, D. J. (1975). Changes in regional blood flow and cardiodynamics associated with electrically and chemically induced epilepsy in the cat. *Brain Res. 90*:115–132.

Elliot, D., Linz, D., and Kane, J. (1982). Electroconvulsive therapy. *Arch. Intern. Med. 142*:979–981.

Faiers, A. A., Calaresu, F. R., and Mogenson, G. J. (1975). Pathway mediating hypotension elicited by stimulation of the amygdala in the rat. *Am. J. Physiol. 228*:1358–1366.

Frysinger, R. C., Marks, J. D., Trelease, R. B., Schechtman, V. L., and Harper, R. M. (1984). Sleep states attenuate the pressor response to central amygdala stimulation. *Exp. Neurol. 83*:604–617.

Galosy, R. A., Crawford, I. L., and Thompson, M. E. (1982). Behavioral stress and cardiovascular regulation: Neural mechanisms. In *Circulation, Neurobiology, and Behavior*, O. A. Smith, R. A. Galosy, and S. M. Weiss (Eds.). Elsevier, New York, pp. 109–120.

Gilchrist, J. M. (1985). Arrhythmogenic seizures: Diagnosis by simultaneous EEG/ECG recording. *Neurology 35*:1503–1506.

Goddard, G. V., McIntyre, D. C., and Leech, C. K. (1969). A permanent change in brain function resulting from daily electrical stimulation. *Exp. Neurol. 25*:295–300.

Goodman, J. H., Homan, R. W., and Crawford, I. L. (1990). Kindled Seizures Elevate Blood Pressure and Induce Cardiac Arrhythmias. *Epilepsia* (in press).

Guyton, A. C. (1948). Acute hypertension in dogs with cerebral ischemia. *Am. J. Physiol. 154*:45–54.

Heinemann, H., Stock, G., and Schaefer, H. (1973). Temporal correlation of responses in blood pressure and motor reaction under electrical stimulation of limbic structures in unanesthetized, unrestrained cats. *Pflügers Arch. 343*:27–40.

Hilton, S. M., and Zbrozyna, A. W. (1963). Amygdaloid region for defense reactions and its efferent pathway to the brainstem. *J. Physiol. 165*:160–173.

Hoff, J. T., and Reis, D. J. (1970). Localization of the regions mediating the Cushing response in CNS of the cat. *Arch. Neurol. 23*:228–240.

Homan, R. W., and Goodman, J. H. (1988). Endurance of the kindling effect is independent of the degree of generalization. *Brain Res. 447*:404–406.

Hopkins, D. A., and Holstege, G. (1978). Amygdaloid projections to the mesencephalon, pons and medulla oblongata in the cat. *Exp. Brain Res. 32*:529–547.

Iwata, J., Chida, K., and LeDoux, J. E. (1987). Cardiovascular responses elicited by stimulation of neurons in the central amygdaloid nucleus in awake but not anesthetized rats resemble conditioned emotional responses. *Brain Res. 418*:183–188.

Johansson, B., and Nilsson, B. (1977). The pathophysiology of the blood brain barrier dysfunction induced by severe hypercapnia and by epileptic brain activity. *Acta Neuropath. 38*:153–158.

Keilson, M. J., Hauser, W. A., Magrill, J. P., and Goldman, M. (1987). ECG abnormalities in patients with epilepsy. *Neurology 37*:1624–1626.

Kiok, M. C., Terrence, C. F., Fromm, G. H., and Lavier, S. (1986). Sinus arrest in epilepsy. *Neurology 36*:115–116.

Kumada, M., Dampney, R. A. L., and Reis, D. J. (1979). Profound hypotension and abolition of the vasomotor component of the cerebral ischemic response produced by restricted lesions of the medulla oblongata in rabbit. *Circ. Res. 45*:63–70.

Lathers, C. M., and Schraeder, P. L. (1982). Autonomic dysfunction in epilepsy: Characterization of autonomic cardiac neural discharge associated with pentylenetetrazol-induced epileptogenic activity. *Epilepsia 23*:633–647.

Lathers, C. M., Schraeder, P. L., and Carnel, S. B. (1984). Neural mechanisms in cardiac arrhythmias associated with epileptogenic activity: The effect of phenobarbital. *Life Sci. 34*:1919–1936.

Lathers, C. M., Schraeder, P. L., and Weiner, F. L. (1987). Synchronization of autonomic neural discharge with epileptogenic activity: The lockstep phenomenon. *Electroencephalogr. Clin. Neurophysiol. 67*:247–259.

Le Doux, J. E., Delbo, A., Tucker, L. W., Harshfield, G., Talman, W. T., and Reis, D. J. (1982). Hierarchic organization of blood pressure responses during the expression of natural behaviors in rat: Mediation by sympathetic nerves. *Exp. Neurol. 78*:121–133.

Leestma, J. E., Kalelkar, M. B., Teas, S. S., Jay, G. W., and Hughes, J. R. (1984). Sudden unexpected death associated with seizures: Analysis of 66 cases. *Epilepsia 25*:84–88.

Mameli, P., Mameli, O., Tolu, E., Padua, G., Giraudi, D., Caria, M. A., and Melis, F. (1988). Neurogenic myocardial arrhythmias in experimental focal epilepsy. *Epilepsia 29*:74–82.

Marshall, D. W., Westmoreland, B. F., and Sharbrough, F. W. (1983). Ictal tachycardia during temporal lobe seizures. *Mayo Clin. Proc. 58*:443–446.

Meldrum, B. S. (1976). Neuropathology and pathophysiology. In *A Textbook of Epilepsy*, J. Laidlaw and A. Richens (Eds.). Churchill-Livingstone, Edinburgh, pp. 314–354.

Meldrum, B. S., and Horton, R. W. (1973). Physiology of status epilepticus in primates. *Arch. Neurol. 28*:1–9.

Meldrum, B. S., Horton, R. W., Bloom, S. R., Butler, J., and Keenan, J. (1979). Endocrine factors and glucose metabolism during prolonged seizures in baboons. *Epilepsia 20*:527–534.

Metz, S. A., Halter, J. B., Porte, D., and Robertson, R. P. (1978). Autonomic epilepsy. *Ann. Intern. Med. 88*:189–193.

Meyer, J. S., Gotch, F., and Favale, E. (1966). Cerebral metabolism during epileptic seizures in man. *Electroencephalogr. Clin. Neurophysiol. 21*:10–22.

Millhouse, O. E. (1969). A Golgi study of the descending medial forebrain bundle. *Brain Res. 15*:341–363.

Mogenson, G. J., and Calaresu, F. R. (1973). Cardiovascular responses to electrical stimulation of the amygdala in the rat. *Exp. Neurol. 39*:166–180.

Petito, C. K., Schaeffer, J. A., and Plum, F. (1977). Ultrastructural characteristics of the brain and blood brain barrier in experimental seizures. *Brain Res. 127*: 251–267.

Pinel, J., and Rovner, L. (1978). Experimental epileptogenesis: Kindling-induced epilepsy in rats. *Exp. Neurol. 58*:190–202.

Plum, F., Posner, J. B., and Troy, B. (1968). Cerebral metabolic and circulatory responses to induced convulsions in animals. *Arch. Neurol. 18*:1–13.

Pritchett, E. L. C., McNamara, J. O., and Gallagher, J. J. (1980). Arrhythmogenic epilepsy: An hypothesis. *Am. Heart J. 100*:683–688.

Racine, R. J. (1972). Modification of seizure activity by electrical stimulation. II. Motor seizure. *Electroencephalogr. Clin. Neurophysiol. 32*:281–294.

Racine, R. J. (1978). Kindling, the first decade. *Neurosurgery 3*:234–252.

Reis, D. J., and Oliphant, M. C. (1964). Bradycardia and tachycardia following electrical stimulation of the amygdaloid region in monkey. *J. Neurophysiol. 27*:893–912.

Schwaber, J. S., Kapp, B. S., and Higgins, G. (1980). The origin and extent of direct amygdala projections to the region of the dorsal motor nucleus of the vagus and the nucleus of the solitary tract. *Neurosci. Lett. 20*:15–20.

Stock, G., Schlor, K. H., Heidt, H., and Buss, J. (1978). Psychomotor behavior and cardiovascular patterns during stimulation of the amygdala. *Pflügers Arch. 376*:177–184.

Suzuki, R., Nitsch, C., Fujiwara, K., and Klatzo, I. (1984). Regional changes in cerebral blood flow and blood brain barrier permeability during epileptic seizures and in acute hypertension in rabbits. *J. Cereb. Blood Flow Metab. 4*:96–102.

Takeuchi, Y., Mclean, J. H., and Hopkins, D. A. (1982). Reciprocal connections between the amygdala and parabrachial nuclei: Ultrastructural demonstration by degeneration and axonal transport of horseradish peroxidase in the cat. *Brain Res. 239*:583–588.

Van Buren, J. M. (1958). Some autonomic concomitants of ictal automatism. *Brain 81*:505–528.

Van Buren, J. M., and Ajmone-Marsan, C. (1960). Correlations of autonomic and EEG components in temporal lobe epilepsy. *Arch. Neurol. 3*:683–703.

Walker, J. E., Mikeska, J. A., and Crawford, I. L. (1981). Cyclic nucleotides in the amygdala of the kindled rat. *Brain Res. Bull. 6*:1–3.

Wasterlain, C. G. (1974). Mortality and morbidity from serial seizures. *Epilepsia 15*:155–176.

Westergaard, E., Hertz, M. N., and Bolwig, T. G. (1978). Increased permeability to horseradish peroxidase across cerebral vessels evoked by electrically-induced seizures in the rat. *Acta Neuropathol. 41*:73–80.

White, P. T., Grant, P., Mosier, J., and Craig, A. (1961). Changes in cerebral dynamics associated with seizures. *Neurology 11*:354–361.

12

Synchronized Cardiac Neural Discharge and Epileptogenic Activity, the Lockstep Phenomenon: Lack of Correlation with Cardiac Arrhythmias

CLAIRE M. LATHERS* *The Medical College of Pennsylvania, Eastern Pennsylvania Psychiatric Institute, Philadelphia, Pennsylvania*

PAUL L. SCHRAEDER *University of Medicine and Dentistry of New Jersey, Robert Wood Johnson Medical School, Camden, New Jersey*

I. INTRODUCTION

In a recent study, cardiac postganglionic sympathetic and vagal nerve discharges were correlated with interictal and ictal discharges (Lathers et al., 1987). The autonomic cardiac neural discharges were intermittently synchronized 1:1 with the epileptogenic discharge; this was designated the lockstep phenomenon (LSP). The LSP was not present during the control period and did not always persist once it was observed.

Dysfunction in the activity of peripheral cardiac autonomic neural discharge is contributory to the production of cardiac arrhythmias (Gillis, 1969; Lathers et al., 1974, 1977, 1978; Weaver et al., 1976) and to sudden death (Lown and Verrier, 1978). Autonomic neural dysfunction and cardiac arrhythmias occur in association with both interictal and ictal epileptogenic activity (Carnel et al., 1985; Lathers and Schraeder, 1982, 1987; Lathers et al., 1984; Penfield and Erickson, 1941; Phizackerly et al., 1954; Schraeder and Lathers, 1983; Walsh et al., 1968). Autonomic dysfunction has been implicated in sudden unexplained death in individuals with epilepsy (Jay and Leestma, 1981; Leestma et al., 1984). The studies referred to suggest that the epileptogenic activity and autonomic dysfunction may be indicative of the disruption of a normal pattern of temporally related intrinsic cortical and autonomic discharges. Thus the purpose

---

Current affiliation: FDA, Rockville, Maryland.

of this study was to examine the LSP to determine whether abnormalities in
the electrocardiogram were correlated with the altered burst discharge patterns
of the autonomic peripheral cardiac nerves synchronized with the electrocorticogram.

II. METHOD

Cats were anesthetized with alpha-chloralose and tracheostomies were done. The
femoral arteries and veins were cannulated to monitor the mean arterial blood
pressure and to administer drugs, respectively. Intermittent intravenous (i.v.)
doses of gallamine (4 mg/kg) maintained paralysis while the cats were on a small-
animal respirator. The lead II ECG was simultaneously monitored. The postganglionic cardiac sympathetic and right cardiac vagal nerve branches were isolated
and the electrical activity was recorded using the technique of Lathers et al.
(1978).

After a 10-minute control period, each cat was administered intravenous
pentylenetetrazol (PTZ) in doses of 10, 20, 50, 100, 200, and 2000 mg/kg at 10-
minute intervals. Interictal spikes (IS) were defined as discrete paroxysmal bilateral spike and/or polyspike and wave complexes. Prolonged ictal discharge
(PI) was defined as continuous polyspike activity lasting 10 seconds or longer.
Brief ictal discharge (BI) consisted of repetitive bilateral bursts of polyspike activity lasting less than 10 seconds per burst interspersed with brief periods of
depression of cerebral activity. For each 10-minute interval the presence or absence of the LSP was determined, i.e., when the neural burst discharge pattern
of postganglionic cardiac sympathetic or cardiac vagal nerves began to be synchronized with the cortical interictal and/or ictal discharges. A count was made
of the number of intradose intervals with interictal lockstep found during the
10 minutes between each dose of PTZ. Similar counts were performed for brief
and prolonged ictal LSP. A count of the number of 10-minute intervals with
each type of abnormality in the ECG was also made. The ECGs abnormalities
evaluated were changes in the P–R intervals, P waves, T waves, and QRS complexes, or the appearance of Q waves, premature atrial contractions, premature
ventricular contractions (PVCs), ventricular tachycardia, atrial fibrillation, ventricular fibrillation, asystole, or cardiovascular collapse. The number of intradose
intervals in which LSP occurred was then correlated across all subjects with the
number of intervals in which each ECG abnormality appeared. The correlations
performed both excluded and included the 2000-mg/kg dose of PTZ since this
dose induced death in all but one cat, which died after 200 mg/kg PTZ. Furthermore, if a variable was constant across subjects, or nearly so, it was not entered
into the correlations.

The relationship between the LSP and the occurrence of a given ECG change
was also analyzed. For each ECG abnormality, a separate 2 × 2 table was created

for each nerve monitored in every cat. Each minute was classified as either containing LSP or not and as exhibiting the ECG abnormality or not. The number of minutes with each of the four possible "yes/no" combinations were the entries in the 2 X 2 table. A separate 2 X 2 table was created for doses 10 and 20 mg/kg i.v. and for doses 50, 100, and 200 mg/kg i.v. PTZ. Since most of the interictal activity occurred 10 and 20 mg/kg PTZ and most of the brief or prolonged ictal activity occurred after 50, 100, and 200 mg/kg PTZ, formation of these two groups allowed comparison of changes in the electrocardiogram associated with interictal and ictal epileptogenic activity. The phi coefficient was computed as a measure of the relationship between the two variables. A +1.0 phi value indicates a perfect relationship; a –1.0 indicates a perfect inverse relationship; and a value of 0 indicates no relationship. These phi values were then averaged for all nerves monitored in each subject. These averages for each subject were then used as the unit of analysis. Although many of the individual 2 X 2 tables have extreme marginal totals, e.g., very few minutes containing a given abnormality, the average of several nerves for each subject is more reliable, especially when averaged across all subjects for reporting.

III. RESULTS

A. Dose of 2000 mg/kg PTZ Excluded

The P-R interval, T wave, P wave, QRS complex, and the occurrence of PVCs had sufficiently different numbers across subjects to be included in this analysis. Eight LSP counts, all involving sympathetic LSP, were analyzed. Of the 40 correlations generated, 3 were significant one tailed. This number is not substantially different from the two that would have been anticipated by chance, so it may be concluded that no relationship between the occurrence of the LSP and the ECG abnormalities has been shown for these data.

B. Dose of 2000 mg/kg PTZ Included

This analysis included the same ECG abnormalities described above as well as the occurrence of ventricular tachycardia, atrial fibrillation, and asystole. The ECG abnormalities were correlated with LSP. Of the 80 correlations, only 3 were significant one tailed in the predicted direction. Several correlations with atrial fibrillation and asystole would have attained significance, but they were negative, suggesting that greater frequency of LSP was related to less frequency of the ECG patterns. These results are probably artifacts due to certain ECG abnormalities occurring mainly at the death dose, when LSP is uncommon and the interval before death is short.

Table 1 indicates the abnormal ECG findings recorded in one cat associated with the epileptogenic activity elicited by each dose of PTZ. Table 2 correlates

Table 1   Abnormal Electrocardiogram Findings Associated with Epileptogenic
Activity Induced by Pentylenetetrazol in One Cat

ECG changes[a]	PTZ (mg/kg i.v.)					
	10	20	50	100	200	2000
P–R interval			X			
T wave	X		X	X	X	X
P wave					X	
QRS complex		X	X	X	X	
Ventricular tachycardia						X
Asystole						X

[a]Q waves, premature atrial contractions, atrial fibrillation, ventricular fibrillation, and
cardiovascular collapse were not observed in this cat.

Table 2   The Occurrence of the Lockstep Phenomenon Associated with
Interictal, Brief Ictal, or Prolonged Ictal Activity Induced by Pentylenetetrazol[a]

	PTZ (mg/kg i.v.)					
	10	20	50	100	200	2000
Sympathetic nerves						
LSP IS	X	X	X	X	X	
LSP BI		X	X	X	X	X
LSP PI		X				
Vagal cardiac nerve						
LSP IS	X					
LSP BI						
LSP PI						

[a]Data were obtained in the same cat whose data are included in Table 1.
Key: IS = interictal; BI = brief ictal; PI = prolonged ictal discharge.

Table 3 2 X 2 Table for Observed Changes in the T Wave for the Combined Doses of 10 and 20 mg/kg i.v. Pentylenetetrazol[a]

	LSP present	LSP absent	
T wave present	1^A	0^B	$1R_1$
T wave absent	13^C	6^D	$19R_2$
	$14C1$	$6C2$	

$$\text{phi coefficient} \quad \frac{AD - BC}{R_1R_2C_1C_2} = \frac{1.6 - 13.0}{1 \times 19 \times 14 \times 6} = 0.16$$

[a]Data were determined for the same cat whose data are included in Tables 1 and 2. The data in this table were obtained from one sympathetic nerve monitored in one cat. Each minute in the 10 one-minute periods after 10 and 20 mg/kg i.v. PTZ was classified as either containing LPS or not and as exhibiting changes in the T wave or not. The number of minutes with each of the four possible "yes/no" combinations are the entries in this 2 X 2 table.

Table 4 Phi Coefficients Obtained for All Eight Cats Exhibiting T Wave Changes Associated with Epileptogenic Activity Induced by Pentylenetetrazol

Experimental date	PTZ (mg/kg)[a]		
	10–20	50, 100, 200	DIF
1-09	0.16	–0.17	0.33
1-24	–0.14	0.11	–0.25
2-27	–0.263	0.003	–0.266
3-03		0.205	
3-05	–0.41	0.115	–0.525
3-10	–0.49	–0.28	–0.21
3-17	0.60	–0.20	0.80
3-19	–0.06	–0.185	0.125
Mean	–0.086	–0.05	0.0006
SE	0.373	0.1807	0.45
N	7	8	7
t vs. ϕ	–0.61	–0.783	< 0.1
p	NS	NS	NS

[a]Neither group of doses of pentylenetetrazol exhibited an average phi different from zero.
Key: NS = not significant.

Table 5 Summary of Changes in the P Wave and QRS Complex Associated
with Epileptogenic Activity Induced by Pentylenetetrazol

	PTZ (mg/kg i.v.)		
Change	10 + 20 vs. ϕ	50–200 vs ϕ	df vs. ϕ
P wave	NS	NS	NS
QRS complex	NS	NS	NS
Brief ictal	NS	NS	NS
Interictal	Positive one-tailed only	NS	NS
Prolonged ictal	NS	$p < 0.05*$	$p < 0.05**$

Key: NS = not significant.
*One-tailed t-test; **one-tailed t-test, more positive relationship at higher doses.

the occurrence of LSP associated with interictal, brief ictal, or prolonged ictal
activity induced by all doses of PTZ. Similar tables (not shown) were constructed for each cat; the findings were similar to those included in Table 1. A 2 X 2
table was created (Table 3) for changes in the T wave associated with discharge
in the first sympathetic branch monitored in this cat at doses of 10 and 20
mg/kg PTZ. The phi coefficient was calculated and was 0.16. The phi value for
the T wave changes occurring after doses of 50, 100, and 200 mg/kg PTZ was
–0.17. Table 4 lists the phi coefficients obtained for all eight cats exhibiting the
T wave changes. The data indicate that neither group of doses of pentylenetetrazol had an average phi coefficient different from zero.

Table 5 is a brief summary of the changes in the P wave and in the QRS complex associated with the three types of epileptogenic activity elicited by the two
groups of PTZ, (1) 10 and 20 and (2) 50, 100, and 200 mg/kg i.v. Most of the
phi values were near zero, indicating the presence of only a few significant phi
values.

IV. DISCUSSION

This study found no relationship between the occurrence of LSP and abnormalities of cardiac depolarization and repolarization in association with PTZ-
induced epileptogenic activity in the absence of an anticonvulsant agent. These
data agree with those obtained in a different group of animals pretreated with
phenobarbital (Dodd-o and Lathers, Chapter 13, this book). The lack of a correlation between the presence of LSP and the occurrence of abnormalities, discussed in this chapter and Chapter 13, should not be confused with the positive

correlation of ECG changes with LSP which was found when the variability of interspike interval was analyzed.

Stauffer et al. (1988) showed that the occurrence of precipitous mean arterial blood pressure changes was correlated with unstable LSP and postulated four possible mechanisms through which LSP may be related to arrhythmia and sudden death in persons with epilepsy:

1. Excessive sympathetic stimulation of a heart that is already electrically unstable due to prior damage (Jay and Leestma, 1981).
2. A nonuniform (simultaneous increases, decreases, or no change) discharge in the postganglionic cardiac sympathetic nerve branches (Lathers et al., 1977, 1978).
3. The parasympathetic nervous system causing sinus arrest and bradycardia during seizures (Kiok et al., 1986; Lathers and Schraeder, 1982).
4. The precipitous blood pressure changes per se.

Evans and Gillis (1978) elicited blood pressure increases by stimulation of the hypothalamus and found that the associated arrhythmias occurred after but not during stimulation and were the result of a sudden surge of parasympathetic activity reflexively evoked by the rapid rise in blood pressure. The proposed four mechanisms that may lead to arrhythmias and sudden death are not mutually exclusive. It is possible that no single mechanism can explain all cases of sudden death in epilepsy. Some cases may result from ventricular fibrillation related to a lowered ventricular fibrillation threshold associated with increased sympathetic discharge. Other cases may result from sinus arrest related to reflex parasympathetic discharge evoked by precipitous blood pressure changes, especially if there is some cardiac damage produced by prior sympathetic stimulation.

Polosa et al. (1971) reported findings similar to the LSP described in this study. They noted spontaneous, rhythmic, synchronized activity of the sympathetic cervical nerve, the cervical phrenic nerve, and small strands of the sciatic nerve after the administration of PTZ. That complex interactions exist between afferent and efferent discharges at central and peripheral levels of the autonomic nervous system is known. What is not known is the exact mechanism of rhythmicity and synchronization in peripheral nerve activity, although central mechanisms are thought to predominate (Polossa et al., 1969, 1970). The activity of populations of preganglionic or postganglionic sympathetic nerves is synchronized into bursts or slow waves that are usually temporally related to the phases of the cardiac and respiratory cycles (Gebber et al., 1980a,b). The oscillations in the discharge of whole sympathetic nerve bundles depict the synchronized firing of a large population of individual preganglionic and postganglionic neuronal units. Factors that determine the number of spontaneously active units at any given moment and the discharge rate of an individual preganglionic sympathetic neuron include the level of the mean arterial blood pressure (via the baroreceptor input), the level of CO_2 (via the chemoreceptor input), the excitability of the neurons, and the degree of synchrony within the driving input to these neurons from the brain stem and from somatic and visceral inputs (Barman et al., 1984).

Dodd-o and Lathers (Chapter 13, this book) found that when stable LSP was lost, precipitous mean arterial blood pressure changes occurred more frequently. This finding supports the fact that changes in the mean arterial blood pressure alter the number of units and the discharge rate of individual preganglionic sympathetic nerves and could be a factor in destabilization of previously stable LSP. When stable LSP was lost, ECG changes occurred more frequently. In addition, specific burst patterns resulting from stimulation of the preganglionic nerve innervating the cat stellate ganglia can increase the number of neurons discharging in the inferior cardiac nerve (Birks et al., 1981), supporting the conclusion that such burst patterns of neural input are a major presynaptic mechanism in the modulation of synaptic transmission in sympathetic ganglia. Thus the central neuronal outflow is an important factor in altering the peripheral efferent discharge to the heart, which can initiate abnormalities in the ECG. The fact that central neuronal outflow alters the peripheral efferent discharge to the heart, resulting in arrhythmias, may explain why the present study did not find a correlation in the occurrence of LSP and the occurrence of abnormalities in the ECG. It may be that the development of LSP precedes the occurrence of changes in the ECG or vice versa. Definitive experiments will have to be done to verify this possibility.

The clinical significance of the lack of correlation of the occurrence of LSP with the occurrence of abnormalities in the ECG may be inferred from a recent discussion by Blumhardt et al. (1986). They reported that in some patients with temporal lobe epilepsy, cardiac acceleration prceded the onset of recognizable rhythmic surface EEG seizure activity and suggested that this sequence may reflect the onset of electrical discharge in deep limbic circuits and in the connections of these structures with the autonomic nervous system. Their study did not find a direct correlation between the occurrence of ECG abnormalities and the development of rhythmical neuronal activity, at least as observable using the previously described recording techniques. Indeed, in some patients arrhythmias were observed at times when there were no seizure discharges on the EEG. These authors also noted that the autonomic effects of temporal lobe epilepsy on heart rate and rhythm may be more severe in untreated, younger patients. This finding agrees with the observation that young epileptic patients are at high risk of sudden unexplained death. In another study, Blumhardt and Oozeer (1982) noted that simultaneous EEG and ECG recordings from patients with established epilepsy have demonstrated the occurrence of nonepileptic and epileptic events on the same tape. They emphasized that the negative findings obtained in some patients must be cautiously interpreted and the outcome established by long-term follow-up studies. We believe that this conclusion and the results of our experimental work herein described suggest the need for more sophisticated electrophysiological monitoring of brain regions involved in autonomic control.

ACKNOWLEDGMENTS

The authors would like to thank Albert Weinhardt and Carol O'Tormey for technical help; Valerie Farris, Isha Agarwal, and Dr. Edward Gracely for statistical analyses; and Darlene Spino for typing the manuscript.

REFERENCES

Barman, S. M., Gebber, G. L., and Cadarexu, F. Q. (1984). Differential control of sympathetic nerve discharge by the brain stem. *Am. J. Physiol. 247*:R513–519.

Birks, R. I., Laskey, W., and Polosa, C. (1981). The effect of burst patterning of preganglionic input on the efficacy of transmission at the cat stellate ganglion. *J. Physiol. (London) 318*:531–539.

Blumhardt, L. D., and Oozeer, R. C. (1982). Simultaneous ambulatory monitoring of the EEG and ECG in patients with unexplained transient disturbances of consciousness. In *ISAM Proceedings of the 4th Gent 1981 Symposium on Ambulatory Monitoring and the 2nd Gent Workshop on Blood Pressure Variability*, F. D. Stott, E. B. Raferty, D. L. Clement, and S. L. Wright (Eds.). Academic Press, New York, 171–182.

Blumhardt, L. D., Smith, P. E. M., and Owen, L. (1986). Electrocardiographic accompaniments of temporal lobe epileptic seizures. *Lancet* May 10:1051–1055.

Carnel, S. B., Schraeder, P. L., and Lathers, C. M. (1985). Effect of phenobarbital pretreatment on cardiac neural discharge and pentylenetetrazol-induced epileptogenic activity in the cat. *Pharmacology 30*:225–240.

Evans, D. E., and Gillis, R. A. (1978). Reflex mechanisms involved in cardiac arrhythmias induced by hypothalamic stimulation. *Am. J. Physiol. 234*: H199–H209.

Gebber, G. L. (1980a). Central oscillators responsible for sympathetic nerve discharge. *Am. J. Physiol. 239*:H143–H155.

Gebber, G. L. (1980b). Bulbospinal control of sympathetic nerve discharge. In *Neural Control of Circulation*, M. J. Hughes and C. D. Barnes (Eds.). Academic Press, New York, pp. 51–80.

Gillis, R. A. (1969). Cardiac sympathetic nerve activity: Changes induced by ouabain and propranolol. *Science 166*:508–510.

Jay, G. W., and Leestma, J. E. (1981). Sudden death in epilepsy. *Acta Neurol. Scand. 63*:1–66.

Kiok, M. C., Terrence, C. F., Fromm, G. H., and Lavine, S. (1986). Sinus arrest in epilepsy. *Neurology 36*:115–116.

Lathers, C. M., and Schraeder, P. L. (1982). Autonomic dysfunction in epilepsy. Characterization of autonomic cardiac neural discharge associated with pentylenetetrazol-induced epileptogenic activity. *Epilepsia 23*:633–648.

Lathers, C. M., and Schraeder, P. L. (1987). Review of autonomic dysfunction, cardiac arrhythmias, and epileptogenic activity. *J. Clin. Pharmacol. 27*:346–356.

Lathers, C. M., Roberts, J., and Kelliher, G. J. (1974). Relationship between the effect of ouabain on arrhythmia and interspike intervals (ISI) of cardiac accelerator nerves. *Pharmacologist 16*:201.

Lathers, C. M., Roberts, J., and Kelliher, G. J. (1977). Correlations of ouabain-induced arrhythmia and nonuniformity in the histamine-evoked discharge of cardiac sympathetic nerves. *J. Pharmacol. Exp. Ther. 203*:467–479.

Lathers, C. M., Kelliher, G. J., Roberts, J., and Beasley, A. B. (1978). Nonuniform cardiac sympathetic nerve discharge: Mechanism for coronary occlusion and digitalis-induced arrhythmia. *Circulation 57*:1058–1065.

Lathers, C. M., Schraeder, P. L., and Carnel, S. B. (1984). Neural mechanisms in cardiac arrhythmias associated with epileptogenic activity: The effect of phenobarbital. *Life Sci. 34*:1919–1936.

Lathers, C. M., Schraeder, P. L., and Weiner, F. L. (1987). Synchronization of cardiac autonomic neural discharge with epileptogenic activity: The lockstep phenomenon. *Electroencephalogr. Clin. Neurophysiol. 67*:247–259.

Leestma, J. E., Kalelkar, M. B., Teas, S. S., Jay, G. W., and Hughes, J. R. (1984). Sudden unexplained death associated with seizure. Analysis of 66 cases. *Epilepsia 25*:84–88.

Lown, B., and Verrier, R. L. (1978). Neural factors and sudden death. In *Perspectives in Cardiovascular Research*, Vol. 2, P. J. Schwartz, A. M. Brown, A. Malliani, and A. Zanchetti (Eds.). Raven Press, New York, pp. 87–98.

Penfield, W., and Erickson, T. C. (1941). *Epilepsy and Cerebral Localization: A Study of the Mechanism, Treatment, and Prevention of Epileptic Seizures.* Thomas, Springfield, Ill., pp. 320–362.

Phizackerly, P. J. R., Poole, E. W., and Whitty, C. W. M. (1954). Sinoauricular heart block as an epileptic manifestation: A case report. *Epilepsia 3*:89–91.

Polosa, C., Rozenberg, P., Mannard, A., Wolkove, N., and Wyszogrodski, I. (1969). Oscillatory behavior of the sympathetic system induced by picrotoxin. *Can. J. Physiol. Pharmacol. 47*:815–826.

Polosa, C., Wyszogrodski, I., and Mannard, A. (1970). Origin of the patterned sympathetic preganglionic neuron discharge undelrying vasomotor waves. In *Proceedings of the Symposium on Interneuronal Transmission in the Autonomic Neuron System.* Igaku Shoin, Tokyo.

Polosa, C., Teare, J. L., and Wyszogrodski, I. (1971). Slow rhythms of sympathetic discharge induced by convulsant drugs. *Can. J. Physiol. Pharmacol. 50*:188–194.

Schraeder, P. L., and Lathers, C. M. (1983). Cardiac neural discharge and epileptogenic activity in the cat: An animal model for unexplained sudden death. *Life Sci. 32*:1371–1382.

Stauffer, A. Z., Dodd-o, J. M., and Lathers, C. M. (1989). The relationship of the lockstep phenomenon and precipitous changes in mean arterial blood pressure. *Electroencephalogr. Clin. Neurophysiol. 72*:340-345.

Walsh, G., Masland, W., and Goldensohn, E. (1968). Paroxysmal cerebral discharge associated with paroxysmal atrial tachycardia. *Electroencephalogr. Clin. Neurophysiol. 24*:187.

Weaver, L. C., Akera, J., and Brody, T. M. (1976). Digoxin toxicity: Primary sites of drug action on the sympathetic nervous system. *J. Pharmacol. Exp. Ther. 197*:1-9.

13

A Characterization of the Lockstep Phenomenon in Phenobarbital-Pretreated Cats

JEFFREY M. DODD-O* and CLAIRE M. LATHERS† *The Medical College of Pennsylvania, Eastern Pennsylvania Psychiatric Institute, Philadelphia, Pennsylvania*

I. INTRODUCTION

Sudden unexplained death (SUD) was defined by Jay and Leestma (1981) as "non-traumatic death occurring in an individual within minutes or hours of the onset of the final illness or ictus." These patients are not previously known to be suffering from any illness that would normally be expected to cause sudden death and no pathologic explanation for their death has been found. Up to a 13% incidence of SUD has been reported in persons with epilepsy, with the epileptic population most at risk for SUD being the young person with a mean age of 32 years (Jay and Leestma, 1981; Krohn, 1977). Many causes for SUD have been postulated, including autonomic dysfunction and its relation to epileptogenic discharge (Jay and Leestma, 1981).

Using diverse models, different investigators have shown evidence of intrinsic activity at various levels in the nervous system. Cortical rhythms, controlled by subcortical neurons (Kiloh et al., 1972b) thought by many to be located in the thalamus (Kiloh et al., 1982a), are the basis for the alpha (8-13 Hz), beta (20-22 Hz), delta (3-4 Hz), etc., rhythms of electroencephalography. Basar (1976) used stereotaxic procedures to demonstrate spontaneous activities from medial geniculate nuclei, inferior colliculus, mesencephalic reticular formation, and dorsal hippocampus. Numerous studies (Barman and Gebber, 1980, 1981; Gebber and Barman, 1981) suggest the existence of an inherent rhythm of sympathetic nerve discharge, possibly originating from the hypothalamus (Barman and Gebber, 1982). The results of Gebber and Barman (1981) indicate that a temporal relationship exists between the intrinsic rhythms of the central and the

Current affiliation:
*University of North Texas, Fort Worth, Texas.
†FDA, Rockville, Maryland.

autonomic nervous systems. Lathers et al. (1977, 1978) reported that changes in the rate of autonomic discharge from postganglionic cardiac sympathetic branches may contribute to cardiac dysrhythmias. Thus it is quite plausible that the association between epileptogenic activity and autonomic dysfunction evidenced in both animal (Lathers and Schraeder, 1982; Meldrum and Brierley, 1973; Meldrum and Horton, 1973; Wasterlain, 1974) and human (Jay and Leestma, 1981; Van Buren, 1958) studies may be a manifestation of the disruption of a normal pattern of temporally related intrinsic cortical and autonomic discharges.

Studies in this laboratory have demonstrated a temporal synchronization between electrocorticogram (ECoG) activity and intrathoracic cardiac postganglionic sympathetic discharge during both ictal and interictal epileptogenic states (Lathers et al., 1987). The purpose of this chapter is to describe this phenomenon in phenobarbital-pretreated cats undergoing epileptogenic activity induced by pentylenetetrazol (PTZ). This relationship between the central nervous system discharges and the autonomic nervous system may prove important in explaining the high incidence of SUD in epilepsy.

II. METHOD

Nine cats were anesthetized with 80 mg/kg intravenous alpha-chloralose. Tracheostomy was performed, and the femoral artery and vein were cannulated. Ventilation was maintained using a small-animal respirator, with intravenous gallamine (4 mg/kg doses, intermittently) being used to maintain paralysis. Arterial blood gases were monitored, and ventilation was altered to maintain the pO_2, pCO_2, and pH values within an acceptable physiological range. A bilateral frontal craniectomy was performed and the dura resected to record ECoG activity. A thoracotomy and right partial pneumonectomy were performed to expose the cardiac postganglionic and right cardiac vagal nerves near the heart. The former were identified as sympathetic by their discharge response to blood pressure drop produced by intravenous (i.v.) injection of 5 μg/kg histamine (Lathers et al., 1978). These nerves were desheathed and nerve activity was recorded in one or more small nerve branches. Mean arterial blood pressure, electrocardiogram (lead II of the ECG), heart rate, and rectal temperature were monitored continuously throughout the experiment. Rectal temperature was maintained between 37.5 and 38.5 degrees centigrade.

A 10-minute control period was monitored before beginning infusion of phenobartital (20 mg/kg i.v.) over 10 minutes. One hour after completing the phenobarbital infusion, six doses of PTZ (10, 20, 50, 100, 200, and 2000 mg/kg) were administered intravenously at 10-minute intervals. The half-life of this drug in the cat is unknown (Knoll Laboratories, personal communications) but has been shown to be 1.4 hours in the dog (Jun, 1976). If one assumes the half-life to be similar in the cat, these doses of PTZ administered were probably cumulative.

Epileptiform discharges were categorized in three degrees, according to duration of discharge. Polyspike discharges continuing for 10 seconds or longer were designated prolonged ictal. Repetitive polyspike bursts of less than 10 seconds duration interrupted by brief periods of baseline cerebral activity were classified as brief ictal. These types of ictal activity are analogous to those seen in the EEG during clinical seizures. Interictal spikes were those bilateral discrete paroxysmal spikes and/or polyspike and wave discharges analogous to the nonictal epileptogenic activity seen routinely in the interictal EEG of patients with a seizure disorder.

In distinguishing interictal discharges from brief ictal activity, spikes occurring more frequently than 3.3/second were not counted as interictal discharges. This maximal rate was decided on after determining that each oscillation of the polygraph pen required at least 100 msec to occur. A 200-msec return to baseline activity was considered evidence distinguishing a series of consecutive interictal spikes from one continuous brief ictal discharge. Spikes occurring more frequently than 3.3/second (or 300 msec between the beginning of any two consecutive spikes) were classified as part of the same polyspike discharge activity.

An interictal ECoG spike was considered to be time locked to a sympathetic discharge only if the latter began within 200 msec of the beginning of the interictal ECoG spike. Each brief ictal discharge was analyzed as a single unit along with its corresponding autonomic activity. The brief ictal and autonomic discharges were considered time locked only if the autonomic activity depicted a single polyspike discharge whose first spike began after the brief ictal discharge began and whose last spike began before the end of the final spike composing the brief ictal discharge. When the ECoG displayed prolonged ictal activity, the autonomic and ECoG discharge during this time period was not considered to be time locked.

When sympathetic and ECoG spikes were time locked for an uninterrupted time period of 10 or more seconds, the total duration of this event was measured. Time-locked discharges were considered to depict LSP when (1) at least two episodes of time-locked autonomic and epileptogenic activity occurred during the 10-second interval, and (2) sympathetic activity occurred more frequently than ECoG activity, or vice versa. In the latter criterion no more than one discharge from the less frequent component was allowed to exist without being time locked. If the sympathetic and ECoG spikes were not consistently time locked over a period of at least 10 seconds (uninterrupted), these spikes were not considered to be exhibiting LSP. If the discharges were time locked for more than 10 seconds and were then interrupted for 4.5 seconds or less, the time-locked discharges were classified as uninterrupted LSP. Interruptions longer than 4.5 seconds indicated that LSP had ended.

The amount of LSP was quantified in terms of incidence and in terms of duration. To quantify incidence, the number of time-locked ECoG and autonomic spikes exhibiting LSP was determined for the 10-minute interval following each dose of PTZ. Next, the total number of sympathetic spikes and of ECoG spikes were determined for each of the nine cats for each of the six doses of PTZ. Also listed were the number of LSP discharges per total number of sympathetic discharges (LSP/S) and ECoG discharges (LSP/E). The value LSP/S is a measure of the proportion of all sympathetic spikes that are locked to ECoG spikes under the conditions of LSP. Likewise, the value LSP/E is a measure of the proportion of all ECoG spikes that are locked to sympathetic spikes under the conditions of LSP.

To quantify duration, the total time (seconds) each cat spent in or out of LSP was determined. This was further classified to depict one of the following situations:

1. The duration of LSP during each minute following administration of PTZ. In this case all doses of PTZ were grouped together and time spent in LSP was determined only as a function of the latency period following administration of PTZ.
2. The duration of LSP during each dose of PTZ administered. In this case duration of LSP was determined for each dose of PTZ regardless of the delay between administration of the drug and beginning of LSP.

One-factor analysis of variance (ANOVA) with repeated measures on time compared the mean proportions of total time that cats displayed LSP following the administration of PTZ. Means were collapsed across doses. A post-hoc Student Newman–Keuls test (alpha = 0.050) was performed when indicated.

Analogous tests compared the observed frequency of LSP during each dose of PTZ. The mean proportions of total time that cats displayed LSP during each 10-minute interval following the administration of each dose of PTZ was examined.

To determine whether the observed incidence of LSP could be due to chance alone, two multiple regressions were performed. In these analyses, the dependent variables were LSP/S and LSP/E. The independent variables were the number of sympathetic and ECoG spikes.

Each spike of the ECoG was associated with two other spikes on the ECoG, one preceding it by 2.8 seconds and one following it by 2.8 seconds, a repeated ECoG interval observed in all cats. The 2.8-second interval could contain other episodes of ECoG activity. Frequently, each episode of ECoG activity contained

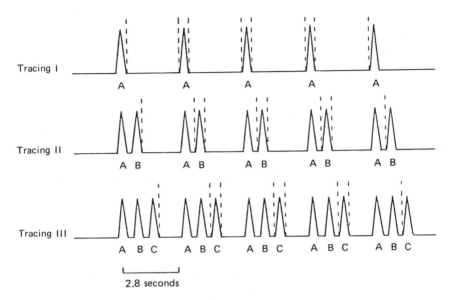

Figure 1   Repeated 2.8-second interval in the electrocorticogram. Tracing I, basic 2.8-second repeated interval. Tracing II, acceptable variation of 2.8-second repeated interval. Tracing III, unacceptable variation. A, B, and C, each a separate subset of interrelated spikes.

within this 2.8-second interval was itself associated with two other ECoG spikes, one preceding it by 2.8 seconds and one following it by 2.8 seconds. The number of spikes contained within this 2.8 second interval varied greatly. However, the 2.8-second repeated ECoG interval was not considered to be present whenever it contained more than one other ECoG discharge within these borders.

Figure 1 is a diagram of these criteria for classification of presence or absence of the repeated ECoG interval. The ordinate displays the amplitude of the spike and the abscissa displays the time interval between spikes. Tracing I displays the basic 2.8-second interval. This interval is actually the duration of the latency period from the end of one spike to the beginning of a spike with which it is associated. All spikes labeled A are related by this 2.8-second latency period. In tracing II, each pair of A spikes related by a 2.8-second interval envelops another B spike. Each B spike is itself related to two other B spikes by a 2.8-second interval. In tracing III, each pair of A spikes related by a 2.8-second repeated ECoG interval envelops two additional (B and C) spikes. Tracing III violates our criteria for categorization as presence of repeated ECoG interval.

Determination was made of the total time (seconds) the repeated ECoG interval was observed. If the repeated ECoG interval (defined above) was present before being interrupted for 4.5 seconds or less, it was considered to be present without interruption, since interruptions longer than 4.5 seconds marked the end of the repeated ECoG interval.

Sympathetic–ECoG activity was classified based on both LSP (presence vs. absnece) and the repeated ECoG interval (presence or absence). The four patterns are: (1) LSP present with repeated ECoG interval present; (2) LSP present with repeated ECoG interval absent; (3) LSP absent with repeated ECoG interval present; and (4) LSP absent with repeated ECoG interval absent.

The cats were evaluated for all doses of LSP, excluding the 2000 mg/kg dose. If artifact rendered segments of either the sympathetic or the ECoG printout unreadable, this segment was deleted.

A paired t-test was used to compare time spent in LSP with repeated ECoG interval present with time spent in LSP with repeated ECoG interval absent. A second paired t-test was performed to compare time spent in LSP with repeated ECoG interval present with time spent with LSP absent with repeated ECoG interval present.

An ANOVA with repeated measures on time and dose and a post-hoc Student Neuman–Keuls test (alpha = 0.050) were performed for each of the following six patterns of ECoG–sympathetic activity: (1) LSP present with repeated ECoG interval present; (2) LSP present with repeated ECoG interval absent; (3) total LSP; (4) LSP absent with repeated ECoG interval present; (5) LSP absent with repeated ECoG interval absent; and (6) total LSP absent.

Precipitous, rather than gradual changes in mean arterial pressure were measured in order to highlight any possible changes in the character of LSP coincident with a change in the mean arterial blood pressure. The mean arterial blood pressure changes occurring in all nine cats were reviewed during the control period, the phenobarbital infusion period, and the PTZ treatment period. Systolic changes of greater than 23 mm Hg over a 10-second interval were never seen during the control period; thus changes greater than 23 mm Hg over a 10-second interval were defined as precipitous. A total of 89 such episodes were analyzed after administration of all doses of PTZ except 2000 mg/kg. This dosage led to death in all cats.

The incidence of precipitous change in mean arterial blood pressure was analyzed using two different methods. Ninety-five percent confidence intervals were constructed around the incidences of precipitous mean arterial blood pressure changes for each minute following the administration of all doses of PTZ. Ninety-five percent confidence intervals were also constructed around the incidences of precipitous mean arterial blood pressure changes at each dose of PTZ.

The ECG of each cat was analyzed during the control period to find any abnormality intrinsic to that particular cat. These were discarded and any new abnormalities occurring after the administration of PTZ were evaluated. Each change was classified according to the time interval during which it occurred and according to the dose during which it occurred. The ECG parameters examined were (1) T wave changes; (2) P wave changes; (3) changes in the QRS complexes; (4) the appearance of a Q wave; (5) premature ventricular contractions; and (6) ventricular tachycardia.

Ninety-five percent confidence intervals were constructed around the incidences of ECG changes for each minute following dosing with PTZ and for each dose of PTZ administered.

III. RESULTS

As depicted in Figure 2, no ECoG spikes were time locked to a sympathetic discharge in the control period (Fig. 2.I) or in the period during the infusion of phenobarbital prior to the administration of PTZ (Figure 2.II). Interictal ECoG spikes were time locked to the sympathetic discharge in Figure 2.III and were designated LSP.

The latency period varied, but the ECoG discharge always preceded the corresponding sympathetic discharge. Sympathetic discharge was observed less frequently than was ECoG discharge. However, in 93% of the time periods during which sympathetic activity was present, the proportion of these discharges which were time locked to ECoG spikes was 0.85 or greater. Further analysis using multiple regressions and bivariate correlations suggested that the incidence of observed LSP was limited more by the incidence of observed sympathetic discharge than by the incidence of observed ECoG discharge.

Table 1 compares, for each cat, the percentage of time that LSP was present (with or without the repeated ECoG interval) with the percentage of time absent. In eight of nine cats LSP was observed to be present during at least 55% of the experiment (LSP present being defined as LSP present with repeated ECoG interval present and with repeated ECoG interval absent). In all cats following all doses of PTZ, LSP was present 66% of the time on average.

The proportion of time each cat demonstrated each pattern is shown in Table 1. As an example, cat 4 demonstrated the pattern LSP present with repeated ECoG interval present for 60% of the time. This was determined by dividing the total number of seconds evaluated (3000 seconds) into the total time the pattern was observed (1801 seconds). Similarly, this cat demonstrated the pattern LSP present with repeated ECoG interval absent 1% of the time, the pattern LSP absent with repeated ECoG interval present 14% of the time, and the pattern LSP absent with repeated ECoG interval absent 26% of the time.

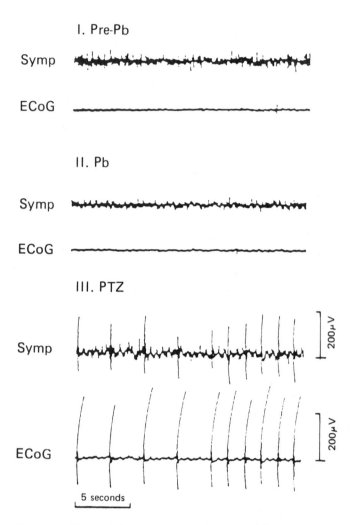

Figure 2 The occurrence of sympathetic and ECoG discharges in a time-locked manner, i.e., the lockstep phenomenon (LSP). Traces in I, II, and III are three different time periods from the same cat: (I) during prephenobarbital control period; (II) 9 minutes, 50 seconds into phenobarbital control period; (III) 8 minutes, 50 seconds into the PTZ 200 mg/kg dosage. Symp = cardiac sympathetic postganglionic neurons. ECoG = electrocorticogram. The horizontal calibration is 5 cm/sec in all cases. The vertical calibration is 200 μV/cm in all cases. The mean arterial blood pressures (not shown)-ECG patterns mean heart rates were: (I) 120-normal-131; (II) 54-normal-112; and (III) 98-normal-152, respectively.

Table 1 Contingency Table Displaying the Presence or Absence of the Lockstep Phenomenon Versus the Presence or Absence of the Repeated Electrocortical Interval

Cat number	LSP present, repeated ECoG interval present (% total for cat)	LSP present, repeated ECoG interval absent (% total for cat)	LSP absent, repeated ECoG interval present (% total for cat)	LSP absent, repeated ECoG interval absent (% total for cat)
1	68	13	15	5
2	40	12	18	31
3	13	1	18	68
4	60	1	14	26
5	41	3	24	33
6	63	3	5	29
7	42	0	26	32
8	46	7	24	22
9	67	3	9	21
Average	49	5	17	30

Table 2 Proportion of Sympathetic and Electrocortical Spike and Proportions of Each in

Cat. No.	PZT 10 mg/kg				PZT 20 mg/kg				PZT 50 mg/kg			
	# Symp	# ECoG	LSP S	LSP E	# Symp	# ECoG	LSP S	LSP E	# Symp	# ECoG	LSP S	LSP E
1	253	313	1.0000	0.8083	354	356	0.9972	0.9916	451	450	0.9956	0.9978
2	48	161	0.9583	0.2857	340	465	0.9882	0.7225	471	582	0.9915	0.9193
3	–	–	–	–	73	308	0.5753	0.1364	224	302	0.8036	0.5960
4	=	=	–	–	204	396	0.5887	0.3682	358	368	0.9915	0.9511
5	–	–	–	–	219	227	1.0000	0.9648	129	641	1.0000	0.2012
6	–	–	–	–	256	390	0.9883	0.6477	337	352	0.9941	0.9517
7	–	–	–	–	239	260	1.0000	0.9192	345	359	1.0000	0.9610
8	139	9	0.0504	0.7778	276	301	0.9746	0.8937	304	310	0.9901	0.9710
9	–	–	–	–	346	374	0.9942	0.9198	298	346	0.9933	0.8555

Note that for the one cat in which LSP was not present during at least 55% of the experiment, the data contained long recording periods which were technically inadequate for quantitative description of the relationship between ECoG and sympathetic spikes. Observation of these periods in cat 8 revealed that they were usually composed of global increases in ECoG activity associated with global increases in sympathetic activity.

Table 2 lists the incidences of sympathetic spikes (# Symp) and ECoG spikes (# ECoG) for the 10-minute period following the administration of a dose of PTZ for each cat. Also listed, in decimal form, are measures of (1) the proportion of sympathetic spikes that occurred time locked to ECoG spikes (TL/S) and (2) the proportion of ECoG spikes that occurred time locked to sympathetic spikes (TL/E). In 40 of the 45 (89%) measured time intervals the ECoG discharges occurred more frequently than did the sympathetic discharges. Also, in 43 of 45 (93%) of the measured time periods, the ratio TL/S was greater than 0.85. This high incidence of ECoG activity occurring more frequently than sympathetic activity, combined with the high proportion ($>$0.85) of observed sympathetic spikes being time locked to ECoG spikes in 93% of the measured time periods, suggests that the incidence of observed sympathetic firings was the limiting factor in the total number of times when time locked activity (and, secondarily, LSP) was observed.

the Lockstep Phenomenon

PZT 100 mg/kg				PZT 200 mg/kg				PZT 2000 mg/kg			
# Symp	# ECoG	LSP S	LSP E	# Symp	# ECoG	LSP S	LSP E	# Symp	# ECoG	LSP S	LSP E
441	429	0.9728	1.0000	318	306	0.9245	0.9608	010	010	1.0000	1.0000
290	335	1.0000	0.8657	124	284	0.9919	0.4331	048	048	1.0000	1.0000
110	125	0.8727	0.7680	262	255	0.8588	0.8824	–	–	–	–
399	430	1.0000	0.9279	392	402	0.9974	0.9726	–	–	–	–
238	328	0.9958	0.7226	211	285	0.8720	0.6456	022	024	0.9091	0.8333
359	395	0.9944	0.9038	225	277	0.9956	0.8087	007	013	1.0000	0.5385
444	443	0.9752	0.9774	347	352	0.9337	0.9204	–	–	–	–
376	432	0.9947	0.8657	158	364	1.0000	0.4341	018	036	1.0000	0.5000
403	398	0.9876	1.0000	359	372	0.9972	0.9624	046	047	1.0000	0.9787

Further evidence that the incidence of LSP is limited by the frequency of sympathetic discharge was that (1) multiple regressions showed no significant predictor where TL/S is dependent; (2) multiple regressions showed TL/E was related to #Symp and to #ECoG (multiple $r = 0.86$ significant to 0.00005); and (3) bivariate correlation of # Symp (0.55, step 1, proportion of variance = 0.30) and # ECoG (0.01, step 2, proportion of variance = 0.73) suggested that ECoG becomes a factor in raising the predictability of ECoG time locked only after sympathetic activity has made its impact.

A certain stability to the neural activity and a high incidence of LSP were associated with the presence of the repeated 2.8-second interval in ECoG. Disruption of this rhythm was associated with a degeneration of LSP. When LSP was present, it was associated an average 74% of the time ($p < 0.01$) with a 2.8-second repeated ECoG interval [13,131 seconds of LSP present with repeated ECoG interval present divided by (13,131 + 4545) seconds of LSP present with and without a repeated ECoG interval present]. Furthermore, when the repeated ECoG interval was present, LSP was absent 9% of the time [1268 seconds repeated ECoG interval present with LSP absent divided by (13,131 + 1268) seconds of repeated ECoG interval present with and without LSP present] ($p < 0.01$). When the repeated ECoG interval was absent, LSP was absent more frequently than present (average 17% LSP without ECoG vs. average 30% LSP absent without ECoG).

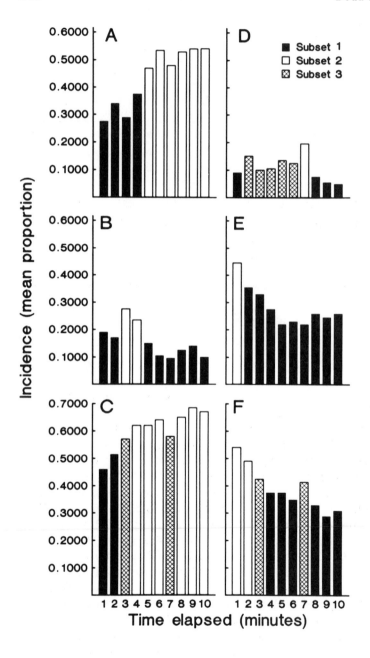

The relative prevalence (seconds) of each sympathetic–ECoG pattern following the administration of PTZ was examined. Figure 3 shows that as the time period after the administration of the most recent dose of PTZ increased, (1) the mean proportion of time that LSP was present with repeated ECoG interval present increased regularly (panel A); (2) the mean proportion of time that LSP was present with repeated ECoG interval absent decreased irregularly (panel B); and (3) the mean proportion of time that LSP was present with or without repeated ECoG interval present increased gradually (panel C). Similarly, panels D, E, and F of Figure 3 show that as the time period after the administration of the most recent dose of PTZ increased, (1) the mean proportion of time that LSP was absent with repeated ECoG interval present increased irregularly over the first seven minutes, then decreased; these changes were not statistically significant: (2) the mean proportion of the time that LSP was absent with repeated ECoG interval absent decreased steadily over the first five minutes, then increased somewhat; minute 1 was significantly greater than all others; and (3) the mean proportion of time that LSP was absent with or without the repeated ECoG interval present decreased progressively, minutes 1 and 2 being significantly greater than the others. Overall, then, the presence of LSP was directly related to the duration of the time interval after the administration of the most

---

Figure 3   Histograms representing the results of the Student Newman–Keuls test for each of the six sympathetic–ECoG patterns as a function of time interval following the administration of PTZ. (A) LSP present with repeated 2.8-second ECoG interval present; (B) LSP present with repeated 2.8-second ECoG interval absent; (C) LSP present whether repeated 2.8-second ECoG interval is present or absent; (D) LSP absent with repeated 2.8-second interval present; (E) LSP absent with repeated 2.8-second ECoG interval absent; and (F) LSP absent whether repeated 2.8-second ECoG interval is present or absent. The ordinate displays the mean proportion (for nine cats) of each one-minute interval following the administration of all doses of PTZ during which the sympathetic–ECoG pattern in question was observed. The abscissa displays the time elapsed interval (in minutes) following the administration of PTZ in all cats. The patterns within the bars distinguish the subsets (minutes) having statistically comparable mean proportions of time during which the sympathetic–ECoG pattern was observed. Subset 1 consists of one-minute intervals having statistically similar mean proportions of time during which the sympathetic–ECoG pattern was observed. Subset 2 consists of one-minute intervals having statistically similar mean proportions of time during which the sympathetic–ECoG pattern was observed. Subset 3 consists of one-minute intervals having mean proportions of time during which the sympathetic–ECoG pattern was observed which is not distinct from either of other two groups.

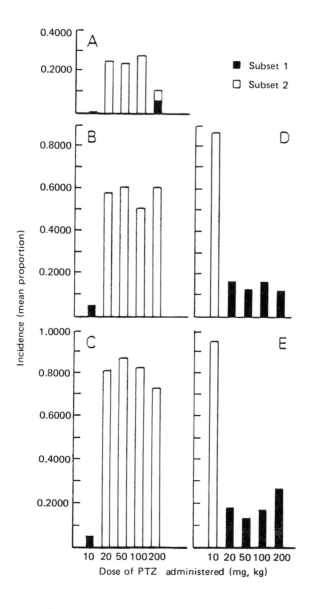

recent dose of PTZ. This relationship is fairly consistent from minute to minute. Similarly, the presence of the repeated ECoG interval was directly related to the duration of the time interval after the administration of the most recent dose of PTZ. This relationship was somewhat inconsistent from minute to minute.

Using repeated-measure ANOVA and Student Newman-Keuls, the relative prevalence of each sympathetic-ECoG pattern in all cats during the entire 10-minute period following the administration of each dose of PTZ was examined.

In one sympathetic-ECoG pattern, LSP absent with repeated ECoG interval present, the mean proportions of time that the pattern existed following each of the five doses of PTZ were statistically comparable. Figure 4A shows the pattern LSP present with repeated ECoG interval present. Two distinct groups were separated, with prevalence following the first dose eliciting none or only minimal interictal epileptogenic activity, significantly less than following any of the subsequent three doses. Prevalence during the final dose, which induced almost no ictal activity and very little interictal activity, was not significantly different from either of the other groups ($p < 0.05$). In a similar manner, the other four ECoG-sympathetic patterns showing varying prevalence are seen in Figure 4 as a function of dose of PTZ administered, i.e., as a function of increasing amounts of epileptogenic activity consisting of more ictal activity and less interictal discharges.

In Figure 5A the incidence of precipitous changes in mean arterial blood pressure for epileptiform discharges induced by all doses of PTZ in all cats was recorded as a function of the time interval after the last administration of PTZ. It

---

Figure 4 Histograms representing the results of the Student Newman-Keuls test for each of the five sympathetic-ECoG patterns as a function of dose of PTZ administered. (A) LSP present with repeated 2.8-second ECoG interval present; (B) LSP present with repeated 2.8-second ECoG interval absent; (C) LSP present whether repeated 2.8-second ECOG interval is present or absent; (D) LSP absent with repeated 2.8-second ECOG interval absent; and (E) LSP absent whether repeated 2.8-second ECoG interval is present or absent. The ordinate displays the mean proportion (for nine cats) of the ten-minute period following the administration of a given dose of PTZ during which the sympathetic-ECoG pattern in question was observed. The abscissa displays the dose of PTZ administered. The patterns within the bars distinguish the subsets (minutes) having statistically comparable mean proportions of time during which the sympathetic-ECoG pattern was observed. Subset 1 consists of one-minute intervals having statistically similar mean proportions of time during which the sympathetic-ECoG pattern was observed. Subset 2 consists of one-minute intervals having statistically similar mean proportions of time during which the sympathetic-ECoG pattern was observed.

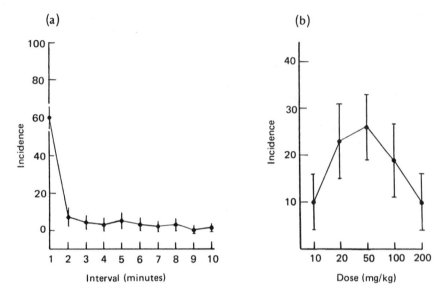

Figure 5 Total incidence of mean arterial blood pressure changes for all nine cats both as a function of time interval since administration of most recent doses of PZT and as a function of dose PZT administered. (a) Total incidence of mean arterial blood pressure changes for all cats vs. minute time interval since most recent administration of PTZ. Vertical bars indicate 95% confidence intervals. No confidence interval can be determined for the values in minute 9. (b) Total incidence of mean arterial blood pressure changes for all cats vs. dose of PTZ administered. Vertical bars indicate 95% confidence intervals.

showed that a statistically greater ($p < 0.05$) incidence of these changes occurred during the minute 1. It held fairly constant during minutes 2 through 10, inclusive.

The incidence of mean arterial blood pressure changes for increasing amounts of epileptogenic activity induced by the increaseing doses of PTZ displayed a bell-shaped distribution (Figure 5B) with a peak following PTZ 50 mg/kg dose. Ninety-five percent confidence intervals showed this incidence to be higher than that following either the PTZ 10 or 200 mg/kg dose.

The incidence of changes in the ECG decreased during the first eight minutes inclusive following the administration of PTZ (Figure 6a). This difference was statistically significant ($p < 0.06$) during minute 1 when compared to minute 7 or 8.

The occurrence of changes in the ECG was least frequent following PTZ 10 mg/kg than following any other dose. This dose of PTZ elicited little or no

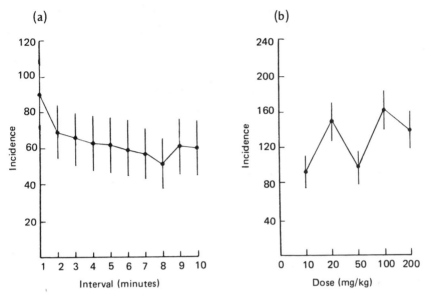

Figure 6   Total incidence of ECG changes for all nine cats both as a function of
time interval since administration of most recent doses of PTZ and as a function
of dose of PZT administered. (a) Totall incidence of ECG changes for all cats vs.
minute interval since most recent administration of PZT. Vertical bars indicate
95% confidence intervals. (b) Total incidence of ECG changes for all cats vs.
dose of PTZ administered. Vertical bars indicate 95% confidence intervals.

interictal activity in most cats and almost no ictal activity. This was a statistically significant difference from the prevalence following all other doses except
PTZ 50 mg/kg. This dose of PTZ elicited primarily ictal activity.

The mean proportion of each minute during which LSP was present, and the
mean proportion of each minute during which the repeated ECoG interval was
observed were directly proportional to the time interval elapsed after the administration of all doses of PTZ. When parameters of autonomic dysfunction
were examined as a function of the time interval since the administration of all
doses of PTZ, the incidence of blood pressure change was significantly greater
(95% confidence interval) during the first minute following the epileptogenic
activity induced by the administration of all doses of PTZ than during any other
minute. Furthermore, the blood pressure became more stable with increasing
time after each dose. Likewise, the incidence of ECG changes decreased over
the first eight minutes following the administration of PTZ and was statistically
greater following minute 1 than following minute 7 or 8, when epileptiform

activity decreased. When this stable LSP was lost, both precipitous mean arterial blood pressure changes and the incidence of ECG changes occurred more frequently.

Just as the mean proportion of time during which LSP was observed was statistically greater after the PTZ 50 mg/kg when maximal numbers of epileptiform discharges were induced, the incidence of mean arterial pressure change was significantly greater after this dose than after the PTZ 10 and 200 mg/kg doses, which were less epileptogenic than the 50 mg/kg doses. No relationship between incidence of ECG changes and LSP, as a function of PTZ dosage, could be found; rather, there seemed to be a correlation with the doses inducing the greatest degree of epileptiform discharge.

IV. DISCUSSION

We examined the temporal sychronization between ECoG and sympathetic spikes that was observed in a PTZ animal model of epilepsy, pretreated with the antiepileptic drug phenobarbital. These temporally synchronized spikes were designated LSP when they occurred consistently over a period of 10 or more uninterrupted seconds. The administration of PTZ to phenobarbital-pretreated cats converted the normal baseline state of desynchronized sympathetic discharges and phenobarbital spindles into a state of hypersynchronized cortical and sympathetic activity.

This laboratory has frequently used PTZ treatment of cats to create an experimental model of epileptogenic activity (Lathers et al., 1978, 1984, 1987; Schraeder and Lathers, 1983). The dosing regimen has been developed to produce all degrees of subconvulsant and convulsant activity (Schraeder and Lathers, 1983). In this way the full spectrum of cortical epileptiform activity can be examined. Phenobarbital was employed by this laboratory as an anticonvulsant in this animal model.

The possibility that this observed temporal synchronization of ECoG and sympathetic spikes represents artifact, originating from either outside or within the cat, was examined first. Possible mechanical artifact from the respirator or the 60-Hz alternating current used to power the polygraph was dismissed for two reasons. First, other experiments undertaken with the same equipment in the same room in the same time period produced no such artifact. Second, these potential sources would produce artifact at a constant rate throughout the entire experiment. Sympathetic spikes, ECoG spikes, and LSP were not observed at a constant rate throughout the entire experiment. In addition, neither sympathetic spikes nor ECoG spikes were observed during either control period.

The possibility of intrinsic artifact from cardiac or skeletal muscle contractions was considered. However, neither the ECoG nor sympathetic spikes bore relationship to the incidence of changes in the ECG. Furthermore, the use of gallamine effectively blocked spontaneous muscle contractions. Analysis with multiple regression showed that the time-locked occurrence of ECoG spikes and sympathetic spikes was not random. This analysis suggested that the incidence of LSP was directly related to the incidence of sympathetic spikes.

Epileptogenic activity induced by PTZ appears to be necessary to allow this phenomenon to express itself. Though in eight of the nine cats LSP was present more often than absent ($>$ 55% of time in seconds) while the cat was under the influence of PTZ, in no cat was this phenomenon present during the control period. Epileptogenic activity induced by PTZ is an experimental model of primary generalized epilepsy. The method of action of this drug, however, is uncertain (Stone, 1972). Three proposed methods of action of PTZ which would allow the LSP to express itself are (1) spatial and temporal summation of neuronal discharges in a subcortical center producing a stimulus strong enough to overcome the cortical and ganglionic threshold (Hahn, 1960); (2) increased synaptic recruitment, resulting in the amplification of subcortical stimuli along their path so that, upon reaching the cortex and sympathetic ganglion, they are capable of causing these neurons to discharge; and (3) increased irritability of all neurons so that subcortical impulses could stimulate cortical and ganglionic neurons (Hahn, 1960). In each case, PTZ effectively creates a hyperirritable state of epileptogenic electrical activity present in the central and autonomic nervous systems. Though phenobarbital can act to minimize this irritability, the effect of this pharmacological agent in this study eventually was overcome by the increased epileptogenic activity.

The 2.8-second repeated ECoG interval, a type of latency period between the end of one spike and the beginning of another associated spike, appeared to convey a stabilizing effect on the presence of LSP. When this repeated ECoG interval was present, LSP was present a significantly greater percentage of time than when LSP was absent. When the repeated ECoG interval was not present, LSP was much less common and the distinct ECoG spikes often degenerated into prolonged ictal activity. Our analysis minimized the degree of association between the repeated ECoG interval and the presence of LSP. Our definition of a repeated ECoG interval excludes periods when two or more additional ECoG spikes are contained within the 2.8-second interval, even if these additional ECoG spikes are time locked to sympathetic spikes. A more liberal definition would result in a more frequent association between LSP and repeated ECoG interval.

The mean proportion of each minute during which LSP was present was directly proportional to the time interval elapsed following the administration of PTZ. The direct relationship reflects the fact that the episodes of epileptogenic activity, and particularly prolonged ictal activity, are most frequently observed shortly after PTZ is administered. Similarly, the incidence of precipitous blood pressure change was significantly greater ($p < 0.05$) during the first minute following the administration of all doses of PTZ than during any other minute. Likewise, the incidence of ECG changes decreased over the first eight minutes following administration of all doses of PTZ, with minute 1 containing a significantly higher incidence compared to minute 7 or 8. Thus the possibility arises of a relationship between the presence of LSP and both a stable mean arterial pressure and a normally functioning autonomic nervous system.

V. SUMMARY

The concept of rhythmic neuronal activity being associated with normal central and autonomic nervous system activity is not new. Normal and abnormal cortical patterns are the basis of the clinical use of electroencephalography. Sympathetic nerve discharge patterns have been characterized by others (Barman and Gebber, 1980; Gebber and Barman, 1980). A temporal relationship between discharge patterns of the central and autonomic nervous system has also been shown previously (Gebber and Barman, 1981). Loss of this rhythmic stability can alter neurotransmitter release (Birks, 1978; Birks et al., 1981) and initiate autonomic dysfunction (Lathers and Schraeder, 1982; Lathers et al., 1977). This chapter characterized LSP and supports the idea of closely related central and autonomic rhythmic activity, which is important in maintaining homeostasis. The data showed that when a stable LSP was lost, both precipitous mean arterial blood pressure changes and the incidence of ECG changes occurred more frequently. This suggests that the LSP, either by its mere presence or by the rhythm at which it occurs, may play a role in the origin of autonomic dysfunction, contributing to the rise of sudden unexplained death in epilepsy.

ACKNOWLEDGMENTS

The authors gratefully acknowledge Dr. Adele Kaplan for her statistical expertise and critical review of the manuscript. We are indebted to Dr. Paul L. Schraeder for his discussions.

REFERENCES

Barman, S. M., and Gebber, G. L. (1980). Sympathetic nerve rhythm of brain stem origin. *Am. J. Physiol. 239 (Regul. Integrative Comp. Physiol. 8)*:R42–R47.

Barman, S. M., and Gebber, G. L. (1981). Brain stem neuronal types with activity patterns related to sympathetic nerve discharge. *Am. J. Physiol. 242 (Regul. Integrative Comp. Physiol. 11)*:R335–R347.

Barman, S. M., and Gebber, G. L. (1982). Hypothalamic neurons with activity patterns related to sympathetic nerve discharge. *Am. J. Physiol. 242 (Regul. Integrative Comp. Physiol. 11)*:R34–R43.

Barman, S. M., and Gebber, G. L. (1984). Spinal interneurons with sympathetic nerve-related activity. *Am. J. Physiol. 247 (Regul. Integrative Comp. Physiol. 16)*:R761–R767.

Basar, E. (1976). Abstract methods of general systems analysis. In *Biophysical and Physiological Systems Analysis*, E. Basar (Ed.). Addison-Wesley, Reading, Mass. pp. 23–47.

Birks, R. I. (1978). Regulation by patterned preganglionic neural activity of transmitter stores in a sympathetic ganglion. *J. Physiol. 280*:559–572.

Birks, R. I., Laskey, W., and Polosa, C. (1981). The effect of burst patterning of preganglionic input on the efficacy of transmission at the cat stellate ganglion. *J. Physiol. 318*:531–539.

Gebber, G. L., and Barman, S. M. (1980). Basis for 2-6 cycle/s rhythm in sympathetic nerve discharge. *Am. J. Physiol. 239 (Regul. Integrative Comp. Physiol. 8)*:R48–R56.

Gebber, G. L., and Barman, S. M. (1981). Sympathetic-related activity of brain stem neurons in baroreceptor-denervated cats. *Am. J. Physiol. 240 (Regul. Integrative Comp. Physiol. 9)*:R348–R355.

Hahn, F. (1960). Analeptics. *Pharmacol. Rev. 12*:447–530.

Jay, G. W. and Leestma, J. E. (1981). Sudden death in epilepsy. A comprehensive review of the literature and proposed mechanisms. *Acta Neurol. Scand. (Suppl. 82)63*:1–66.

Jun, H. W. (1976). Pharmacokinetic studies of pentylenetetrazol in dogs. *J. Pharmacol. Sci. 65*:1038–1041.

Kiloh, L. G., McComas, A. J., and Osselton, J. W. (1972a). The neural basis of the EEG. In *Clinical Encephalography*, L. G. Kiloh, A. J. McComas, and J. W. Osselton (Eds.). Butterworths, London, pp. 21–34.

Kiloh, L. G., McComas, A. J., and Osselton, J. W. (1972b). Normal findings. In *Clinical Encephalography*, L. G. Kiloh, A. J. McComas, and J. W. Osselton (Eds.). Butterworths, London, pp. 52–70.

Krohn, W. (1977). Causes of death among epileptics. *Epilepsia 4*:315–321.

Lathers, C. M., and Schraeder, P. L. (1982). Autonomic dysfunction in epilepsy: Characterization of autonomic cardiac neural discharge associated with pentylenetetrazol-induced epileptogenic activity. *Epilepsia 23*:633–647.

Lathers, C. M., Roberts, J., and Kelliher, G. J. (1977). Correlation of ouabain-induced arrhythmia and nonuniformity in the histamine-evoked discharge of cardiac sympathetic nerves. *J. Pharmacol. Exp. Ther. 203*:467–479.

Lathers, C. M., Kelliher, G. J., Roberts, J., and Beasley, A. B. (1978). Nonuniform cardiac sympathetic nerve discharge. Mechanisms for coronary occlusion and digitalis-induced arrhythmia. *Circulation 57*:1058–1065.

Lathers, C. M., Schraeder, P. L., and Carnel, S. B. (1984). Neural mechanism in cardiac arrhythmia associated with epileptogenic activity: The effect of phenobarbital in the cat. *Life Sci. 34*:1919–1936.

Lathers, C. M., Schraeder, P. L., and Weiner, F. L. (1987). Synchronization of cardiac autonomic neural discharge with epileptogenic activity: The lockstep phenomenon. *Electroencephalogr. Clin. Neurophysiol. 67*:247–259.

Meldrum, B. S., and Brierley, J. B. (1973). Prolonged epileptic seizures in primates. *Arch. Neurol. 28*:10–17.

Meldrum, B. S., and Horton, R. W. (1973). Physiology of status epilepticus in primates. *Arch. Neurol. 28*:1–9.

Schraeder, P. L., and Lathers, C. M. (1983). Cardiac neural discharge and epileptogenic activity in the cat: An animal model for unexplained death. *Life Sci. 32*:1371–1382.

Stone, W. E. (1972). Systemic chemical convulsants and metabolic derangements. In *Experimental Models of Epilepsy. A Manual for the Laboratory Worker*, D. P. Purpura, J. K. Perry, D. Tower, D. M. Woodbury, and R. Walter (Eds.). Raven Press, New York, pp.407–433.

Van Buren, J. M. (1958). Some autonomic concomitants of ictal automatism. A study of temporal lobe attacks. *Brain 81*:505–528.

Wasterlain, C. G. (1974). Mortality and morbidity from serial studies. An experimental study. *Epilepsia 15*:155–176.

14

Relationship of the Lockstep Phenomenon and Precipitous Changes in Blood Pressure

AMY Z. STAUFFER*, JEFFREY M. DODD-O†, and CLAIRE M. LATHERS‡
The Medical College of Pennsylvania, Eastern Pennsylvania Psychiatric Institute, Philadelphia, Pennsylvania

I. INTRODUCTION

Sudden unexplained death (SUD) is defined as "non-traumatic" death occurring in an individual within minutes or hours of the onset of the final illness or ictus" (Jay and Leestma, 1981). No anatomic cause of death can be demonstrated at autopsy. The prevalence of SUD in persons with epilepsy has been estimated to be between 1 death in 525 epileptic persons and 1 per 2100 (Leestma et al., 1984). Autonomic dysfunction occurring in conjunction with epileptogenic activity and causing fatal cardiac arrhythmia and/or arrest has been postulated as an explanation for the increased prevalence of SUD in persons with epilepsy (Leestma et al., 1984).

Lathers and Schraeder (1982; Schraeder and Lathers, 1983) demonstrated that autonomic dysfunction occurs during ictal and interictal epileptogenic activity induced by pentylenetetrazol (PTZ). Lathers et al. (1987) defined the lockstep phenomenon (LSP), during which postganglionic cardiac sympathetic neural discharge occurs as if time locked to electrocorticographic epileptiform discharges (Figure 1). The purpose of this study is to determine whether the LSP in any of its patterns is related to sudden alterations in autonomic function as manifested by precipitous changes in mean arterial blood pressure. A better

Current affiliation:
*University of Connecticut, Farmington, Connecticut.
†University of North Texas, Fort Worth, Texas.
‡FDA, Rockville, Maryland.

understanding of the LSP and how it correlates with changes in physiological parameters such as mean arterial blood pressure, cardiac neural discharge, and cardiac rate and rhythm will help to delineate mechanisms that may contribute to sudden death in the epileptic person. Such an understanding should then allow one to develop better drugs and/or combination of drugs to prevent the physiologic changes that may result in a fatal event.

II. METHOD

Nine cats were intravenously (i.v.) anesthetized with 80 mg/kg alpha-chloralose. Tracheostomies were performed and the femoral arteries and veins were cannulated. The animals were ventilated with a small-animal respirator, maintaining pO_2, PCO_2, and pH within an acceptable physiological range. Intermittent doses of gallamine (2 mg/kg i.v.) maintained paralysis. After bilateral frontal craniectomy, the dura was resected to allow placement of electrodes for recording of the electrocardiogram (ECoG). A thoracotomy and right partial pneumonectomy were performed in order to expose the cardiac postganglionic sympathetic and right cardiac vagal nerves. Sympathetic nerves were identified by their response to a blood pressure drop induced by histamine (5 µg/kg i.v.). The activity of sympathetic nerves, ECoG, ECG (lead II), and the mean arterial blood pressure were recorded and stored on magnetic tape. Rectal temperature was maintained at 37.5–38.5 degrees centigrade.

Each cat received 20 mg/kg intravenous phenobarbital infused over 10 minutes after a 10-minute control period. One hour after completion of the infusion of phenobarbital, the animals received six doses (10, 20, 50, 100, 200, and 2000 mg/kg) of pentylenetetrazol (PTZ) intravenously at 10-minute intervals. Although the half-life of PTZ in the cat is unknown (Knoll Laboratories, personal communication), it has been shown to be 1.4 hours in the dog (Jun, 1976). If the assumption is made that the half-life of PTZ in the cat is similar to that in the dog, then the doses of PTZ were cumulative.

Three categories of epileptiform discharges were defined according to duration. Polyspike discharges of 10 or more seconds were classified as prolonged ictal. Repetitive polyspike discharges of less than 10 seconds duration that were interrupted by periods of depression of cerebral activity were classified as brief ictal. Prolonged ictal and brief ictal activity are analogous to the activity seen in the EEG during clinical seizures. Discrete paroxysmal spikes and/or polyspike and wave discharges, which are analogous to the nonictal epileptogenic activity seen in the interictal EEG of patients with a seizure disorder, were classified as interictal spikes.

The term lockstep phenomenon (LSP) is used to describe the occurrence of sympathetic postganglionic discharge and various types of epileptogenic ECoG activity in a time-locked fashion (Dodd-o and Lathers, Chapter 13, this book; Lathers et al., 1987). In the present experiment, the parameters used to define the occurrence of LSP are those utilized by Dodd-o and Lathers. When an inter-

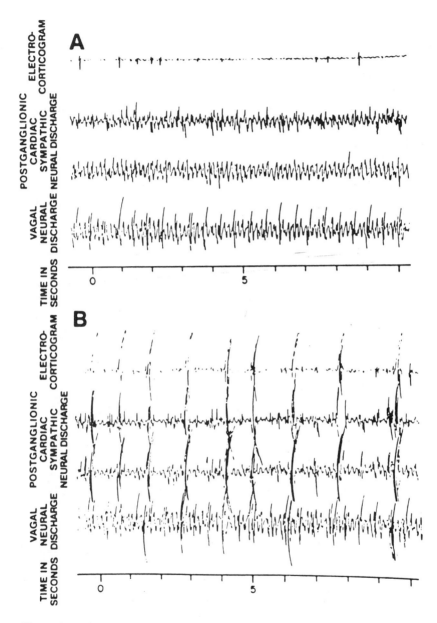

Figure 1 Electrocorticographic and autonomic cardiac neural discharge monitored in one cat. The records in each panel, from top to bottom, illustrate the ECoG and neural discharge for two sympathetic postganglionic and the vagal cardiac nerves, respectively. Panel A was obtained during the control period; panel B was recorded 43 seconds after the administration of PTZ of 10 mg/kg i.v. [From Lathers et al. (1987), reproduced with permission.]

ictal ECoG spike occurred, it was said to be time locked to a sympathetic spike only if the sympathetic spike began within 200 msec of the beginning of the interictal ECoG spike. If the ECoG activity was brief ictal in type, it was considered as a single event and was analyzed with the sympathetic neural activity occurring during the corresponding time interval. The LSP was said to exist if and only if the first spike of the sympathetic polyspike discharge began after the corresponding brief ictal discharge began, and if the last spike of the sympathetic polyspike discharge began before the final spike of the brief ictal discharge ended. Time periods during which the ECoG displayed prolonged ictal activity were not considered to contain LSP.

The total amounts of time that the LSP was present and absent were analyzed. The LSP was considered to be present only when the previously mentioned criteria were fulfilled for an uninterrupted time interval of 10 or more seconds. During this 10-second interval, at least two episodes of time-locked sympathetic postganglionic and ECoG discharges had to exist. When the incidences of sympathetic and ECoG discharges were not equal over the 10-second interval, a closer look was taken at the characteristics of the less frequently occurring discharge. If more than one of the less frequently occurring discharges appeared alone, the LSP was considered to be absent. If the LSP was interrupted after being present for an uninterrupted time interval of greater than 10 seconds, the LSP was considered to have ended if the period of interruption was greater than 4.5 seconds. If, however, the interruption in LSP lasted 4.5 seconds or less, the LSP was considered to exist without interruption.

The repeated 2.8-second ECoG interval is the interspike time interval found in a previous study to exist most frequently between ECoG spikes when LSP was present (Dodd-o and Lathers, Chapter 13, this book). The time interval is measured from the end of one ECoG spike to the beginning of another ECoG spike. Contained within this 2.8-second interval may be another ECoG spike. This third ECoG spike need not be related to either of the spikes that bound the 2.8-second interval in question. This third spike is, however, related to another ECoG spike which begins 2.8 seconds after the third ECoG spike ends.

The duration of time (in seconds) the 2.8-second interval was present was determined as follows. To be considered to exist, the foregoing criteria had to be fulfilled for at least three consecutive 2.8-second intervals. Once present, the 2.8-second interval was considered to be present without interruption only if it continued without any interval of disruption lasting more than 4.5 seconds. If the repeated 2.8-second interval was present but was then interrupted for more than 4.5 seconds, the repeated 2.8-second interval was said to have ended.

In an effort to explore the importance of LSP stability in maintaining blood pressure, a more specific classification of LSP was developed. First, four categories of LSP were created. The first of these, no LSP, included all of those time intervals in which the ECoG–sympathetic discharge pattern was such that conditions for the existence of LSP were not fulfilled. If the condition for LSP were present, the rate of LSP was classified as either stable or unstable. The term stable LSP was used to describe all uninterrupted time periods of 10 or more seconds during which the time interval between sympathetic spikes was unchanged. If the interspike interval was constant but then changed for no more than one interspike interval, stability was considered to be maintained. Two categories of stable LSP were observed: (1) stable LSP in which the repeated 2.8-second interval was present and (2) stable LSP in which the repeated 2.8-second interval was absent.

If the interspike interval was altered on two consecutive occasions, stability of LSP was considered to be lost. The term unstable LSP was used to describe all time intervals of 10 or more seconds during which LSP existed but the criteria for "stable LSP" were absent. The four categories (no LSP, stable LSP with 2.8-second interval, stable LSP without 2.8-second interval, and unstable LSP) were analyzed and then the unstable category was divided into unstable LSP with increasing rate and unstable LSP with decreasing rate. The term unstable LSP with increasing rate was used to describe periods of unstable LSP in which the duration of interspike interval decreased between consecutive spikes. The term unstable LSP with decreasing rate was used to describe those periods of unstable LSP in which the duration of the interspike interval increased between consecutive spikes. These two types of unstable LSP were analyzed along with the other three LSP patterns (no LSP, stable LSP with 2.8-second interval, and stable LSP without 2.8-second interval) to determine if direction, i.e., an increasing or decreasing rate, had any effect on blood pressure changes. In summary, the LSP patterns were:

1. LSP absent.
2. Stable LSP with 2.8-second interval.
3. Stable LSP without 2.8-second interval.
4. Unstable LSP (a) with increasing rate and (b) with decreasing rate.

Mean arterial blood pressure changes were reviewed. After examination of the control period and the PTZ treatment period, it was found that mean arterial blood pressure changes of 23 mm Hg over a 10-second interval never occurred during the control period. This rate of change, i.e., 23 mm Hg over a 10-second period, was termed a precipitous blood pressure change. The occurrence and incidence of such changes were examined in all cats after the administration of each dose of PTZ except for the dose of 2000 mg/kg. This latter dose led to death in all cats, and thus it was decided not to analyze characterization of this event with the rest of the experiment.

III. STATISTICAL ANALYSIS

For all cats, the amount of time in seconds that was spent in each LSP pattern was recorded. The number of precipitous blood pressure changes was also determined. Since each precipitous blood pressure change occurred over a 10-second period, the amount of time in seconds that was spent in precipitous blood pressure changes is equal to the number of precipitous blood pressure changes multiplied by 10.

For each LSP pattern (no LSP, stable LSP with 2.8-second interval, stable LSP without 2.8-second interval, and unstable LSP) the proportion of time spent in precipitous blood pressure changes was calculated by dividing the amount of time spent in precipitous blood pressure changes by the total amount of time spent in that LSP pattern. This was done for each cat. To determine if any of the LSP patterns were associated with a significantly higher mean proportion of time in precipitous blood pressure changes, a one-way repeated-measures analysis of variance (ANOVA) was performed. LSP pattern was used as the independent variable and mean proportion of time spent in precipitous blood pressure changes was used as the dependent variable. The Biomedical Program Package (BMDP) was used. To determine which of the LSP patterns was significantly different from the others, a post-hoc Newman–Keuls test was performed if significance of the F-ratio ($p < 0.05$) was found. Because the observations for each cat were proportions, the variances and means of the comparison groups were not independent of one another. Therefore, square root transformation ($X = \sqrt{x + 10}$) was applied to all data points before analysis. This strategy is suggested by Winer (1971) to stabilize the variances. The log transformation, $X' = \log (x + 1.0)$ was also applied (Winer, 1971). Neither strategy made a significant impact on variance heterogeneity. Since equal-sized groups weaken the impact of variance heterogeneity on alpha, the untransformed values were used, but Huynh–Feldt degrees of freedom were applied to correct for heterogeneity of variance.

To determine if any significant differences existed between unstable LSP with increasing rate and unstable LSP with decreasing rate, the unstable LSP category was divided into unstable LSP with increasing rate and unstable LSP with decreasing rate. The previous analysis was repeated.

The next question was whether a significantly different mean proportion of precipitous blood pressure changes occurred during any of the LSP patterns. For each LSP pattern, the number of precipitous blood pressure changes occurring with that LSP pattern was divided by the total number of precipitous blood pressure changes in that cat. To adjust for the fact that more time was spent in some LSP patterns than in others, this proportion was divided by the proportion of time spent in that LSP pattern, i.e., the amount of time spent in that LSP pattern divided by the total time analyzed for that cat. This adjustment was done separately for each of the nine cats. A one-way repeated-measures ANOVA was performed, using LSP pattern as the independent variable and proportion of precipitous blood pressure changes as the dependent variable. The unstable LSP category was then divided into unstable LSP with increasing rate and unstable

LSP with decreasing rate. The analysis was repeated to determine if there was a significant difference between unstable LSP with increasing rate, unstable LSP with decreasing rate, LSP absent, stable LSP with a 2.8-second interval, and stable LSP without a 2.8-second interval in terms of mean proportion of precipitous blood pressure changes. The difference between this analysis and the previous one lies in the fact that this analysis was limited to the time during which there were precipitous blood pressure changes, whereas the previous analysis took into account all time analyzed for each cat.

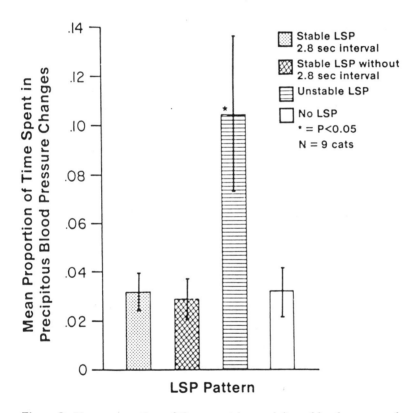

Figure 2 Mean proportion of time spent in precipitous blood pressure changes as a function of the LSP pattern ($N = 9$ cats). The one-way repeated-measure ANOVA showed borderline significance of the F-ratio (Huynh–Feldt probability = 0.056), indicating that a significantly different mean proportion of time was spent in precipitous pressure changes in one or more of the LSP patterns. The post-hoc Newman–Keuls test showed that the unstable LSP pattern was significantly higher than all other patterns in terms of mean proportion of time spent in precipitous blood pressure changes.

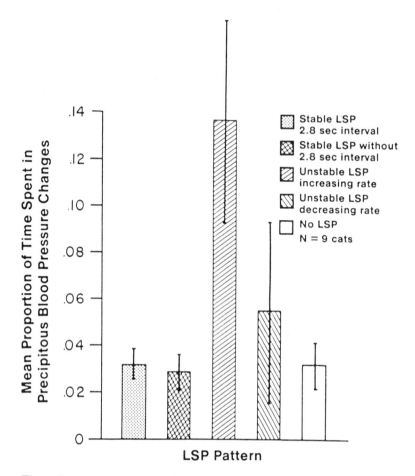

Figure 3 Mean proportion of time spent in precipitous blood pressure changes as a function of LSP pattern (N = 9 cats). This analysis is identical to the one presented in Figure 2, except that the unstable LSP category is divided into unstable LSP with increasing rate and unstable LSP with decreasing rate. Although there were no statistically significant differences among the LSP patterns (Huynh–Feldt probability = 0.068), the observed pattern was that unstable LSP with increasing rate contributed the highest mean proportion of time in precipitous blood pressure changes.

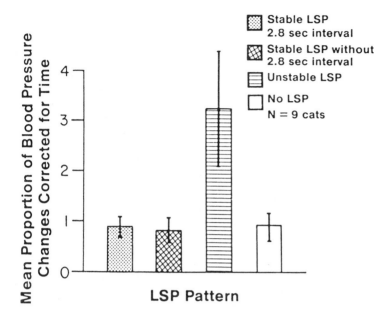

Figure 4 Mean proportion of precipitous blood pressure changes (corrected for time) as a function of LSP pattern (N = 9 cats). The one-way repeated-measures ANOVA was not significant (Huynh–Feldt probability = 0.093), indicating that there were no statistically significant differences among the LSP patterns in terms of mean proportion of precipitous blood pressure changes. The observation can be made, however, that unstable LSP had the highest mean proportion of precipitous blood pressure changes.

V. RESULTS

A. LSP Pattern Versus Mean Proportion of Time Spent in Precipitous Blood Pressure Changes

In comparing the mean proportion of time spent in precipitous blood pressure changes for each LSP pattern, the one-way repeated-measures ANOVA showed borderline significance of the F-ratio (Huynh-Feldt probability, p = 0.056). This indicated that a significantly different mean proportion of time was spent in precipitous blood pressure changes in one or more of the LSP patterns. The post-hoc Newman-Keuls test showed that the unstable LSP pattern was significantly higher than all of the other LSP patterns in terms of mean proportion of time spent in precipitous blood pressure changes (Figure 2).

When the unstable LSP category was divided into unstable LSP with increasing rate and unstable LSP with decreasing rate and the analysis was repeated,

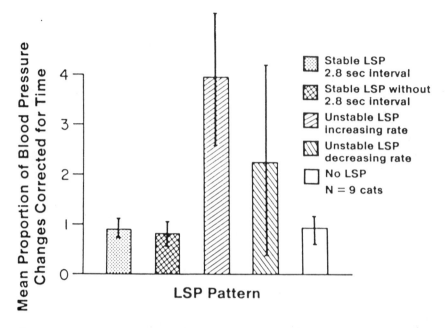

Figure 5 Mean proportion of precipitous blood pressure changes (corrected for time) as a function of LSP pattern. Unstable LSP is divided into unstable LSP with increasing rate and unstable LSP with decreasing rate. The one-way repeated-measures ANOVA showed no statistically significant differences among the LSP patterns in terms of mean proportion of precipitous blood pressure changes (Huynh–Feldt probability = 0.2105), but it can be observed that unstable LSP with increasing rate contributed the highest mean proportion of precipitous blood pressure changes. It can also be seen that the mean proportion of precipitous blood pressure changes for unstable LSP with decreasing rate was higher than the other three patterns.

the corrected (Huynh–Feldt) probability was 0.068. The observed pattern was that unstable LSP with increasing rate contributed the highest mean proportion of time in precipitous blood pressure changes, but the difference was not great enough to achieve statistical significance (Figure 3).

B. LSP Pattern Versus Mean Proportion of Precipitous Blood Pressure Changes

When comparing the mean proportions of precipitous blood pressure changes occurring during each of the LSP patterns (no LSP, stable LSP with 2.8-second interval, stable LSP without 2.8-second interval, and unstable LSP), the one-way repeated-measures ANOVA was not significant (Huynh–Feldt probability, $p = 0.0926$). This indicated that there were no statistically significant differences among the LSP patterns in terms of mean proportion of precipitous blood pressure changes. However, the observation can be made (Figure 4) that the unstable LSP pattern had the highest mean proportion of precipitous blood pressure changes, although this difference was not statistically significant.

When the unstable LSP category was divided into unstable LSP with increasing rate and unstable LSP with decreasing rate, the ANOVA was also not significant (Huynh–Feldt probability, $p = 0.2105$). Although there were no statistically significant differences among the LSP patterns in terms of mean proportion of precipitous blood pressure changes, it can be observed that unstable LSP with increasing rate contributed the highest mean proportion of precipitous blood pressure changes. It was also found that the mean proportion of precipitous blood pressure changes for unstable LSP with decreasing rate was higher than the other three LSP patterns (Figure 5).

V. DISCUSSION

It is important to consider the autonomic neuroanatomical pathways that may be the basis for the LSP, since epileptogenic activity originating in the cortex could be transmitted to the hypothalamus and to the brain stem to alter autonomic neural control of blood pressure and cardiac rate and rhythm (Figure 6). The hypothalamus exerts control over the autonomic nervous system; the anterior and medial hypothalamus regulate parasympathetic function and the posterior and lateral hypothalamus regulate sympathetic function. Direct projections exist from the hypothalamus to the preganglionic sympathetic neurons of the intermediolateral cell column and to the parasympathetic nuclei of the brain stem (Saper et al., 1976). The mammillotegmental tract connects the hypothalamus with the reticular formation, which contains multisynaptic descending pathways linking the hypothalamus with autonomic areas in the brain stem and spinal cord. The medullary reticular formation contains cardiovascular areas that can produce changes in heart rate and blood pressure. These areas produce their effects through reticulospinal connections to the intermediolateral cell column and through connections to preganglionic parasympathetic neurons (Willis and Grossman, 1981). The intermediolateral cell column also receives input from the following regions of the medulla: A1 (norepinephrine-containing) neurons; C1 area (epinephrine-containing neurons); raphe; and the nucleus tractus solitarius. The nucleus tractus solitarius receives afferent projections from the arterial baroreceptors. Aside from its medullary input, the intermediolateral cell column receives projections from the A5 area, a group of norepinephrine-containing neurons that is located in the pons (Natelson, 1985). The hypothalamus is also connected to the brain stem by the medial forebrain bundle, which projects to

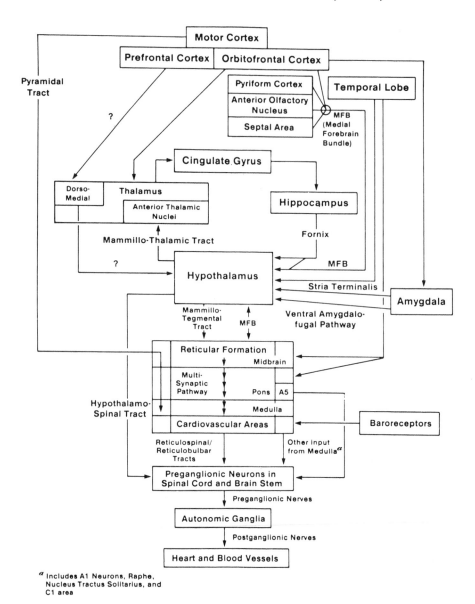

Figure 6 Numerous neuroanatomical pathways exist by which epileptogenic activity may be transmitted to the autonomic nervous system, resulting in LSP and associated autonomic changes.

the midbrain reticular formation, providing another pathway for descending control over the autonomic nervous system. The medial forebrain bundle connects the hypothalamus with structures in the forebrain, such as the septal area, anterior olfactory nucleus, and the pyriform cortex. The medial forebrain bundle also contains fibers from the fornix and the orbitofrontal cortex. The orbitofrontal cortex projects to the thalamus and the amygdala (Korner, 1979), which is connected to the hypothalamus by the stria terminalis and the ventral amygdalofugal pathway.

A close link between the hypothalamus and the limbic system exists through the Papez circuit. Papez (1937) postulated that information from the cortex travels by way of the cingulate gyrus to the hippocampus, which projects to the hypothalamus via the fornix. The mamillothalamic tract connects the mammillary bodies to the anterior nuclei of the thalamus. The circuit is completed by a pathway connecting the thalamus and the cingulate gyrus. Electrical stimulation of the hypothalamus or other structures in the Papez circuit results in autonomic responses. Autonomic responses also occur as a result of stimulation of other areas of the cortex. Wall and Davis (1951) described three cortical areas in monkeys in which blood pressure changes of greater than 10–20 mm Hg could be produced with electrical stimulation. The first of these areas is the sensorimotor cortex, the descending pathway from this area is independent of the hypothalamus and closely related to the pyramidal tract. A direct corticospinal pathway that is independent of the hypothalamus was also described by Landau (1953). The second area is the orbitofrontal cortex; the pathway that begins in this area passes through the hypothalamus. The third of the areas described by Wall and Davis is the anterior temporal lobe; the pathway from this area of the cortex is partially dependent on the hypothalamus and partially direct to the tegmentum and pons. Although it has not been established that neocorticohypothalamic connections exist in man, the possibility has been raised that the dorsomedial nucleus of the thalamus, which connects with the prefrontal cortex, has projections to the hypothalamus (Breusch, 1984).

exist through which epileptogenic activity originating in the cortex could reach the hypothalamus and brain stem, resulting in discharge from the autonomic nervous system and phenomena such as blood pressure changes and cardiac arrhythmia. Electrical stimulation of the cerebral cortex in man and animals results in autonomic responses such as changes in blood pressure (Chapman et al., 1950; Hoff and Green, 1936), changes in heart rate, and dilatation of the pupil (Hoff and Green, 1936). Blood pressure changes have been evoked through stimulation of various regions of the cortex, including tips of the temporal lobes (Chapman et al., 1950), motor cortex, premotor cortex, parietal cortex, and cingulate gyrus (Hoff and Green, 1936). Furthermore, autonomic changes, including alterations in blood pressure, have been associated with epileptogenic activity.

The precipitous blood pressure changes observed in our experiments were not consistent in terms of direction; there was a total of 46 increases and 48 decreases observed during the 60-minute periods monitored in each of the nine cats. Experiments involving electrical stimulation of the cortex have shown similar blood pressure changes in terms of direction. Wall and Davis (1951) and Delgado (1960) found both increases and decreases in blood pressure upon stimulation of the cortex. Kaada et al. (1949) also elicited both increases and decreases in blood pressure with electrical stimulation of the cortex, as well as biphasic responses in which an increase in blood pressure was followed by a secondary decrease or a decrease in blood pressure was followed by a secondary increase. In our experiments, biphasic responses (defined for the purpose of this discussion as two precipitous blood pressure changes of opposite direction occurring within 10 seconds of each other) were seen nine times in four cats.

Hoff and Green (1936) demonstrated pressor and depressor points in the cortex which are located 2-4 mm from each other. This observation may help to explain the inconsistency of the direction of precipitous blood pressure changes, the relationship of blood pressure changes to unstable LSP, and why the direction of blood pressure changes was not related to the direction of unstable LSP (increasing rate or decreasing rate). If, for example, predominantly pressor areas were being stimulated by epileptogenic activity and the frequency of the epileptogenic activity increased, the blood pressure might increase; if the frequency of the epileptogenic activity decreased, the blood pressure might decrease. If, however, predominantly depressor areas were stimulated by the epileptogenic activity, the blood pressure might decrease with increasing epileptogenic activity and increase with decreasing epileptogenic activity.

The question that remains is how the mean arterial blood pressure can decrease in the presence of an increased rate of postganglionic cardiac sympathetic discharge. In cats treated with ouabain, Lathers et al. (1977) demonstrated "nonuniformity" of postganglionic cardiac sympathetic discharge; i.e., some cardiac sympathetic branches showed increased activity, some showed decreased activity, and some branches showed no change in activity. This nonuniform discharge was associated with ouabain-induced arrhythmia (Lathers et al., 1977). Lathers and Schraeder (1982) found a similar nonuniform sympathetic discharge in cats treated with PTZ. If two or three branches of postganglionic cardiac sympathetic nerves exhibit this nonuniform discharge pattern, then the possibility exists that the discharge from the sympathetic nerves that innervate the blood vessels and control blood pressure may not be uniform. In this case, blood pressure could decrease even though discharge in some cardiac sympathetic branches was increased.

This discussion has concentrated mainly on epileptogenic activity originating in the cortex because one of the factors associated with sudden unexplained death (SUD) is the presence of structural lesions of the brain that are thought to cause seizures. In one study, autopsies of 60% of epileptic persons who died suddenly revealed structural lesions of the brain, including old contusions of the frontal and temporal lobes, brain tumors, cortical malformations, evidence of craniotomy, focal atrophy or hemiatrophy, Wernicke's encephalopathy, and cryptic vascular malformation (Leestma et al., 1984). In another study (Freytag and Ingraham, 1964), 63% of cases of SUD associated with epilepsy were found to have structural brain lesions. However, epileptic persons without such lesions may also die suddenly; furthermore, autonomic symptoms occur in association with generalized epilepsy. It is thought that the thalamus and the midbrain reticular formation are involved in generalized epilepsy, perhaps as a site of origin for the seizure activity (Kiloh et al., 1980). The thalamus, being part of the Papez circuit and having connections to the cortex, is capable of transmitting epileptogenic activity to the hypothalamus, resulting in autonomic manifestations. The reticular formation contains the multisynaptic pathways that connect the hypothalamus with the autonomic areas in the brain stem and spinal cord. Seizure activity occurring in the reticular formation could be transmitted to the autonomic areas of the brain stem and spinal cord by these pathways.

VI. SUMMARY

The results of this study show that autonomic changes, i.e., precipitous blood pressure changes, are associated with the unstable LSP patterns. These findings indicate that the LSP (and its patterns) should be investigated further to determine its relationship to cardiac arrhythmias and epilepsy-related SUD. At least three mechanisms can be postulated through which LSP may be related to arrhythmia and SUD in persons with epilepsy. The first of these is excessive sympathetic stimulation of a heart that is already electrically unstable due to prior damage. It is the opinion of Jay and Leestma (1981) that this is the case; they describe pathological changes in the myocardium that several investigators have found in patients with epilepsy who died suddenly. The pathological changes are consistent with repeated high levels of catecholamines and resemble those produced in experimental animals by sympathetic stimulation. Jay and Leestma have suggested that this damage to the heart provides a locus where fatal arrhythmias can begin when the heart is again stimulated by sympathetic discharge. The LSP may be the link between the epileptogenic activity in the brain and sympathetic stimulation of the heart.

The second possible mechanism involves nonuniform discharge of the postganglionic sympathetic nerve branches, which is associated with arrhythmias caused by administration of ouabain (Lathers et al., 1977). As mentioned earlier, Lathers and Schraeder (1982) found a similar nonuniform sympathetic discharge pattern in cats treated with PTZ. In the latter study, the nonuniform cardiac neural discharge was associated with epileptogenic activity and changes in the autonomic parameters of mean arterial blood pressure and cardiac rhythm. It was suggested that these changes may contribute to SUD.

The third mechanism is especially relevant to this study; precipitous blood pressure changes per se may be a factor in the development of arrhythmia in persons with epilepsy. In a study by Allen (1931), premature systolic arrhythmias followed increases in blood pressure induced by stimulation of the superior colliculus in rabbits. The arrhythmias were not observed when blood pressure was maintained at a constant level during stimulation of the superior colliculus; the conclusion was made that the arrhythmias could be attributed to the blood pressure changes. Evans and Gillis (1978) elicited blood pressure increases by stimulation of the hypothalamus and concluded that the arrhythmias that occurred after (not during) such stimulation were the result of a sudden surge of parasympathetic activity reflexly evoked by the rise in blood pressure.

A case reported by Kiok et al. (1986) describes a 23-year-old male who had sinus arrest lasting up to nine seconds, as well as bradycardia of 40- to 50-bpm, during clinically observed seizures. The authors suggest that the parasympathetic nervous system may be involved in the production of some cases of arrhythmia in epileptic persons. Although the blood pressure remained stable during the seizures in this particular case, the autonomic manifestations do suggest parasympathetic involvement. Interestingly, the patient described in the report was found by computer tomography to have right temporal lobe atrophy and had subtherapeutic blood levels of anticonvulsant drugs. According to Jay and Leestma (1981), structural abnormalities of the brain and subtherapeutic levels of anticonvulsants are two factors associated with epilepsy-related SUD.

The three mechanisms leading to arrhythmia and SUD that are outlined in this discussion are by no means mutually exclusive. It is quite possible that no single mechanism can explain all cases of SUD in epileptic persons. Perhaps some cases are caused by ventricular fibrillation related to a lower ventricular fibrillation threshold associated with increased cardiac sympathetic discharge, whereas other cases are caused by sinus arrest related to reflex parasympathetic discharge evoked by precipitous blood pressure changes (especially if there is some cardiac damage produced by prior sympathetic stimulation). The association of autonomic events with the LSP indicates that further investigation in this direction is warranted.

ACKNOWLEDGMENTS

The authors gratefully acknowledge Dr. Adele Kaplan for statistical analyses and Carol Harwick, Darlene Spino, and Don Stauffer for typing the manuscript.

Special thanks to Dr. Paul L. Schraeder for consultation. The research was funded by NIH grant BRSGRR-04518. A. Z. Stauffer received a 1986 Medical Student Research Fellowship from the Epilepsy Foundation of America.

REFERENCES

Allen, W. F. (1931). An experimentally produced premature systolic arrhythmia (pulsus bigeminus) in rabbits. *Am. J. Physiol. 98*:344–351.

Breusch, S. R. (1984). Anatomy of the human hypothalamus. In *The Hypothalamus*, J. R. Givens (Ed.). Year Book Medical, Chicago, p. 13.

Chapman, W. P., Livingston, K. E., and Papper, J. L. (1950). Effect upon blood pressure of electrical stimulation of tips of temporal lobes in man. *J. Neurophysiol. 13*:65–71.

Delgado, J. M. R. (1960). Circulating effects of cortical stimulation. *Physiol. Rev. 40*(54):146–171.

Evans, D. E., and Gillis, R. A. (1978). Reflex mechanisms involved in cardiac arrhythmias induced by hypothalamic stimulation. *Am. J. Physiol. 234*(2): H199–H209.

Freytag, J. R., and Ingraham, F. D. (1964). 295 medical autopsies in epileptics. *Arch. Pathol. 78*:274–286.

Hoff, E. C., and Green, H. G. (1936). Cardiovascular reactions induced by electrical stimulation of the cerebral cortex. *Am. J. Physiol. 117*:411–422.

Jay, G. W., and Leestma, J. E. (1981). Sudden death in epilepsy. *Acta Neurol. Scand. (Suppl. 82)63*:1–66.

Jun, H. W. (1976). Pharmacokinetic studies of pentylenetetrazol in dogs. *J. Pharmacol. Sci. 65*:1038–1041.

Kaada, B. R., Pribram, K. H., and Epstein, J. A. (1949). Respiratory and vascular responses in monkeys from temporal lobe pole, insula, orbital surface and cingulate gyrus. *J. Neurophysiol. 12*:347–356.

Kiloh, L. G., McComas, A. J., and Osselton, J. W. (1980). *Clinical Electroencephalography*. Butterworths, London.

Kiok, M. C., Terrence, C. F., Fromm, G. H., and Lavine, S. (1986). Sinus arrest in epilepsy. *Neurology 36*:115–116.

Korner, P. I. (1979). Central nervous control of autonomic cardiovascular function. In *Handbook of Physiology – The Cardiovascular System*, Vol. 1, R. M. Berne, N. Sperelaskis, and S. R. Geiger (Eds.). American Physiological Society, Bethesda, Md., pp. 691–739.

Landau, W. M. (1953). Autonomic responses mediated via the corticospinal tract. *J. Neurophysiol. 16*:299–311.

Lathers, C. M., and Schraeder, P. L. (1982). Autonomic dysfunction in epilepsy: Characterization of autonomic cardiac neural discharge associated with pentylenetetrazol-induced epileptogenic activity. *Epilepsia 23*:633–647.

Lathers, C. M., Roberts, J., and Kelliher, G. J. (1977). Correlation of ouabain-induced arrhythmia and nonuniformity in the histamine-evoked discharge of cardiac sympathetic nerves. *J. Pharmacol. Exp. Ther. 203*:467–479.

Lathers, C. M., Schraeder, P. L., and Weiner, F. L. (1987). Synchronization of cardiac autonomic neural discharge with epileptogenic activity: The lockstep phenomenon. *Electroencephalogr. Clin. Neurophysiol.* 67:247–259.

Leestma, J. E., Kalelkar, M. B., Teas, S. S., Jay, G. W., and Hughes, J. R. (1984). Sudden unexpected death associated with seizures: Analysis of 66 cases. *Epilepsia* 25(1):84–88.

Natelson, B. H. (1985). Neurocardiology: An interdisciplinary area for the 80's. *Arch. Neurol.* 42:178–184.

Papez, J. W. (1937). A proposed mechanism of emotion. *Arch. Neurol. Psychiatr.* 38:725–743.

Saper, C. B., Loewy, A. D., Swanson, L. W., and Cowan, W. M. (1976). Direct hypothalamoautonomic connections. *Brain Res.* 117:305–312.

Schraeder, P. L., and Lathers, C. M. (1983). Cardiac neural discharge and epileptogenic activity in the cat: An animal model for unexplained death. *Life Sci.* 32:1371–1382.

Wall, P. D., and David, G. D. (1951). Three cerebral cortical systems affecting autonomic function. *J. Neurophysiol.* 14:507–517.

Willis, W. L., and Grossman, R. G. (1981). *Medical Neurobiology.* C. V. Mosby, St. Louis, p. 405.

Winer, B. J. (1971). *Statistical Principles in Experimental Design*, 2nd ed., McGraw-Hill, New York, p. 399.

15

Interspike Interval Histogram Characterization of Synchronized Cardiac Sympathetic Neural Discharge and Epileptogenic Activity in the Electrocorticogram of the Cat

DANIEL K. O'ROURKE and CLAIRE M. LATHERS* *The Medical College of Pennsylvania, Eastern Pennsylvania Psychiatric Institute, Philadelphia, Pennsylvania*

I. INTRODUCTION

This is one of a series of articles (Lathers et al., 1987; also Chapters 12-14, this book) attempting to characterize one potential mechanism in an animal model which may, in part, explain unexpected death in the epileptic patient. Since many of the mechanisms of death at the time of clinically observable seizures are known, our emphasis has been to determine one potential factor that may be a contributory mechanism behind unexplained interictal death. Our model has utilized the anesthetized cat infused intravenously with pentylenetrazol (PTZ). This chemical is known to produce seizures (Hahn, 1960; Lathers et al., 1984).

Our model has utilized the anesthesized cat infused intravenously with pentylenetetrazol (PTZ). This chemical is known to produce seizures (Hahn, 1960; Lathers et al., 1984). It is important to note that the majority of epileptic patients who die unexpectedly are found on autopsy to have cortical lesions, which probably served as seizure foci during life (Leestma et al., 1984).

The lockstep phenemonon (LSP) theory may help explain sudden unexpected death in this population. It is defined by the occurrence of a one to one synchronization of the electrocorticogram (ECoG) discharge patterns with the discharge patterns of the peripheral autonomic nerves innervating the heart. An example of LSP is seen in Figure 1. We theorize that the lockstep phenomenon

---

Current affiliation: FDA, Rockville, Maryland.

239

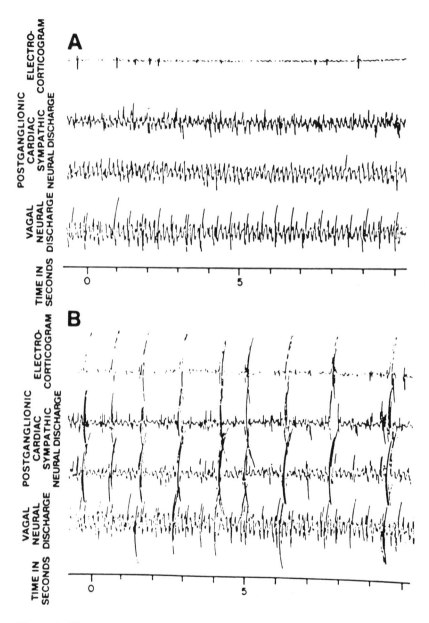

Figure 1 Electrocorticogram and two postganglionic cardiac sympathetic neural discharge patterns monitored simultaneously. (A) Pattern of neural discharges recorded during the control period, i.e., the period just prior to the first dose of PTZ administration. (B) Example of the lockstep phenomenon. The ECoG neural burst discharge patterns are seen to be correlated one-to-one with those of both postganglionic cardiac sympathetic neural discharge patterns.

occurs when the oscillatory driver of the interictal cortical focus becomes linked to the oscillatory driver of the autonomic cardiac nerves. The actual cause of death is hypothesized to be dependent on the function of the neural discharge, which would then be driven at the rate of the interictal focus. Since these are autonomic nerves innervating the heart, the finely tuned electrical depolarization system of the heart could be disturbed. This autonomic dysfunction may directly produce cardiac arrhythmias. These and other theories are discussed and analyzed in terms of the science of chaos. Chaos is a concept in physics that is applicable in modeling these observed natural phenomena and aids in the interpretation of our data. Chaos identifies pattern and regularity in seemingly disorganized events (Winfree, 1987). The science is most useful in predicting the activity of nonlinear, noncyclical functions, such as the plot of the intervals between depolarizations in an EEG showing LSP or in the plot of ventricular depolarizations in atrial fibrillation monitored by an ECG. The principles of chaos help to substantiate the association of LSP and sudden unexpected death in epilepsy.

Our goal in this series of papers is to demonstrate that the lockstep phenomenon occurs and then to characterize LSP and its effects. This study demonstrated that, by the use of the interspike interval (ISI) technique, the discharges noted in the ECoG are correlated in several important ways with the simultaneous discharges occuring in two postganglionic sympathetic nerves monitored in the same cat.

II. METHODS

The animal preparation used in this experiment has been described previously (Carnel et al., 1985; Dodd-o and Lathers, Chapter 13, this book; Lathers et al., 1977, 1984). Briefly, nine cats were intravenously (i.v.) anesthetized with 80 mg/kg i.v. alpha-chloralose. Gallamine 4 mg/kg i.v. was used to maintain paralysis. Leads were placed to monitor several postganglionic sympathetic nerves, the vagus nerve, the ECoG, and the ECG. A 20-mg/kg i.v. dose of phenobarbital administered over 10 minutes was followed by a 60-minute period of stabilization before the experiment was begun. Pentylenetetrazol was administered intravenously at 10, 20, 50, 100, 200, and 2000 mg/kg with a 10-minute interval between each dose. Differential amplitude discriminators (DAD) were used to produce a better signal-to-noise ratio. The output from the DADs was stored on magnetic tape and printed on a polygraph.

The data on the magnetic tapes were played back and fed into a Nuclear Chicago model 7100 Data Retrieval computer, which analyzed the discharge patterns for the time between each depolarization (interspike interval). The tape was played from the time PTZ was first administered until the next dose was given. The summed ISIs were plotted as a histogram. An oscilloscope was used to monitor the patterns being displayed and to adjust the discriminator of the computer. A variable-pulse generator was used to standardize the dis-

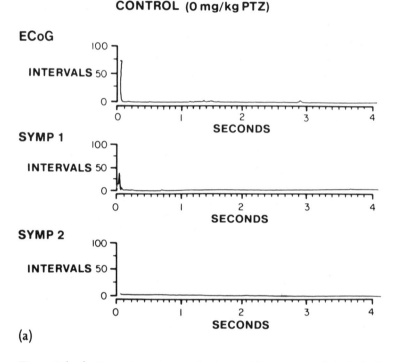

CONTROL (0 mg/kg PTZ)

Figure 2 (a-g) Ten minute interspike interval histograms of the ECoG and two postganglionic sympathetics from representative cats.

criminator and later to provide a standard peak on the ISI histogram. This was used to extrapolate the number of intervals in the unknown peaks by comparing the areas beneath the ISI histogram curve.

The ISI histograms were characterized by recording the number of peaks, height, mode, and least and greatest intervals. The area of the peak was approximated by assuming a triangle formed by the highest point (the mode) and the two baseline extremes. The area was then used to calculate the number of occurrences of that interval in seconds under the curve by comparing its number to the area of a known curve. Graphs of these data are illustrated in Figure 2. A one-way ANOVA was calculated for the modes of the intervals.

One cat was excluded from the computation of the statistical analysis because the ISIs showed no useful information. The signal-to-noise ratio was small enough that the discriminator on the computer could not be set to discern the interictal spikes from that of the background information. This appears to have been due to equipment failure of one of the second-stage amplifiers. All statistics were computed excluding this cat.

10 mg/kg PTZ

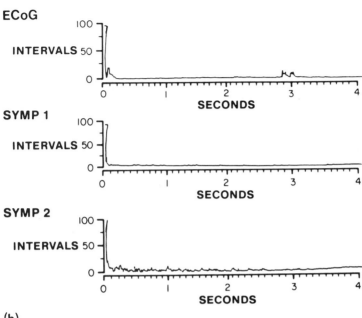

(b)

20 mg/kg PTZ

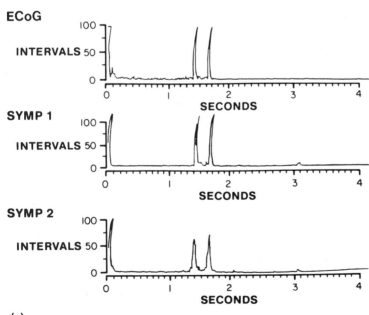

(c)

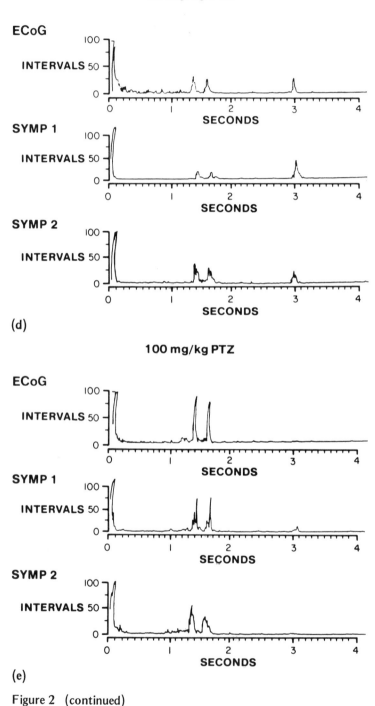

(d)

(e)

Figure 2 (continued)

200 mg/kg PTZ

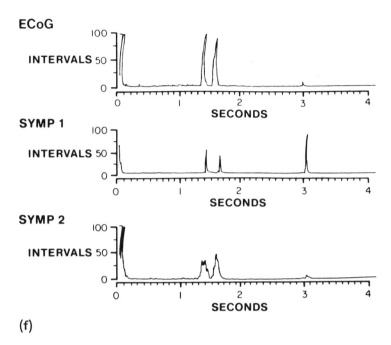

(f)

2000 mg/kg PTZ

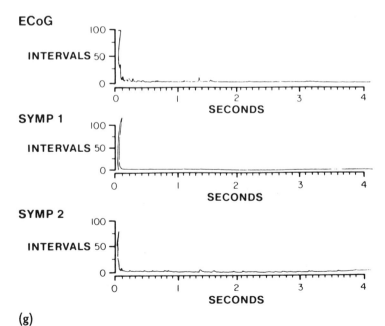

(g)

Table 1 Time Intervals for the ECoG and Two Postganglionic Sympathetic
Cardiac Neural Discharge Patterns

Peak	ECoG	Symp 1	Symp 2
1	1.38	1.38	1.38
2	1.54	1.64	1.58
3	2.82	2.85	2.98
F value for one-way ANOVA with 2 degrees of freedom:			
	1399*	1755*	177*

*$p < 0.01$.

III. RESULTS

Three characteristic time intervals seen on the ISI histograms are summarized in
Table 1. Their average modes were approximately the same and their lengths
were constant with respect to PTZ dose administered (see Figs. 9–11).

The neural and ECoG discharge data produced in each experiment are shown
in Figure 1. We analyzed these data using the techniques discussed above and
produced the ISIs shown in Figure 2. Note that as the dose of PTZ is increased,
two characteristic peaks are seen. A third peak can be seen to occur at an interval of about three seconds. These peaks, which represent sums of intervals, were
found to be statistically different with $p < 0.01$. In the control (Figure 2a) and
at the lethal dose of 2000 mg/kg PTZ, there are no histogram peaks seen because at these points the LSP does not occur. A peak at less than 0.1 second
occurs on each of the histograms. This reflects the ictal activity that occurs
immediately after a dose of PTZ is given and represents the ISI histogram in
ictus. The data from one cat are shown here for illustration but eight cats were
used in the computations and statistical analysis.

Figures 3, 4, and 5 should be reviewed together. They were constructed by
adding the total number of intervals that occurred at any of the three characteristic time intervals and plotting this against the dose of PTZ. These graphs
show a rapid incline and then a plateau. In physiologic terms, the LSP occurs
at fairly characteristic time intervals, producing a similar number of intervals,
independent of the dose of PTZ once the threshold dose was given. This is similar for the ECoG and for the two representative postganglionic sympathetic
nerves.

The number of intervals seen in each peak rose quickly with increasing PTZ
dose and then plateaued. The implication is that the number of time intervals
which constituted the three characteristic peaks of the ISI histogram rose until

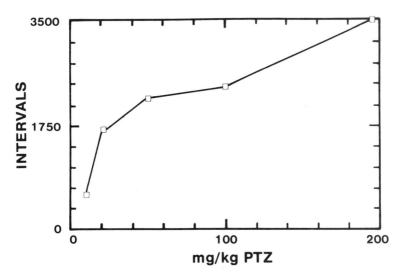

Figure 3 Summed interspike intervals for the ECoG vs. PTZ dose-8 cats included. The total number of time intervals which produced the three characteristic peaks of the ECoG ISI were summed and plotted against the dose of PTZ administered. The number of intervals increases rapidly with increasing dose of PTZ until 50 mg/kg of PTZ is reached. There is a plateau period between 50 and 100 mg/kg PTZ. The increase in the total number of intervals between 100 and 200 mg/kg PTZ occurs only in the ECoG and represents no increase in the time spent in the lockstep phenomenon. Compare with Figures 4 and 5.

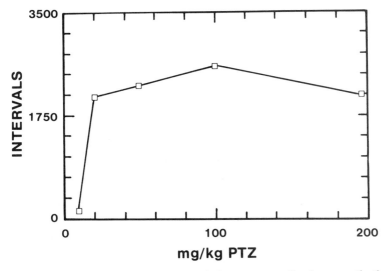

Figure 4 Summed interspike intervals for a postganglionic sympathetic nerve (# 1) vs. PTZ dose-8 cats included. There is a sharp rise at low doses of PTZ and a plateau of PTZ doses greater than 50 mg/kg, which is probably the natural occurrence of this phenomenon.

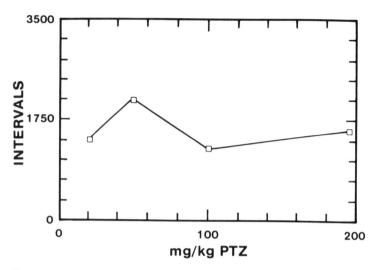

Figure 5 Summed interspike intervals for a postganglionic sympathetic nerve (#2) vs. PTZ dose-8 cats included. There is a sharp rise until 50 mg/kg PTZ then a dip to lower numbers of intervals with increasing doses of PTZ. Although the number of intervals is less than in Figures 3 and 4, the shape of the curve approximates that of the other postganglionic sympathetic cardiac nerve.

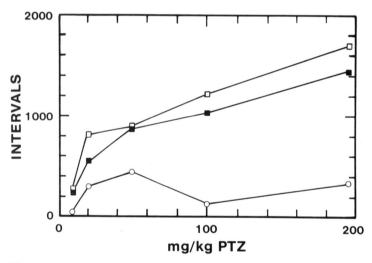

Figure 6 Summed interspike intervals for the three peaks seen on the ECoG vs. PTZ dose-8 cats included. ECoG interspike interval number increases for each peak after the PTZ dose of 100 mg/kg PTZ. This trend is not repeated by the sympathetic nerves monitored. This increase represents intervals that do not appear to contribute to LSP. Average modes are 1.38 seconds (open square), 1.54 seconds (closed square), and 2.82 seconds (open circle).

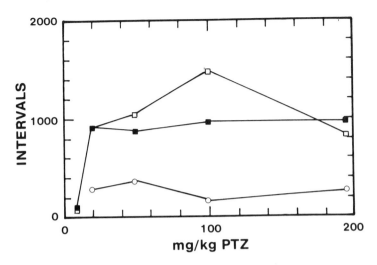

Figure 7 Summed interspike intervals for the three peaks seen from one post-ganglionic sympathetic nerve (# 1) vs. PTZ dose-8 cats included. The plot with the 1.64-second average mode (closed square) curve represents what we surmise to be typical of LSP, i.e., there is a rapid increase in the number of intervals representing LSP beginning. A plateau thereafter signifies the maintenance of LSP. The other average modes are 1.38 seconds (open square) and 2.85 seconds (open circle).

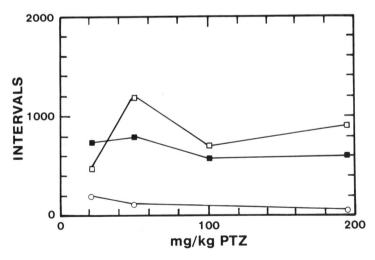

Figure 8 Summed interspike intervals for the three peaks seen from one post-ganglionic sympathetic nerve (# 2) vs. PTZ dose-8 cats included. Number of intervals increases with increasing PTZ dose until a critical value of PTZ is reached. The plots then begin to plateau. Average modes are 1.38 seconds (open square), 1.58 seconds (closed square), and 2.98 seconds (open circle). Compare this graph with Figures 6 and 7.

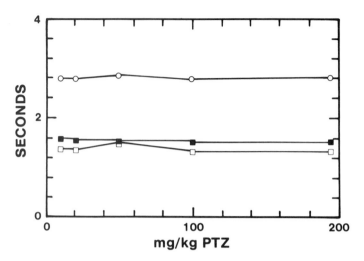

Figure 9 The mode of the interspike interval histogram in seconds for the three peaks seen on the ECoG vs. PTZ dose-8 cats included. This plot demonstrates the consistency of the interval length in seconds of the lockstep phenomenon. Average modes are 1.38 seconds (open square), 1.54 seconds (closed circle), and 2.82 seconds (open circle).

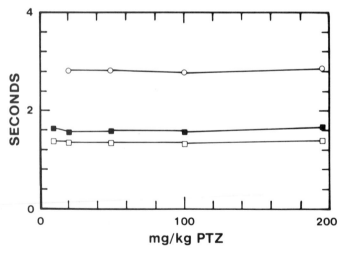

Figure 10 The mode of the interspike interval histogram in seconds for the three peaks seen on one postganglionic sympathetic nerve discharge pattern (# 1) vs. PTZ dose-8 cats included. The average mode is very constant over all doses of PTZ. While the number of intervals changes with increasing PTZ dose, the length of the interval, as demonstrated here, does not change. Average modes are 1.38 seconds (open square), 1.64 seconds (closed circle), and 2.85 seconds (open circle).

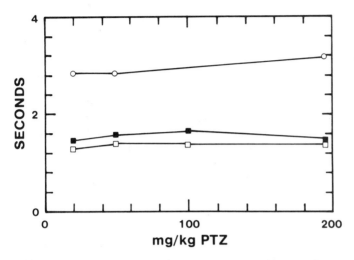

Figure 11   The mode of the interspike interval histogram in seconds for the three peaks seen on one postganglionic sympathetic nerve discharge pattern (#2) vs. PTZ dose-8 cats included. Average modes are 1.38 seconds (open square), 1.58 seconds (closed square), and 2.98 seconds (open circle). (Compare with Figures 9 and 10.)

a certain plasma concentration was reached. Increasing the plasma concentration beyond this level did not increase the number of intervals at the three characteristic time intervals. The ECoG showed an increase in the number of intervals from 100 to 200 mg/kg PTZ. This was not associated with a concomitant rise in the number of intervals seen in either of the sympathetic nerves. There was therefore no further contribution to LSP for the increased number of intervals in this range.

Figures 6 to 8 are similar to Figures 3 to 5 except that the individual histograms from each ISI plot are shown separately, summed over eight cats. This plot was used to demonstrate that each of the individual peaks follows the general trend of rising sharply to 50 mg/kg and then leveling to a plateau. In other words, when the LSP occurred, the number of intervals produced at each dose of PTZ remained fairly constant regardless of the dose of PTZ. Further, it occurred at one of three characteristic time intervals. The LSP occurred at one of the shorter two time intervals more commonly then it did at the longer interval.

Figures 9 to 11 are plots of modes of time intervals in seconds versus dose of PTZ administered. Note that the length of the time interval in seconds is very nearly constant. A series of straight, nonintersecting, horizontal lines in this graph indicates that the modes of the ISI peaks are completely independent of PTZ dose. Note that the time interval with a mode at three seconds did not occur in every cat and at some doses of PTZ it did not occur at all, thus producing few data points.

IV. DISCUSSION

Figure 12I is a representation of the anatomical location of the three oscillatory drivers of concern in LSP and cardiac arrhythmias: the cortex, the cardiac medullary center, and the sinoatrial (SA) node of the heart. In our experiment the cardiac accelerator nerve was recorded to assess the partial output from the cardiac center in the medulla. The pathways involved in the brain between the cortex and the medullary centers were described by Stauffer et al. (Chapter 14, this book).

Figure 12II depicts schematically the normal association of the oscillatory drivers in the brain: the interictal activity in the cortex, the cardiac medullary center in the medulla, and the SA node of the heart. Note that springs have been used to represent the interaction between the centers. The centers influence each other but the depolarizations are not synchronized one to one. In Figure 12III a solid bar is used to depict the association between the interictal focus and the cardiac medullary center during LSP because there is a one-to-one association between the depolarizations of these two centers. In other words, the interictal discharge is driving the cardiac medullary center. A spring still depicts the connection between the medullary centers and the heart because the association is never one to one. When the first two drivers in the brain move in synchrony, their effect is translated to the SA node to produce a change in the depolarization of the heart. A change in rate, rhythm, or aberration results.

The ISI histograms in this study show the dichotomy of LSP, i.e., it is either on or off. The discharge pattern characteristic of LSP, once present, was not altered appreciably by increasing the dose of PTZ until the lethal dose was given. This is demonstrated by Figures 9 to 11. The intervals were shown to be distinct from one another by a one-way ANOVA with $p < 0.01$.

We suggest that the operative mechanism in the LSP may be that the cortex fires constantly, during both the ictal and interictal periods. In the ictal period the interictal depolarizations overwhelm the nearby cells and thus the seizure discharges spread becoming clinically noticeable. In the interictal period the cells may continue to depolarize. If these cells fire with an electrical potential strong enough and at the proper frequency to overtake another group of cells, then the rate of depolarization of the latter group of cells will be driven to seizure activity which will serve as the pacemaker for the second group of cells. In this experiment the second group of cells was the nucleus of the sympathetic nerves located in the cardiac centers of the medulla. These nerves innervate the heart and exhibit both chronotropic and inotropic effects; excessive stimulation will cause cardiac arrhythmias (Randall et al., 1978).

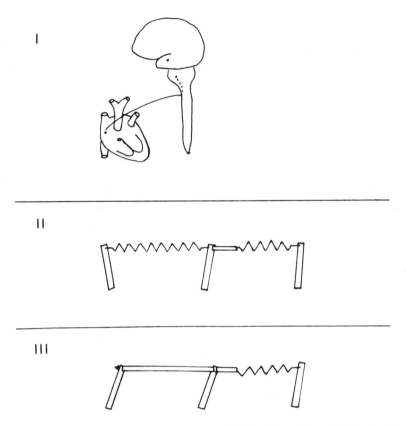

Figure 12 A model for the interaction of the brain and heart in the lockstep phenomenon.

The spread of seizure activity to variable sites involves more than simply the intensity of the interictal discharge. Proximity to specialized tracts may also be of concern. During the ictal period the intensity of the depolarization originating at the focus is strong enough to spread to areas of the brain which elicit clinically noticeable phenomena. In a generalized seizure the spread is so extensive that the reticular activating system is involved and the patient loses consciousness. The former dichotomy proposed for the seizure focus—i.e., it is intense enough either to cause a full-blown seizure or to be completely inoperative—seems incorrect. Interictal activity enables it to capture areas of the brain in close proximity by direct continuity and in distant areas by involvement of tracts that efficiently carry the impulses long distances. The clinical expression of these dynamics is a link between the oscillatory drivers of the focus and that of, for instance, the medullary cardiac centers. Figure 12 diagrammatically shows our concept of the interaction among the cortex focus, the medullary cardiac center, and the heart. The SA node is a pacemaker which is influenced by the discharge of the parasympathetic and sympathetic autonomic nerves that innervate it; this neural connection between the medullary centers and the heart is represented by a spring. These centers have the ability to influence the activity of the SA node but not to directly drive it, just as a spring potentiates movement but does not directly drive it (Guyton, 1981). In the normal state the rate of firing of the SA node, and thus the rate of the heart, and the depolarizations of the nerves reaching the heart will not be correlated one to one since the heart has its own automatic pacemaker. However, it appears that with the development of interictal and ictal discharge and the occurrence of LSP, cardiac arrhythmias may occur in an unpredictable manner. These arrhythmias may contribute to sudden death.

Many systems in nature are linked in a similar fashion to the proposed LSP link. The phenomenon is called entrainment or mode locking by physicists. Gleick (1987) uses the example of the relationship of the moon to the earth to demonstrate this point. In the orbit of the moon around the earth, one lunar surface is always presented to the earth. This is because the orbit of the moon is locked to the rotation of the earth. The rotation of the earth and the orbit of the moon are locked just as the oscillators of the epileptic focus and the medullary cardiac centers are locked one to one during the state of what we call the lockstep phenomenon, or what physicists call mode locking.

The occurrence of a very regular oscillator in the brain is theoretically dangerous, regardless of its mechanism of known effect. The science called chaos which has arisen in the last few decades is of great use in explaining the phenomenon of linked drivers. Ary Goldberger, a prominent physiologist and chaostician, has written: "Fractal processes associated with scaled, broad-band spectra are 'information-rich.' Periodic states, in contrast, reflect narrow-band spectra and are defined by monotonous repetitive sequences, depleted of information content" (Goldberger et al., 1985). The fractal processes of which he speaks, ubiquitous in biological systems including the brain, are those systems that convey different information, depending on how closely you look at them. A commonly used example is that of the Mona Lisa. At a great distance, the outside borders of its frame form a rectangle, and this is all that is conveyed to the observer. At an intermediate distance the beauty of the woman may be appreciated. At a closer distance, the mastery of the artist can be known in terms of each brush stroke. Each of the observations is unique, but together they form the treasured masterpiece. The electrical depolarizations of the brain are an example of such a fractal process. The complexity of a fractal process may at times depreciate into a simple periodic process representing decay of the system and a dramatic change. The key message conveyed by the application of the science of chaos is that simple systems, such as periodic ones, are easily perturbed and less able to return to the preperturbed state. Therefore, seeing a periodic rhythm in the brain, where there is normally rich complexity, implies a susceptibility to failure of the system, i.e., death.

The ultimate cause of sudden unexpected death in this population is thought to be cardiac because at autopsy no obvious cause of death can be found. The only two possible causes are failure of one of the two major electrical systems of the body, the brain and the heart. If the brain fails to send out the impulses from the respiratory centers, then respiratory failure will be the immediate cause of death. If the brain sends a message to the heart that causes it to enter a fatal arrhythmia, or if the heart enters an arrhythmia on its own, then once again sudden death will occur. It is probable that other associated factors play a role in the disturbance of the normal healthy state, such as a fixed lesion in the heart, which alone would not explain death and/or autonomic dysfunction, as has been published by several labs including ours (Stauffer et al., Chapter 14, this book; Van Buren, 1958). Central respiratory failure and arrhythmia are the only obvious etiologies that would leave no signs at autopsy (Jay and Leestma, 1981). Arrhythmia is much more likely, given the findings of this experiment. The perturbation of the electrical depolarization of the heart may have several mechanisms, any or several of which may be operational. Further investigation is necessary to sort out the causes. The difficulty in doing a study of this, however, may mandate empirical treatment. We must first have plausible mechanisms from which models can be built.

The specific mechanism of death in this population may be more complex than the sympathetic discharge rate, although even this theory has merit. An area of damage to the electrical stimulation system of the heart, i.e., the His-Purkinje system, may be caused by continual stimulation of the beta receptors by the sympathetic nerves innervating these receptors; this stimulation might produce a fixed microscopic lesion, which alone would be harmless but sufficient to cause this portion of the myocardium to be less flexible in its response to other insults, e.g., excessive sympathetic discharge. A second possibility concerns the arrangement of the receptors in the ventricle. Beta receptors in the ventricles are arranged in a pattern such that their highest density is in the apex with a gradually decreasing density near the base (Lathers et al., 1986). Downregulating of the beta receptors from continual sympathetic discharge might disturb this gradation, producing a potentially arrhythmic situation. A pattern of increased sympathetic depolarization could be the fatal step in a two-stage process.

A third possibility is that of a forbidden sequence of sympathetic depolarizations, i.e., a pattern of depolarizations from the sympathetics, which can interrupt the regular electrical depolarization. Art Winfree (1987) has begun to characterize these processes in terms of chaos modeling of the heart. More work needs to be performed to identify which of these theories or combination of theories is active in the epileptic patient who dies of sudden unexpected death. Mathematical models like those developed for the heart by Jose Jalife and colleagues (Salata and Jalife, 1985) will facilitate our understanding and provide a basis for continued investigation.

Our model for the demonstration of the interictal activity of LSP is, of course, only an approximation of the human with epilepsy. There are, however, the following important similarities. The focal lesions which have been demonstrated in the brains of patients who have succumbed to interictal unexplained death have shown cortical lesions in as many as 60% of those patients autopsied (Leestma et al., 1984). Moreover, the cat has a more highly developed cortex than many other animals proposed for such models, e.g., the rat, which makes the cat model more likely to represent human epilepsy. The inadequacies of any animal model demonstrate clearly why future research must be coupled with mathematical modeling to maintain good correlation and to add direction for future study.

The possibility exists that our model produces the LSP in a way that does not simulate the natural phenomenon. First, epilepsy in our model was caused by intravenous administration of a chemical, PTZ, which has access to parts of the brain in proportion to their perfusion with blood. Although many areas of the cortex are exposed to the drug, probably one one area eventually becomes the pacemaker of interictal discharge activity.

The study used pretreatment with phenobarbital in order to dampen the epileptogenic activity of PTZ to allow a greater amount of time spent in interictal activity, i.e., to prevent status epilepticus. This allowed us to maximize the time spent in the interictal period. Recall that our objective was to study the possible mechanism of interictal death, not ictal death. In a previous study (Lathers et al., 1987) which did not use phenobarbital, we showed that phenobarbital is not directly involved in the production of LSP.

The interspike interval technique is a novel way of analyzing LSP. It is a rapid method of analyzing the complex discharge patterns generated by a nerve and the brain. When computing an ISI much information is lost; only an instantaneous picture is produced. It is rather like taking the first derivative of a function: the information obtained is valuable but it is now only a useful trend of the original, more complex function. Therefore, the ISI will never serve as the sole measure of LSP, but rather as a very useful indirect measure of the occurrence of LSP.

The computation of mean ISI and the calculation of the area from the ISI peaks were accomplished by approximating the patterns with a triangle. Several errors can be introduced in this operation. First, the area will almost always be underestimated; thus it is more difficult to show statistical significance, making any results all the more valid. Second, the standard that was used to calculate the area-to-interval number was based on the area noted in the standard peak histograms, which were added to each ISI histogram. Since this area would also probably be underestimated, the calculated number of intervals would be greater than the actual number of intervals that created the histogram. We consider the actual difference to be negligible.

Sudden unexplained death in the epileptic patient may prove to have many causes, but it seems important to understand the possible mechanisms that have been discussed here and to contemplate their treatment. It seems practical to think that the administration of a pharmacologic agent to an identified population at risk might be an effective means of prevention. To go about proving this we must first have a valid animal model. Second we must be able to quantitate very closely the degree of LSP occurring, enabling the comparison of various pharmacological agents in the prevention of LSP. The technique of using ISIs to examine the characteristic intervals is a rapid-assessment technique that could be used to analyze the effect of a pharmacological agent. Several authors have used the ISI to characterize discharge patterns, for example, the action of ouabain on autonomic nerves (Lathers et al., 1977).

The future application of this technique is intriguing. An ambulatory EEG monitor coupled with an ambulatory ECG monitor could be used to record the electrical events for 24 hours. Given that the characteristic intervals for LSP have been identified, a statistical analysis of the EEG using the ISI technique could rapidly identify these characteristic intervals and pinpoint the precise time at which they occurred. Next, the ECG could be analyzed for aberrations. A statistical correlation would be sought for those time periods found to be suspect in the EEG with the aberrations noted in the ECG. This would eliminate the need for direct recording of the postganglionic cardiac stimulator nerve, as has been done in this experiment, since it is quite impractical in the human.

V. SUMMARY

The association between epileptogenic activity in the ECoG and aberrations in cardiac activity was investigated by further characterizing the lockstep phenomenon. The pattern of neuronal discharges from several postganglionic cardiac sympathetic branches with simultaneous recordings of the ECoG and the ECG monitored in nine anesthetized cats in which epileptogenic activity was induced with PTZ was analyzed on the basis of time intervals between action potentials in the ECoG. A similar analysis was made of the time intervals between action potentials in the nerves innervating the heart.

Time intervals for both ECoG and cardiac sympathetic discharge were summed and plotted as ISI histograms using a data retrieval computer. The ISIs obtained for the ECoG and the cardiac accelerator nerve tracings were compared. Analysis and comparison of these ISIs demonstrated the occurrence of LSP. The intervals found to be most characteristic of the LSP when monitoring the ECoG were 1.38, 1.58, and 2.85 seconds. These intervals were found to be statistically different with $p < 0.01$.

The implications of our findings were discussed in terms of the science of chaos. The data suggest that the discharge patterns from the ECoG and the sympathetic nerves are synchronized. This abberent discharge pattern may be associated with changes in the ECG, which may ultimately contribute to understanding the mechanism of sudden unexpected death in persons with epilepsy.

REFERENCES

Carnel, S. B., Schraeder, P. L., and Lathers, C. M. (1985). Effect of phenobarbitol pretereatment on cardiac neural discharge and pentylenetetrazol-induced epileptic activity in the cat. *Pharmacology 30*:225-240.

Gleick, J. (1987). *Chaos: Making a New Science*. Viking, New York.

Goldberger, A. L., Bhargava, V., and West, B. J. (1985). Nonlinear dynamics of the heart beat. *Physica 17D*:207-214.

Guyton, A. C. (1981). Rhythmic excitation of the heart. In *Textbook of Medical Physiology*, A. C. Guyton (Ed.). Saunders, Philadelphia, pp. 165-175.

Hahn, F. (1960). Analeptics. *Pharmacol. Rev. 12*:447-530.

Jay, G. W., and Leestma, J. E. (1981). Sudden death in epilepsy. *Acta Neurol. Scand. (Suppl. 82) 63*:1-66.

Lathers, C. M., Levin, R. M., and Spivey, W. H. (1986). Regional distribution of myocardial receptors. *Europ. J. Pharmacol. 130*:111-117.

Lathers, C. M., Roberts, J., and Kelliher, G. J. (1977). Correlation of ouabain-induced arrhythmia and nonuniformity in the histamine-evoked discharge of cardiac sympathetic nerves. *J. Pharmacol. Exp. Ther. 203*:467-479.

Lathers, C. M., Schraeder, P. L., and Carnel, S. B. (1984). Neural mechanisms in cardiac arrhythmias associated with epileptogenic activity: The effect of phenobarbitol. *Life Sci. 34*:1919-1936.

Lathers, C. M., Schraeder, P. L., and Weiner, F. L. (1987). Synchronization of cardiac autonomic neural discharge with epileptogenic activity: The lockstep phenomenon. *Electroencephalogr. Clin. Neurophysiol. 67*:247-259.

Leestma, J. E., Kalelkar, M. B., Teas, S. S., Jay, G. W., and Hughes, J. R. (1984). Sudden unexpected death associated with seizures: Analysis of 66 cases. *Epilepsia 25*:84-88.

Olsen, R. W. (1981). The GABA postsynaptic membrane receptor-ionophore complex site of action of convulsant and anticonvulsant drugs. *Mol. Cell. Biochem. 39*:261–279.

Randall, W. C., Thomas, J. X., Euler, D. E., and Rosanski, G. L. (1978). Cardiac dysrhythmias associated with autonomic nervous system imbalance in the conscious dog. In *Perspectives in Cardiovascular Research*, Vol. 2, *Neural Mechanisms in Cardiac Arrhythmias*, P. J. Shwartz, A. M. Brown, A. Malliani, and A. Zanchetti (Eds.). Raven Press, New York, pp. 123–138.

Salata, J. J., and Jalife, J. (1985). "Fade" of hyperpolarizing response to vagal stimulation at the sinoatrial and atrioventricular nodes of the rabbit heart. *Circ. Res. 56*(5):718–727.

Van Buren, J. M. (1958). Some autonomic concomitants of ictal automatism. *Brain 81*:505–528.

Winfree, A. T. (1987). *When Time Breaks Down: The Three-Dimensional Dynamics of Electrochemical Waves and Cardiac Arrhythmias*. Princeton University Press, Princeton, N.J.

16

Power Spectral Analysis: A Procedure for Assessing Autonomic Activity Related to Risk Factors for Sudden and Unexplained Death in Epilepsy

STEPHEN R. QUINT, JOHN A. MESSENHEIMER, and MICHAEL B. TENNISON *School of Medicine, University of North Carolina, Chapel Hill, North Carolina*

I. INTRODUCTION

Sudden death of unknown etiology has been an active area of research for the past two decades (DeSilva and Lown, 1978; Falconer and Rajs, 1976; Gordon et al., 1984, 1986; Guilleminault et al., 1984; Hirsch and Martin, 1971; Jay and Leestma, 1981; Kiok et al., 1986; Leestma et al., 1984; Myers et al., 1986; Neuspiel and Kuller, 1985; Schraeder and Lathers, 1983; Terrence et al., 1975). Sudden unexplained death (SUD) in epileptic persons comprises an inordinately large subpopulation of this group in relation to its occurrence in the general population (Jay and Leestma, 1981; Neuspiel and Kuller, 1985; Wannamaker, 1985). Abnormalities in the autonomic nervous system, particularly in its regulatory function of the cardiovascular system, have been postulated as central to the causes of death (Gordon et al., 1984, 1986; Guilleminault et al., 1984; Hirsch and Martin, 1971; Jay and Leestma, 1981; Kiok et al., 1986; Leestma et al., 1984; Myers et al., 1986; Neuspiel and Kuller, 1985; Schraeder and Lathers, 1983; Terrence et al., 1975; Wannamaker, 1985).

The implications of autonomic involvement in SUD are particularly significant in epilepsy in that even minimal epileptogenic activity can cause profound alteration of autonomic activity and balance, with associated alterations in cardiorespiratory parameters including ECG changes, blood pressure, respiration, and vasomotor tone (Hirsch and Martin, 1971; Lathers and Schraeder, 1982;

Schraeder and Lathers, 1983; Wannamaker, 1985). ECG effects commonly observed in experimental epilepsy include heart rate changes, arrhythmias, conduction blocks, altered ECG morphology, and QT interval changes (Lathers and Schraeder, 1982, 1987; Lathers et al., 1987; Mameli et al., 1988; Schraeder and Lathers, 1983). Heart rate changes without arrhythmias have been reported during seizures in patients with epilepsy (Blumhardt et al., 1986; Keilson et al., 1987; Marshall et al., 1983). Additionally, many drugs used in the treatment of epilepsy have direct autonomic or cardiac effects. This may have some significance in the observation that in almost all cases of SUD in epileptics, the level of prescribed anticonvulsant is found to be subtherapeutic or absent (Hirsch and Martin, 1971; Jay and Leestma, 1981; Leestma et al., 1984; Neuspiel and Kuller, 1985; Terrence et al., 1975). The incidence of SUD in epilepsy is not uncommon, with estimates varying from 1/1100 to 1/500 or more frequent (Jay and Leestma, 1981; Leestma et al., 1984). Identification of this subpopulation of epileptics at risk for SUD may be possible through a detailed understanding of autonomic activity under circumstances peculiar to epilepsy. Of particular benefit would be a procedure that would enable quantification of autonomic activity dynamically, with a methodology not requiring a perturbation of the system for the purpose of measurement.

The specific autonomic nervous system dysfunction that may be a critical factor in the genesis of sudden death in epileptics is uncertain (Lathers and Schraeder, 1982, 1987; Lathers et al., 1987; Mameli et al., 1988; Wannamaker, 1985). Jay and Leestma (1981) postulate that this catastrophic and unpredictable event is a result of fatal ventricular arrhythmia due to sympathetic stimulation. Taken as support of this hypothesis is the finding of focal myocarditis-like lesions in the hearts of epileptic patients who experienced SUD (Falconer and Rajs, 1976), as similar lesions have been produced in animal models by intense sympathetic stimulation of the heart.

Cardiovascular homeostasis is maintained by both the sympathetic and parasympathetic portions of the autonomic nervous system, with their effects being modulated by the renin–angiotensin system. Valsalva's maneuver, ocular compression, carotid sinus massage, and other transient perturbations to the cardiorespiratory control system have traditionally been used to evaluate the functional status of the autonomic nervous system. These techniques are cumbersome, perturb the system that is being assessed, and do not lend themselves to steady-state evaluation of autonomic function. In animal models, fluctuations in heart rate have been investigated by power spectral analysis and have been shown to correlate with the activity of the autonomic nervous system.

Three peaks in the power spectrum have been described, in dogs (Akselrod et al., 1981), to correlate with respiration (high frequency), the baroreceptor reflex (midfrequency), and changes in vasomotor tone related to the thermo-

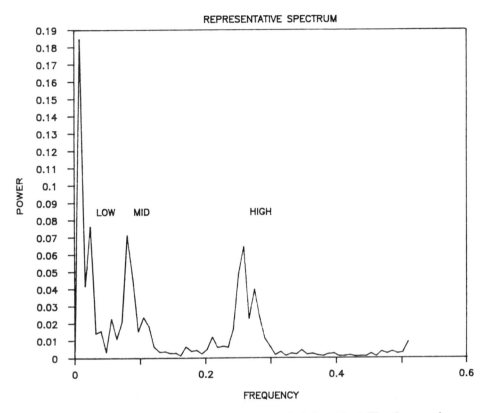

Figure 1 Power spectrum of HPV from a normal adult subject. The three peaks illustrate the frequency bands where spectral power is typically concentrated, which correspond to frequencies of oscillation in the heart period under autonomic control.

regulation system (low frequency). This distribution in spectral power, from a normal human subject, is illustrated in Figure 1. The high-frequency peak (centered at the frequency of respiration) is generally recognized to be mediated solely by the parasympathetic system (Eckberg, 1983; McCabe et al., 1984; Pomeranz et al., 1985; Porges, 1986), although sympathetic activity has been implicated in respiratory arrhythmias (Pagini et al., 1986). The midfrequency peak, often referred to as the low-frequency peak in recent studies (Pagani et al., 1986; Pomeranz et al., 1985), is centered at approximately 0.1 Hz and is mediated at rest by the parasympathetic system alone in the supine position (Akselrod et al., 1981; Pagani et al., 1986; Pomeranz et al., 1985) and by the combined sympathetic-parasympathetic autonomic system in the sitting and standing postures (Pagani et al., 1986; Pomeranz et al., 1985). The mid-frequency peak is prominent in an upright posture and the high-frequency peak is augmented in the supine position (Baselli et al., 1987; Pagani et al., 1986; Pomeranz et al., 1985). Pagani and colleagues (1986) suggested a ratio of the mid- to high-frequency components as an indicator of relative sympathetic-parasympathetic balance. The low-frequency peak (at approximately 0.03 Hz) has both sympathetic and parasympathetic components (Akselrod et al., 1981) and is attenuated by the renin-angiotensin system. Power in the low-frequency band was not found significant by Myers et al. (1986) in comparing groups of patients at risk and not at risk for sudden cardiac death, and they found this peak to be very sensitive to postural changes and other activity. This peak is often ignored (Pagani et al., 1986) or possibly included with the mid-frequency component (Pomeranz et al., 1985).

Spectral analysis of heartbeat variability in several patient populations has been used to identify groups at risk for sudden infant death, cardiac patients at risk for sudden cardiac death, and patients with autonomic disorders and to study the influence of vagal tone on early development (Baselli et al., 1987; Gordon et al., 1984, 1986; Nugent and Finley, 1983; Pagani et al., 1986; Pomeranz et al., 1985; Porges, 1986; Zwiener, 1978). At present this method has proven valuable in understanding the relationship of the autonomic system to normal and abnormal conditions rather than as predictive of patient outcome. We are unaware of the application of this method, other than our preliminary reports (Messenheimer et al., 1987; Quint et al., 1987; Tennison et al., 1987), to the study of autonomic function in epilepsy. Epileptic patients frequently undergo intensive monitoring with routine collection of ECG, EEG, and video data, providing an ideal opportunity to study the involvement of the autonomic nervous system in this disease. Heart period variability (HPV) data are therefore readily available for analysis and correlation with seizure type, sleep/wake state, and antiepileptic drug level. To the extent that the ECG is recorded in analog form in epileptic patients who suffer unexplained death, it is possible to use this method to investigate SUD in epilepsy.

II. THEORY

A. Spectral Concepts

There are many methods for estimation of the spectral content of a signal, including maximum likelihood, maximum entropy, spectral filtering procedures, and Fourier analysis. The most generally used of these is Fourier analysis, with the fast Fourier transform (FFT) used as an efficient algorithm for computer determination of the discrete Fourier transform.

1. Spectral Decomposition of a Data Record

The premise of Fourier transformation is that an arbitrary waveform may be represented by a sum of sinusoids or, equivalently, by a sum of complex exponentials. For waveforms of discrete variables, either finite sequences of lenght N or periodic sequences with N elements in each period,

$$x(n) = x(0) + x(1) + \cdots + x(N-1) \quad 0 < n < N$$

the waveform may be decomposed into a sum of N complex exponentials (or sine and cosine waves) in N multiple harmonics of the fundamental frequency.

$$x(n) = \frac{1}{N} \sum_{k=0}^{N-1} X(k) e^{j\left(\frac{2\pi}{N}\right)nk}$$

with

$$e^{j 2\pi f_1 nk} = \frac{1}{2} [\cos(2\pi f_1 nk) + j\sin(2\pi f_1 nk)]$$

and fundamental frequency

$$f_1 = \frac{1}{N}$$

The fundamental frequency is the inverse of the duration of a finite sequence, or one period of a periodic sequence. The weighting factor $X(k)$ of the exponential for each harmonic (Fourier coefficient) gives the relative presence of this frequency in the waveform. The set of N Fourier coefficients, which represents the decomposition of the waveform into its spectral components, is generally made up of complex numbers that can be presented as real and imaginary numbers in a rectilinear coordinate system $(a + jb)$ or as magnitude and phase in a polar coordinate system $(r$ angle $\theta)$. The autospectrum is the magnitude squared $[r^2$ or $(a^2 + b^2)]$, which is an estimate of the power present at each frequency component (or power spectrum).

The estimate of autospectra differs from the true power spectrum due to the presence of both random and bias errors which are either present in the data or introduced through computation of the estimate due to finite register-length effects. The mean value of the data is the zero frequency component in the corresponding spectral estimate. This term may be treated independently of the dynamic portion of the data, and it is advantageous to subtract this term before computation of the spectral estimate.

The power spectrum determined from a single record of time data is termed an inconsistent estimate because the random error at each spectral point is constant regardless of the sample size. Each spectral component has 2 degrees of freedom, independent of the number of data points in the time record. Averaging the spectral estimates of sequential records at each frequency increases the degrees of freedom at each spectral point in proportion to the number of records averaged, so that the random error approaches zero for large sample sizes. This process produces a consistent estimate of the power spectrum. However, spectral averaging will only produce a reliable estimate of the true spectra if the data are stationary.

2. Stationarity of a Data Record

Stationarity of a time record is satisfied provided sequential records have the same averaged properties (all moments are equal). A data set is weakly stationary if its mean and autocorrelation function do not vary with time in the set. This condition can be met, in practice, only as a matter of degree. Although various tests are available to assess the stationarity of data sets, weak stationarity is often judged qualitatively by visually comparing sequential data records for transients and by comparing the Fourier transforms of the autocorrelation functions. Because heart rate is influenced by a multitude of inputs (exercise, anxiety, body position, etc.), it is essential to keep the environment as constant as possible during collection of heart period data to minimize nonstationarities. When transients and other nonstationarities appear in a data record it is possible to remove them under some circumstances with filtering and other procedures (Bendat and Piersol, 1986; McCabe et al., 1984; Porges, 1986). More generally, however, the portion of the record containing the nonstationarities is omitted from the analysis (Akselrod, 1981; Baselli et al., 1987; Myers et al., 1986; Pagani et al., 1986).

3. Aliasing

For the determination of the spectral content of a signal by discrete computational procedures, the data set representing the signal must be both finite and represented by discrete numbers. A finite discrete data set may be obtained from a continuous signal by sampling at a regular interval for a finite number of representative values. The sample rate must be fast enough to capture all of the information in the data, or, in terms of the sample interval, the time between samples must be short enough to represent all of the variation in the data. Fluctuations present in the data at a frequency faster than half the sample frequency will be represented at a slower frequency (aliasing).

4. Windowing

Truncation of the data set at the end points introduces frequency components that may not properly represent the spectral content of the data. Windowing has the effect of tapering, rather than truncating, the mean–zero data to zero at both ends of the record. The resulting distortion of the data in the frequency domain corresponds to convolving the autospectrum of the heart period data with the autospectrum of the window.

5. Scaling of Spectral Data

When presented in graph form the autospectrum (or power spectrum) is commonly scaled logarithmically, linearly, or as a square root. Both square-root scaling (also called an amplitude spectrum) and logarithmic scaling of the autospectrum have the advantage of compressing a large range of data for presentation on a single graph. However, for visual interpretation, this compression causes moderate variations in the spectral data to become indistinct. Linear scaling of the autospectra is best suited for visual distinction of the amplitude variations of interest in HPV data. However, this may require matching the scale of the vertical axis to the actual data.

Detailed presentations on the theory of discrete Fournier analysis and the analysis of random data can be found in Oppenheim and Schafer (1975) and Bendat and Piersol (1986).

B. Spectral Analysis of the ECG

1. Heart Rate Versus Heart Period

Because the dynamic activity of the autonomic nervous system is most directly reflected in the time between successive heartbeats, spectral analysis is generally performed on the fluctuations in time or frequency between successive beats rather than on the ECG waveform itself. Although many investigators use instantaneous heart rate (the inverse of heart period) as the independent variable, we use heart period, which is a direct measure of time. Analysis of either measure of fluctuation between beats yields qualitatively similar results. The time between successive beats of the heart, generally measured as the R-R interval, is a discrete random variable. Obviously, it is necessary to obtain a measure of this variable before further analysis is possible.

2. Heart Rate Detectors

The most convenient method to obtain a discrete representation of heart rate is to sample the analog output of a clinical heart rate detector at a rate near the heart rate. There are several problems with this technique. First of all, the ECG is subject to noise from a variety of sources (Friesen et al., 1990), and long

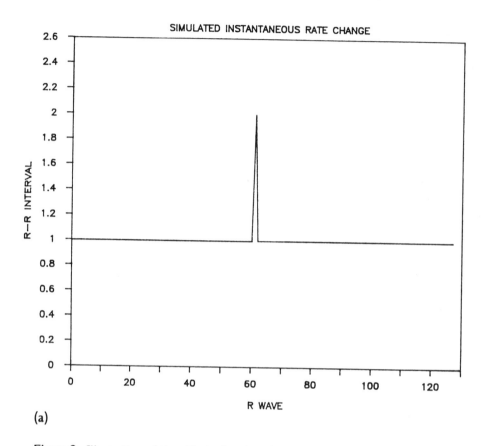

(a)

Figure 2   Illustration of the effect of an impulse on the power spectrum. (a) Simulated heart period data with 128 beats at 1 bps, with a single two-second interval between beats 63 and 64.

records of constant high signal-to-noise measurements are rare under all but the best of circumstances. The algorithm for detection of the R wave used in the clinical detector is generally unknown to the user, and all algorithms for heart event detection are subject to both missed and false beats (Friesen et al., 1990). There are erroneous data, which introduce a positive or negative impulse to the data set, are then present in the sample heart period data for spectral analysis without a procedure for observation or correction of the error. An impulse (or scaled unit sample in discrete signal-processing terminology) contributes equal power to all frequencies of the power spectrum (Figure 2). In generating an analog output for sampling, the heart rate detector introduces a data hold char-

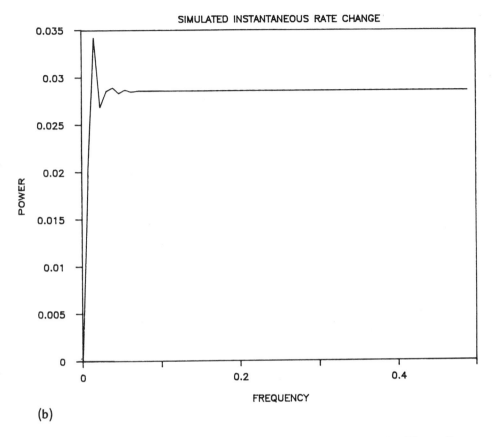

Figure 2 (continued) (b) Power spectrum of the unit sample impulse. The oscillatory effect at low frequency is due to the mean removal and windowing of the time sequence data.

acteristic (generally first order) into the signal, with associated random and bias errors.

Selection of the sample rate for the instantaneous heart rate output is another problem that can introduce error in the data. Sampling too slow will introduce aliasing and sampling too fast generates redundant data and ultimately reduces the significance in the data (less than 2 degrees of freedom per spectral point). Because the very characteristic of interest in the data is the dynamic variation of heart rate, there is no completely satisfactory solution to the problem of sample rate selection with this technique.

3. Spectral Analysis of the Heart Event Series

As an event series, the heart period (or heart rate) data are in the proper format for discrete Fourier analysis. However, there are both practical and theoretical problems with estimating the power spectra directly from the event series. The practical difficulty is, again, the problem of reliable and verifiable detection of heart period. A procedure is required for determining the R-R interval from long records of noise-contaminated ECG without missing or falsely detecting an event. By digitizing the ECG waveform it is possible to use a detection algorithm to mark events and then rapidly review the marked waveform with an editing facility to correct errors.

Spectral analysis of the discrete event series has the advantage of not introducing the errors related to converting the discrete data to an analog signal and then sampling it at a regular interval. In particular, the random and bias errors associated with estimation of regularly spaced samples are avoided, and because the data are discrete there is no aliasing. However, this approach has two theoretical problems. First, the frequency dimensions are in cycles per event rather than hertz. This variable may be converted to hertz by multiplying by the mean event rate, with an error related to the amount of variability in the data. This approximation of radian frequency to Hertz is generally considered reasonably good for heart event series (De Boer et al., 1984; Mohn, 1976), and this direct procedure for estimation of the spectral content of the heart (or rate) is widely used (Akselrod et al., 1981; Haddad et al., 1984). However, because of the indirect relationship of the event series to time it is difficult to determine the cross-correlation or cross-spectra between this variable and other physiological measures not directly tied to the heart event. For investigations of the interaction between the heart period (or rate) and most other time-related variables it is necessary to convert the event series to a time series with regularly occurring samples. Procedures for this conversion are presented by De Boer et al. (1984) and Berger et al. (1986). An excellent presentation of theoretical considerations for spectral analysis of heart rate is given by Sayers (1980).

III. PROCEDURES

A. Clinical and Experimental Protocol

Data are collected from a variety of patients and experimental subjects. Recording of the ECG is always included in our epilepsy monitoring procedures. The ECG is recorded with two chest leads, placed to accentuate the QRS amplitude and minimize the T wave. Data from volunteer subjects were collected in the Clinical Research Unit of the North Carolina Memorial Hospital, in patients admitted for evaluation of epilepsy, and in epileptic patients monitored at home.

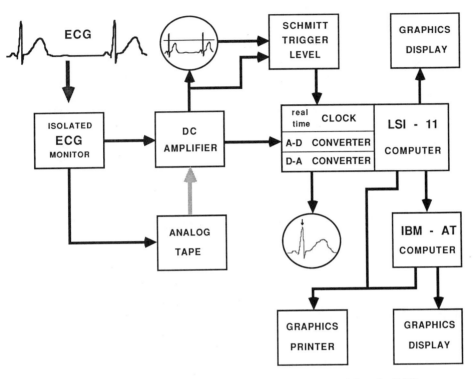

Figure 3 Schematic diagram showing the procedure for digitizing the ECG, detection of R–R intervals, and processing of the resultant heart period data.

The physiological signals monitored in addition to the ECG, as well as the recording procedures, vary as appropriate to the circumstances.

1. Anticonvulsant Studies

In studying the effects of anticonvulsants on the autonomic activity in normal subjects we record only the ECG, through on-line computer digitization of this waveform. The ECG is recorded from subjects at rest in a standing or supine position in a quiet room. The ECGs recorded in each volunteer subject continuously for 10 minutes in the absence of the drug (control) and again following administration of the anticonvulsant, coincident with its peak concentration in the blood. The anticonvulsants we have studied to data are carbamazepine, administered orally (600 mg), and phenytoin given intravenously in a single 250-mg dose. Anticonvulsant serum concentrations are obtained corresponding to the time that the data for HPV are collected.

2. Epilepsy Studies

All inpatients and outpatients undergoing diagnostic or presurgical epilepsy monitoring are studied using a commercially available (Telefactor) 16-channel radio telemetry–based system (CCTV/EEG). Montages which include an EEG channel and up to 15 channels of EEG are recorded on videotape (Figure 5) along with a video image of the subject. Recorded seizures which are technically acceptable are selected and replayed, with EEG and ECG hard copy printed and the ECG digitized and stored by the computer system. Separate preictal, ictal, and postictal segments are then evaluated. The hard copy record is used to relate the onset of seizure activity, as determined from the EEG and/or behavioral state noted from the video signal, to the corresponding location in the digitized record stored in a computer file.

A commercially available eight-channel recording system (Oxford), with one channel dedicated to ECG, is used in outpatient ambulatory monitoring. Selected segments from these cassette tapes are analyzed in a manner similar to the procedure used in CCTV/EEG monitoring. The absence of a video picture as a behavioral correlate to the ECG and fewer channels of EEG are disadvantages of this type of monitoring. We tested both the CCTV/EEG and ambulatory recording systems and verified that neither has tape speed fluctuations that contribute to the time measured between heartbeats (less than 1 msec/sec).

B. Data Collection and Spectral Estimation

We extract the heart period from the ECG through a process of digitizing the ECG, detecting the R wave of each QRS complex in the ECG, and measuring each successive R-R interval (Figure 3). Spectra are determined from stationary records of heart period data.

1. ECG Digitization and Heart Period Determination

The amplified ECG is displayed on an oscilloscope (Tektronix R5113) along with a potentiometer-adjusted threshold level, either on-line from a Hewlett Packard 7830A isolated ECG monitor or off-line from video or cassette tape. This analog waveform is sampled using a Digital 11/73 computer system, with the position of the threshold crossing of each QRS wave stored along with the digitized waveform (Figure 4A). During data processing sequential 500-point records of the waveform are recalled from disk and rapidly displayed on a digital oscilloscope (Hatachi V131), with the threshold crossing points moved to the local peak (R wave) and marked with an arrow (Figure 4B). The number of points between arrows (R-R interval) is written to a file along with the sample rate. A heart period sequential plot is generated from this file and displayed on the terminal screen; it may also be printed (Figure 6). Missed beats

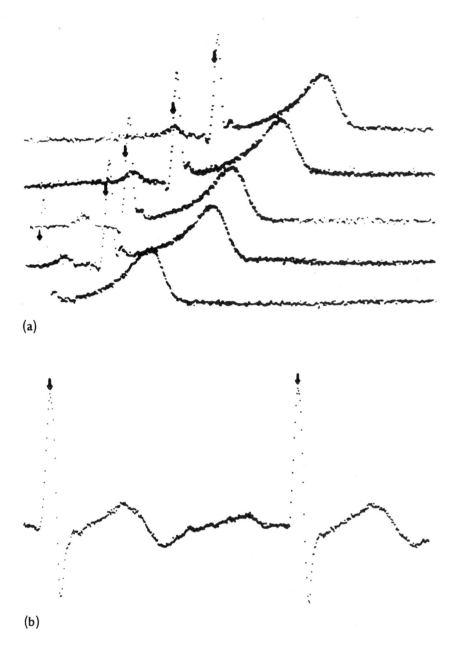

(a)

(b)

Figure 4 Digitization and threshold detection of the QRS complex, and R–R interval determination. (a) The continuously digitized ECG is displayed as five sequential traces on the digital storage scope, after which the screen is erased and the process repeated. Threshold crossings are marked with an arrow. (b) During processing sequential 500-point records of the digitized ECG are recalled from disk and displayed on the digital scope with the threshold crossings moved to the local peak (R wave). A file is simultaneously created which contains the times between arrows (heart period).

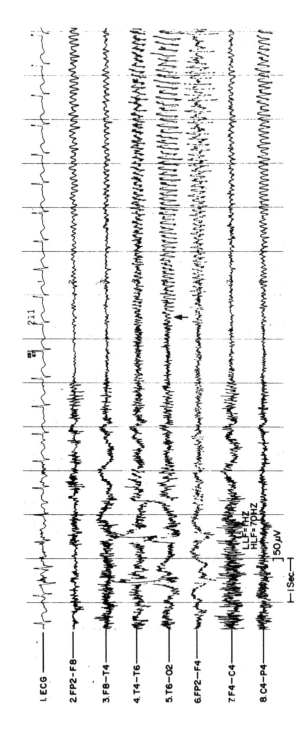

Figure 5 Strip chart tracing of the ECG and seven channels of EEG at the onset of an ictal episode in a patient with partial complex seizures localized to the right posterior temporal region (see Case 1, Section IV.B). The electrographic ictal onset is marked with an arrow in channel 5. Marked changes in the rhythmicity of the ECG (see Figure 7) preceded the EEG changes by approximately 16 beats (10 seconds).

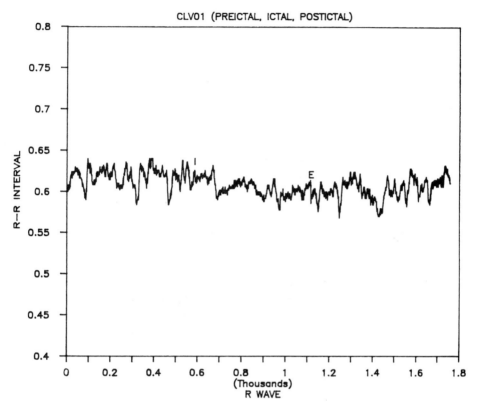

Figure 6 Heart period plotted sequentially for the seizure of Figure 5 with the ictal onset marked I and the end of the ictus marked E. These data represent the R–R interval for approximately five minutes preceding the ictus, five minutes of the ictus, and five minutes of the postictal period. Each period was divided into 4 records of 128 beats each, and the power spectra for these 16 records is presented in the three-dimensional plot of Figure 7.

and/or spurious noise erroneously marked as beats are easily recognized in this display as unit spikes of double or half height respectively, and they are noted for editing. Individual 500-point records of the digitized ECG may be randomly accessed and displayed on the digital scope for editing purposes (Figure 4B), and arrows marking the R wave may be inserted, removed, or positioned within the record as appropriate. This editing feature is essential regardless of the R wave detection technique (threshold crossing or pattern detection algorithm), due to the prevalence of many types of noise in the ECG even under the best of circumstances (Friesen et al., 1990). The spike introduced by a single missed

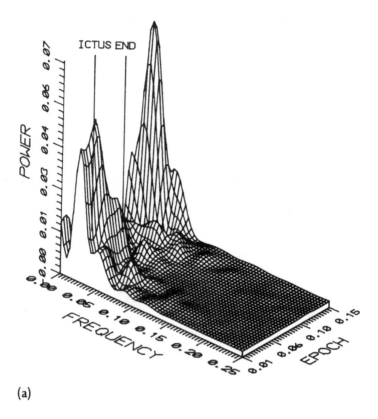

(a)

Figure 7 Three-dimensional representation of the power spectra corresponding to the heart period data of Figure 6. Power spectra for 16 records of 128 beats each, from the preictal through postictal periods, were smoothed across frequency and records to create this power spectra surface.

or falsely detected beat essentially contaminates all frequencies of the spectrum with erroneous power (Figure 2).

2. Power Spectra Estimation

Once we are satisfied that the heart period sequential plot accurately represents the R–R interval sequence of the ECG, the data are normalized by subtracting the mean of 128 consecutive R–R intervals from each heart period within that record and then dividing each by the mean. This data set is then multiplied by a modified super-Gaussian window ($P = 6, E = 0.0005$), which tapers the beginning and end of the record to the mean. From the normalized mean-zero data, spectra are generated, displayed, and printed for each sequential 128-beat record.

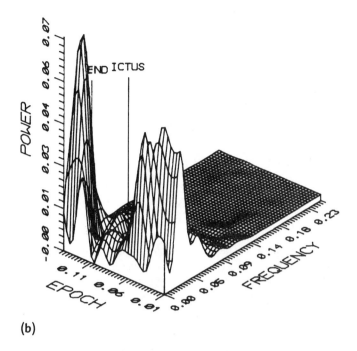

(b)

Figure 7 (continued) The electrographic ictal onset (marked ICTUS) followed the marked drop in HPV power by about 16 beats, and spectral power gradually recovered over approximately 20 beats following the electrographic end (marked END) of the seizure.

We use linear scaling of the autospectra with the range of the vertical axis automatically matched to the data. Spectral records that are judged absent of significant nonstationarities, based on the time interval and spectral records, are averaged to form an estimate of the power spectrum. We consider an estimate determined from three to four records to represent a good compromise of the time required to maintain the subject in a constant environment, the nonstationarities which transiently appear in the ECG under these circumstances, and the need for averaging many records to obtain a reliable (consistent) estimate of the power spectrum.

3.   Data Evaluation and Presentation

Although the Digital 11/73 is an extraordinary computer for data acquisition and processing, there is a paucity of cost-effective and convenient software and hardware available for statistical analysis and generation of quality graphics. The R-R interval and power spectral data are therefore ported to an IBM-AT computer for statistical quantification, drawing of three-dimensional surfaces (Figure 7), and generation of publication-quality heart period and spectral plots (Figures 2 and 6). Spectral data are tested for significance (F-test for equal variance within subjects, with nonparametric comparison of these results between subjects) in each of the three spectral bands that have been shown to characterize specific autonomic activity. Our computer-software system for collecting, processing, and evaluating HPV data is presented in detail sequence (Quint et al., 1989).

IV. PRELIMINARY FINDINGS

Both seizure activity and anticonvulsant therapy are postulated to be related to sudden and unexplained death in epilepsy through autonomic effects (Hirsch and Martin, 1971; Jay and Leestma, 1981; Leestma et al., 1984; Terrence et al., 1975). For this reason we are interested in the effect of anticonvulsants and epileptogenesis on autonomic regulation. The interaction of anticonvulsant therapy and the basic mechanisms of epilepsy are almost certainly more complex than the effect of either alone is on the autonomic nervous system. However, in studying their effects on autonomic regulation we hope to understand the relationship of seizures, anticonvulsant therapy, and autonomic activity to sudden death. Through the noninvasive procedure of spectral analysis of HPV, autonomic activity may be observed indirectly through its relationship to the dynamic variability in the interval between successive heartbeats. These studies are in progress, and the data are presented as examples of application of the method rather than as evidence of a specific effect of seizures or an anticonvulsant drug on autonomic activity.

A. Anticonvulsant Effects

We have obtained preliminary HPV data from normal subjects receiving carbamazepine or phenytoin while participating in pharmacokinetic studies. Data from subjects ($N = 6$) receiving carbamazepine (600 mg orally four times daily) were collected at the predicted peak serum concentration. Ten minutes of ECG data were collected under controlled conditions with subjects supine and standing. Baseline measurements from each subject, obtained prior to the administration of the drug, were used as control data for each subject. Data from subjects receiving phenytoin ($N = 12$) were obtained from the supine position only. ECG data were collected at baseline, at the end of infusion of 250 mg of phenytoin and again one hour after the end of infusion. The baseline measurements for each subject were used as control data.

Data from both carbamazepine and phenytoin subjects were examined by comparing the spectral data in each of the three major frequency bands between the control and drug condition.

1. Carbamazepine

Of the six subjects in the carbamazepine study, four had significant changes in one or more frequency bands. In the supine position two subjects had significant decreases in power at all three frequency bands while one subject had a significant increase and one had a significant decrease limited to the high-frequency band (0.2–4.0 Hz). In the standing position, one subject had decreases at the low-frequency and mid-frequency bands while one subject had an increase at the mid-band and one had a decrease at the high-frequency band. Overall, significant changes were seen in 12 bands in four subjects. Of the 12 changes, 10 were decreases in power.

2. Phenytoin

Data from the subjects receiving phenytoin were more variable. Significant changes occurred in 18 bands for 7 of the 12 subjects at the end of infusion and in 16 bands for 10 subjects one hour after the end of infusion. Most of the changes were increases in power (14/18 at the end of infusion and 11/16 one hour after infusion). This is contrasted with reductions in power observed with carbamazepine.

These results are preliminary and insufficient to draw meaningful conclusions. They do suggest, however, that phenytoin and carbamazepine have very different effects on HPV. Since the data for each drug were obtained under different circumstances, we cannot be certain that the differences in HPV are attributable to drug alone.

B. Seizures

In addition to the normal variation in HPV between subjects, there is a considerable difference in the effects on HPV exerted by seizures both within and between subjects. Because uninterrupted records are required for spectral analysis, it is generally difficult to follow HPV through the ictus with spectral techniques due to movement artifact associated with the seizure. Data are presented for three patients with partial complex or generalized seizures, in which the R-R interval was detectable in the ECG through the ictus, to illustrate the variety and similarities of the effects of seizures on HPV.

1. Case I

This patient had repeated partial complex seizures which were localized in onset to the right posterior temporal region. The seizures consisted of left head and eye deviation and hallucinations in a hemianopic left visual field. The patient was monitored with the CCTV/EEG system, in the supine position. Figure 5 is a tracing of the ECG and selected channels of the EEG. The R-R interval sequential plot was determined for a period extending from approximately five minutes

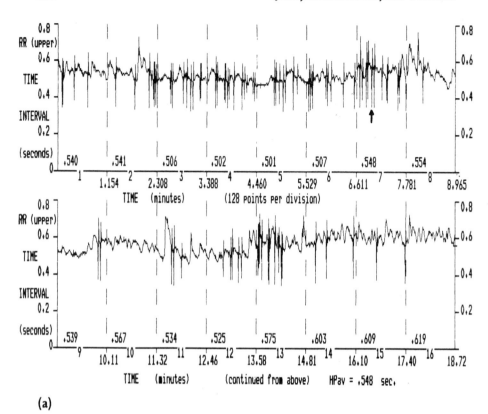

(a)

Figure 8   (a) Heart period plotted sequentially from approximately nine minutes preictally through nine minutes of the postictus (see Case 2, section IV. B), organized into 16 records of 128 beats each. Characterized by a short R-R interval, PACs appear as a downward impulse followed by an upward impulse (compensatory pause), except in the short ictal period (electrographic ictal onset approximately at minute 9 and ending at minute 9.7 in the record.

preictally, through the ictus (five minutes), and for approximately five minutes postictally (Figure 6). Little variation was evident in the preseizure portion of the R-R interval plot, probably related to a combination of the patient's postural position during recording (Pagani et al., 1986) and the cumulative effect of repeated seizures (Wannamaker, 1985) or anticonvulsants (carbamazepine and phenytoin). As evident from this figure, the mean heart period during the ictus did not differ from the preictal or postictal period. The power spectrum was determined for each successive 128-beat record from these data, in the manner described above, and these spectra are presented in a three-dimensional plot in

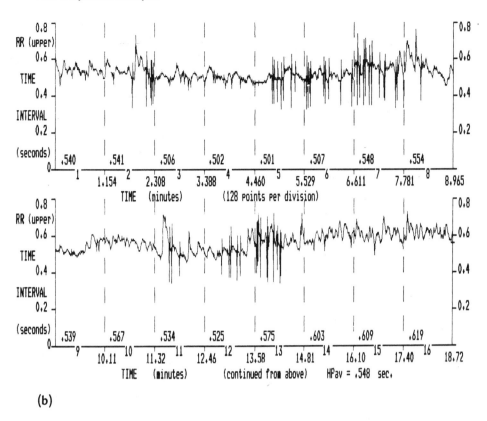

(b)

Figure 8 (continued) (b) Same heart period plot with negative/positive impulses due to PACs averaged in preictal records 1, 3, and 4 and in postictal records 14 and 15. Because these PACs occur as nonphasic events (unrelated to rate regulation), they may be averaged to reveal the underlying rhythmicity of heart rate. The power spectra may then be determined without introducing broad spectrum artifacts due to impulses in the data (see Figure 3).

Figure 7. During the ictal period the power fell throughout the spectrum in this subject, with the low-frequency power loss most obvious due to its predominance in the preictal period. This effect actually preceded the onset of the ictus as detected in the EEG (Figure 5). Accompanying 3 of 10 seizures recorded in this patient there were occasional sudden and brief heart rate changes in the postictal period (not seen in this record), which did not occur preictally and are generally not seen in normal subjects. These impulse rate changes had the appearance of those seen in the postictal period for Case III (Figure 11).

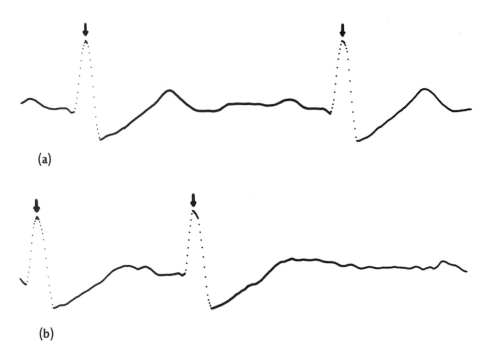

(a)

(b)

Figure 9   Digitized ECG showing normal rhythm and a premature atrial contraction from the preictal period of Figure 9a (see Case 2, section IV B). (a) Two QRS complexes from a normal section of ECG with the arrows marking the R waves separated by 568 msec. (b) Two QRS complexes with the P wave of the second beat occurring on the T wave of the first. The arrows are separated by 342 msec corresponding to the R-R interval marked by the arrow in Figure 9a.

2. Case II

Partial complex seizures occurred approximately once per day in this patient, localized in the left temporal regions. Seizures were accompanied by aphasia and abdominal pain. Records of the ECG and EEG during seizure activity were obtained with home ambulatory monitoring. In one of these records repeated instantaneous heart period changes were present in the ECG, as shown in the R-R interval sequential plot in Figure 8A. In this case (Figure 9) these events are characterized by a short R-R interval caused by a premature atrial contraction (PAC) followed by a compensatory long heart period, seen as a negative-positive impulse pair in Figure 8A. These impulses in the heart period record were suppressed during the ictus and gradually reappeared with increasing frequency following the seizure. Because there is a compensatory pause following each of these premature beats, it is possible to use the editing procedure to average each

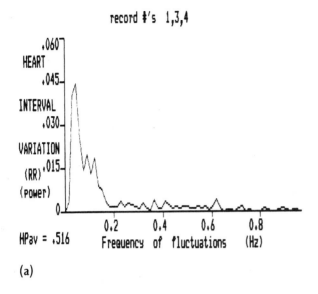

(a)

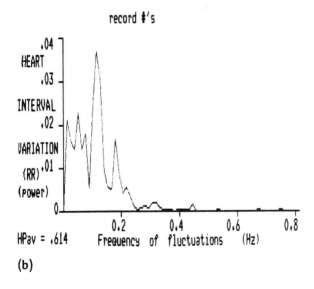

(b)

Figure 10 Power spectra averages for heart period data from selected records in Figure 9b, with PACs removed. (a) Preictal records 1, 3, and 4; (b) postictal records 15 and 16. From the preictal to the postictal periods there is a modest reduction in power in the low-frequency band and a corresponding increase in power in the mid-frequency band. The ictal period was too short, in this case, to determine its spectral content.

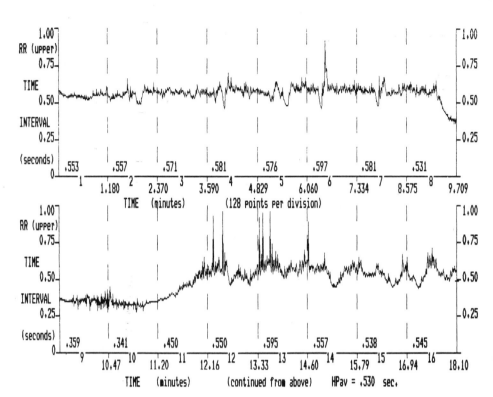

Figure 11 Heart period plot from an ECG preceding, during, and following an ictal episode (see Case 3, section IV.B), organized as 16 consecutive records of 128 R-R intervals per record. The ictal onset occurs in record 8 with the precipitous fall in heart period, and the postictal period begins in record 11 with a gradual return of heart period to the preictal level. The high-frequency fluctuations in heart period in the ictal period (records 9 and 10) are due to error in precisely identifying the R wave in the ECG. Positive impulses, which appear in the early postictal period and correspond to brief profound heart slowing, represent phasic events in heart rate regulation.

impulse pair and obtain a spectrum of the underlying heart period variability (Figure 8b). There is a slight shift in power from the low-frequency band preictally to the mid-frequency band postictally (Figure 10). Although HPV does appear to be reduced during the ictal period, the ictus in this case is too short for its spectrum to be determined with the present version of our software. The mean heart period is only slightly less during the seizure than in the preictal or postictal period.

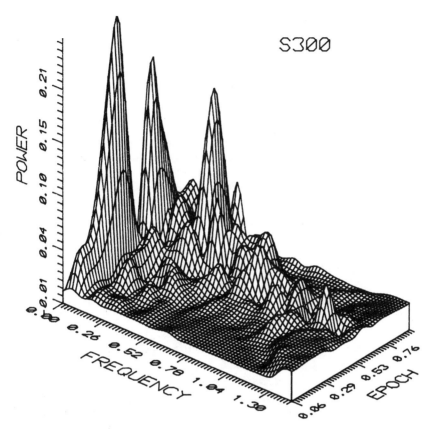

Figure 12 Three-dimensional surface plot from the 16 heart period records of
Figure 11. The transition from the preictal to ictal period is represented by an
average of the autospectra of records 7 and 9, and the transition from ictal to
postictal period is represented by averaging the autospectra for records 10 and
12. Smoothing was performed across frequency and records (epochs) to generate
this surface. The broad-spectrum low-amplitude power in the ictal period of this
plot is artifact due to random error in locating the R wave in the ECG during
seizures.

Because these heart period impulses were present at least an hour preceding
this seizure and not present during most other seizures in this patient, we are
uncertain if the PACs were related to this seizure. However, their suppression
during the ictus and slow reappearance postictally clearly indicate some interaction between the seizure and the origination of the PACs.

3. Case III

This 4-year-old experienced frequent generalized seizures, having developed a severe hypersensitivity reaction to phenobarbitol, phenytoin, and carbamazepine. As an interim measure prior to beginning valproic acid therapy, the child was maintained on a ketogenic diet and lorazepam. Eight to twelve generalized tonic-clonic seizures, 60–90 seconds in duration, were noted daily. ECG and EEG data were recorded in this patient, in a supine position, with CCTV monitoring from his hospital room. From the R–R interval plot, HPV is seen to gradually increase in the preictal period, greatly diminish in the ictal period, and become pronounced postictally (Figure 11). In the three-dimensional spectral plot of these data (Figure 12), this variability develops as increasing power in the low-frequency and mid-frequency bands in the preictal period, is reduced in these bands during the ictus, and is large in the low-frequency band postictally. A respiratory component (high-frequency band) also becomes prominent in the postictal period. The mean heart period during the ictus is considerably less than the preictal or postictal period in this case. Instantaneous rate changes appear in the R–R interval plot immediately after the seizure, followed by the appearance of large oscillations. These instantaneous rate changes are similar to those often present in the ictal and postictal period for the patient in Case I and differ from the negative/positive impulses of Case II in that in Case III they appear postictally and as single positive impulses only. These positive impulses are seen in the ECG to be isolated beats with extended time from the Q wave of one beat to the P wave of the next beat, not preceded by any type of premature beat. This sudden slowing suggests a strong parasympathetic influence, also indicated by the high-frequency peak. Although we did not monitor respiration, the large oscillation in the postictal period, which coincides with the very large low-frequency spectral peak (0.03 Hz) and the appearance of the respiratory peak, are probably due to periodic breathing with an envelope of 0.03 Hz.

V. DISCUSSION

The spectral changes in HPV which we have observed in relation to seizures are indicative of a significant change in cardiac autonomic regulation. Although recordings obtained during ictal episodes are often short or difficult to analyze due to movement noise and artifact, there appears to be a consistent decrease in power over the entire spectrum during ictal periods compared to either the preictal or postictal periods. At times this power loss preceded the EEG ictal onset (Figure 7). This is in agreement with observations of Blumhardt et al. (1986) and Van Buren and Ajmone-Marsan (1960) that autonomic effects of seizures may be the very first manifestation of seizure activity.

More variable changes observed in the postictal period include increases and deacreases in power in the different frequency bands compared to the preictal period. These variations in the postictal spectra were seen in analyzing repeated seizures within a single patient as well as between patients. This variability of seizure effects from patient to patient and even within the same patient are not surprising. Van Buren and Ajmone-Marsan (1960) documented the importance of the baseline autonomic state in determining the type and direction of changes in autonomic activity which accompany a seizure.

The consistently reduced power we observed in the ictal period was often associated with tachycardia. Keilson et al. (1987) and Blumhardt et al. (1986) reported sinus tachycardia as the most frequent accompaniment to ictal episodes. In addition to spectral and mean rate changes associated with seizures, we frequently observed precipitous or instantaneous heart slowing, rarely occurring in normal subjects, in the late ictal or postictal period. These episodes of transient heart slowing were associated with extended R-R and normal QT intervals in an otherwise unremarkable ECG. Keilson et al. (1987) and Blumhardt et al. (1986) similarly observed sudden transient changes in heart rate in some patients in both the ictal and postictal periods, not associated with cardiac arrhythmias. These short periods of bradycardia differed from those reported by Mameli et al. (1988) in an experimental epilepsy model using decerebrate rats, in which brief periods of heart slowing during ictal and interictal episodes were frequently observed in conjunction with cardiac arrhythmias.

When a sequential plot of heart period is generated, with heart period defined as the time separating every systole whether of sinus node, atrial, or ventricular origin, there is a characteristic difference between records containing arrhythmias and those without. Extrasystoles, resulting from either PACs or PVCs, are generally followed by a compensatory pause. This pause is such that the total time from the beat preceding the extrasystole to the following beat is equivalent to two normal heart periods. In the heart period plot the arrhythmia appears as a negative impulse followed immediately by a positive impulse (Figure 8A), such that when this impulse pair is replaced by its average there is no evidence of a transient change in the heart period data (Figure 8B, records 1, 3, 4, 14, 15). In records containing impulse (one beat) or transient (several beats) changes in heart period without the presence of arrhythmias (Figure 11), there is a fundamentally different process involved, and these cannot be removed from the record by averaging. Arrhythmias characterized by premature beats followed by a compensatory pause are not associated with a change in the autonomic influence to the sinus node, as neither mean rate nor HPV is altered. This is a nonphasic event, and the system which regulates rate is not involved in the extrasystole. This is in contrast to profound transient rate changes of the type seen in Figure 11, which are a consequence of the rate-regulating system and must be effected through a transient change in autonomic influence on the sinus node.

This is a phasic event, equivalent to a phase shift in heart period with respect to other dynamic physiologic parameters.

Lathers and Schraeder (1982, 1983, 1987) and Lathers et al. (1987) demonstrated an imbalance in sympathetic and parasympathetic activity in experimental epilepsy, both during ictal activity and with interictal spike activity. This autonomic imbalance was characterized by alterations in heart rate and mean arterial pressure with a disruption in the physiological relationship between these variables. Cardiac arrhythmias (both PACs and PVCs) and other ECG effects were also observed in relation to nonuniform cardiac sympathetic neural discharge associated with epileptogenic activity. Disruption in the physiological relation between mean arterial blood pressure and heart rate, along with ECG changes, also occurred with the lockstep phenomenon (synchronization between cortical, cardiac sympathetic, and to a lesser extent vagal discharges; Lathers et al., 1987). The general loss of power in the heart period spectrum with varying increases in heart rate which we have observed during seizures is in agreement with nonuniform autonomic discharge or increased activity with loss of rhythmicity in the cardiac sympathetic discharge. The most common ECG effect associated with seizures which we have observed, profound brief heart slowing in the late ictal and postictal periods, may occur through a mechanism similar to the lockstep phenomenon described by Lathers et al. (1987), although we have not seen EEG discharges in synchrony or arrhythmias with these remarkable transient events. These transient events could also result from short periods of nonuniform (dysfunctional) cardiac sympathetic activity during which the sinus node is dominated by parasympathetic input.

It is important to recognize that not all changes in HPV which appear to be related to seizure activity can be detected or quantified by spectral analysis. In many instances, and in particular in association with epilepsy, records of the R-R interval contain profound transient changes in heart period as well as shifts in the mean. It is often possible to remove these nonstationarities from the heart period record by filtering or other procedures and obtain the spectral distribution of the underlying variability, but important information may be discarded in the process. Transients in the record, especially in epilepsy, may be indicative of dysfunctional autonomic activity and should be analyzed in the time domain. To fully characterize and quantify changes in HPV in epilepsy both frequency and time domain procedures should be used. We are currently evaluating several nonspectral techniques for use in quantifying transient features in heart period data.

REFERENCES

Akselrod, S., Gordon, D., Ubel, F. A., Shannon, D. C., Barger, D. C., and Cohen, R. J. (1981). Power spectrum analysis of heart rate fluctuation: A quantitative probe of beat-to-beat cardiovascular control. *Science 213*:220–222.

Baselli, G., Cerutti, S., Civardi, S., Lombardi, F., Malliani, A., Merri, M., Pagini, M., and Rizzo, G. (1987). Heart rate variability signal processing: A quantitative approach as an aid to diagnosis in cardiovascular pathologies. *Int. J. Bio-Med. Comput. 20*:51-70.

Bendat, J. S., and Piersol, A. G. (1986). *Random Data: Analysis and Measurement Procedures.* Wiley, New York.

Berger, R. D., Akselrod, A., Gordon, D., and Cohen, R. J. (1986). An efficient algorithm for spectral analysis of heart rate variability. *IEEE Trans. Biomed. Eng. 33*:900-904.

Blumhardt, L. D., Smith, P. E. M., and Owen, L. (1986). Electrocardiographic accompaniments of temporal lobe epileptic seizures. *Lancet 1*:1051-1056.

DeBoer, R. W., Karemaker, J. M., and Strackee, J. (1984). Comparing spectra of a series of point events particularly for heart rate variability data. *IEEE Trans. Biomed. Eng. 31*:384-387.

DeSilva, R., and Lown, J. (1978). Ventricular premature beats, stress and sudden death. *Psychosomatics 19*:649-661.

Eckberg, D. L. (1983). Human sinus arrhythmia as an index of vagal cardiac outflow. *J. Appl. Physiol. 54*:961-966.

Falconer, B., and Rajs, J. (1976). Postmortem findings of cardiac lesions in epileptics: A preliminary report. *J. Forensic Sci. 8*:63-71.

Friessen, G. M., Jannett, T. C., Afify, M., Yates, S., Quint, S. R., and Nagel, H. T. (1990). A comparison of the noise sensitivity of nine QRS detection algorithms. *IEEE Trans. Biomed. Eng. 37*:85-98.

Gordon, D., Cohen, R. J., Kelly, D., Akselrod, S., and Shannon, D. C. (1984). Sudden infant death syndrome: Abnormalities in short term fluctuations in heart rate and respiratory activity. *Pediatr. Res. 18*:921-926.

Gordon, D., Southall, D. P., Kelly, D. H., Wilson, A., Akselrod, S., Richards, J., Kenet, B., Kenet, R., Cohen, R. J., and Shannon, D. C. (1986). Analysis of heart rate and respiratory patterns in sudden infant death syndrome victims and control infants. *Pediatr. Res. 10*:680-684.

Guilleminault, G., Pool, P., Motta, J., and Gillis, A. M. (1984). Sinus arrest during REM sleep in young adults. *N. Engl. J. Med. 306*:1006-1010.

Haddad, G. G., Jeng, H. J., Lee, S. H., and Lai, T. L. (1984). Rhythmic variations in R-R interval during sleep and wakefulness in puppies and dogs. *Am. J. Physiol. 247*:H67-H73.

Hirsch, C. S., and Martin, L. M. (1971). Unexpected death in young epileptics. *Neurology 21*:682-690.

Jay, W. J., and Leestma, J. E. (1981). Sudden death in epilepsy. *Acta Neurol. Scand. (Suppl. 82)63*:1-66.

Keilson, M. J., Hauser, W. A., Magrill, J. P., and Goldman, M. (1987). ECG abnormalities in patients with epilepsy. *Neurology 37*:1624-1626.

Kiok, M. C., Terrence, C. F., Fromm, G. H., and Lavine, S. (1986). Sinus arrest in epilepsy. *Neurology 36*:115-116.

Lathers, C. M., and Schraeder, P. L. (1982). Autonomic dysfunction in epilepsy: Characterization of autonomic cardiac neural discharge associated with pentylenetetrazol-induced epileptogenic activity. *Epilepsia 23*:633-647.

Lathers, C. M., and Schraeder, P. L. (1987). Review of autonomic dysfunction, cardiac arrhythmias, and epileptogenic activity. *J. Clin. Pharmacol. 27*:346-356.

Lathers, C. M., Schraeder, P. L., and Weiner, F. L. (1987). Synchronization of cardiac autonomic neural discharge with epileptogenic activity: The lockstep phenomenon. *Electroenceph. Clin. Neurophysiol. 67*:247-259.

Leestma, J. E., Kalelkar, M. B., Teas, S. S., Jay, G. W., and Hughes, J. R. (1984). Sudden unexpected death associated with seizures: Analysis of 66 cases. *Epilepsia 25*:84-88.

Mameli, P., Mameli, O., Tolu, E., Padua, G., Giraudi, D., Caria, M. A., and Melis, F. (1988). Neurogenic myocardial arrhythmias in experimental focal epilepsy. *Epilepsia 29*:74-82.

Marshall, D. W., Westmoreland, B. F., and Sharbrough, F. W. (1983). Ictal tachycardia during temporal lobe seizure. *Mayo Clin. Proc. 58*:443-446.

McCabe, P. M., Yongue, B. G., Porges, S. W., and Ackles, P. K. (1984). Changes in heart period, heart period variability, and a spectral analysis estimate of respiratory sinus arrhythmias during aortic nerve stimulation in rabbits. *Psychophysiology 21*:149-158.

Messenheimer, J. A., Quint, S. R., Tennison, M. B., Corcoran, M. C., and Keaney, P. (1987). Changes in heart period variability during repeated complex partial seizures. *Epilepsia 28*:635.

Mohn, R. K. (1976). Suggestions for the harmonic analysis of point process data. *Comp. Biomed. Res. 9*:521-530.

Myers, G. A., Martin, G. J., Magid, N. M., Barnett, P. S., Schadd, J. W., Weiss, J. S., Lesch, M., and Singer, D. H. (1986). Power spectral analysis of heart rate variability in sudden cardiac death: Comparison to other methods. *IEEE Trans. Biomed. Eng. 33*:1149-1156.

Neuspiel, D. R., and Kuller, L. H. (1985). Sudden and unexpected natural death in childhood and adolescence. *J. Am. Med. Assoc. 254*:1321-1325.

Nugent, S. T., and Finley, J. P. (1983). Spectral analysis of periodic and normal breathing in infants. *IEEE Trans. Biomed. Eng. 30*:672-675.

Oppenheim, A. V., and Schafer, R. W. (1975). *Digital Signal Processing.* Prentice Hall, Englewood Cliffs, N.J.

Pagani, M., Lombardi, F., Guzzetti, S., Rimoldi, O., Furlan, R., Pizzinelli, P., Sandrone, G., Malfatto, G., Dell'Orto, S., Piccaluga, E., Turiel, M., Baselli, G., Cerutti, S., and Malliani, A. (1986). Power spectral analysis of heart rate and arterial pressure variabilities as a marker of sympatho-vagal interaction in man and conscious dog. *Circ. Res. 59*:178-193.

Pomeranz, B., Macaulay, R. J., Caudill, M. A., Kutz, I., Adam, D., Gordon, D., Kilborn, K. M., Barger, A. C., Shannon, D. C., Cohen, R. J., and Benson, H. (1985). Assessment of autonomic functions in humans by heart rate spectral analysis. *Am. J. Physiol. 248*:H151-H153.

Porges, S. W. (1986). Respiratory sinus arrhythmia: Physiological basis, quantitative methods, and clinical implications. In *Cardiorespiratory and Cardiosomatic Psychophysiology*, P. Grossman, K. Janssen, and D. Vaitl (Eds.). Plenum, New York, pp. 101-115.

Quint, S. R., Messenheimer, J. A., Tennison, M. B., and Corcoran, M. C. (1987). A procedure for assessing autonomic activity related to risk factors for sudden and unexplained death in epileptics. *Epilepsia 28*:610.

Quint, S. R., Messenheimer, J. A., Tennison, M. B., and Nagel, H. T. (1990). Assessing autonomic activity from the EKG related to seizure onset detection and localization. Proceedings of the Second IEEE Symposium on Computer-Based Medical Systems, pp. 2–9.

Sayers, B. (1980). Signal analysis of heart-rate variability. In *The Study of Heart Rate Variability*, R. I. Kitney and O. Rompelman (Eds.). Clarendon Press, Oxford, pp. 27–58.

Schraeder, P. L., and Lathers, C. M. (1983). Cardiac neural discharge and epileptogenic activity in the cat: An animal model for unexplained death. *Life Sci. 32*:1371–1382.

Tennison, M. B., Quint, S. R., Messenheimer, J. A., Corcoran, M. C., and Keaney, P. (1987). Autonomic effects of seizures assessed by power spectral analysis of heart period variability. *Epilepsia 28*:612.

Terrence, C. F., Wisotzkey, H. M., and Perper, J. A. (1975). Unexpected, unexplained death in epileptic patients. *Neurology 25*:594–598.

Van Buren, J. M., and Ajmone-Marsan, C. (1960). A correlation of autonomic and EEG components in temporal lobe epilepsy. *Arch. Neurol. 3*:683–703.

Wannamaker, B. B. (1985). Autonomic nervous system and epilepsy. *Epilepsia (Suppl. 1)26*:31–39.

Zwiener, U. (1978). Spectral analyses of blood pressure, heart rate and respiration rhythms in different postures of healthy individuals and patients with neurovegetative disorders. *Acta Biol. Med. Ger. 37*:1461–1469.

17

GABA Neurotransmission, Epileptogenic Activity, and Cardiac Arrhythmias

ROCHELLE D. SCHWARTZ   *Duke University Medical Center, Durham, North Carolina*

CLAIRE M. LATHERS*   *The Medical College of Pennsylvania, Eastern Pennsylvania Psychiatric Institute, Philadelphia, Pennsylvania*

I. INTRODUCTION

Gamma-aminobutyric acid (GABA) is the major inhibitory neurotransmitter in the central nervous system. It binds to a receptor-gated chloride ion channel ($GABA_A$ receptor) resulting in an increase in membrane chloride permeability, neuronal hyperpolarization or depolarization, and an inhibition of neuronal firing (for review, Schwartz, 1988). Thus GABA has a prominent role in maintaining control over neuronal excitability. Not surprisingly, there is much evidence to demonstrate that impairment of GABAergic neurotransmission is associated with the etiology and pathophysiology of convulsive disorders such as epilepsy (Meldrum, 1975).

Compounds that inhibit GABA synthesis (3-mercaptoproprionic acid, isoniazid) (Killam and Bain, 1957) and receptor antagonists that block $GABA_A$ recognition sites (bicuculline) or the chloride channel directly (pictotoxin, pentylenetetrazol) (Schwartz, 1988) induce seizures (Rastogi and Ticku, 1986). In humans, drugs known to facilitate GABAergic neurotransmission are clinically effective anticonvulsants (i.e., benzodiazepines, barbiturates). In addition, these agents prevent or reverse convulsant activity in animal models of epilepsy such as electroconvulsive shock (Rastogi and Ticku, 1985), kindling (McNamara et al., 1987), and pentylenetetrazol-, picrotoxin-, and bicuculline-induced seizures (Rastogi and Ticku, 1986). Anticonvulsant activity is also afforded by agents which facilitate GABAergic transmission by inhibiting GABA metabolism (Iadarola and Gale, 1981).

Current affiliation: FDA, Rockville, Maryland.

GABA neurotransmission is also important in regulating the central control of cardiovascular function. GABAergic transmission arising in forebrain structures such as the periventricular hypothalamus directly reduces sympathetic outflow to the cardiovascular system (for review, Gillis et al., 1988). However, GABA-ergic mechanisms in the forebrain increase parasympathetic outflow by exerting an influence on hindbrain structures to control heart rate (Gillis et al., 1988). In the hindbrain, GABAergic control of both sympathetic and parasympathetic outflow is more complex. Sympathetic outflow can be both increased and decreased. For example, the medullary nucleus tractus solitarius (NTS), the termination for baroreceptor afferents, controls sympathetic outflow to regulate heart rate and blood pressure. This nucleus contains high levels of GABA (Dietrich et al., 1982; Gale et al., 1980; Maley and Newton, 1985; Siemers et al., 1972). GABA uptake (Siemers et al., 1972), release (Kubo and Kihara, 1987), and binding sites (Gale et al., 1980) are also present in the NTS. Application of GABA to the ventral surface of the medulla, the NTS, and the nucleus ambiguus, another ventrolateral medullary nucleus that participates in parasympathetic control of cardiovascular function, produces a bicuculline-sensitive decrease in heart rate and arterial blood pressure (DiMicco et al., 1979; Keeler et al., 1984; Kubo and Kihara, 1987; Machado and Brody, 1988). Inhibition of CNS GABA-ergic tone using picrotoxin or bicuculline results in an enhanced sympathetic outflow to the heart, leading to increased coronary resistance and arrhythmias (Segal et al., 1984). Prior administration of the $GABA_A$ agonist muscimol into the cerebroventricles prevents these cardiac alterations.

These kinds of studies clearly indicate that the neuronal excitability/inhibitory state in the CNS is an important factor in the development of seizures and of cardiovascular abnormalities such as arrhythmias. Therefore, many investigators have examined how alterations in GABAergic neurotransmission lead to changes in neuronal excitability. The modulation of GABAergic neurotransmission can occur by alteration of a variety of processes: (1) GABA synthesis, (2) GABA release from the nerve terminal, (3) GABA uptake or metabolism, and (4) $GABA_A$ receptor sensitivity (leading to neuronal hypoactivity or hyperactivity). This chapter discusses several factors that regulate two of these processes, presynaptic GABA release and $GABA_A$ receptor sensitivity. Theories as to how regulation of these processes might play a role in the interruption of normal GABA-ergic tone and the development of neuronal excitability are also discussed.

II. REGULATION OF $GABA_A$ RECEPTOR SENSITIVITY AND FUNCTION

The $GABA_A$ receptor is a multimeric protein complex which contains GABA recognition sites and allosteric modulatory sites for anticonvulsants and sedative/hypnotics such as benzodiazepines and barbiturates and for convulsants such as

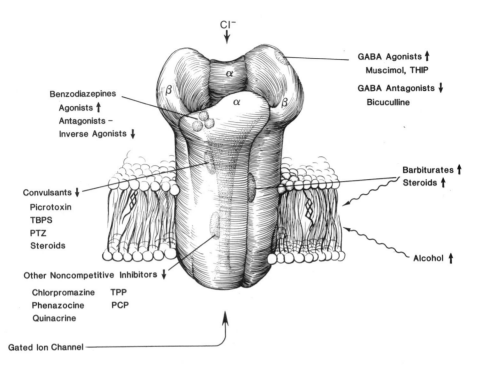

Cl⁻

GABA Agonists ↑
Muscimol, THIP

GABA Antagonists ↓
Bicuculline

Benzodiazepines
Agonists ↑
Antagonists –
Inverse Agonists ↓

Barbiturates ↑
Steroids ↑

Convulsants ↓
Picrotoxin
TBPS
PTZ
Steroids

Alcohol ↑

Other Noncompetitive Inhibitors ↓

Chlorpromazine   TPP
Phenazocine   PCP
Quinacrine

Gated Ion Channel

Figure 1 Schematic model of the GABA$_A$ receptor complex. This model is
not meant to indicate the subunit assembly or the location and stoichiometry of
the various recognition sites associated with the subunits. Although only four
subunits are shown, current evidence predicts the presence of a fifth subunit.
Arrows indicate the enhancement (↑) or inhibition (↓) of GABAergic function
by various agents. THIP = 4, 5, 6, 7-tetrahydroisoxazolo[5,4-c]pyridin-3-ol;
PTZ = pentylenetetrazole; TPP = tetraphenylphosphonium; and PCP = phencyclidine; and TBPS = t-butylbicyclophosphate. [From Schwartz (1988), reproduced with permission.]

picrotoxin (Schwartz, 1988). (See Figure 1 for a schematic representation.)
The subunits form an anion channel through which chloride ions can enter with
the concentration gradient. GABA-activated increases in chloride permeability
are enhanced by benzodiazepines, barbiturates, and alcohol and inhibited by the
GABA receptor antagonist bicuculline and other convulsants such as picrotoxin
and pentylenetetrazol (Schwartz, 1988). These compounds have been used as
pharmacologic tools to study the biochemical and functional characteristics of
the GABA$_A$ receptor.

In addition to these pharmacologic agents, various endogenous substances
also affect GABA$_A$ receptor function. Under certain conditions, the generation

and release of endogenous substances can be enhanced, leading to a disturbance in tonic GABAergic transmission and to neuronal hyperexcitability or hypoexcitability. Examples of endogenous substances that have been found to alter $GABA_A$ receptor sensitivity are discussed in this section.

A. Endogenous Benzodiazepine Ligands

For many years investigators have searched for endogenous ligands which bind to the benzodiazepine recognition sites associated with the $GABA_A$ receptor. Although early studies indicated possible candidates such as purines, purine nucleosides, nicotinamide, and beta-carbolines (cf. Sangameswaran and De Blas, 1985), there has been no evidence to show that these compounds act as endogenous benzodiazepine ligands. However, more recently, two groups identified endogenous ligands at the benzodiazepine site (diazepam-binding inhibitor, Alho et al., 1985; butyl-β-carboline-3-carboxylate, Pena et al., 1986); both have anxiogenic or proconvulsant activity (Alho et al., 1985; Novas et al., 1988). In contrast, benzodiazepine-like molecules that can act as agonists have been isolated in brain, using monoclonal antibodies (Sangemeswaran and De Blas, 1985). If these substances are synthesized and released in brain to regulate $GABA_A$ receptor function, they can provide another level for control of neuronal excitability. We currently await studies to support this hypothesis.

B. Steroids

The effects of steroids on neuronal excitability are complex in nature. Steroids such as progesterone and deoxycorticosterone have CNS depressant properties and increase seizure threshold, while cortisol and corticosterone increase neuronal excitability and lower seizure threshold (for review, Majewska, 1987). To determine the mechanism(s) for steroid-induced alterations in neuronal excitability, researchers have examined the interaction of steroids with the GABA receptor complex. Metabolites of progesterone and deoxycorticosterone (3α-hydroxyprogesterone and 5α-tetrahydrodeoxycorticosterone, respectively) interact with the GABA receptor–like hypnotic barbiturates. Like barbiturates, these compounds enhance benzodiazepine and muscimol ($GABA_A$ agonist) binding to rat brain membranes and inhibit t-butylbicyclophosphate (TBPS) binding to "convulsant sites" associated with the GABA-gated Cl^- channel (Majewska et al., 1986). In addition, these neuroactive steroids induce Cl^- uptake in brain vesicles in a picrotoxin-sensitive manner (Majewska et al., 1986), potentiate GABA-activated Cl^- permeability (Harrison et al., 1987; Morrow et al., 1987), and enhance GABA-mediated neuronal inhibition (Smith et al., 1987).

Conversely, pregnenolone sulfate, a 3α-hydroxy steroid synthesized de novo in brain (Corpechot et al., 1983), produces neuronal excitation (Carette and

Paulain, 1984). This neurosteroid, a precursor of progesterone, was recently shown to compete with TBPS for convulsant sites on the GABA$_A$ receptor complex and inhibit GABA-induced Cl$^-$ permeability (Majewska and Schwartz, 1987). Thus pregnenolone sulfate acts as an endogenous antagonist of the GABA$_A$ receptor (Majewska and Schwartz, 1987), providing a basis for the convulsant properties of 3α-hydroxy steroids (Atkinson, 1965).

C. Unsaturated Free Fatty Acids

Cleavage of membrane phospholipids by endogenous phospholipases has been shown to alter the binding characteristics of several neurotransmitter receptors and regulate receptor–effector coupling (for review, Schwartz et al., 1987). Exogenously applied phospholipase A$_2$ (PLA$_2$) enhances muscimol binding (Fujimoto and Okabayashi, 1983; Yoneda et al., 1985); and inhibits the binding of TBPS to GABA-associated Cl$^-$ channels in brain membranes (Havoundjian et al., 1986). Since PLA$_2$ inhibits both barbiturate- and muscimol-induced Cl$^-$ flux, uncoupling of the receptor/effector system is possible (Schwartz et al., 1987).

The major fatty acid generated by PLA$_2$ is arachidonic acid. Studies have shown that the effect of PLA$_2$ on GABA receptors is due to generation of arachidonic acid (and other unsaturated fatty acids) but not lysophospholipids or saturated fatty acids (Schwartz et al., 1987; Yoneda et al., 1985). Since unsaturated free fatty acids are highly susceptible to peroxidation, the generation of fatty acid peroxides might also regulate GABA receptor sensitivity. This is supported by evidence that generation of superoxide radicals inhibits GABA-mediated Cl$^-$ flux (Schwartz et al., 1987), and oxygen radical scavengers reverse the effects of arachidonic acid and PLA$_2$ on GABA receptors (Schwartz et al., 1987; Yoneda et al., 1985).

PLA$_2$ activation and arachidonic acid generation are hypothesized to be associated with brain hypoxia and ischemia (probably due to increased intracellular calcium levels) (Imaizumi et al., 1988). In addition, recent studies have shown that excitatory amino acids which are released during hypoxia/ischemia activate PLA$_2$ by increasing intracellular calcium, as discussed later (Dumuis et al., 1988). There is some evidence to suggest that the generation of fatty acids and their peroxides contributes to the increased neuronal excitability and seizure activity that often accompany hypoxic/ischemic neuronal damage (Bazan, 1970; Rodriquez de Turco et al., 1983; Willmore and Rubin, 1981; for review, Somjen, 1988).

D. Calcium

In addition to the activation of PLA$_2$, increases in intracellular calcium lead to activation of numerous biochemical processes. Among these are the activation of other enzymes such as protein kinases and protein phosphatases, which are known to regulate the sensitivity of several neurotransmitter receptor systems. Although early studies did not indicate that calcium was particularly important for regulating $GABA_A$ receptors, recent studies demonstrated that calcium reduces GABA-activated Cl⁻ conductance (Inoue et al., 1986; Schwartz and Mindlin, 1988). Like its action at nicotinic receptors, calcium may promote desensitization of the $GABA_A$ receptor with a resultant decrement in ion channel function (Schwartz and Mindlin, 1988). The loss in GABA receptor function associated with desensitization can lead to increased neuronal excitability and the development of seizures (Ben-Ari et al., 1979; Thalmann and Herskowitz, 1985).

Calcium can enter neurons through cation channels that are gated by excitatory amino acids such as glutamate (MacDermott and Dale, 1987). As with loss of GABA neurotransmission, activation of excitatory amino acid receptors produces neuronal excitation (MacDermott and Dale, 1987). As mentioned earlier, the spread of neuronal excitation occurs during or after hypoxic/ischemic damage to the CNS, when large amounts of excitotoxic amino acids are released and intracellular calcium levels rise (Somjen, 1988). In regions where $GABA_A$ and glutamate receptors (N-ethyl-D-aspartate sensitive) reside on the same cellular target, the glutamate-induced influx of calcium may also attenuate $GABA_A$ receptor sensitivity, adding to the neuronal hyperexcitability.

E. Cyclic Nucleotides

Various neurotransmitter- and voltage-gated ion channels are regulated by intracellular second messengers such as cyclic nucleotides (Huganir and Greengard, 1983; Rossie and Catterall, 1987). Regulation of ion channel function by cAMP or cGMP often involves phosphorylation of receptor and/or ion channel proteins (Huganir and Greengard, 1983; Rossie and Catterall, 1987). Analysis of the amino acid sequence of the $GABA_A$ receptor subunits suggests the presence of a cAMP-dependent phosphorylation site on the beta subunit (Schofield et al., 1987). More recently, phosphorylation of the beta subunit by cAMP-dependent protein kinase has been demonstrated (Kirkness et al., 1989). In support of the structural findings, functional studies have shown that cAMP analogs inhibit GABA-mediated Cl⁻ flux although the role of cAMP-dependent phosphorylation is still unknown (Heuschneider and Schwartz, 1989).

Several studies suggest a role of cyclic nucleotides in the pathophysiology of seizure disorders (Ferrendelli, 1986). Both electrically and chemically induced convulsions result in elevated cAMP levels in several brain regions (Ferrendelli et al., 1980; Sattin, 1971). Similarly, cAMP levels in cerebrospinal fluid have been reported to be elevated in patients up to three days following a seizure (Myllyla et al., 1975). Although Ferrendelli et al. (1980) suggest that the seizure-induced rise in cAMP levels may terminate seizure activity, several studies have demonstrated that cerebrocortical or intracerebral application of cAMP derivatives induces seizure activity (Gessa et al., 1970; Ludvig and Moshe, 1987; Purpura and Shofer, 1972). Whether the convulsant properties of cAMP are mediated (in part) by inhibition of GABAergic transmission is still to be determined.

F. Conclusions About Changes in GABA$_A$ Receptor Sensitivity

The endogenous substances described above all have the ability to modulate the function of the GABA$_A$ receptor and disrupt GABAergic neurotransmission. Any number of physiologic, pharmacologic, or environmental stimuli could trigger the release or accumulation of these substances which subsequently promote neuronal excitability. The ultimate central and peripheral consequences, such as convulsant or cardiac arrhythmic activity, respectively, depend on the specific brain region, pathway, or nucleus in which GABAergic transmission is interrupted.

III. MODULATION OF PRESYNAPTIC GABA RELEASE: POSSIBLE EXPLANATIONS FOR ARRHYTHMIAS AND/OR SUDDEN DEATH IN EPILEPTIC PERSONS

Suter and Lathers (1984), Kraras et al. (1987), and Lathers et al. (1988) have speculated on one possible mechanism that may be involved in the development of cardiac arrhythmias and/or sudden unexplained death in some epileptic patients (Figure 2). Prostaglandin E$_2$ (Suter and Lathers, 1984) or enkephalins (Frenk et al., 1978; Snead et al., 1983) injected into the central nervous system elicit seizure activity. PTZ increases PGE$_2$ or enkephalin levels in the central nervous system (Suter and Lathers, 1984; Vindrola et al., 1984). It has been suggested that these changes induced by PTZ within the central autonomic centers led to the production of epileptogenic activity and autonomic dysfunction in the experiments of Lathers and Schraeder (1982). The metenkephalins may act within the central nervous system by interfering with the K$^+$- and Ca^{2+}-dependent mechanisms of GABA release (Bixby and Spitzer, 1983; Brennan et al., 1980). Enkephalins may act on central opiate receptors to inhibit GABA release since the actions of these agents are blocked by opioid antagonists such as naloxone (Brennan et al., 1980; Laubie et al., 1977; Yukimura et al., 1981). This inhibition of the release of GABA is important since decreased GABA levels are thought to contribute to the initiation of epileptogenic activity (Krnjevic, 1980; Ribak et al., 1979).

Inhibition of GABA release in anesthetized cats also leads to increased sympathetic and parasympathetic neural outflow and the enhancement of central reflex-induced vagal bradycardia (DiMicco et al., 1979; Gillis et al., 1980). The resultant increased parasympathetic central outflow and enhancement of the

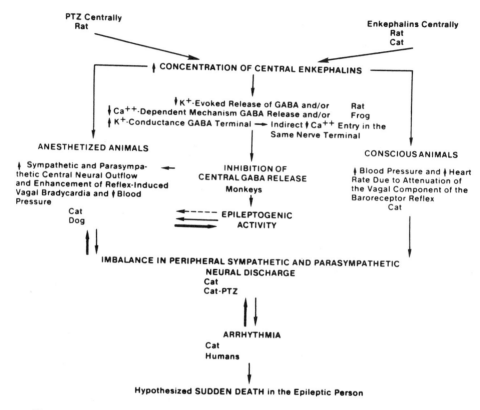

Figure 2 Hypothesized biochemical and autonomic mechanisms involved in the development of cardiac arrhythmias and/or sudden unexplained death in persons with epilepsy. [From Lathers et al. (1988), reproduced with permission.]

central reflex-induced vagal bradycardia via the enkephalin-induced inhibition of GABA release (Figure 2) may explain the fall in heart rate observed after the intracerebroventricular (i.c.v.) injection of (D-Ala^2) methionine-enkephalin-amide (DAME). The data of Gillis et al. (1980) suggested that an increase in blood pressure should occur in anesthetized cats. However, i.c.v. administration of DAME in the experiments of Lathers et al. (1988) and the injection of DAME into the cisterna magna in anesthetized dogs produced a fall in blood pressure (Laubie et al., 1977). Lathers et al. (1988) hypothesized that the unanticipated fall in blood pressure was due to the ability of the epileptogenic activity to produce autonomic dysfunction, as suggested by the studies of Lathers and Schraeder (1982) Schraeder and Lathers (1983) and indicated by the broken arrow in

Figure 2. The altered central parasympathetic and sympathetic neural outflow may induce an imbalance within each division as well as an imbalance between both peripheral autonomic divisions that innervate the heart, resulting in the production of arrhythmia (Lathers et al., 1977, 1978) and/or sudden unexplained death in the epileptic person (Carnel et al., 1985; Lathers et al., 1984; Schraeder and Lathers, 1983, 1989).

In alpha-chloralose anesthetized cats, the i.c.v. administration of DAME also produced a marked decrease in blood pressure with a decrease in heart rate occurring in most animals (Lathers et al., 1988). Schaz et al. (1980) reported a dose-dependent increase of blood pressure and heart rate after the administration of DAME in conscious cats. Yukimura et al. (1981) observed similar changes when they injected DAME i.c.v. into conscious cats. A maximal change in blood pressure occurred approximately 15 minutes before the greatest increase in heart rate. The experiments of Lathers et al. (1988) also showed a change in blood pressure followed approximately 20 minutes later by a change in heart rate. Since differences have been observed in the physiological effects of DAME, depending on whether a conscious or anesthetized preparation is used, one must question whether the presence of the anesthetic agent alpha-chloralose explains the differences found in the two different experimental models. Alpha-chloralose is a good anesthetic agent for neurological studies since many reflexes, including the baroreceptors, are present and, in fact, enhanced (Clifford and Soma, 1969). This anesthetic also causes minimal change in the amount of epinephrine present in the adrenal glands of cats and does not depress cardiac neural discharge (Clifford and Soma, 1969; Cox et al., 1936). These data inicate that the baroreceptor mechanism was intact in the anesthetized animals receiving alpha-chloralose and centrally administered DAME in the study of Lathers et al. (1988) and in the study of Laubie et al. (1977).

Epileptogenic activity occurred in conscious cats five minutes after the administration of DAME and ended before the changes in cardiovascular parameters had concluded (Schaz et al., 1980). In the experiments of Lathers et al. (1988), epileptogenic activity was also observed, although it began during the first several minutes after the administration of DAME and continued throughout the duration of the experiment. Since the epileptogenic activity began after the cardiovascular changes (Schaz et al., 1980), it was concluded that the epileptogenic activity was independent of the autonomic changes. However, there are studies that support the concept that autonomic cardiovascular changes may occur initially and be followed by the development of epileptogenic activity. Indeed, in the studies by Schott et al. (1977) and Schraeder et al. (1983), seizure activity in patients was abolished when cardiac arrhythmias were eliminated with the insertion of pacemakers or with the initiation of antiarrhythmic agents. The possibility that cardiac arrhythmias may result in the development of seizure activity via impaired peripheral cardiac neural discharge going back to the central nervous system is depicted in Figure 2 by the heavy arrows beginning with arrhythmia. In addition, other studies (Carnel et al., 1985; Lathers and Schraeder, 1982, 1987; Lathers et al., 1984; Schraeder and Lathers, 1983) found that epileptogenic activity may indeed lead to cardiovascular dysfunction in animals. These findings substantiate earlier observations made in humans. As early as 1941, Penfield and Erickson reported a patient with temporal lobe seizures and episodes of tachycardia. Additional studies by Mulder et al. (1954), Phizackerly et al. (1954), White et al. (1961), and Walsh et al. (1968) reported changes in the electrocardiogram in humans which were associated with epileptogenic activity. In summary, Figure 2 illustrates how epileptogenic activity may initiate an enhanced autonomic central neural outflow which impairs peripheral cardiac neural discharge and may then result in the production of arrhythmia. For further details of the proposed mechanism, see the recent reviews by Lathers and Schraeder (1987) and Schraeder and Lathers (1988).

IV. SUMMARY

In this chapter we presented two mechanisms for interference of GABA neurotransmission which might lead to initiation of arrhythmias or epileptogenic activity in epileptic persons. This chain of events may produce sudden death. It is possible that alterations at any of the other sites involved in GABA neurotransmission may also be important in the production of seizures and arrhythmias. Additional experiments in whole animals will be needed to ascertain which of these processes are predominantly responsible for the simultaneous initiation of epileptogenic and arrhythmic activity.

REFERENCES

Alho, H., Costa, E., Ferrero, P., Fujimoto, M., Cosenza-Murphy, D., and Guidotti, A. (1985). Diazepam-binding inhibitor: A neuropeptide located in selected neuronal populations of rat brain. *Science 229*:179–182.

Atkinson, R. M. (1965). Action of some steroids on the central nervous system of the mouse. *Pharmacol. Med. Chem. 8*:426–432.

Bazan, N. G., Jr. (1970). Effects of ischemia and electroconvulsive shock on free fatty acid pool in the brain. *Biochem. Biophys. Acta 218*:1–10.

Ben-Ari, Y., Krnjevic, K., and Reinhardt,W. (1979). Hippocampal seizures and failure of inhibition. *Can. J. Physiol. Pharmacol. 57*:1462–1466.

Bixby, J. L., and Spitzer, N. C. (1983). Enkephalin reduces quantal content at the frog neuromuscular junction. *Nature 301*:431–432.

Brennan, M. J. W., Cantrill, R. C., and Wylie, B. A. (1980). Modulation of synaptosomal GABA release by enkephalin. *Life Sci. 27*:1097–1101.

Carette, B., and Paulain, P. (1984). Excitatory effects of dehydroepiandrosterone, its sulfate and pregnenolone-sulfate, applied by iontophoresis and pressure on single neurones in the septo-optic area of guinea pig brain. *Neurosci. Lett.* 45:205-210.

Carnel, S. D., Schraeder, P. L., and Lathers, C. M. (1985). The effect of phenobarbital pretreatment on cardiac neural discharge and pentylenetetrazol-induced epileptogenic activity. *Pharmacology* 30:225-240.

Clifford, P. H., and Soma, L. R. (1969). Feline anesthesia. *Fed. Proc. 28*: 1479-1499.

Corpechot, C., Synguelakis, M., Tulna, S., Axelson, M., Sjoval, J., Vihco, R., Baulieu, E. E., and Robel, P. (1983). Pregnenolone and its sulfate in the rat brain. *Brain Res. 270*:119-125.

Cox, W. V., Lewiston, M. E., and Robertson, H. F. (1936). The effect of stellate ganglionectomy on the cardiac function of intact dogs (and its effect on the extent of myocardial infarction and on cardiac function following coronary artery occlusion). *Am. Heart J. 12*:285-300.

Dietrich, W. D., Lowry, O. H., and Loewy, A. D. (1982). The distribution of glutamate, GABA and aspartate in the nucleus tractus solitarius of the cat. *Brain Res. 237*:254-260.

DiMicco, J. A., Gale, K., Hamilton, B., and Gillis, R. A. (1979). GABA receptor control of parasympathetic outflow to the heart: Characterization and brainstem localization. *Science 204*:1106-1109.

Dumuis, A., Sebben, M., Haynes, L., Pin, J.-P., and Bockaert, J. (1988). NMDA receptors activate the arachidonic acid cascade system in striatal neurons. *Nature 336*:68-70.

Ferrendelli, J. A. (1986). Roles of biogenic amines and cyclic nucleotides in seizure mechanisms. *Adv. Neurol. 44*:393-400.

Ferrendelli, J. A., Blank, A. C., and Gross, R. A. (1980). Relationships between seizure activity and cyclic nucleotide levels in brain. *Brain Res. 200*:93-103.

Frenk, N., Urca, G., and Liebeskind, J. C. (1978). Epileptic properties of leucine- and methionine-enkephalin: Comparison with morphine and reversibility by naloxone. *Brain Res. 147*:327-337.

Fujimoto, J., and Okabayashi, T. (1983). Influence of phospholipase treatments on ligand bindings to a benzodiazepine receptor–GABA receptor–chloride ionophore complex. *Life Sci. 32*:2302-2400.

Gale, K., Hamilton, B. L., Brown, S. C., Norman, W. P., Souza, J. D., and Gillis, R. A. (1980). GABA and specific GABA binding sites in brain nuclei associated with vagal outflow. *Brain Res. Bull. (Suppl. 2)5*:325-338.

Gessa, G. L., Krishna, G., Forn, J., Tagliamonte, A., and Brodie, B. B. (1970). Behavioral and vegetative effects produced by dibutyryl cyclic AMP injected into different areas of the brain. *Adv. Biochem. Psychopharmacol. 3*: 371-381.

Gillis, R. A., DiMicco, J., Williford, D., Hamilton, B. L., and Gale, K. (1980). Importance of the CNS GABAergic mechanisms in the regulation of cardiovascular function. *Brain Res. Bull. (Suppl. 2)5*:303-315.

Gillis, R. A., Quest, J. A., and DiMicco, J. (1988). Central regulation of autonomic function by GABA receptors. in *GABA and Benzodiazepine Receptors*, Vol. 2, R. F. Squires (Ed.). CRC Press, Boca Raton, pp. 47–62.

Harrison, N. L., Majewska, M. D., Harrington, J. W., and Barker, J. L. (1987). Structure-activity relationships for steroid interaction with the α-aminobutyric acid$_A$ receptor complex. *J. Pharmacol. Exp. Ther. 241*:346–353.

Havoundjian, H., Cohen, R. M., Paul, S. M., and Skolnick, P. (1986). Differential sensitivity of "central" and "peripheral" type benzodiazepine receptors to phospholipase A_2. *J. Neurochem. 46*:804–811.

Heuschneider, G., and Schwartz, R. D. (1989). cAMP and forskolin decrease α-aminobutyric acid-gated chloride flux in rat brain synaptoneurosomes. *Proc. Nat. Acad. Sci. 86*:2938–2942.

Huganir, R. L., and Greengard, P. (1983). cAMP-dependent protein kinase phosphorylates the nicotinic acetylcholine receptor. *Proc. Nat. Acad. Sci. 80*: 1130–1134.

Iadarola, M., and Gale, K. (1981). Cellular compartments of GABA in brain and their relationship to anticonvulsant activity. *Mol. Cell. Biochem. 39*:305–330.

Imaizumi, S., Tominaga, T., Uenohara, H., Kinouchi, H., Yoshimoto, T., and Suzuki, J. (1988). In *Mechanisms of Cerebral Hypoxia and Stroke*, G. G. Somjen (Ed.). Plenum, New York, pp. 321–335.

Inoue, M., Oomura, Y., Yakushiji, T., and Akaike, H. (1986). Intracellular calcium ions decrease the affinity of the GABA receptor. *Nature 324*:156–158.

Keeler, J. R., Schults, C. W., Chase, T. N., and Helke, C. J. (1984). The ventral surface of the medulla in the rat: Pharmacologic and autoradiographic localization of GABA-induced cardiovascular effects. *Brain Res. 297*:217–224.

Killam, K. F., and Bain, J. A. (1957). Convulsant hydrazides. I. In vitro and in vivo inhibition by convulsant hydrazides of enzymes catalyzed by vitamin B_6. *J. Pharmacol. Exp. Ther. 119*:255–262.

Kirkness, E. F., Bovenkerk, C. F., Ueda, T., and Turner, A. J. (1989). Phosphorylation of α-aminobutyrate (GABA)/benzodiazepine receptors by cyclic AMP-dependent protein kinase. *Biochem. J. 259*:613–616.

Kraras, C. M., Tumer, N., and Lathers, C. M. (1987). The role of neuropeptides in the production of epileptogenic activity and autonomic dysfunction: Origin of arrhythmia and sudden death in the epileptic patient? *Med. Hypotheses 23*:19–31.

Krnjevic, K. (1980). Principles of synaptic transmission. In *Anti-Epileptic Drugs: Mechanisms of Action*, G. Glaser, J. Penry, and D. Woodbury (Eds.). Raven Press, New York, p. 127.

Kubo, T., and Kihara, M. (1987). Evidence for the presence of GABAergic and glycine-like systems responsible for cardiovascular control in the nucleus tractus solitarii of the rat. *Neurosci. Lett. 74*:331–336.

Lathers, C. M., and Schraeder, P. L. (1982). Autonomic dysfunction in epilepsy. Characterization of autonomic cardiac neural discharge associated with pentylenetetrazol-induced epileptogenic activity. *Epilepsia 23*:633–647.

Lathers. C. M., and Schraeder, P. L. (1987). Review of autonomic dysfunction cardiac arrhythmias, and epileptogenic activity. *J. Clin. Pharmacol. 27*:346-356.

Lathers, C. M., Roberts, J., and Kelliher, G. J. (1977). Correlation of ouabain-induced arrhythmia and nonuniformity in the histamine-evoked discharge of cardiac sympathetic nerves. *J. Pharmacol. Exp. Ther. 203*:467-479.

Lathers, C. M., Kelliher, G. J., Roberts, J., and Beasley, A. B. (1978). Nonuniform cardiac sympathetic nerve discharge: Mechanism for coronary occlusion and digitalis-induced arrhythmia. *Circulation 57*:1058-1065.

Lathers, C. M., Schraeder, P. L., and Carnel, S. B. (1984). Neural mechanisms in cardiac arrhythmias associated with epileptogenic activity: The effect of phenobarbital. *Life Sci. 34*:1919-1936.

Lathers, C. M., Tumer, N., and Kraras, C. M. (1988). The effect of intracerebroventricular D-Ala^2-methionine enkephalinamide and naloxone on cardiovascular parameters in the cat. *Life Sci. 43*:2287-2298.

Laubie, M., Schmitt, H., Vincent, M., and Remond, G. (1977). Central cardiovascular effects of morphinomimetic peptides in dogs. *Eur. J. Pharmacol. 46*:67-71.

Ludvig, N., and Moshe, S. L. (1987). Cyclic AMP derivatives injected into the inferior colliculus induce audiogenic seizure-like phenomena in normal rats. *Brain Res. 437*:193-196.

MacDermott, A. B., and Dale, N. (1987). Receptors, ion channels and synpatic potentials underlying the integrative actions of excitatory amino acids. *Trends Neurosci. 10*:280-283.

Machado, B. H., and Brody, M. J. (1988). Role of the nucleus ambiguus in the regulation of heart rate and arterial pressure. *Hypertension 11*:602-607.

Majewska, M. D. (1987). Steroids and brain activity. Essential dialogue between body and mind. *Biochem. Pharmacol. 36*:3781-3788.

Majewska, M. D., and Schwartz, R. D. (1987). Pregnenolone-sulfate: An endogenous antagonist of the α-aminobutyric acid receptor complex in brain? *Brain Res. 404*:355-360.

Majewska, M. D., Harrison, N. L., Schwartz, R. D., Barker, J. L., and Paul, S. M. (1986). Steroid hormone metabolites are barbiturate-like modulators of the GABA receptor. *Science 232*:1004-1007.

Maley, B., and Newton, B. W. (1985). Immunohistochemistry of α-aminobutyric acid in the cat nucleus tractus solitarius. *Brain Res. 330*:364-368.

McNamara, J. O., Bonhaus, D. W., Shin, C., Crain, B. J., Gellman, R. L., and Giacchino, J. L. (1987). The kindling model of epilepsy: A critical review. *CRC Crit. Rev. Neurobiol. 1*(4):341-389.

Meldrum, B. S. (1975). Epilepsy and gamma-aminobutyric acid-mediated inhibition. *Int. Rev. Neurobiol. 17*:1-36.

Morrow, A. L., Suzdak, P. D., and Paul, S. M. (1987). Steroid hormone metabolites potentiate GABA receptor-mediated chloride ion flux with nanomolar potency. *Eur. J. Pharmacol. 142*:483-485.

Mulder, D. W., Daly, D., and Bailey, A. A. (1954). Visceral epilepsy. *Arch. Intern. Med. 93*:481-493.

Myllyla, V. V., Heikkinen, E. R., Vapaatalo, H., and Hokkanen, E. (1975). Cyclic AMP concentration and enzyme activities of cerebrospinal fluid in patients with epilepsy or central nervous system damage. *Eur. Neurol.* *13*:123–130.

Novas, M. L., Wolfman, C. L., Medina, J. H., and De Robertis, E. (1988). Proconvulsant and "anxiogenic" effects of *n*-butyl-β-carboline-3-carboxylate, an endogenous benzodiazepine binding inhibitor. *Pharmacol. Biochem. Behav.* *30*:331–336.

Pena, C., Medina, J. H., Novas, M. L., Paladini, A. C., and De Robertis, E. (1986). Isolation and identification in bovine cerebral cortex of *n*-butyl-β-carboline-3-carboxylate, a potent benzodiazepine binding inhibitor. *Proc. Nat. Acad. Sci.* *83*:4952–4956.

Penfield, W., and Erickson, T. C. (1941). *Epilepsy and Cerebral Localization.* Springfield, Ill., Thomas, p. 111.

Phizackerly, P. J. R., Poole, E. W., and Whitty, C. W. M. (1954). Sinoauricular heart block as an epileptic manifestation: A case report. *Epilepsia 3*:89–91.

Purpura, D. P., and Shofer, R. J. (1972). Excitatory action of dibutyryl cyclic adenosine monophosphate on immature cerebral cortex. *Brain Res. 38*:179–181.

Rastogi, S. K., and Ticku, M. K. (1985). Involvement of a GABAergic mechanism in the anticonvulsant effect of pentobarbital against maximal electroshock-induced seizures in rats. *Pharmacol. Biochem. Behav. 22*:141–146.

Rastogi, S. K., and Ticku, M. K. (1986). Anticonvulsant profile of drugs which facilitate gabaergic transmission on convulsions mediated by a gabaergic mechanism. *Neuropharmacol. 25*:175–185.

Ribak, C. E., Harris, A. B., Vaughn, J. E., and Roberts, E. (1979). Inhibitory GABAergic nerve terminals decrease at sites of focal epilepsy. *Science 205*: 211–214.

Rodriguez de Turco, E. B., Morelli de Liberti, S., and Bazan, N. G. (1983). Stimulation of free fatty acid and diacylglycerol accumulation in cerebrum and cerebellum during bicuculline-induced status epilepticus. Effect of pretreatment with α-methyl-p-tyrosine and p-chlorophenyl alanine. *J. Neurochem. 40*:252–259.

Rossie, S., and Catterall, W. A. (1987). Cyclic AMP-dependent phosphorylation of voltage-sensitive sodium channels in primary cultures of rat brain neurons. *J. Biol. Chem. 262*:12735–12744.

Sangameswaran, L. and De Blas, A. L. (1985). Demonstration of benzodiazepine-like molecules in the mammalian brain with a monoclonal antibody to benzodiazepines. *Proc. Natl. Acad. Sci. USA 82*:5560–5564.

Sattin, A. (1971). Increase in the content of adenosine 3′, 5′-monophosphate in mouse forebrain during seizures and prevention of the increase by methylxanthines. *J. Neurochem. 18*:1087–1096.

Schaz, K., Stock, G., Simon, W., Schlor, K., Unger, T., Rockhold, R., and Ganten, D. (1980). Enkephalin effects on blood pressure, heart rate and baroreceptor reflex. *Hypertension 2*:395–407.

Schofield, P. R., Darlison, M. G., Fujita, N., Burt, D. R., Stephenson, F. A., Rodriquez, H., Rhee, L. M., Ramachandran, J., Reale, V., Glencourse, T. A., Seeburg, P. H., and Barnard, E. A. (1987). Sequence and functional expression of the GABA$_A$ receptor shows a ligand-gated receptor super-family. *Nature 328*:221–227.

Schott, G. C., McLeod, A. A., and Jewitt, D. E. (1977). Cardiac arrhythmias that masquerade as epilepsy. *Brit. Med. J. 1*:1454–1457.

Schraeder, P. L., and Lathers, C. M. (1983). Cardiac neural discharge and epileptogenic activity in the cat: An animal model for unexplained sudden death. *Life Sci. 32*:1371–1382.

Schraeder, P. L., and Lathers, C. M. (1989). Paroxysmal cardiovascular dysfunction and epileptogenic activity. *Epilepsy Res. 3*:55–62.

Schraeder, P. L., Pontzer, R., and Engel, T. R. (1983). A case of being scared to death. *Arch. Intern. Med. 143*:1793–1794.

Schwartz, R. D. (1988). The GABA$_A$ receptor-gated ion channel: Biochemical and pharmacological studies of structure and function. *Biochem. Pharmacol. 37*:3369–3375.

Schwartz, R. D., and Mindlin, M. C. (1988). Inhibition of the GABA receptor-gated chloride ion channel in brain by noncomparative inhibitors of the nicotinic receptor-gated cation channel. *Mol. Pharmacol. 244*:963–970.

Schwartz, R. D., Skolnick, P., and Saul, S. M. (1987). Regulation of α-aminobutyric acid/barbiturate receptor-gated chloride ion flux in brain vesicles by phospholipase A$_2$: Possible role of oxygen radicals. *J. Neurochem. 50*:565–571.

Segal, S. A., Jacob, T., and Gillis, R. A. (1984). Blockade of central nervous system GABAergic tone causes sympathetic-mediated increases in coronary vascular resistance in cats. *Circ. Res. 55*:404–415.

Siemers, E. R., Rea, M. A., Felton, D. L., and Aprison, M. H. (1972). Distribution and uptake of glycine, glutamate and α-aminobutyric acid in the vagal nuclei and eight other regions of the rat medulla oblongata. *Neurochem. Res. 7*:455–468.

Smith, S. S., Waterhouse, B. D., and Woodward, D. J. (1987). Locally applied progesterone metabolites alter neuronal responsiveness in the cerebellum. *Brain Res. Bull. 18*:739–747.

Snead, O. C. (1983). Seizures induced by carbachol, morphine, leucine-enkephalin: A comparison. *Ann. Neurol. 13*:445–451.

Somjen, G. G. (1988). Basic mechanisms in cerebral hypoxia and stroke. In *Mechanisms of Cerebral Hypoxia and Stroke*, G. G. Somjen (Ed.). Plenum, New York, pp. 447–466.

Suter, L., and Lathers, C. M. (1984). Modulation of presynaptic gamma aminobutyric acid release by prostaglandin E$_2$: Explanation for epileptogenic activity and dysfunction in autonomic cardiac neural discharge leading to arrhythmias. *Med. Hypotheses 15*:15–30.

Thalmann, R. H., and Herskowitz, N. (1985). Some factors that influence the decrement in the response to GABA during its continuous iontophoretic application to hippocampal neurons. *Brain Res. 342*:219–233.

Vindrola, O., Asai, M., Zubieta, M., Talavera, E., Rodriquez, R., and Linares, G. (1984). Pentylenetetrazol kindling produces a long lasting elevation of IR-met-enkephalin but not IR-leu-enkephalin in rat brain. *Brain Res. 297*: 121–125.

Walsh, G., Masland, W., and Goldensohn, E. (1968). Paroxysmal cerebral discharge associated with paroxysmal atrial tachycardia. *Electroencephalogr. Clin. Neurophysiol. 24*:187.

White, P. T., Grant, P., Mosier, J., and Craig, A. (1961). Changes in cerebral dynamics associated with seizures. *Neurology 11*:354–361.

Willmore, L. J., and Rubin, J. J. (1981). Antiperoxidant pretreatment and iron-induced epileptiform discharges in the rat: EEG and histopathologic studies. *Neurology 31*:63–69.

Yoneda, Y., Kuriyama, K., and Takahashi, M. (1985). Modulation of synaptic GABA receptor binding by membrane phospholipids: Possible role of active oxygen radicals. *Brain Res. 333*:111–122.

Yukimura, T., Stock, G., Stumpf, H., Unger, T., and Ganten, D. (1981). Effects of (D-Ala^2)-methionine-enkephalin in blood pressure, heart rate, and baroreceptor reflex sensitivity in conscious rats. *Hypertension 3*:528–532.

18

Role of Neuropeptides in the Production of Epileptogenic Activity and Arrhythmias

CLAIRE M. LATHERS* *The Medical College of Pennsylvania, Eastern Pennsylvania Psychiatric Institute, Philadelphia, Pennsylvania*

I. INTRODUCTION

Pentylenetetrazol (PTZ)-induced interictal and ictal epileptogenic activity associated with autonomic dysfunction—i.e., changes in autonomic cardiac neural discharge, mean arterial blood pressure, and heart rate and rhythm—has been reported in the cat (Lathers and Schraeder, 1982). If the autonomic dysfunction, including the development of arrhythmias, also occurs in humans, it may be a contributory factor to sudden unexplained death in the person with epilepsy. Elevation of immunoreactive (IR) met-enkephalin content in the septum, hypothalamus, amygdala, and hippocampus of rats occurs after PTZ-induced convulsions (Vindrola et al., 1984). This elevation may ultimately change central sympathetic neural discharge to the heart, resulting in the development of arrhythmias. Indeed, numerous reports indicate that neuropeptides may produce epileptic seizures (Elazor et al., 1979; Frenk et al., 1978). Resolution of the question of whether enkephalins elicit epileptogenic activity and autonomic dysfunction via an action to inhibit the release of GABA (Brennan et al., 1980; Snead and Bearden, 1980) is important, since an understanding of this mechanism should eventually allow the design of pharmacologic agents to prevent the epileptogenic activity and autonomic dysfunction.

A. PTZ-Induced Increased Concentrations of Central Enkephalins and Epileptogenic Activity

PTZ-induced kindling was associated with a longlasting elevation in brain content of immunoreactive IR met-enkephalin in the septum, hypothalamus, amy-

---

*Current affiliation: FDA, Rockville, Maryland.

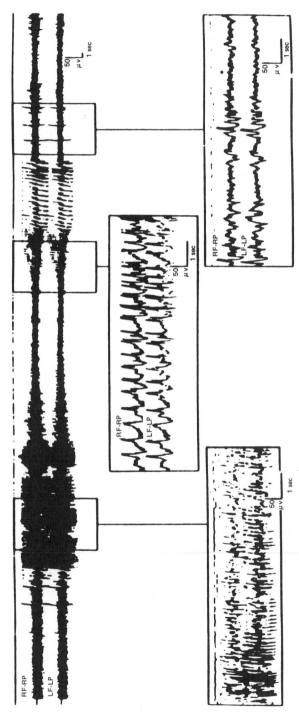

Figure 1 ECoG changes produced by 100 μg of leu-enkephalin injected i.c.v. The insets show a faster time trace. RF and RP = right frontal and parietal leads; LF and LP = left frontal and parietal leads. The rat was immobile during this paroxysmal electrical activity. The first change in the ECoG occurred within 1 minute of administration and was a paroxysm of spikes at a frequency of 7–9 Hz lasting 30–40 seconds. This tapered off to 2–3 Hz slow-wave activity, which was followed by 20–25 seconds of low-voltage fast activity. A few seconds of 1-Hz high-voltage slow-wave activity then built up to 25–30 seconds of low-voltage activity. Finally, a prolonged period of high-voltage single spikes occurred at a rate of 1 paroxysm/5 seconds. [From Snead and Bearden (1980), reproduced with permission.]

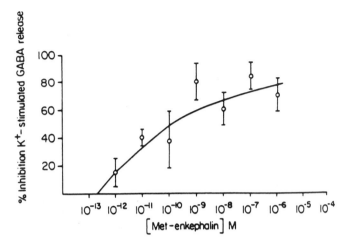

Figure 2 A dose–response curve for the inhibition of K^+ (55 mM)-induced GABA release by met-enkephalin. Each point is the mean percentage of inhibition ± S.D. (N = 5). Basal release of GABA was 7651 ± 980 dpm (N = 46). [From Brennan et al. (1980), reproduced with permission.]

gdala, and hippocampus of rats (Vindrola et al., 1984). Kindling was produced by the administration of intraperitoneal (i.p.) injections of 40 mg/kg PTZ every 24 hours for 10 days. The control group received an equivalent volume of saline on the same schedule. Every animal was observed for one hour after each injection for the appearance of convulsions. IR met-enkephalin was quantified in several brain areas 16 days after the last injection of PTZ in both the control and experimental groups. Additional rats received a PTZ dose on day 16 and were sacrificed 1 and 24 hours later. Brain tissue was prepared and enkephalin content was assayed by radioimmunoassay. A longlasting elevation in amygdala, septum, hypothalamus, and hippocampus IR met-enkephalin content occurred in animals subjected to kindling and sacrificed 16 days after the last dose of PTZ. A decrease in IR met-enkephalin occurred 1 hour after the PTZ-induced seizure but increased to newly elevated levels 24 hours later. Thus PTZ-induced kindling increased levels of enkephalins which were temporally related to the appearance of seizures.

B. Central Neuropeptide-Induced Epileptogenic Activity

In addition to the findings of increased brain concentrations of enkephalins after induction of seizures by PTZ, injection of these agents has been shown to elicit seizure activity. Specifically, the intracerebroventricular (i.c.v.) injection of leu-

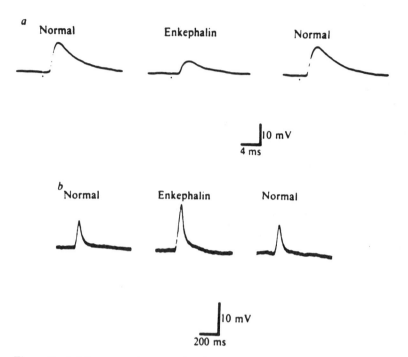

Figure 3 (a) Compound nerve stimulation with a suction electrode elicits an endplate potential that is reduced by focal puffer application of 20 μM met-enkephalin. Saline contained 0.8 mM Ca^{2+} and 8.0 mM Mg^{2+}. (b) Responses to iontophoretically applied acetylcholine; the amplitude of the response is increased by focal application of 20 μM met-enkephalin. Note that the response with enkephalin is longer as well as larger. [From Bixby and Spitzer (1983); reproduced with permission.]

enkephalin (Urca and Frenk, 1983) and hippocampal injection of leu-enkephalin (Elazor et al., 1979) induced seizures in rats and cats. Snead and Bearden (1980) also found that neuropeptides administered into the central nervous system induced epileptogenic activity in rats. Intraventricular leu-enkephalin produced a consistent dramatic paroxysmal electrical response within the first 60 seconds of administration (Figure 1), which persisted for up to 6 minutes. The enkephalin-induced paroxysms increased the 3- to 6-Hz band of the EEG spectrum. This indicated that enkephalin is directly involved in the production of epileptogenic activity (Snead and Bearden, 1980).

C. Enkephalin Modulation of GABA Release

Met-enkephalin inhibited K^+ depolarization-induced release of ^3H-GABA from rat synaptosomes in a dose-dependent fashion (Brennan et al., 1980). The concentration of met-enkephalin which inhibited 50% of the K^+-stimulated release was approximately 5×10^{-10} M (Figure 2). In every instance, the reduction of GABA release was prevented by naloxone, suggesting that met-enkephalin may interact with opiate receptors in order to modulate the release of GABA.

D. Met-Enkephalin Modulation of Acetylcholine Release

Met-enkephalin reversibly and specifically reduces the quantal content of acetylcholine release from peripheral nerve terminals in the frog cutaneous pectoris muscle by blocking voltage-dependent Ca^+ channels (Bixby and Spitzer, 1983). It is likely that met-enkephalin also blocks the release of Ca^{2+}-dependent neurotransmitters, such as GABA, from central synapses. Bixby and Spitzer applied met-enkephalin (10-30 μM) by pressure ejection through a "puffer" pipette to the presynaptic terminals of frog neuromuscular junctions before compound nerve stimulation with a suction electrode. Met-enkephalin was also applied in the presence of 15 μM naloxone. Application of saline to the presynaptic terminals before stimulation served as a control. Finally, puffer application of enkephalin was employed on the postsynaptic membrane, followed by both iontophoretic application of acetylcholine and nerve stimulation. Application of met-enkephalin to the presynaptic membrane led to a consistent decrease in the size of the evoked response (Figure 3a). The decrease, which averaged 40%, was not seen when met-enkephalin was applied in the presence of 15 μM naloxone or when normal saline substituted for enkephalin. In addition, met-enkephalin not only did not reduce but slightly increased the size of response to iontophoretically applied acetylcholine on the postsynaptic membrane (Figure 3b). Thus the opiate appear to be exerting its effect presynaptically, possibly by blocking the Ca^{2+} channels. When these channels are blocked there is decreased release of acetylcholine from nerve terminals in the frog cutaneous pectoris muscle (Bixby and Spitzer, 1983). GABA release in the central nervous system has been reported to be Ca^{2+}-dependent (DeBelleroche and Bradford, 1972). Therefore, met-enkephalin may be able to inhibit GABA release in the central nervous system by preventing Ca^{2+} influx into the presynaptic nerve terminal in a manner similar to that by which met-enkephalin reduces the presynaptic release of acetylcholine.

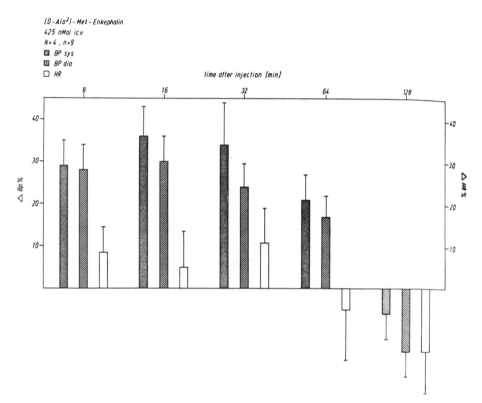

Figure 4   Changes in blood pressure and heart rate (given as percent change of the corresponding control values) elicited by i.c.v. injection of DAME, 425 nmol, in freely moving cats. Data are expressed as means ±SEM and have been obtained at different time intervals following the injections of (D-Ala^2)met-enk. Nine experiments were performed in four cats. In control experiments, using i.c.v. injections of the same volumes of 0.9% NaCl, changes in arterial blood pressure did not exceed 5–10 mm Hg. Pretreatment values of blood pressure and heart rate were 92 ± 3 mm Hg and 145 ± 3 bpm, respectively. [From Schaz et al. (1980), reproduced with permission.]

II. CENTRAL CARDIOVASCULAR AND NEUROLOGICAL EFFECTS OF ENKEPHALINS

A. Action on Mean Arterial Blood Pressure, Heart Rate, and Brain Electrical Activity in Conscious Cats

The administration of neuropeptides elicits cardiovascular changes as well as epileptogenic activity in conscious male cats (Schaz et al., 1980). After i.c.v. application of [(D-Ala^2) methionine-enkephalinamide (DAME)] at a dose of 425 nmol in the cat, arterial systolic and diastolic blood pressures increased, suggesting that (D-Ala^2)met-enk may produce a centrally mediated vasopressor response (Figure 4). A small increase in heart rate occurred. The maximal cardiovascular response was seen 16 minutes after i.c.v. injection and was attenuated after 64 minutes. A 170-nmol dose of DAME had no effect on blood pressure and heart rate. A dose of 850 nmol increased arterial pressure and produced catatonia-like behavior during the first 30 minutes; this was followed by an excitatory behavior that lasted up to 2 hours. Spike-wave complexes occurred within the amygdala and hippocampus after 850 nmol. The time course of electrical activity changes did not exactly follow the hemodynamic changes (Figure 5). Spike-wave complexes appeared 5 minutes after the changes in hemodynamic parameters and lasted only 40 minutes (Schaz et al., 1980).

Yukimura et al. (1981) studied the i.c.v. injection of 5, 10, 25, 50, and 100 nmol DAME in cats. In additional experiments, 500 nmol of naloxone was injected i.c.v. three minutes before DAME to test the effects of the opioid antagonist on enkephalin action. DAME induced dose-dependent increases in systolic blood pressure and heart rate. Doses of 50 nmol or less produced a maximal increase in blood pressure within 15 minutes; heart rate did not reach maximum until 30 minutes. For more than two hours after 50 and 100 nmol of DAME, sharp waves were seen in the hippocampus recording; theta activity was attenuated. Seizures were not observed. Naloxone given prior to the injection of 25 nmol of DAME blocked all cardiovascular responses (Table 1). A 50-nmol dose blocked only the blood pressure responses; the heart rate increases and baroreceptor reflex attenuations were unaltered. The baroreceptor reflex was attenuated for 15–60 minutes after DAME; higher doses were effective for a longer time (Table 1). Naloxone administered prior to enkephalin injection produced no changes in central electrical activity. It was concluded that enkephalins may play a role in central mechanisms of cardiovascular control by interacting with opiate receptors in the brain (Yukimura et al., 1981).

B. Action on Mean Arterial Blood Pressure, Heart Rate, and Brain Electrical Activity in Anesthetized Animals

The injection of DAME into the cisterna magna of anesthetized dogs induced a short period of moderate hypertension followed by a marked and prolonged

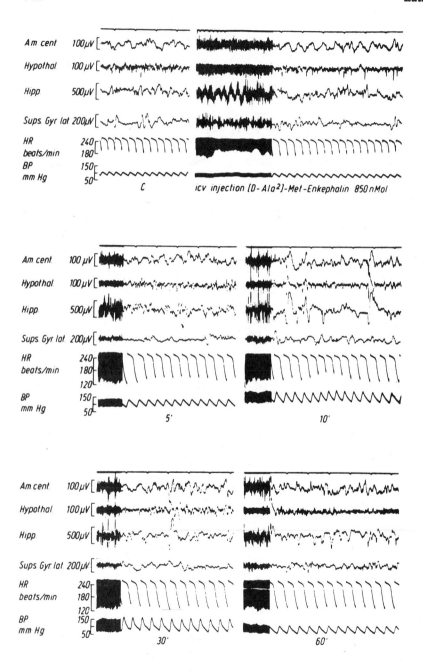

decrease in blood pressure, heart rate, and splanchnic nerve discharge (Laubie et al., 1977). Intravenous naloxone produced a transient increase in all three parameters and antagonism of DAME, which was extended by a subsequent injection of naloxone (Figure 6). It was concluded that the opioid peptides may be involved in central cardiovascular control. The i.c.v. injection of DAME (500 μg/kg) has been shown to produce hypotension, bradycardia, and seizure activity when administered to anesthetized cats (Kraras et al., 1987; Lathers et al., 1988). In general, i.v. naloxone (100 μg/kg) reversed the effects of DAME on blood pressure and heart rate while eliminating seizure activity.

Figure 7 illustrates the effect of DAME in one cat. Although the mean arterial blood pressure fell from the control value of 108 mm Hg to 93 mm Hg, the heart rate increased to 132 bpm 18 minutes after the administration of DAME compared to the control interval rate of 108 bpm (Figure 7B). The subsequent administration of 100 μg/kg i.v. naloxone to this cat then decreased the heart rate elevated by the administration of DAME; a further decrease in blood pressure occurred after naloxone. The epileptogenic activity induced by DAME was decreased but not abolished by naloxone (Figure 7C).

DAME also produced brief ictal activity beginning several minutes postadministration in most cats. Brief ictal activity consists of repetitive bilateral bursts of polyspike activity, each lasting less than 10 seconds, interspersed with brief periods of depression of cerebral activity. Administration of naloxone (100 μg/kg, i.v.) eliminated brief ictal activity in some cats within four minutes of its administration, whereas in other cats the seizure activity was somewhat depressed although still present. DAME-induced depression of heart rate and blood pressure was generally reversed by naloxone.

Figure 5 Recordings of the electrical activity of the central amygdala (Am. cent.); hypothalamus (Hypothal.); hippocampus (Hipp.); and lateral suprasylvian gyrus (Subs. Gyr. lat.); of heart rate (HR), instantaneously recorded as intervals between two heartbeats; and of arterial blood pressure (BP) before, immediately after, and 5, 10, 30, and 60 minutes after i.c.v. injection of (D-Ala^2)met-enk 850 nmol, in a freely moving cat. The paper speed can be seen by the continuous marks on the top of each panel: each point represents 1 second. Five minutes (5′) after application of the peptide, there is an increase in arterial pressure by approximately 20 mm Hg. At 10′, arterial pressure is markedly increased by 30 mm Hg, and in the subcortical recordings, there are hypersynchronous waves and spike–wave complexes. At 60 minutes after i.c.v. application of (D-Ala^2) met-enk, electrical recordings are not different from the control period: however, arterial blood pressure is still elevated by 35 mm Hg. [From Schaz et al. (1980), reproduced with permission.]

Table 1 Effects of DAME on Blood Pressure, Heart Rate, and Baroreceptor Reflex Sensitivity in Conscious Cats[a]

Treatment	Control	15 min	30 min	60 min	120 min
Systolic blood pressure (mm Hg)					
25 nmol DAME	133 ± 8	154 ± 14*	149 ± 13	144 ± 11	134 ± 13
naloxone + 25 nmol DAME	133 ± 11	124 ± 17	133 ± 18	118 ± 14	125 ± 18
50 nmol DAME	143 ± 9	168 ± 15*	163 ± 12	148 ± 11	129 ± 7
naloxone + 50 nmol DAME	136 ± 9	150 ± 10	153 ± 9	148 ± 21	146 ± 25
Heart rate (bpm)					
25 nmol DAME	154 ± 12	182 ± 12*	188 ± 13*	164 ± 10	146 ± 12
naloxone + 25 nmol DAME	149 ± 24	164 ± 21	158 ± 20	158 ± 27	172 ± 23
50 nmol DAME	147 ± 6	166 ± 8*	193 ± 9*	160 ± 9	142 ± 6
naloxone + 50 nmol DAME	144 ± 5	193 ± 29*	180 ± 20*	146 ± 9	149 ± 10

[a]Data are expressed as means ± SEM.

$*p < 0.05$.

Source: Yukimura et al. (1981), reproduced with permission.

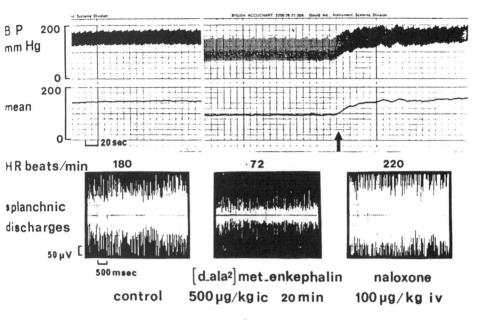

Figure 6 The inhibitory effect of (D-Ala^2)met-enk (500 μg/kg) injected into the cisterna magna on blood pressure, heart rate, and splanchnic neural discharges on a dog anesthetized with alpha-chloralose and the reversal produced by naloxone (100 μg/kg i.v.). [From Laubie et al. (1977), reproduced with permission.]

III. DISCUSSION

In the studies of Lathers and Schraeder (1982; Schraeder and Lathers, 1983), in the control period, the mean heart rate increased with a decrease in the mean arterial blood pressure in anesthetized cats. This relationship did not always occur with the development of epileptogenic activity induced by the intravenous administration of PTZ. The autonomic cardiac nerves did not always respond in a predictable manner to changes in blood pressure after the development of epileptogenic activity. In contrast, during the control period, all postganglionic cardiac sympathetic nerves exhibited an increased discharge as blood pressure fell following the administration of a vasodilating test dose of histamine. Discharge in the parasympathetic cardiac nerves followed the changes in the mean arterial blood pressure. These relationships of cardiac neural discharges (sympathetic and parasympathetic) to blood pressure changes represent the normal physiological function (Bronk et al., 1936). With the development of interictal activity, the variability of mean neural discharge for the parasympathetic nerves began to

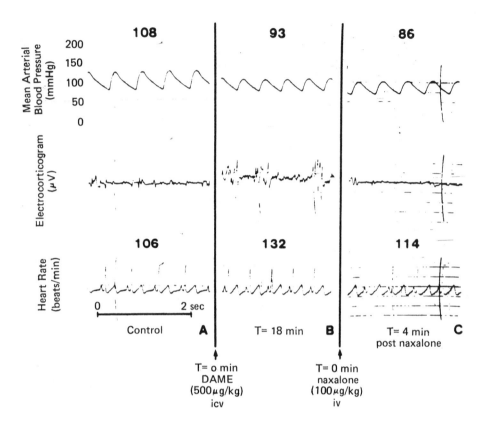

Figure 7 Brief ictal activity produced by DAME and eliminated by naloxone in cats anesthetized with alpha-chloralose. Heart rate and blood pressure changes are also shown. [From Kraras et al. (1987), reproduced with permission.]

increase, as demonstrated by an increase in the standard deviation. With greater degrees of epileptogenic activity, the standard deviation continued to increase; that is, the variability in the discharge among the parasympathetic nerves monitored became larger. A neural variability, again evidenced by a large standard deviation, also occurred in the mean postganglionic cardiac sympathetic discharge. The variability observed for the mean sympathetic discharge developed subsequent to that occurring in the parasympathetic discharge. Thus autonomic cardiac neural dysfunction was observed within both divisions of the autonomic cardiac nervous systems and between the two divisions. The altered cardiac neural discharge was associated with minimal epileptogenic activity (i.e., interictal discharges) and the development of cardiac arrhythmias. The proposed mecha-

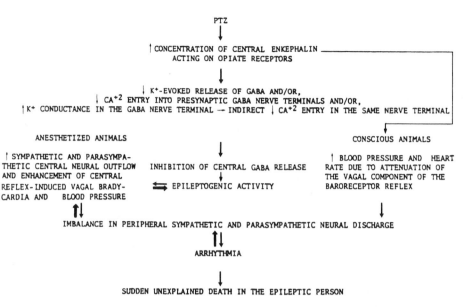

Figure 8 Postulated mechanism by which central enkephalins could antagonize GABA, resulting in autonomic dysfunction, epileptogenic activity, and sudden death. [From Kraras et al. (1987), reproduced with permission.]

nisms involved in the development of these arrhythmias and the possible role of enkephalins in the induction of sudden unexplained death in some epileptic patients are summarized in Figure 8 and are discussed below.

The injection of enkephalins into the central nervous system elicits seizure activity (Frenk et al., 1978; Snead, 1983). Intraperitoneal administration of PTZ produced increases in enkephalin content of the amygdala, striatum, and septum (Vindrola et al., 1983). An increase in the level of enkephalin in the amygdala may have initiated seizure activity since the amygdala is extensively interconnected with the hypothalamus; indeed, it is considered to have a higher order modulating influence on the hypothalamus. Furthermore, almost any visceral or somatic activity, including cardiovascular and respiratory changes, elicited by stimulating the amygdala can also be elicited by stimulating various areas within the hypothalamus (Nolte, 1981). Seizure activity originating in the amygdala may have induced changes in the discharge to the hypothalamus; disturbances in hypothalamic function may result in autonomic dysfunction. PTZ (i.p.) has also been shown to induce an increase in enkephalin levels within the hypothalamus (Vindrola et al., 1984). Since the hypothalamus contains autonomic centers, it may be that the PTZ-induced increases in central enkephalin levels led to the production of epileptogenic activity and autonomic dysfunction in the experiments of Lathers and Schraeder (1982).

A central mechanism by which increased concentrations of enkephalins inhibit K^+-dependent GABA release may exist, since met-enkephalin has been shown to inhibit the release of GABA from rat brain synaptosomes (Brennan et al., 1980). There is also evidence suggesting that increased concentrations of enkephalins directly decrease the entry of Ca^{2+} into the presynaptic GABA nerve terminals (Bixby and Spitzer, 1983). Met-enkephalin reduced the amount of acetylcholine released at the frog neuromuscular junction, most likely by blocking voltage-dependent Ca^{2+} channels in the presynaptic terminal. However, it is also possible that enkephalin reduced Ca^{2+} entry indirectly, by increasing K^+ conductance in the terminal. Nevertheless, it may be that met-enkephalin acts within the central nervous system by interfering with the K^+- and/or Ca^{2+}-dependent mechanism of GABA release (Figure 8). Decreased GABA levels are thought to initiate epileptogenic activity (Krnjevic, 1980; Ribak et al., 1979).

Enkephalins may inhibit the release of GABA by acting on central opiate receptors. Inhibition of GABA release by met-enkephalin was prevented by administration of naloxone (Brennan et al., 1980). Pretreatment with i.c.v. naloxone also prevented DAME from inducing changes in blood pressure and heart rate as well as producing seizure activity in conscious cats (Yukimura et al., 1981). Administration of i.v. naloxone after DAME reversed the effects of DAME on heart rate and blood pressure (Laubie et al., 1977). Naloxone (i.v.) had the same action on heart rate and blood pressure and either eliminated or depressed DAME-induced seizure activity in anesthetized cats in the experiments of Kraras et al. (1987) and Lathers et al. (1988). Thus it may be that enkephalins act on central opiate receptors to inhibit GABA release since the actions of these agents are blocked by opioid antagonists such as naloxone.

Inhibition of GABA release in anesthetized cats produces increased sympathetic and parasympathetic neural outflow and the enhancement of central reflex–induced vagal bradycardia (DiMicco et al., 1979; Gillis et al., 1980). The resultant increased parasympathetic central outflow and enhancement of central reflex–induced vagal bradycardia via the enkephalin-induced inhibition of GABA release, as depicted in Figure 8, may explain the decrease in heart rate observed after the i.c.v. injection of DAME in the experiments of Kraras et al. (1987) and Lathers et al. (1988). The data of Gillis et al. (1980) suggested that an increase in blood pressure should occur in anesthetized cats after removal of the tonically active GABAergic system present in the brain. However, the i.c.v. injection of DAME in our experiments and the injection of DAME into the cisterna magna in anesthetized dogs (Laubie et al., 1977) to inhibit the release of GABA produced hypotension. We hypothesize that the unanticipated fall in blood pressure is due to the ability of the epileptogenic activity to produce autonomic dysfunction, as suggested by the studies of Lathers and Schraeder (1982; Schraeder and Lathers, 1983) and as indicated by the broken arrow in Figure 8. Altered central parasympathetic and sympathetic neural outflow may induce an imbalance within each division as well as an imbalance between both peripheral autonomic divisions that innervate the heart. This imbalance may result in the production of arrhythmia (Laters et al., 1977, 1978) and/or sudden unexplained death (Carnel et al., 1985; Lathers and Schraeder, 1982, 1987; Lathers et al., 1984, 1988; Suter and Lathers, 1984).

The cardiovascular effects of enkephalins in the central nervous system vary in a dose-dependent manner and according to the state of the animal, that is, conscious vs. anesthetized. Met-enkephalin had no effect after i.c.v. injection in dogs anesthetized with alpha-chloralose; met-enkephalin has a half-life of several seconds and the lack of a visible effect may be due to its rapid inactivation. However, DAME, a synthetic analogue of met-enkephalin that is metabolically more stable than the natural peptide, produced prolonged hypotension and bradycardia in alpha-chloralose–anesthetized dogs when injected into the cisterna magna (Laubie et al., 1977). In alpha-chloralose–anesthetized cats, the i.c.v. administration of DAME also produced a marked decrease in blood pressure with a decrease in heart rate occurring in most animals (Kraras et al., 1987; Lathers et al., 1988). In contrast, a dose-dependent increase of blood pressure and heart rate was induced by administration of (D-Ala^2)met-enk in conscious cats (Schaz et al., 1980). Similar changes were reported by Yukimura et al. (1981) when they injected DAME i.c.v. into conscious cats. Maximal increases in blood pressure occurred approximately 15 minutes before the greatest increase in heart rate. Blood pressure increased 20 minutes before the increase in heart rate occurred (Kraras et al., 1987; Lathers et al., 1988).

The observation of differences in the physiological effects of DAME, depending on whether a conscious or anesthetized preparation is used, raises the question of whether the presence of the anesthetic agent alpha-chloralose explains the differences found in the two experimental models. Alpha-chloralose has been shown to be a good anesthetic agent for neurological studies since many reflexes, including the baroreceptors, are present and, in fact, enhanced (Clifford and Soma, 1969). This anesthetic also causes minimal change in the amount of epinephrine present in the adrenal glands of cats and does not depress cardiac renal discharge (Clifford and Soma, 1969; Cox et al., 1936). These data indicate that the baroreceptor mechanism was intact in the anesthetized animals receiving alpha-chloralose and centrally administered DAME in the studies of Kraras et al. (1987), Lathers et al. (1988), and Laubie et al. (1977).

The occurrence of epileptogenic activity in conscious cats began five minutes after the administration of (D-Ala^2)met-enk and ended before the changes in cardiovascular parameters (Schaz et al., 1980). Epileptogenic activity was also observed in anesthetized cats to which DAME was administered (Kraras et al., 1987; Lathers et al., 1988), although it began during the first several minutes after the administration of DAME and continued throughout the duration of the experiments. Since the epileptogenic activity began after the cardiovascular changes in experiments of Schaz et al. (1980), they concluded that the epileptogenic activity was independent of the autonomic changes. However, there are studies that support the concept that autonomic cardiovascular changes may occur initially and be followed by the development of seizure activity. Indeed, seizure activity in patients was abolished when cardiac arrhythmias were eliminated with the insertion of pacemakers or with the initiation of antiarrhythmic agents (Schott et al., 1977). The possibility that cardiac arrhythmias may result in the development of seizure activity via impaired peripheral cardiac neural discharge going back to the central nervous system is depicted in Figure 8 by the heavy arrows beginning with arrhythmia. In addition, the studies of Lathers and Schraeder (1982) and Schraeder and Lathers (1983) found that epileptogenic activity may lead to cardiovascular dysfunction in animals and substantiate earlier observations made in humans. As early as 1941, Penfield and Erickson reported a patient with temporal lobe seizures and episodes of tachycardia. Additional studies by Mulder et al. (1954), Phizackerly et al. (1954), White et al. (1961), and Walsh et al. (1968) reported changes in the electrocardiogram in humans which were associated with epileptogenic activity. Thus Figure 8 illustrates how epileptogenic activity may initiate an enhanced autonomic central neural outflow which impairs peripheral cardiac neural discharge and results in the production of arrhythmia.

Further experiments are needed to determine whether enkephalins elicit epileptogenic activity and autonomic dysfunction in both conscious and anesthetized animal preparations. It will be important to determine whether enkephalins impair autonomic dysfunction via an inhibition of the release of GABA from the nerve terminal since delineation of this mechanism will allow the design of experiments to evaluate the ability of pharmacologic agents to prevent the enkephalin-induced epileptogenic activity and autonomic dysfunction. Suppression of progression to cardiac arrhythmias induced by the autonomic dysfunction should ultimately decrease the incidence of sudden unexplained death in the epileptic patient.

IV. SUMMARY

Autonomic dysfunction, including arrhythmias, is often associated with epileptogenic activity. This study examines the potential role for enkephalins in this process. Brennan et al. (1980) reported a greater percentage of inhibition of K^+-stimulated GABA release with increasing concentrations of met-enkephalin. Snead and Bearden (1980) found that leu-enkephalin in the central nervous system may induce epileptogenic activity. In addition, DAME has been shown to produce a centrally mediated vasopressor response as well as attenuation of the baroreceptor reflex in conscious cats (Schaz et al., 1980) possibly leading to autonomic imbalance. The latter may precipitate arrhythmias and be a contributor to sudden unexplained death in the epilepsy. Resolution of the question of whether enkephalins elicit epileptogenic activity and autonomic dysfunction via inhibition of GABA release is important since an understanding of this mechanism should eventually allow the design of pharmacologic agents to prevent the epileptogenic activity, autonomic dysfunction, and associated sudden death.

REFERENCES

Bixby, L., and Spitzer, C. (1983). Enkephalin reduces quantal content at the frog neuromuscular junction. *Nature 301*:431–432.

Brennan, M., Cantrill, R. C., and Wylie, B. A. (1980). Modulation of synaptosomal GABA release by enkephalin. *Life Sci. 27*:1097–1101.

Bronk, D. W., Ferguson, R., and Margaria, R. (1936). The activity of the cardiac sympathetic center. *Am. J. Physiol. 117*:237–249.

Carnel, S. B., Schraeder, P. L., and Lathers, C. M. (1985). The effect of phenobarbital pretreatment on cardiac neural discharge and pentylenetetrazol-induced epileptogenic activity. *Pharmacology 30*:225–240.

Clifford, D. H., and Soma, L. R. (1969). Feline anesthesia. *Fed. Proc. 28*:1479–1499.

Cox, W. V., Lewiston, M. E., and Robertson, H. F. (1936). The effect of stellate ganglionectomy on the cardiac function of intact dogs (and its effect on the extent of myocardial infarction and on cardiac function following coronary artery occlusion). *Am. Heart J. 12*:285–300.

DeBelleroche, J., and Bradford, J. (1972). Metabolism of beds of mammalian cortical synaptosomes: Response to depolarizing influences. *J. Neurochem. 19*:585–602.

DiMicco, J., Gale, K., Hamilton, B. L., and Gillis, R. A. (1979). GABA receptor control of parasympathetic outflow to heart: Characterization and brainstem localization. *Science 204*:1106–1109.

Elazor, F., Motles, E., Elv, Y., and Simantov, R. (1979). Acute tolerance to the excitatory effect of enkephalin microinjections into hippocampus. *Life Sci. 24*:541–548.

Frenk, H., Urca, G., and Leibeskind, J. C. (1978). Epileptic properties of leucine- and methionine-enkephalin: Comparison with morphine and reversibility by naloxone. *Brain Res. 147*:327–337.

Gillis, R. A., DiMicco, J., Williford, D., Hamilton, B. L., and Gale, K. (1980). Importance of the CNS GABAergic mechanisms in the regulation of cardiovascular function. *Brain Res. Bull. (Suppl. 2) 5*:303–315.

Kraras, C. M., Tumer, N., and Lathers, C. M. (1987). The role of neuropeptides in the production of epileptogenic activity and autonomic dysfunction:

Origin of arrhythmias and sudden death in the epileptic patient? *Med. Hypothesis* 23:19–31.

Krnjevic, K. (1980). Principles of synaptic transmission. In *Advances in Neurology*, Vol. 27, *Antiepileptic drugs: Mechanisms of action*, G. Glaser, J. Penry, and D. Woodbury (eds.). Raven Press, New York, p.127.

Lathers, C. M., and Schraeder, P. L. (1982). Autonomic dysfunction in epilepsy: Characterization of autonomic cardiac neural discharge associated with pentylenetetrazol-induced epileptogenic activity. *Epilepsia* 27:633–647.

Lathers, C. M., and Schraeder, P. L. (1987). Review of autonomic dysfunction, cardiac arrhythmias, and epileptogenic activity. *J. Clin. Pharmacol.* 27:346–356.

Lathers, C. M., Roberts, J., and Kelliher, G. J. (1977). Correlation of ouabain-induced arrhythmia and nonuniformity in the histamine-evoked discharge of cardiac sympathetic nerves. *J. Pharmacol. Exp. Ther.* 203:467–479.

Lathers, C. M., Kelliher, G. J., Roberts, J., and Beasley, A. B. (1978). Nonuniform cardiac sympathetic nerve discharge: Mechanism for coronary occlusion and digitalis-induced arrhythmias. *Circulation* 57:1058–1065.

Lathers, C. M., Schraeder, P. L., and Carnel, S. B. (1984). Neural mechanisms in cardiac arrhythmias associated with epileptogenic activity: The effect of phenobarbital. *Life Sci.* 34:1919–1936.

Lathers, C. M., Tumer, N., and Kraras, C. M. (1988). The effect of intracerebroventricular D-Ala^2 methionine enkephalinamide and naloxone on cardiovascular parameters in the cat. *Life Sci.* 43:2287–2298.

Laubie, M., Schmitt, H., Vincent, M., and Remond, G. (1977). Central cardiovascular effects of morphinomimetic peptides in dogs. *Eur. J. Pharmacol.* 46: 67–71.

Mulder, D. W., Daly, D., and Bailey, A. A. (1954). Visceral epilepsy. *Arch. Intern. Med.* 93:481–493.

Nolte, J. (1981). Olfactory and limbic systems. In *The Human Brain: An Introduction to Its Functional Anatomy*, J. Lotz (Ed.). C. V. Mosby, St. Louis, p. 304.

Penfield, W., and Erickson, I. C. (1941). *Epilepsy and Cerebral Localization*. Thomas, Springfield, Ill., pp. 320–362.

Phizackerly, P. J. R., Poole, E. W., and Whitty, C. W. M. (1954). Sinoauricular heart block as an epileptic manifestation: A case report. *Epilepsia* 3:89–91.

Ribak, C. E., Harris, A. B., Vaughn, J. E., and Roberts, E. (1979). Inhibitory GABAergic nerve terminals decrease at sites of focal epilepsy. *Science* 205: 211–214.

Schaz, K., Stock, G., Simon, W., Schlor, K., Unger, T., Rockhold, R., and Ganten, D. (1980). Enkephalin effects on blood pressure, heart rate and baroreceptor reflex. *Hypertension* 2(4):395–407.

Schott, G. D., McLeod, A. A., and Jewitt, D. E. (1977). Cardiac arrhythmias that masquerade as epilepsy. *Br. Med. J.* 1:1454–1457.

Schraeder, P. L., and Lathers, C. M. (1983). Cardiac neural discharge and epileptogenic activity in the cat: An animal model for unexplained death. *Life Sci.* 32:1371–1382.

Schraeder, P. L., and Lathers, C. M. (1989). Paroxysmal cardiovascular dysfunction and epileptogenic activity. *Epilepsy Res. 3*:55–62.

Snead, O. C. (1983). Seizures induced by carbachol, morphine, leucine-enkephalin: A comparison. *Ann. Neurol. 13*:445–451.

Snead, O. C., and Bearden, L. J. (1980). Anticonvulsants specific for petit mal antagonist epileptogenic effect of leucine enkephalin. *Science 210*:1031–1033.

Suter, L. E., and Lathers, C. M. (1984). Modulation of presynaptic gamma aminobutyric acid release by prostaglandin E_2 : Explanation for epileptogenic activity and dysfunction in autonomic cardiac neural discharge leading to arrhythmias? *Med. Hypothesis 15*:15–30.

Urca, G., and Frenk, H. (1983). Intracerebral opiates block the epileptic effect of intracerebroventricular (I.C.V.) leucine-enkephalin. *Brain Res. 259*:103–110.

Vindrola, O., Asai, M., Zubieta, M., and Linares, G. (1983). Brain content of immunoreactive (leu[5])enkephalin and (met[5])enkephalin after pentylenetetrazol-induced convulsions. *Eur. J. Pharmacol. 90*:85–89.

Vindrola, O., Asai, M., Zubieta, M., Talavera, E., Rodriquez, R., and Linares, G. (1984). Pentylenetetrazol kindling produces a long lasting elevation of IR-met-enkephalin but not IR-leu-enkephalin in rat brain. *Brain Res. 297*:121–125.

Walsh, G., Masland, W., and Goldensohn, E. (1968). Paroxysmal cerebral discharge associated with paroxysmal atrial tachycardia. *Electroencephalogr. Clin. Neurophysiol. 24*:187.

White, P. T., Grant, P., Mosier, J., and Craig, A. (1961). Changes in cerebral dynamics associated with seizures. *Neurology 11*:354–361.

Yukimura, J., Stock, G., Stumpf, H., Unger, T., and Ganten, D. (1981). Effects of (D-Ala[2])-methionine-enkephalin in blood pressure, heart rate, and baroreceptor reflex sensitivity in conscious cats. *Hypertension 3*(5):528–533.

19

Alcohol, Arrhythmias, Seizures, and Sudden Death

ARTHUR W. K. CHAN *Research Institute on Alcoholism and State University of New York, Buffalo, New York*

CLAIRE M. LATHERS* *The Medical College of Pennsylvania, Eastern Pennsylvania Psychiatric Institute, Philadelphia, Pennsylvania*

JAN E. LEESTMA *Chicago Neurosurgical Center, Columbus Hospital, Chicago, Illinois*

I. INTRODUCTION

In a recent discussion of sudden death mechanisms in the alcoholic person, Massello (1984) noted that chronic alcoholism is associated with multisystem degenerative disorders which result from chronic alcohol abuse. These degenerative disorders include hepatic cirrhosis, acute and chronic pancreatitis, anemias, and nervous system degenerations. Since alcohol is a poison when consumed in excessive amounts, respiratory depression and death may occur. Death associated with alcohol use may also be due to motor vehicle accidents, crime, and accidental head injuries. In addition, the use of alcohol is associated with sudden unexpected nontraumatic deaths. Medical examiners generally find these cases to be deaths in relatively young persons who have no well-documented medical history of any alcohol-related pathology. Death is usually very quick, much in the same fashion as deaths due to cardiac arrhythmias. Physical examination of the body is unrevealing and an autopsy may be negative or reveal nothing more than the fatty change in the liver. Postmortem blood levels will be negative or well below those levels that are normally thought to be lethal. In short, the medical examiner will be able to conclude only that the decreased was a hard and steady drinker or an alcoholic. The death certificate may become an enigma unless the medical examiner is aware that the alcoholic is a high-risk candidate for sudden unexpected death that can occur through a variety of pathophysiological mechanisms (Mas-

Current affiliation: FDA, Rockville, Maryland

sello, 1984). These interrelated pathophysiological mechanisms may include alcohol-associated cardiac disorders, the alcohol withdrawal syndrome, alcohol-induced hypoglycemia, and alcohol fatty liver.

This chapter begins with a discussion of the arrhythmogenic effects of alcohol on the heart, followed by evidence indicating that alcohol has the capability to lower the seizure threshold and problems associated with alcohol consumption in the person with epilepsy. This discussion will indicate why the use of alcohol in the person with epilepsy may also place that person at risk for unwanted cardiac arrhythmias and/or sudden death. These introductory sections of the chapter will be followed by a discussion of the occurrence of seizures during alcohol withdrawal, the relationship between alcoholism and epilepsy, and a comparison of the neurochemical mechanism involved in alcohol withdrawal seizures and in the genesis, maintenance, and cessation of epileptic seizures. In summary, this chapter will include evidence that alcohol, acutely or chronically in normal individuals without epilepsy, can induce cardiac arrhythmias that may result in an unexpected death. Thus the use of alcohol in the person with epilepsy may also place that person at risk for unwanted cardiac arrhythmias and/or sudden death. An understanding of the neurochemical changes involved in seizure initiation, in the presence or absence of alcohol, may ultimately allow the design of preventative treatment to obviate the occurrence of seizures, which when coupled with cardiac arrhythmias may result in sudden unexpected death.

II. CARDIAC CHANGES INDUCED BY ALCOHOL
CONSUMPTION

The acute ingestion of alcohol has been demonstrated to have adverse cardiac effects (Lang et al., 1985; Segel et al., 1984). However, this chapter focuses primarily on the chronic effects of alcohol on the heart and on seizures associated with alcohol withdrawal. Near the middle of the nineteenth century, a disease designated alcohol cardiomyopathy, characterized by cardiomegaly and congestive failure, was reported. No abnormalities in the coronary arteries, valves, septum, or myocardial wall were noted (Talbott, 1976). With the advent of electron microscopy and invasive cardiovascular techniques, previously undetected alcohol-induced alterations in both structure and function of the presumably normal heart were found. Talbott suggested that primary alcoholic heart disease consists of three separate clinical entities—nutritional, toxic, and conductive—each the result of a different etiological mechanism.

Nutritional or beriberi primary alcoholic heart disease may present with dyspnea, orthopnea, paroxysmal nocturnal palpitations, and occasionally angina. Eventually peripheral neuritis may develop. Dietary therapy, vitamin supplements, with emphasis on B complex and C, and abstinence from alcohol are essential to recovery. This disorder can be fatal if not treated.

Toxic primary alcoholic heart disease may occur with the frequent consumption as little as 3 ounces of alcohol over a period of five years or longer (Gunnar and Sutton, 1971). It may present with fragmented or destroyed myofibers, altered or lost contractile elements, swollen mitochondria and edema fluid, irregular accumulation and deposition of glycogen, altered membrane permeability, increased lipid deposition, vacuolinization with hydrophilic fatty and hyalin degeneration, focal areas of inflammatory response, and resultant fibrous scarring accompanied by at least partial loss of compliance in the ventricle, especially on the left side. These structural alterations can become profound and of hemodynamic importance before clinical symptoms are apparent. Initial clinical symptoms are limited to pulmonary function, including dyspnea precipitated and aggravated by exercise, labored breathing with rales as fluid accumulates in the lungs, and an elevated pulse and blood pressure. Eventually signs of right heart failure appear: edema, an enlarged liver, and venous distention in the neck. Absence of arrhythmia is evidence against conductive primary alcoholic heart disease and in favor of the toxic type. The ECG in a patient with the toxic type of cardiac disease may lack Q waves in leads II, III, and atrioventricular fibrillation; may have tall, peaked T waves appearing in V_2 and V_3; and the combination of the phonocardiogram and the ECG may reveal a prolonged left ventricular conduction time, reflecting decreased ventricular compliance due to the structural changes. In the later stages of the disease, ventricular hypertrophy may appear. The toxic disorder is treated with abstinence from alcohol, bed rest for several months, digitalis, a diuretic, and a high-protein diet. Detection during the early stages may prevent the onset of cardiac failure; later detection is generally associated with irreversible structural damage.

Conductive primary alcoholic heart disease is associated with an altered electrolyte balance that affects the conductivity of the heart and results in arrhythmia. The disorder is primarily within the conductive system since no abnormalities of ventricular wall competence, contractility, or ejection time develop, except as they relate to the alcohol-induced arrhythmia. The arrhythmias, roughly in order of incidence, include auricular fibrillation, supraventricular tachycardia, ventricular premature beats, and nodal rhythm. Patients with severe arrhythmias may develop convulsive seizures secondary to the Wolff-Parkinson-White arrhythmia (Sataline, 1973; Talbott and Gander, 1974). Talbott (1976) noted that magnesium administration usually controls these secondary seizures, since they are of cardiac rather than cerebral origin.

Talbott (1976), using Holter monitoring in patients undergoing alcoholic detoxification, reported sinus tachycardia with hypertension, ventricular and/or auricular premature contractions, nodal tachycardia, varying degrees of intraventricular and sinoventricular block, and ventricular tachycardia, in decreasing order of incidence. The prolonged and often progressive fatigue that accompanies detoxification can produce potentially catastrophic events such as cardio-

Table 1 Duration of Chronic Alcohol Intake in
the 36 Patients Studied

Duration (years)	Number of patients
< ½	0
½–1	1
1–5	1
5–10	4
10–40	30
Total	36

Reproduced with permission from Abbasakoor et al.
Ann NY Acad Sci 173:364–370, 1976.

genic shock, ventricular fibrillation or flutter, left-sided failure, or cardiac stand-still. Any of these symptoms could result in sudden death. It is also suggested that conductive primary alcoholic heart disease is the chief pathological mecha-nism causing the high mortality sometimes reported with the withdrawal syn-drome. Talbott (1976) controlled and/or prevented arrhythmias by administer-ing high doses of magnesium and potassium in a fructose base. The patient was transferred to coronary monitoring if ventricular flutter or tachycardia was pres-ent. Oral or intravenous diazepam was used to control vomiting and convulsions.

Cardiac arrhythmias and other changes in the ECG have been described in both acute and chronic alcoholism. A correlation between excessive alcohol con-sumption and heart disease has been established (Abbasakoor et al., 1976). T wave abnormalities, in particular, have been related to chronic cardiomyopathy (Blankenhorn, 1945; Bridgen and Robinson, 1964; Evans, 1964; Fowler et al., 1961; Frederiksen and Hed, 1945; Sanders, 1970) or to acute withdrawal from

Table 2 Duration of Acute Alcohol Intake in the
36 Patients Studied

Duration (days)	Number of patients
3–7	9
8–48	18
49–84	3
> 84	6
Total	36

Reproduced with permission of Ann NY Acad Sci 173:
364–370, 1976.

Table 3 Incidence of All Dysrhythmias in the 36 Patients Studied

Dysrhythmia	Number of patients	Percentage of patients
Sinus tachycardia	31	86%
Atrial or nodal premature beats	3	8%
Ventricular premature beats	14	39%
T wave changes	20	56%
Normal ECG	3	8%

Reproduced with permission from Abbasakoor et al., Ann NY Acad Sci 173:364–370, 1976.

ethanol (Vetter et al., 1967). Abbasakoor et al. (1976) utilized 12-hour recordings of ECG in 50 acutely intoxicated male patients (average age 45; range of 33–61 years) with no prior history of cardiovascular disease. Patients taking any antiarrhythmic drugs, including phenytoin, were not included in the study. As seen in Table 1, the history of alcohol intake ranged from 6 months to 40 years. Daily alcoholic beverage consumption ranged from three days to several months in duration prior to admission into the group of patients studied (Table 2). Three patients were excluded from the study because measurement of blood alcohol levels did not confirm the clinical diagnosis of acute ethanol intoxication.

The arrhythmias recorded in the 36 patients are listed in Table 3. An examination of the incidence of atrial arrhythmias revealed that 31 patients (86%) had sinus tachycardia some time during the ECG recording; 27 (74%) exhibited persistent sinus tachycardia; 2 (6%) patients had atrial premature beats; and 1 (3%) manifested nodal premature beats. Examination of the incidence and nature of ventricular arrhythmias indicated that 12 (33%) patients had ventricular premature beats originating from a single ectopic focus. One patient had multifocal ventricular premature beats and one had a run of ventricular tachycardia for 28 consecutive beats which terminated spontaneously. Seventeen patients exhibited peaked T wave changes and three showed a shifting T wave vector.

The blood alcohol levels obtained on admission ranged from 240 to 520 mg%. The mean blood alcohol concentration in those persons with ventricular arrhythmias was 347 mg%; those with no arrhythmias had a mean level of 373 mg%. The difference between the levels was not significant (NS).

The serum potassium concentration was above 4 meq/L in 20 patients, between 3.5 and 3.9 meq/L in 18 patients, and below 3.4 meq/L in 1 patient. Of 14 patients with ventricular arrhythmias 7 had levels in the range of 3.5–3.9 meq/L (mean of 3.93 meq/L). The mean potassium level in those with a normal ventricular rhythm was 4.12 meq/L (NS).

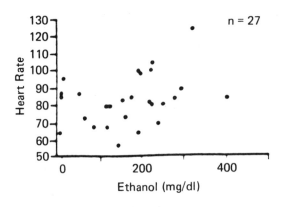

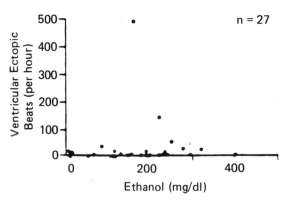

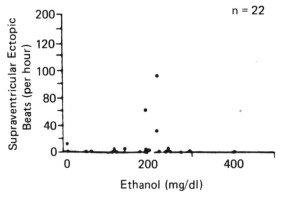

Figure 1 Correlation of serum ethanol levels with heart rate and arrhythmias. Upper, Mean heart rate obtained on the first 24-hour ambulatory monitoring on the vertical axis plotted against the admission serum concentration of ethanol on the horizontal axis ($r = 0.30$, $p < 0.07$). Middle and lower, Mean rate of ventricular ectopic beats per hour and supraventricular ectopic beats per hour likewise plotted against ethanol concentration (r, $= 0.34$, $p < 0.05$, and $r = 0.40$, $p < 0.008$, respectively). Reproduced with permission from Buckingham et al., Am. Ht. J. 110:961–965, 1985.

Table 4   Arrhythmias Documented on Initial 24-Hour ECG in 38 Patients

Arrhythmia	Number of patients	Percentage of patients
Persistent sinus bradycardia	1	3
Persistent sinus tachycardia	6	16
Ventricular ectopic beats	24	63
Frequent ventricular ectopic beats (> 30/hr)	5	13
Ventricular couplets	9	24
Nonsustained ventricular tachycardia	5	13
Atrial fibrillation	5	13
Supraventricular ectopic beats	26	79

Reproduced with permission from Buckingham et al. Am. Ht. J. 110:961–965, 1985.

This study found that sinus tachycardia was the most common cardiac rhythm, a not surprising result in view of the common clinical observations of this phenomenon. Furthermore, catecholamine levels are increased in chronic alcoholic patients during intoxication and after cessation of consumption. This increase was associated with a sinus tachycardia of 25% in 66 patients with alcoholic cardiomyopathy (Alexander, 1968) and suggested a role for catecholamines in the initiation of arrhythmias in those who chronically consume alcohol.

Sereny (1971) reported that the percentage of abnormal changes in the ECG varied with the time between the consumption of the last drink and the ECG recording. ECGs obtained within 24 hours of admission found 49% with sinus tachycardia; the incidence fell to 5% at 48 hours. This author attributed the sinus tachycardia to the action of alcohol and/or its metabolite acetaldehyde. These data suggest the acetaldehyde may contribute to the cardiac rhythm changes induced by alcohol.

Ventricular premature beats are the most common form of arrhythmia, both in normal persons and in association with disease (Abbasakoor et al., 1976). An incidence of 0.8% was reported for 122,000 asymptomatic Air Force personnel (range of 16–50 years; Hiss and Lamb, 1962). Ventricular premature beats in the form of bigeminy may persist for years in some apparently normal individuals. Hinkle et al. (1969) examined 301 active working males (median age 55 years) using Holter monitoring and found that 62% had one or more ventricular premature beats and 8.8% had more than 10 beats/1000; 19.4% exhibited 1–10 beats/ 1000; and 33.2% of the records exhibited extrasystoles that originated from more than one focus. These arrhythmias were thought to be associated with the presence of coronary artery disease. The study of Abbasakoor et al. (1976) reported an incidence of 39% for ventricular arrhythmias; this was probably lower

Table 5 Comparison of Arrhythmias in 38 Patients with and without Organic
Heart Disease

Arrhythmia	With OHD (N = 10)	Without OHD (N = 28)	p Value
VEBs	9 (90)	16 (57)	NS
> 30/hr VEBs	3 (30)	2 (7)	NS
Ventricular couplets	5 (50)	4 (14)	NS
Nonsustained VT	4 (40)	1 (4)	$p < 0.05$
SVEBs	10 (100)	21 (75)	NS
Atrial fibrillation	5 (50)	0 (0)	$p < 0.001$
Mean age	64 ± 9	47 ± 13	$p < 0.002$
Mean heart rate	88 ± 18	83 ± 14	NS
Mean rate of VEBs/hr	70 ± 153	9 ± 27	$p < 0.01$
Mean rate of SVEBs/hr	97 ± 160	8 ± 31	NS

Key: OHD = organic heart disease; VEBs = ventricular ectopic beats; VT = ventricular
tachycardia; SVEBs = supraventricular ectopic beats; NS = not significant. Numbers in
parentheses are percentages. Reproduced with permission from Buckingham et al., *Am. Ht.
J., 110*:961–965, 1985.

than the incidence reported above since they excluded patients with known
heart disease. However, the 39% incidence was higher than the 0.8% incidence
reported for the Air Force personnel (Hiss and Lamb, 1962). This may be due to
the fact that the Air Force population represented one that was prescreened to
detect individuals with obvious health problems. Abbasakoor et al. (1976) suggested that the incidence of premature ventricular beats in acutely intoxicated
patients with no known heart disease appears to be higher than that in the general population without heart disease and concluded that a much larger number
of patients would have to be studied to prove this hypothesis. Buckingham et al.
(1985) also noted that this question has yet to be resolved.

Abbasakoor et al. (1976) were surprised not to find a higher incidence of
hypokalemia, given that hyperaldosteronism may be associated with acute alcohol
intoxication and with chronic alcoholic liver disease. They noted that the incidence of 8% for atrial arrhythmias was similar to the 12% reported by Vetter et
al. (1967) and that this type of arrhythmia is much more common in alcoholic
cardiomyopathy. They were unable to demonstrate any correlation between the
alcohol levels on admission and the subsequent incidence of arrhythmia.

Buckingham et al. (1985) examined changes in cardiac rhythm in 38 patients
admitted to an acute alcoholic detoxification center, using 24-hour Holter ambulatory ECG monitoring with 24 hours of admission and at the time of patient
discharge. The study found a mild correlation between the serum ethanol level

(samples were drawn within 12 hours of admission) and the mean heart rate of ventricular ectopic beats per hour ($p < 0.05$; Figure 1). Nonsustained ventricular tachycardia and atrial fibrillation were more common in those with underlying organic heart disease (Tables 4 and 5). Repeat 24-hour Holter monitoring revealed no changes in the occurrence of arrhythmias two weeks after alcohol consumption had stopped. The authors recognized that their study lacked a control group and that not all patients were examined upon discharge. In addition, since they classified patients as those with and those without organic heart disease based only on the clinical history, physical examination, and ECG, it was not possible to detect subclinical organic heart disease. Furthermore, many of the patients with organic heart diseases were older, which may in part explain why they had more arrhythmias. The data suggest an increased risk with increasing age. Nevertheless, Buckingham et al. concluded that alcohol can induce cardiac arrhythmias in patients who are predisposed to them by virtue of the underlying organic heart disease but that alcohol does not necessarily cause arrhythmias in apparently healthy persons.

III. PROPOSED MECHANISM FOR ARRHYTHMIAS, SEIZURES, AND DEATH ASSOCIATED WITH ALCOHOL CONSUMPTION

Fisher and Abrams (1977) reported the initial appearance of premature ventricular contractions in a 46-year-old chronic alcoholic, followed six hours later with a ventricular tachycardia that immediately degenerated into ventricular fibrillation (Figure 2), which responded to resuscitation efforts. Since both potassium and magnesium levels were low, they were replaced and intravenous lidocaine was administered. Ventricular tachycardia again occurred and required countershock. Additional potassium and procainamide were given and no additional arrhythmias were noted. This case report emphasizes the observation that hypokalemia and possible hypomagnesemia are important factors in the development of ventricular ectopy and that persons with delirium tremens require close monitoring and aggressive therapy to prevent life-threatening arrhythmias in the presence of electrolyte imbalance.

Smile (1984) reported a 47-year-old male with a known history of alcohol abuse who underwent a severe alcohol withdrawal complicated by seizures, hallucinations, hypertension, and supraventricular tachycardia. Intravenous diazepam (70 mg over 30 minutes) failed to exert an effect. Three 0.5-mg increments of propranolol were then given intravenously, which immediately converted the supraventricular tachycardia to sinus tachycardia and reduced the blood pressure from 210/130 to 130/80 mm Hg. The patient had no history of supraventricular tachycardia or cardiomyopathy and had normal electrolytes with the exception of a magnesium level that was slightly below normal. The combination of post-

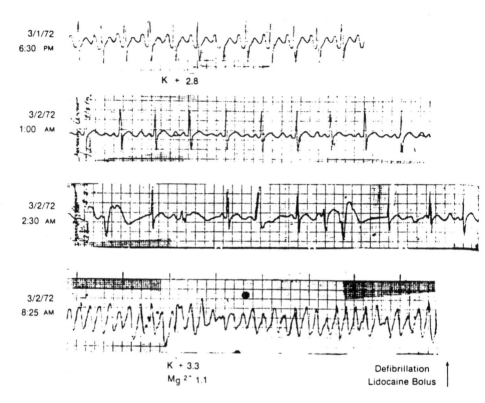

Figure 2 Serial monitor strips taken in Medical Intensive Care Unit. Top two tracings reveal sinus mechanism. At 2:30 AM, bursts of premature ventricular contractions are noted. These were not treated. Shortly before 8:25 AM, ventricular tachycardia developed that immediately degenerated into ventricular fibrillations, as seen in fourth rhythm strip. (Monitor strips have been retouched.) Reproduced with permission from Fisher and Abrams: Arch Intern Med 137:1240, 1977.

ictal hypoxia and circulating catecholamine excess may have contributed to the initiation of supraventricular tachycarrhythmia. The use of a beta-adrenergic blocking agent was based on the studies demonstrating elevated plasma and urinary catecholamines during withdrawal (Carlsson and Haggendal, 1967; Ogata et al., 1971). Smile (1984) concluded that intravenous beta-adrenergic blocking agents have proven beneficial in patients withdrawing from alcohol consumption if there is no history of asthma, congestive heart failure, insulin-dependent diabetes, or sympathetic hyperactivity resulting in tachyarrhythmias, hypertension, and hypertensive encephalopathy.

The arrhythmogenic effects of alcohol consumption have been suggested to be due to the positive inotropic and chronotropic actions of acetaldehyde (Mc-Cloy et al., 1974). Alpha- and beta-adrenergic blocking agents eliminate the arrhythmias, suggesting that the positive inotropic and chronotropic actions of acetaldehyde may result from the release of catecholamines (Nakano and Prancan, 1972). Acetaldehyde may indirectly release catecholamines during intoxication with alcohol and withdrawal, since urinary excretion of epinephrine and norepinephrine is increased up to 50% when alcohol is being consumed by alcoholic persons and remains elevated for several days after intake has stopped (Cooper and Sellers, 1974).

Abbasakoor et al. (1976) reported that one patient developed ventricular tachycardia during alcohol withdrawal, suggesting that the tendency to develop ventricular arrhythmias in association with alcohol withdrawal may not be innocuous. Although the incidence of ventricular tachycardia in a large group of alcoholic patients is unknown, it could quite possibly be the mechanism of death in some. Since the increased concentrations of circulating catecholamines may be a contributory factor to the initiation of arrhythmias, the usefulness of beta-adrenergic blocking agents such as propranolol as part of the treatment for the abstinence syndrome deserves investigation.

Alcohol taken in excess over a period of years may damage a normal heart, causing a condition called primary alcoholic heart disease (Talbott, 1976). The deleterious effects of excessive consumption of alcohol on the abnormal heart (Conway, 1968; Gould et al., 1972; Wilson et al., 1970) has been called secondary alcoholic heart disease (Talbott, 1976). In this context, ingestion of alcohol has been reported as the direct cause of sudden and unexpected death by cardiac arrest (Laurie, 1971; Nevins and Lyon, 1972).

Small amounts of alcohol may lower the seizure threshold in a susceptible patient without epilepsy (Mucha and Pinel, 1979). Seizures can be precipitated in both idiopathic and posttraumatic epilepsy after an episode of social drinking (Victor and Brausch, 1967; Victor and Laureno, 1978). In addition, all of the studies cited above indicate that alcohol, acutely or chronically ingested by normal individuals without epilepsy, can induce cardiac arrhythmias that may result in an unexpected death. Thus the use of alcohol in the person with epilepsy may also place that person at risk for unwanted cardiac arrhythmias and/or sudden death.

From a pathological perspective, which often has forensic implications, the effect of alcohol on the heart by itself or on the heart and central nervous system jointly bring about sudden and unexpected death in certain individuals. To be sure, there are individuals who suffer sudden and catastrophic collapse due to the apparent intrinsic effects of alcohol on heart action, but there are others in whom other acute or chronic effects of alcohol on the nervous system and/or

liver interplay to produce a fatal outcome. Such cases are especially complicated when a known seizure disorder and/or psychiatric symptoms have been
treated with tricyclic antidepressants or phenothiazines. Each of these types
of psychoactive agents has its own well-known effects on the heart. Many of
these subjects are discussed elsewhere in this book.

The phenomenon of sudden death in alcoholics is well known to forensic
pathologists and is a common enough problem that significant difficulty is often
found in developing a cause of death following autopsy (Camps, 1976; Polson
et al., 1985). Such deaths may occur with or without apparent morphological
changes in the heart. In sudden deaths in individuals who are not apparently
chronic alcoholics but die during or after excessive alcohol consumption, the
heart may appear entirely normal in gross appearance but probably would show,
if examined, ultrastructural changes in muscle fibers which can be observed in
acute alcohol toxicity in experimental animals. In such cases there may also be
some element of respiratory failure and hypoxia due to suppression of the respiratory drive by alcohol, aspiration of vomitus, and/or brain stem edema or
herniation secondary to alcohol-induced cerebral edema, whose effects on the
heart may be difficult to separate from those due solely to alcohol (Leestma,
1988). Other possibilities include some direct effect of alcohol on coronary arterial perfusion (Altura et al., 1983). Any or all of these effects, of course, can
be synergistic to extraordinary loads placed on the heart by seizure activity,
metabolic abnormalities, or preexisting disease.

In the chronic alcoholic, so-called alcoholic cardiomyopathy can cause sudden death. The pathology of the hearts of such victims is usually that of an enlarged, flabby heart, which may show focal myocardial fibrosis usually of the
left ventricular wall in the absence of significant coronary artery disease and
hypertension, though hypertension is often known to have been present. There
is usually myocardial cellular hypertrophy, sometimes vacuolation of fibers, and
usually extensive fatty infiltration of the heart, which may extend to all portions
including papillary muscles (Camps, 1976; Polson et al., 1985; Richards, 1964).
Precisely why such findings would cause sudden cardiac collapse is not at all
clear. Possibly the dilated and flabby heart has affected the cardiac conduction
system, thus setting the stage for a fatal arrhythmia triggered by other factors
such as intrinsic myocardial effects of alcohol, vascular spasm, metabolic or electrolyte abnormalities, vitamin deficiency (B complex), or abnormal autonomic
reflexes (Altura et al., 1983). Of course, if there are underlying disease conditions of the heart such as chronic valvular disease, infective endocarditis, "floppy"
mitral valves, coronary artery disease, or myocarditis, the added burden of alcohol may have a fatal effect.

IV. UNDERLYING AND EXOGENOUS FACTORS IN SEIZURES IN ALCOHOLIC INDIVIDUALS

The neurochemical environment of the brain, as affected by the abuse of and withdrawal from alcohol, must invariably interact with structural pathology as well as chemical alterations of the metabolism caused by coexisting disease states, the manifestations of the alcoholic state in nonneural organs, and exogenous drug and other substance use, in the production of the alcohol withdrawal seizure. The precise analysis of the contributions of each of these other factors to the seizure state is difficult to accomplish at best. The fact that each of the following conditions, in the absence of apparent alcohol abuse, can produce or facilitate seizures implies that when one or more are present in addition to the alcoholic state, facilitation of seizures would logically occur. Whether such interactions contribute to or cause sudden unexpected death, by whatever mechanism, remains to be shown.

A. Brain Lesions in Alcoholic Individuals

Though it is seldom included in the pathology of alcohol abuse, cerebral trauma is a major, if not the most commonly encountered intracranial lesion in a chronic alcoholic population (Craig et al., 1980; Leestma, 1988; Torvik et al., 1982). In the alcoholic population with seizures, it is the most commonly encountered form of brain pathology (more than a third of cases): in the nonalcoholic adult individual presenting with seizures, following "no known cause" and cerebrovascular disease, brain trauma is found in about 16% of cases (Hillbom, 1980). Most often the traumatic lesions are not acute and take the form of cortical contusions alone or in combination with chronic subdural hematoma and/or some other traumatic lesion (Leestma, 1988).

The role of cortical contusions in facilitating or causing seizures is not precisely understood and involves a number of controversial areas in epileptology, such as the phenomenon of kindling (Racine and McIntyre, 1986). The cortical contusion, apparently a simple lesion grossly, is a highly complex lesion histologically and functionally. Whereas the center of the contusion is devoid of viable neurons, the margins present a transitional zone, or "penumbra," between normal and damaged brain. Here some, but not all neurons are damaged or absent. Some, but not all interneuronal connections and longer connections are severed or damaged. In the repair process, which included gliosis, revascularization, repair of the blood–brain barrier, and reordering and replacement of synaptic connections, vital homeostatic mechanisms may be out of balance. For example, facilitory connections can be reestablished or undamaged while inhibitory connections to the neuronal field are lacking. The neurochemical environment of the traumatic lesion can foster abnormal discharges rather than suppress them, and/or the ability of a nearby population of neurons to correctly process impulses can be altered (Engle, 1983; Leestma, 1988; Meldrum and Corsellis, 1984; Ward, 1969).

In light of the fact that many cortical contusions morphologically undercut nearby apparently intact cortical regions, it is logical to assume that recurrent collateral inhibitory connections are probably damaged, and that this along with some or all of the foregoing phenomena serve to set the stage for potential irritative foci, which can become epileptogenic. When these lesions are located in portions of the cortex that are known to have a lower threshold of excitability than other cortical regions, the added potential for epileptogenesis is present.

By far the most common region for traumatic cortical contusions is the base of the brain, specifically the orbital portion of the frontal lobes as well as inferior and basal temporal lobes (Engle, 1983; Jay and Leestma, 1981; Laidlaw and Richens, 1976; Meldrum and Corsellis, 1984). All these regions, perhaps because of their proximity to the hippocampal formation, are known to have lower thresholds of excitability than more lateral or rostral cortical regions. Stimulation of such regions in experimental animals can induce hypothalamic-autonomic effects, some of which involve alterations of cardiac function (Jay and Leestma, 1981). Such autonomic cardiac interaction with the epileptic state forms much of the theoretical basis of the sudden unexpected death syndrome in epileptics (SUDEP) to which this book is devoted.

The fact that uncal herniation and grooving are very common in any form of brain swelling, especially that due to brain trauma and/or subdural hematoma, increases the chance that ischemia due to pressure against the tentorial edge may produce damage and eventual sclerosis of portions of the mesial temporal lobe, a lesion thought to be both a cause and a symptom of the epileptic state (Falconer, 1974; Meldrum and Corsellis, 1984).

Most traumatic contusions, especially in the chronic alcoholic, are multiple and often widely spaced. This results from the tendency for repeated trauma, usually due to a backward, unguarded fall, in which both contracoup and "gliding" contusions of the basal brain cortex are commonly seen (Leestma and Grcevic, 1988; Lindenberg and Freytag, 1957). The additive effect of multiple cortical lesions as a contribution to epileptogenesis would seem to be obvious.

Other traumatic lesions in the alcoholic involve more diffuse, deeper lesions (diffuse axonal injury, inner cerebral trauma) of long axons of passage due to a shear force and rotational strain injury (Adams et al., 1982). The effect of such lesions is usually evident clinically in the postconcussive syndrome, in parameters of higher cortical function such as memory, learning, emotion management, and associations (Alves and Jane, 1985). To be sure, some brain-injured individuals, apparently in the absence of cortical contusions, develop posttraumatic epilepsy (Laidlaw and Richens, 1976), but the precise mechanism for such an eventuality is not clearly defined.

Complications of head trauma which may produce neuroanatomical changes that cause or enhance epileptogenesis include subarachnoid hemorrhage, intraventricular hemorrhage, meningitis, and the presence of metallic or other foreign bodies in the brain, which may induce scarring or inflammatory reactions (Leestma and Grcevic, 1988).

B. Nontraumatic Brain Lesions in the Alcoholic

Some lesions in the brain which are classically considered to be associated with alcoholism are known to cause or occur with seizures. These include some cases of Wernicke's encephalopathy (Harper, 1979; Torvik et al., 1982), some individuals with alcoholic cerebellar degeneration, and those very rare individuals who suffer from Marchiafava–Bignami disease (Leestma, 1988). Whether individuals who apparently suffer from alcoholic brain atrophy in the absence of trauma suffer seizures definably related to the atrophy is not clear. Those individuals with central pontine myelinolysis alone, related to alcoholism, apparently have no particular propensity to suffer seizures, except on a withdrawal basis.

Of some interest in alcoholic cerebellar degeneration is the consideration that given the degree of cerebellar atrophy, one must wonder if the loss of inhibitory influence of the cerebellum at higher centers has an effect on seizure threshold. In the case of intractable epileptics who have a diffuse, nonalcoholic type of cerebellar degeneration due to chronic seizures and/or phenytoin toxicity (Leestma, 1988; Meldrum and Corsellis, 1984), a case could be made for some impact of the atrophy on seizure severity and frequency.

Whether the contribution to brain atrophy and/or seizure development in the alcoholic is made by some alcohol-mediated change in cerebral and/or cardiac vascular perfusion is not clear but has been suggested, to further complicate an already confusing phenomenon (Altura et al., 1983).

C. Exogenous and Other Factors in Seizures in Alcoholics

Alcoholics frequently are not single drug users and may abuse a number of other drugs. Many of these (e.g., narcotics, cannabis) are inhibitors of seizure activity, but one must be mindful that deprivation and withdrawal from these agents can set into motion events that are similar to alcohol withdrawal and may unmask a seizure state, though the neuropharmacology is far less well understood than is alcohol withdrawal.

Though it is not commonly encountered, or well studied, individuals who consume large quantities of caffeine-containing beverages (coffee, colas, and other soft drinks) or take caffeine in some other form (such as No-Doz) may suffer seizures, sometimes with fatal result, presumably as a result of their caffeine use (Leestma et al., 1989). Such cases have been encountered in long-term observation of epileptic individuals who suffer SUDEP. Similar seizure-enhancing or causing drugs of abuse, such as amphetamines and PCP, are often encountered in alcoholics and nonalcoholic individuals who suffer seizures with or without fatal result. Again, there has been limited investigation into these agents and how they facilitate or cause seizures.

The list of conditions that are exacerbated or caused by the abuse of alcohol is lengthy (Craig et al., 1980; Harper, 1979; Leestma, 1988; Torvik et al., 1982), with many of them involved in the production or facilitation of seizures and/or sudden death. The list includes cirrhosis and liver failure, pulmonary infection and abscess with or without brain abscess and meningitis, cardiomyopathy, and electrolyte abnormalities. Of particular interest is hepatic and cardiac pathology in relation to sudden death. The finding of fatty liver of significant degree is common in any alcoholic, and sometimes, in the absence of any other obvious anatomic finding and when it is extensive, this is invoked by the coroner's pathologist as a cause for sudden unexpected death, though the precise mechanism is rarely defined (Polson et al., 1985). One has to wonder if the biochemical abnormalities of amino acid metabolism which exist in incipient liver failure, and which may or may not be present in severe fatty liver, could not translate into a neurochemical disorder of the sorts that are discussed above, which could result alone or in combination with alcohol withdrawal to produce seizures, some possibly fatal.

V. OCCURRENCE OF SEIZURES DURING ALCOHOL WITHDRAWAL

The occurrence of seizures in the alcoholic is common, presumably most often due to processes occurring during alcohol withdrawal (Naranjo and Sellers, 1986). To be sure, most episodes of seizures differ little in outcome from those in the general epileptic population, but the observation of sudden unexpected death in chronic alcoholics who had a history of epileptic attacks is not uncommon (Freytag and Lindenberg, 1964; Leestma et al., 1984). This leads to the suggestion that, since most individuals have no detectable blood level of ethanol, alcohol withdrawal may have played a role in the precipitation of premortem seizures which may have caused death by mechanisms discussed extensively in this book.

About 2-15% of alcoholics in withdrawal develop seizures, and this estimate may be higher in alcoholics who have a history of withdrawal seizures or who will develop delirium tremens (Brown et al., 1988; Chan, 1985; Naranjo and Sellers, 1986). The affected individuals may present the following seizure histories:

1. No prior personal or familial history of epilepsy, with alcohol withdrawal seizures occurring for the first time.

2. No preexisting personal or familial history of epilepsy, but recurrent alcohol withdrawal seizures.
3. Those belonging to (1) or (2) who later develop epilepsy with or without relapse of alcohol abuse.
4. Epileptic persons who have their first alcohol withdrawal seizures.
5. Epileptic persons who have recurrent alcohol withdrawal seizures.
6. Those belonging to categories (4) and (5) who have a familial history of epilepsy.
7. Those who have presumably acquired epilepsy secondary to traumatic lesions of the brain which were, in turn, caused by falls, fights, or other episodes in connection with their alcoholism.
8. Those with traumatic lesions with any of the previous categories.

Although it is well known that children of alcoholics have an increased risk of becoming alcoholics (Goodwin, 1987), no data are available to indicate that these people are more likely than those without familial history of alcoholism to have seizures during alcohol withdrawal.

Many factors alone or in addition to alcohol abuse can potentially trigger seizures during alcohol withdrawal. These include traumatic lesions involving the cortex such as contusions, focal scarred regions beneath old epidural or subdural hematomas where burr holes may have been placed, old or recent subcortical traumatic streak and ball hemorrhages, and diffuse or multifocal traumatic lesions such as shear force injuries as in "diffuse" axonal injury (Adams et al., 1982) or "inner" cerebral trauma (Grcevic, 1988; Leestma and Grcevic, 1988). Nontraumatic brain lesions which can also provide epileptogenic foci include old or recent ischemic lesions, cortical infarcts, vascular malformations, subcortical lacunas, old or recent sequelae of infection (herpes simplex and other viral encephalitides, bacterial, mycobacterial or fungal meningitis, brain abscess, or parasitic disease of the brain) (Leestma, 1988; Torvik et al., 1982). Cerebral vasculitis and related autoimmune processes are also seen. In spite of the plethora of etiologies for an epileptic state, it has been suggested that alcohol withdrawal is the most common single precipitating factor for the development of status epilepticus, and probably for most seizures in the alcoholic (Chan, 1985; Pilke et al., 1984).

Several reviews have summarized literature dealing with the relationship between alcoholism and epilepsy (Brennan and Lyttle, 1987; Chan, 1985; Espir and Rose, 1987; Johnson, 1985; Little and Gayle, 1980; Scollo-Lavizzari, 1983). The term alcoholic epilepsy has been used with varying definitions in different reports (Chan, 1985; Tartara et al., 1983). This has contributed to the uncertainty concerning the prevalence of epilepsy among alcoholics and of alcoholism among epileptic patients. Another reason for such an uncertainty is that there is a scarcity of population-based epidemiological studies of these statistics (Chan, 1985; Little and Gayle, 1980). Therefore, more investigations are needed to confirm or refute the suggestion that the prevalence of epilepsy among alcoholics is at least triple that in the general population and that alcoholism may be more prevalent among epileptic patients than in the general population (Chan, 1985; Little and Gayle, 1980). Recently, Hauser (1988) suggested that the prevalence of alcohol abuse among cases of epilepsy did not appear to be elevated above that of the general population. Strictly speaking, an isolated occurrence of alcohol withdrawal seizure without a prior history and/or subsequent recurrence of epileptic seizures does not meet the definition of epilepsy.

Many biochemical, neurochemical, and endocrinological changes are associated with the alcohol withdrawal syndrome. Some of the neurochemical changes may actually be important triggering factors for precipitating seizures in susceptible individuals. Much of this information has been derived from animal models of alcohol dependence (Cicero, 1980; Friedman, 1980; Goldstein, 1978, 1986). Studies of biochemical correlates of alcohol withdrawal in humans have largely been confined to analyses of blood or, under special circumstances, cerebrospinal fluid (CSF) or postmortem brain samples (Airaksinen and Peura, 1987; Wilkins and Gorelick, 1986). Although the exact mechanisms for the development of alcohol withdrawal reactions are still not fully understood, several CNS models of alcohol withdrawal have been suggested (Wilkins and Gorelick, 1986). These assumed that during withdrawal one or more of the following systems are perturbed: neurotransmitter synthesis and/or receptor binding; facilitation of specific neural pathways; or changes in neuronal membranes, which in turn affect neuronal functions (Wilkins and Gorelick, 1986). The basic underlying theory is that during chronic alcohol exposure the CNS attempts to compensate for the depressant effects of ethanol through neurochemical and neurophysiological adaptations. When alcohol is withdrawn abruptly, the "overcompensation" is unmasked in the form of a hyperexcitable state. Thus, in general, most neurochemical changes associated with alcohol withdrawal are in opposite directions to those elicited by acute ethanol treatment.

The rest of this chapter reviews the neuropharmacological aspects of alcohol withdrawal. These are compared to neurochemical mechanisms that have been postulated to be involved in the genesis, maintenance, and cessation of epileptic seizures. As a first approximation, if the neurochemical changes associated with alcohol withdrawal are the causes, rather than the results, of withdrawal seizures, they should at least be similar to those proposed to be the mechanisms for initiation of epileptic seizures. However, there are limitations to this kind of reasoning, as outlined in the next section. Since the acute and chronic effects of ethanol have been thoroughly reviewed (Hoffman and Tabakoff, 1985; Hunt, 1985; Pohorecky and Brick, 1988; Tabakoff and Hoffman, 1980, 1983), readers are referred to these articles for detailed listings of the voluminous literature on these subject matters. Only leading references are cited and cursory summaries are given for the broad subjects of neurochemical mechanisms of epileptic seizures.

Some of the pathological and neuropathological consequences of alcohol abuse which cause or in some way interact with the epileptic state and with alcohol withdrawal are also discussed. These include neurotrauma, infection, malnutrition and hepatic dysfunction, polydrug use, and noncompliance with anticonvulsant medication.

A. Methodological Issues

Interpretation of neurochemical correlates of alcohol withdrawal seizures are hampered by our incomplete knowledge of the mechanisms of epileptic seizures and the neurochemical bases of ethanol tolerance and physical dependence. Other methodological concerns are summarized below.

1. It is often difficult to determine whether the neurochemical changes associated with alcohol withdrawal are the cause or the result of the withdrawal hyperexcitability. The difficulty can be compounded by inadequate information concerning when the samples used for neurochemical studies were taken relative to the time of the last dose of alcohol (Tabakoff and Hoffman, 1980). Therefore, the data are difficult to interpret with respect to whether the neurochemical changes are due to the acute, chronic, or withdrawal effects of alcohol. Similarly, in experimental models of epilepsy, it may be difficult to distinguish whether an observed neurochemical change is the cause or result of seizures. Long lasting neurochemical changes can exist in animals that have had seizures previously.

2. Biochemical correlates of human alcohol withdrawal reactions may sometimes be confounded if the alcoholic subjects are on medications to prevent or treat the symptoms. Although animal models have the advantage in that the effects of alcohol per se can be studied under controlled conditions, studies of the human alcohol withdrawal reactions are complicated by the frequent occurrence of multiple interacting factors mentioned previously.

3. In general, the time courses of withdrawal reactions in rodents are shorter than those in humans. Rodent models of alcohol withdrawal also lack the complete array of symptoms seen in humans (Friedman, 1980). In humans, seizures during alcohol withdrawal are primarily of the generalized tonic-clonic or grand mal type (Chan, 1985; Victor and Brausch, 1967). Although spontaneous tonic-clonic seizures have been reported in rodent models of alcohol withdrawal, seizures in these models were often induced by audiogenic stimuli or by handling such as picking up the animal by the tail (Goldstein, 1986). A substantial body of neurochemical data on experimental models of epilepsy have come from the

kindling model. The relevance of kindling and related processes to human epileptogenesis was recently reviewed by Schmutz (1987). He concluded that there are similarities between kindling and certain aspects of human epilepsy. There has also been speculation that repeated episodes of alcohol withdrawal may contribute to the development of kindling (Gorelick and Wilkins, 1986; Pinel, 1980; Wilkins and Gorelick, 1986). Recently, Brown and colleagues (1988) reported that the number of detoxifications appeared to be an important variable in the predisposition to withdrawal seizures. Therefore, it is deemed appropriate to compare the neurochemical correlates of alcohol withdrawal with those of kindling seizures, even though much remains to be investigated about the relationship between kindling and human epilepsy.

4. In animal studies, there can be differences in neurochemical changes associated with alcohol withdrawal because of differences in the duration and/or method of alcohol administration (Hoffman and Tabakoff, 1985; Hunt, 1985; Pohorecky and Brick, 1988). Many in vitro studies of brain preparations from animals undergoing withdrawal used rather high ethanol concentrations ($>$ 100 mM or $>$ 400 mg/dl). Thus there is doubt about the physiological significance of the findings.

5. For practical reasons most studies of alcohol withdrawal examine only one particular neurochemical parameter. However, the dynamic and complex interactions among the various systems of neurotransmitters and neuromodulators need to be considered. Unfortunately, many of these complex interactions have yet to be understood. The same difficulty exists in the interpretations of neurochemical mechanisms of epileptic seizures. The time courses of neurochemical changes postulated to be involved in the genesis of withdrawal signs, e.g., seizures, may or may not be parallel to those of occurrence of withdrawal seizures. Studies with samples taken at several time periods during withdrawal would be more informative than studies involving only one time period.

We next consider specific neurochemical correlates of alcohol withdrawal and epileptic seizures.

B. GABA Systems

Table 6 compares neurochemical changes affecting the GABA systems during alcohol withdrawal with those postulated to be involved in the mechanisms of epileptic seizures. It is evident that for several parameters the changes are similar in both symptoms. More detailed discussion of these data follows.

1. GABA Levels

One difficulty in interpretation of data generated from measurements of brain GABA levels is that the data do not distinguish between the metabolic and the neurotransmitter pools of GABA in the CNS (Hoffman and Tabakoff, 1985).

Table 6   GABA Systems in Alcohol Withdrawal and Epileptic Seizures

Parameter	Alcohol withdrawal	Epileptic seizures
GABA levels	[↓], ↑ in brain ↓ or NC in CSF	[↓] in epileptic foci and CSF
GABA inhibitor injection	Exacerbate seizure scores	Induce seizures
GABA agonists injection	Antagonize seizures	Antagonize seizures
Sodium valproate treatment	Antagonize seizures	Antagonize seizures
GABA receptor binding	$[↓]B^{max}$ and/or K^d; $↑B^{max}$	↑, ↓, or NC depending on brain regions or types of seizures
BZD receptor binding	Central type NC Peripheral type $↑B^{max}$; NC K^d	[↓] in seizure-sensitive animals Central type [↑] or NC after seizures Peripheral type $↑K^d$ after seizures

Key: ↑ = increase; ↓ = decrease; NC = no change. Highlighted changes (in brackets) are those deemed more likely to occur.

Reports have appeared which showed either increased or decreased levels of GABA in the brain during or after alcohol withdrawal (Hoffman and Tabakoff, 1985; Pohorecky and Brick, 1988). For example, a maximal decrease in GABA levels in mouse brain at hour 8 after alcohol withdrawal was reported to coincide with the occurrence of peak withdrawal symptoms (Pohorecky and Brick, 1988). However, in another study (Chan et al., 1982), decreased GABA levels were found in mice at hour 4, but not at hour 8, after ethanol withdrawal even though handling-induced seizures occurred for at least up to hour 10. Alcoholics who had seizures during withdrawal had lower GABA levels in the CSF than those who had no seizures, but control subjects who did not have seizures also had low CSF GABA levels; in another study, GABA levels in CSF were not changed in alcohol withdrawal (Pohorecky and Brick, 1988). Other investigators have reported that alcoholics had lower plasma GABA levels compared to control subjects (Coffman and Petty, 1985). The plasma samples were obtained 24–48 hours after admission. Thus, the alcoholic subjects would still have been undergoing withdrawal. These investigators assumed that plasma GABA levels reflected brain GABA activity, but such an assumption may not be justified.

Injections of GABA inhibitors, such as picrotoxin, exacerbated seizure scores (a numerical system to quantitate the severity of withdrawal seizures), while injections of GABA agonists, such as aminooxyacetic acid and muscimol, attenuated seizure scores (Fadda et al., 1985; Pohorecky and Brick, 1988; Wilkins and Gorelick, 1986). Likewise, compounds that elevated GABA levels, such as the anticonvulsant N-dipropylacetate (sodium valproate), had the same effect on seizures. The fall of GABA levels (18%) in the brain stem during withdrawal could be antagonized by ethanol (Pohorecky and Brick, 1988).

Several investigators have reviewed the literature indicating that increases in GABA levels led to seizure protection and decreases in GABA levels elicited convulsive activity in human and experimental models of epilepsy (Fariello, 1985; Gale, 1985; Sherwin and Van Gelder, 1986). Gale (1985) showed that the ability of GABA-elevating agents to protect against maximal electroshock seizures was directly correlated with an increase in GABA specifically in the nerve-terminal compartment of substantia nigra. In amygdala-kindled rats, GABA synthesis was reduced in the stimulated amygdala and in corpus striatum and substantia nigra (Loscher and Schwark, 1987). Similarly, in the rat kindling model of epilepsy a significant decrease in the number of GABA immunoreactive positive cell bodies was found in the stimulated CA1 region of the rat hippocampus compared to the contralateral unstimulated side (Kamphuis et al., 1986). A single convulsion induced by electroshock or flurothyl resulted in an inhibition of GABA release, which, in turn, inhibited GABA synthesis (Green et al., 1987b,c).

2. GABA Receptors

Most animal studies reported a decrease in number and/or affinity of GABA receptors in selective brain areas after chronic alcohol treatment and/or withdrawal (Hoffman and Tabakoff, 1985; Hunt, 1985). The decrease in binding appeared to coincide with the maximal severity of withdrawal symptoms. These changes could lead to a decrease in efficacy of GABA transmission. Elevated GABA binding was reported in postmortem samples from alcoholics compared to controls (Pohorecky and Brick, 1988).

Olsen and colleagues (1986) summarized the following evidence concerning the involvement of GABA receptors in epileptic seizures. In a monkey model of epilepsy, brain lesions induced by alumina cream had lower GABA receptor binding compared to that in the unlesioned side. Surgical biopsy samples containing epileptic foci had lower GABA binding than nonfocal samples. GABA receptor binding was lower in mice (DBA/2J) that are susceptible to audiogenic seizures when compared to nonsusceptible mice (C57BL/6). Analogously, the same finding was reported in certain brain regions of the genetically epilepsy-prone rats. In amygdala-kindled rats GABA receptor binding was decreased in amygdala and substantia nigra but significantly increased in the striatum (Loscher and Schwark, 1987); the neurochemical changes found in this study were from animals that had had their final seizure one week earlier. Therefore, these changes were unlikely to be due to postictal events, but rather they were relevant to kindling itself.

In the cobalt-induced epileptic focus, GABA receptor binding was decreased, but not in the perifocal area (Pitkanen et al., 1987). In contrast, GABA receptor binding was reported to be increased in one area of the hippocampus 24 hours after the last kindled seizure (Shin et al., 1985). This finding may reflect a strengthening of the endogenous anticonvulsant process in the refractory period (Loscher and Schwark, 1987). Recently, Santori and Collins (1988) reported that cortical kindling which triggered sensorimotor seizures did not alter GABA receptor binding within local and long circuits connected to the focus. Failure of the subjects to display "mature" seizures was cited as one of the reasons for the negative finding.

3. Benzodiazepine Receptors

Very few studies examined benzodiazepine (BZD) binding during ethanol withdrawal, or, in particular, during withdrawal seizures. A study of currently drinking alcoholics showed that these subjects had a significant reduction in the density of peripheral-type BZD binding sites in platelets, as measured by the ligand PK 11195 (Suranyi-Cadotte et al., 1988). This effect disappeared following abstention from alcohol, but no information was available on the same parameter in alcoholics undergoing alcohol withdrawal. Nevertheless, mice and rats that had developed physical dependence on ethanol showed increases in B_{max} but not dissociation constant (K_d) in the binding of the peripheral-type receptors in different brain regions (Syapin and Alkana, 1988; Tamborska and Marangos, 1986); the increases were also seen during withdrawal, and in one study the effects persisted for three days after cessation of ethanol administration (Tamborska and Marangos, 1986). In these studies, there were no changes in the binding of central-type BZD receptors. An increase in BZD receptor binding material was found in urine from alcoholics during withdrawal (Sandler et al., 1984). This led investigators to suggest that the substance may be an endogenous BZD inverse agonist, which could account for the alcohol withdrawal syndrome. If this were true, the BZD antagonist Ro15-1788 would be expected to decrease the severity of alcohol withdrawal reactions. However, investigators were unable to demonstrate an effect of Ro15-1788 on alcohol withdrawal seizures in animals (Adinoff et al., 1986; Little et al., 1985).

A 30% deficit in BZD receptor binding was observed in the midbrain of seizure-sensitive gerbils relative to normal controls (Olsen et al., 1986). This was shown by autoradiography to involve a decrease in the number of binding sites in the substantia nigra and periaqueductal gray areas. Several studies (reviewed by Morin and Wasterlain, 1983) have shown that BZD receptor binding was increased (B_{max} increase) 15 minutes after a single electroshock or pentylenetetra-zol-induced seizure and 24 hours after a large number of electroshock seizures. However, no change in BZD binding was observed in a mouse model of status epilepticus (Morin and Wasterlain, 1983). Likewise, BZD receptor binding was found to be unaltered when human epileptic foci from the cortex were compared with nonspiking cortex (Sherwin et al., 1986). Using a rat model of spontaneous petit mal–like seizures, Hariton and colleagues (1988) found no difference in the binding of the central-type BZD receptors in the cortex, cerebellum, and hippocampus between epileptic and nonepileptic animals. However, there were increases (125–150%) in the Kd of the peripheral-type BZD receptors in the same brain regions of epileptic rats.

C. Glutamate

Physiologically relevant concentrations ($<$ 50 mM) of ethanol stimulated binding to glutamate receptors, but binding was decreased at higher concentrations (Hoffman and Tabakoff, 1985; Hunt, 1985). Chronic exposure to ethanol also resulted in enhanced glutamate binding, irrespective of whether the measurements were made before or one day after withdrawal (Hunt, 1985). In mice, handling-induced seizures during alcohol withdrawal were attenuated by the glutamate receptor antagonist glutamate diethyl ester. During withdrawal, the mice were more sensitive to seizures induced by kainic acid (a glutamate agonist) than those induced by pentylenetetrazol (Hunt, 1985). These data suggest that chronic ethanol treatment caused the mice to develop supersensitivity to glutamate (Hunt, 1985).

Farriello (1985) reviewed evidence (summarized below) linking glutamate to seizures. Some of the evidence is indirect; for example, systemic or topical application of glutamate induced seizures in animals. Glutamate antagonists exerted anticonvulsant effects in experimental models of epilepsy. Kainic acid, which binds to receptors for excitatory amino acid, induced prolonged status epilepticus in animals. Excessive release of glutamate had been demonstrated in the genesis of partial seizures in the cobalt model. This might cause a decrease in tissue content of glutamate, which was observed in human epileptogenic foci. Glutamic acid dehydrogenase activity was increased in the spiking cortex of epileptic patients (Sherwin et al., 1986). The hypothesis that a hyperfunctioning glutamate system is involved in the genesis of seizures needs to be further investigated.

D. Catecholamines

1. Dopamine

Conflicting data have been reported on dopamine (DA) receptor binding following chronic ethanol administration, with reports of no change, increase, and decrease (Hoffman and Tabakoff, 1985; Hunt, 1985; Pohorecky and Brick, 1988). Differences in duration of ethanol treatment could have contributed to the conflicting data. In one study, chronic ethanol treatment for 21 days, but not for 14 days, caused a significant increase in B_{max} but not K_d of both D_1 and D_2 DA receptors (Hruska, 1988). The changes did not correlate with tolerance development and were not reversed after 24 hours of alcohol withdrawal. The relevance of this finding to the neurochemical basis of alcohol withdrawal seizures remains to be determined. Several studies have suggested that dopaminergic subsensitivity developed after chronic ethanol treatment and withdrawal (Dar and Wooles, 1984; Hoffman and Tabakoff, 1985; Hunt, 1985). However, increased DA turnover and supersensitivity have also been reported. Alcoholics showing withdrawal symptoms had reduced CSF levels of homovanillic acid (HVA), the major metabolite of DA, compared to those not having symptoms (Hoffman and Tabakoff, 1985). However, alcoholics having delirium tremens had increased CSF levels of HVA (Banki and Molnar, 1981). A correlation between CSF levels of HVA and clinical symptoms of alcohol withdrawal in humans has been reported (Borg et al., 1986); however, HVA levels in alcoholics were not different from those of controls between days 2 and 8 of alcohol withdrawal. The use of medication in alcoholics might have masked any existing difference. Mixed results have also been reported regarding the effects of bromocriptine, a DA agonist, on alcohol withdrawal signs, with report of amelioration and no change (Burroughs et al., 1985; Hoffman and Tabakoff, 1985; Hunt, 1985; Pohorecky and Brick, 1988). Serum DA beta-hydroxylase activity did not correlate with the severity of withdrawal symptoms (Bagdy and Arato, 1987).

Data concerning a role of DA in the regulation of seizure disorders are at best circumstantial (reviewed by Burley and Ferrendelli, 1984; Killam and Killam, 1984; Marrosu et al., 1983; McNamara, 1984). Chlorpromazine, a potent DA antagonist, induced EEG activation in epileptic patients and increased the incidence and severity of seizures in epileptic baboons. However, this drug also affected other neurotransmitter systems. Conflicting data exist concerning the ability of DA agonists (e.g., apomorphine) to block different kinds of epileptic seizures.

2. Norepinephrine

It has been suggested that the hyperexcitability state during alcohol withdrawal may in part be due to increases in the turnover of norepinephrine (NE) in both brain and peripheral tissues (Hoffman and Tabakoff, 1985; Pohorecky and Brick, 1988). During alcohol withdrawal, alcoholics had elevated CSF levels of NE and 3-methoxy-4-hydroxyphenyl glycol (MHPG), a primary metabolite of NE (Hawley et al., 1985; Pohorecky and Brick, 1988; Wilkins and Gorelick, 1986). Plasma MHPG levels were also elevated (Nutt et al., 1988). It remains to

be investigated whether the adrenergic hyperactivity seen during alcohol withdrawal is a determinant of severity of withdrawal or a simple reflection of the
stress of withdrawal. The former possibility is favored by some investigators
(Airaksinen and Peura, 1987). However, pharmacological studies in animals have
shown that the severity of handling seizures during withdrawal was increased by
drugs that decrease noradrenergic function (e.g., propranolol). In contrast, in
alcoholics propranolol and atenolol were found to decrease some but not all
withdrawal symptoms (Gottlieb, 1988; Kraus et al., 1985; Pohorecky and Brick,
1988). Similarly, the alpha$_2$-adrenoceptor agonist clonidine was efficacious in
treating some symptoms of alcohol withdrawal in humans (Baumgartner and
Rowen, 1987; Manhem et al., 1985; Pohorecky and Brick, 1988; Wilkins et al.,
1983) and animals (Parale and Kulkarni, 1986; Wilkins and Gorelick, 1986).

Data on the effect of lesions of the noraderenergic system on severity of
ethanol withdrawal seizures were conflicting, with reports of no effect or increased seizure activity (Clemmesen et al., 1985). Valverius and colleagues
(1987) stressed that ethanol may produce changes in beta-adrenergic receptor
number by a mechanism other than an increase in NE turnover; the effect of
ethanol on the interaction of guanine nucleotide-binding protein (Gs) with the
beta-adrenergic receptor needs to be considered (Saito et al., 1987). These investigators found that after chronic ethanol diet treatment and at the time of
ethanol withdrawal the beta-adrenergic receptors were "uncoupled" from Gs.
Their results indicate that after seven days of chronic ethanol intake, mice
showed a small but significant decrease in agonist-binding sites without a concomitant change in the number of antagonist-binding sites.

Many studies have shown that the central noradrenergic system normally retards the development of different types of seizures (Barry et al., 1987; Burley
and Ferrendelli, 1984; Killam and Killam, 1984; McNamara, 1984). Innate deficits in NE may be one of the causes of seizures in genetically determined epilepsy-prone rats (Laird et al., 1984). Rats were made hypersensitive to hippocampal kindling by lesion of the central catecholamine system; when a suspen-
sion of NE-rich cells from the locus coeruleus region of rat fetuses was grafted
bilaterally into the hippocampus, the onset and progression of kindling-induced
epilepsy were markedly suppressed (Barry et al., 1987). Depletion of NE in
selected parts of the brain by agents such as 6-hydroxydopamine or reserpine
increased the incidence and susceptibility to seizures (Burley and Ferrendelli,
1984; Racine and McIntyre, 1986). Phentolamine, an antagonist of alpha-NE-
receptors, lowered the threshold for maximal electroshock seizures, while propranolol, an antagonist of beta-NE receptors, decreased thresholds of pentylenetetrazol seizures (Burley and Ferrendelli, 1984). Elevation of brain NE
levels by pharmacological manipulations appeared to elevate seizure thresholds
for certain types of epilepsy, but the data were equivocal because the agents

used also affected DA levels (Burley and Ferrendelli, 1984). Nevertheless, more recent data indicates that the NE system is more important than the DA system in modulating kindling rates (Racine and McIntyre, 1986). Other data also seem to support the concept that increased NE influence in the CNS has an anticonvulsant effect (reviewed by Burley and Ferrendelli, 1984). A reduction in the number of alpha$_1$-adrenoceptors has been found in human epileptogenic foci and in frontal cortex of interictal genetically epilepsy-prone rats (Nicoletti et al., 1986; Sherwin et al., 1986).

E. Acetylcholine

After chronic ethanol treatment rats showed an increase in stimulated acetylcholine (ACh) release, a decreased inhibitory response to ethanol, and reduced brain ACh levels (Hoffman and Tabakoff, 1985; Pohorecky and Brick, 1988). The binding of quinuclidinyl benzylate (QNB), an antagonist to muscarinic ACh receptors, was increased in the hippocampus and cortex but not in the striatum of ethanol-treated mice at the time of withdrawal and at hour 8 after withdrawal (Hoffman and Tabakoff, 1985). These changes may have been related to certain signs of physical dependence on ethanol (Hoffman and Tabakoff, 1985). Other studies did not find any change in QNB binding after chronic treatment; the length of ethanol exposure might have been a determining factor (Hunt, 1985). In one study where an increase in striatal ACh receptors was observed during ethanol withdrawal, rats that had withdrawal seizures had less of an increase than those that had no seizures (Hoffman and Tabakoff, 1985). Intrahippocampal injection of the cholinesterase inhibitor physostigmine in rats that otherwise only showed mild alcohol withdrawal signs elicited seizure activity in 80% of the animals. In contrast, seizure activity was elicited in only 30% of control animals (Gonzalez, 1985). The data suggest that some of the symptoms of ethanol withdrawal may be related to an increase in sensitivity of hippocampal neurons to cholinergic stimulation. Rats with alcohol withdrawal seizures were very sensitive to nicotine tremor (Airaksinen and Peura, 1987). Long-term ethanol treatment resulted in a decrease in the number of binding sites for nicotine ACh receptors in the hippocampus but an increase of nicotine binding sites in the hypothalamus and thalamus (Hoffman and Tabakoff, 1985; Pohorecky and Brick, 1988). The significance of these changes needs to be further investigated. In postmortem brain samples of alcoholics there was no change in nicotinic receptors, but a decline in the number of muscarinic receptors compared to control samples (Pohorecky and Brick, 1988).

Data from topical epilepsy indicate that ACh may be involved in seizure disorders (reviewed by Craig, 1984). For example, decreased levels of ACh, choline acetyltransferase (CAT), and acetylcholinesterase (AChE) were found in the tissue adjacent to focal epilepsy. Inhibitors of choline esterase have anticonvulsant effects. Intrastriatal injection of a subconvulsive dose of carbachol, a cholinergic agonist, decreased the seizure threshold in premotor cortical seizures (Ono et al., 1987). In the kindling model of epilepsy, the rate of development of amygdaloid kindling was retarded by atropine, a muscarinic antagonist (McNamara, 1984). Muscarinic ACh receptors were decreased transiently in numbers in the brains of kindled rats, but no long-term alterations in B_{max} and K_d have been found (McNamara, 1984; Morin and Wasterlain, 1983). McNamara (1984) suggested that the kindling phenomenon cannot be accounted for by modifications of cholinergic neuronal communication.

F. Serotonin

No coherent picture has emerged regarding the chronic effects of ethanol on serotonin (5-HT) (Hunt, 1985; Pohorecky and Brick, 1988). Hunt (1985) postulated that supersensitivity of 5-HT-2 receptors may occur after chronic ethanol treatment. The hypothesis was based on the similarity between symptoms of behavioral hyperactivity (e.g., tremor and aberrant head movements) resulting from stimulation of 5-HT-2 receptors and those observed in animals during ethanol withdrawal. More investigations are needed to test this hypothesis. Pharmacological manipulations of the 5-HT system have produced conflicting results regarding whether such treatments affected ethanol withdrawal. For instance, methysergide, a 5-HT antagonist, increased the number of handling-induced seizures during alcohol withdrawal in one study but not in others (Hunt, 1985). Another study reported that head twitches occurring during withdrawal were antagonized by 5-HT antagonists (Hunt, 1985; Pohorecky and Brick, 1988). In humans, disorientation and hallucination during delirium tremens seemed to be determined mostly by elevation of CSF levels of 5-hydroxy-indoleacetic acid (5HIAAA), a major metabolite of 5-HT (Banki and Molnar, 1981). However, it is not certain whether CSF 5HIAA levels correlated with the occurrence of withdrawal seizures.

Pharmacological and pathophysiological investigations support the hypothesis that serotonergic defects are determinants of both seizure severity and susceptibility in the genetically epilepsy-prone rat (reviewed by Jobe et al., 1986). For instance, drugs that induced 5-HT decrements enhanced seizure severity, whereas those that caused 5-HT increments reduced seizure severity. Similarly, depletion of 5-HT or blockade of 5-HT receptors caused a marked decrease in maximal electroshock (MES) seizure thresholds. The precursor to 5-HT, 5-hydroxytryptophan, could elevate MES and PTZ seizure thresholds (McNamara, 1984) but had no anticonvulsant effects in epileptic gerbils and amygdaloid-kindled rats (Loscher and Czuczwar, 1985). The anticonvulsant effect of 5-hydroxytryptophan against electroconvulsions in rats could be attenuated by the 5-HT-2 receptor antagonist ketanserin (Loscher and Czuczar, 1985). These data suggest that

5-HT-2 receptors may be involved in this anticonvulsant effect. A single electro-convulsive shock (ECS) in rats did not elicit any change in either the spontaneous or K^+-evoked release of 5-HT from cortex slices either 30 minutes or 24 hours later (Green et al., 1987a). In contrast, after repeated ECS and 24 hours after the last treatment, K^+-evoked release of 5-HT was inhibited by 84%. Green and colleagues (1987a) suggested that the 5-HT changes might be involved in the enhanced 5-HT-receptor function seen after repeated ECS.

G. Calcium

Adaptations involving the calcium (Ca) system have been proposed as biochemical bases for the development of tolerance to, and physical dependence on, ethanol (Dolin et al., 1987; Hudspith et al., 1987; Littleton, 1984; Lynch et al., 1986; Messing et al., 1986). For example, an adaptive change was to increase the sensitivity of the neurotransmitter release process to Ca^{2+}, opposing the inhibitory effect of ethanol on Ca^{2+} entry. Another example was an increase in the number of voltage-operated Ca^{2+} channels, which would tend to decrease extracellular Ca^{2+} levels. When ethanol is suddenly withdrawn, the decreases in extracellular Ca^{2+} may precipitate epileptic seizures (Heinemann and Hamon, 1986). Ca^{2+} channel antagonists such as nitrendipine and verapamil had significant attenuating effects on alcohol withdrawal seizures (De Sarro et al., 1988; Little et al., 1986). Another Ca^{2+} channel blocker, caroverine, was found to be as effective as meprobamate in treating acute alcohol withdrawal (Koppi et al., 1987).

Literature dealing with the role of Ca in the genesis of epileptic seizures has been reviewed (Heinemann and Hamon, 1986; Heinemann et al., 1986). Basically, both acutely induced and chronic epilepsies are associated with an increased Ca^{2+} uptake into neurons. This leads to a decrease in extracellular Ca^{2+} and a rise in extracellular potassium, which may facilitate the initiation and spreading as well as the maintenance of ictal activity. The Ca^{2+} channel blocker caroverine is reputed to be effective against some forms of epileptic seizures (Koppi et al., 1987). Oral administration of nimodipine, a Ca^{2+} antagonist, arrested seizures induced by several methods in rabbits (Meyer et al., 1987).

H. Adenosine

A possible role of adenosine (Ad) in the CNS actions of ethanol has been suggested (Dar et al., 1983). For example, pretreatment of mice with theophylline, an antagonist of Ad, before acute ethanol administration markedly reduced the duration of ethanol sleep time and also decreased the intensity and duration of motor incoordination (Dar et al., 1983). Similar results were obtained with dipyridamole, a blocker of Ad re-uptake. When cultured neuroblastoma–glioma hybrid cells were exposed chronically to ethanol, the cells developed tolerance to the ethanol-induced increase in Ad receptor-stimulated cAMP levels; "physical dependence" was evident by reduced Ad-stimulated cAMP levels in the absence of ethanol (Gordon et al., 1986). The same two phenomena were also demonstrated in lymphocytes from alcoholics (Diamond et al., 1987). After chronic ethanol treatment (10 days) in rats, there was an apparent increase (28%) in the number of brain Ad receptors, but the result was not statistically significant. The number of Ad receptors and the dissociation constant were reduced 40% at hours 24 and 48 after withdrawal and returned to prewithdrawal levels at hour 72 (Dar et al., 1983). It is not certain whether these changes were partly responsible for the hyperexcitable state during alcohol withdrawal.

Data are available to indicate that Ad may act as an endogenous anticonvulsant (Ault and Wang, 1986; Burley and Ferrendelli, 1984). For instance, injection of Ad prolonged the refractory period between the first and second MES. Dipyridamole, an Ad uptake inhibitor, has the same effect as Ad. Stable analogues of Ad could delay the onset of PTZ seizures, and theophylline, an Ad antagonist, enhanced the incidence of seizures with subconvulsant doses of PTZ (Burley and Ferrendelli, 1984). Rosen and Berman (1987) found that the phenylisopropyl derivative of Ad (PIA) had potent anticonvulsant effects on kindled seizures in the amygdala, hippocampus, and caudate nucleus, but the N-ethylcarboxyindo derivative of Ad (NECA) had an effect only in the caudate nucleus. They suggested that PIA probably acted via the A_1-Ad receptors, while NECA acted via the A_2-Ad receptors.

I. Sodium- and Postassium-Activated Adenosine Triphosphatase

The inhibition of sodium- and potassium-activated adenoside triphosphate (Na^+/K^+-ATPase) activity by ethanol was enhanced in the presence of very low concentrations of NE (Hoffman and Tabakoff, 1985; Pohorecky and Brick, 1988). Chronic ethanol exposure reduced the sensitivity of Na^+/K^+-ATPase to NE (Swann, 1987). Conflicting results have been reported for the effect of chronic ethanol treatment on Na^+/K^+-ATPase, with some studies reporting no change and other studies reporting increased activity (Pohorecky and Brick, 1988). The enzyme activity was elevated during ethanol withdrawal (12–48 hours after termination of ethanol treatment), with peak increase at 24 hours. This increase in ATPase activity has been postulated to be secondary to NE release as a result of stress during ethanol withdrawal (Pohorecky and Brick, 1988).

Since one of the vital functions of Na^+/K^+-ATPase is to maintain the ionic gradients for both Na^+ and K^+ across neuronal membranes, this enzyme is expected to be affected by seizure activities. Thus, Na^+/K^+-ATPase has been found to be decreased in actively spiking human cerebral cortex (Sherwin and Van Gelder, 1986). Extracellular concentrations of K^+ rose after repetitive electrical stimulation, a change that has been suggested to contribute to the generation and spread of epileptic activity (Heinemann et al., 1986). The anticonvulsant phenytoin inhibited Na^+/K^+-ATPase when given acutely in rats; chronic administration of phenytoin markedly increased glial Na^+/K^+-ATPase, but slightly decreased neuronal ATPase (White et al., 1985).

J. Opiates and Hormones

1. Opioid Peptides

There have been reports of increased or decreased synthesis and release of beta-endorphin–like peptides from the pituitary after chronic ethanol treatment (Hoffman and Tabakoff, 1985; Pohorecky and Brick, 1988). The conflicting data may be due to factors such as different means of ethanol administration, which impart different levels of stress to the animals, inconsistencies in analytical methods, and limitations imposed by in vitro studies of neuropeptides. Conflicting results have also been reported for plasma levels of beta-endorphins in chronic alcoholics, with data showing normal, high, or low levels (Brambilla et al., 1988). Reduced CSF levels of beta-endorphin and possibly a trend toward lower CSF levels of enkephalin have been reported in chronic alcoholics (Hoffman and Tabakoff, 1985). The opioid antagonist naloxone or naltrexone has been reported to block the effects of ethanol on locomotor activity and duration of loss of righting reflex, but not other ethanol-induced behavioral decrements (Hoffman and Tabakoff, 1985; Hunt, 1985). However, some studies did not confirm these findings (Hatch and Jernigan, 1988). Similarly, conflicting results have been reported regarding the effectiveness of these two opiate antagonists in reversing ethanol-induced coma or preventing the symptoms of ethanol intoxication (Hoffman and Tabakoff, 1985; Hunt, 1985).

The effects of naloxone on the severity of ethanol withdrawal reactions have been investigated, with reports of no effect and reduction of withdrawal seizures (Hunt, 1985; Kotlinska and Langwinski, 1986, 1987). More consistent results were obtained if naloxone was administered daily during the development of ethanol dependence and also at the time of ethanol withdrawal; under these conditions, withdrawal seizures were reduced significantly (Berman et al., 1984; Kotlinska and Langwinski, 1987). Audiogenic seizures during ethanol withdrawal could be blocked by delta opioid agonists such as [leu] -enkephalin and a synthetic analogue of [met] -enkephalin (Kotlinska and Langwinski, 1986). A neuropeptide, delta sleep-inducing peptide (DSIP), which has been postulated to possess an agonistic activity on opiate receptors, was efficacious in diminishing some clinical signs of opiate and alcohol withdrawal in humans (Dick et al., 1984). However, no data are available to indicate that DSIP is useful in preventing withdrawal seizures.

In general, in vitro ethanol decreased binding to delta receptors (high affinity for enkephalin), increased mu receptor binding (high affinity for morphine), and did not affect kappa receptor binding (Hoffman and Tabakoff, 1985; Hunt, 1985; Pohorecky and Brick, 1988). The changes in binding have been attributed to alterations in affinity for ligands or in the number of receptors (Hoffman and Tabakoff, 1985). The time course of the changes in mμ receptor affinity and the changes in function of opiate receptors in control of DA release did not correlate well with that of overt withdrawal symptoms (Hoffman and Tabakoff, 1985). Most in vitro studies involved very high ethanol concentrations (100–1000 mM). Therefore, the significance of the data for in vivo situations is questionable.

Bajorek et al. (1984) suggested that a general role of endogenous opioid peptides in the epilepsies is their release following seizures in the gerbil and kindling models, which tends to limit further seizures and excitability. A recent review summarized data which indicate that postictal motor deficits following amygdaloid-kindled seizures may be mediated by mμ and kappa opioid receptors (Caldecott-Hazard and Engel, 1987). Additionally, kindling-induced postictal seizure suppression may be mediated by kappa receptors and perhaps also by mμ receptors. The predominant actions of exogenously applied opiates and opioid-like peptides are their anticonvulsant effects (Bajorek et al., 1984; Gale, 1985).

2. Hormones

Alcoholics undergoing withdrawal often show changes in blood levels of several hormones (Camerlingo et al., 1986; Wilkins and Gorelick, 1986). For example, there have been reports of increases in adrenal-corticotropic hormone (ACTH), cortisol, and vasopressin, as well as decreases in prolactin, the thyroid-stimulating hormone (TSH) response to thyrotropin-releasing hormone (TRH), and the growth hormone (GH) response to insulin-induced hypoglycemia. Blunted responses of GH to seizures (Culebras et al., 1987), clonidine (Nutt et al., 1988), apomorphine (Balldin et al., 1985), and L-tryptophan (Nutt et al., 1988) have also been reported. The hormonal changes are probably due to the brain's responses to the chronic effects of ethanol and to the stress of alcohol withdrawal. Some of these changes are longlasting; e.g., the blunted response of TSH to TRH has been reported to be still detectable after two years of abstinence from alcohol (Wilkins and Gorelick, 1986). Therefore, these changes are not likely to be the causes of the appearance of withdrawal signs.

Hormone levels of GH, cortisol, and prolactin were significantly increased within 1 hour postictally of generalized convulsions, with recovery to control levels within 24 hours (Culebras et al., 1987). These elevations in hormonal levels were significantly higher than the stress-induced increases in cortisol and prolactin; there was no stress-induced increase in GH (Culebras et al., 1987).

ACTH is well known for its use in the treatment of infantile spasm. It has also been found to have anticonvulsant effects in kindling seizures and, to a certain extent, in the gerbil model of epilepsy (Bajorek et al., 1984). Recently, Matsumoto and colleagues (1987) reported that TRH may also be used to treat infantile spasms. These data are in line with the finding that intracerebroventricular administration of TRH suppressed seizure development of amygdaloid kindling (Kajita et al., 1987). The same investigators found that immunoreactive TRH increased markedly in the amygdaloid/pyriform cortex and hippocampus 24 and 48 hours after the last kindled seizure and returned to control levels three weeks later. There were also longlasting (21 days) increases in striatal TRH binding sites within 24 hours after seizures stopped. The investigators suggested that these changes might be related to susceptibility to kindled seizures. Contrary to the reported anticonvulsant effect of TRH, intraventricularly injected TRH has been shown to have a convulsant effect in the gerbil model of epilepsy (Bajorek et al., 1984). The relationship of TRH and ACTH to different seizure states needs to be further investigated.

K. Cyclic Nucleotide System

1. Cyclic AMP

In general, acute ethanol treatment in animals and alcohol ingestion in alcoholics resulted in a decrease in brain cyclic AMP (cAMP) levels (Hoffman and Tabakoff, 1985; Pohorecky and Brick, 1988). Chronic ethanol treatment resulted in either increased or decreased levels of cAMP and the same phenomena persisted during ethanol withdrawal (Hoffman and Tabakoff, 1985; Hunt, 1985). These findings may be related to changes of the cAMP system in response to increases in NE turnover during alcohol withdrawal (Wilkins and Gorelick, 1986). However, a direct relationship between brain or CSF levels of cAMP and withdrawal seizures has not been established. Alcoholics undergoing delirium tremens had reduced CSF levels of cAMP (Hoffman and Tabakoff, 1985). During this phase of alcohol withdrawal occurrence of seizures is uncommon (Naranjo and Sellers, 1986).

2. Cyclic GMP

Acute ethanol treatment generally decreased cyclic GMP (cGMP) levels, especially in the cerebellum, and the levels remained reduced during chronic ethanol intake (Hoffman and Tabakoff, 1985; Hunt, 1985; Pohorecky and Brick, 1988). Alcoholics undergoing delirium tremens had increased CSF levels of cGMP (Hoffman and Tabakoff, 1985). Dibutyryl cGMP, when injected into the ventricular system of the brain, enhanced ethanol withdrawal–induced twitches in mice, but a similar injection of dibutyryl cAMP reduced the head twitches (Hunt, 1985).

Several convulsant drugs and stimuli elevated CNS levels of cAMP and/or cGMP (Ferrendelli, 1983). Seizures also produced elevations in cyclic nucleotides, with increases of cAMP occurring only after the onset of epileptiform EEG discharges or clinically evident seizures, and elevations of cGMP occurring prior to the onset of seizures. Antiepileptic drugs such as phenytoin and phenobarbital blocked the seizure-induced or depolarization-induced accumulation of both cAMP and cGMP (Ferrendelli, 1983). The seizure-induced increase in cAMP was probably the result of activation of adenylate cyclases by NE and Ad which were released by seizure discharges. On the other hand, the accumulation of cGMP was probably due to activation of guanylate cyclase by the increases in intracellular Ca^{2+} during seizure discharges (Ferrendelli, 1983).

VI. SUMMARY

Although our knowledge of the mechanisms of epileptic seizures is still incomplete, several neurochemical parameters, outlined in this chapter, have been proposed as being involved in mediating the development, maintenance, and cessation of seizures. The relationship between the phenomenon of sudden unexplained death in epilepsy and the use of alcohol is unknown. However, it is known that alcohol use is associated with an increased risk of autonomic dysfunction and seizure. It is also clear that no single neurochemical system can adequately explain the complex nature of epileptic seizures. The same conclusion applies to the neurochemical mechanisms of alcohol withdrawal reactions. This is because there are complex dynamic interactions among the neurotransmitter and neuromodulator systems in the brain. Interpretations of neurochemical correlates of withdrawal seizures are hampered by our incomplete knowledge of these complex interactions, the neurochemical bases of tolerance and physical dependence, and the mechanisms underlying the genesis of epileptic seizures. Another complicating factor is that occurrence of withdrawal seizures is only one component of the withdrawal syndrome. The challenge is to separate the neurochemical changes that may trigger seizures from those that are the result of seizures or other withdrawal reactions, particularly those caused by stress. Since only 2-15% of alcoholics in withdrawal develop seizures, it is unlikely that the probability of having withdrawal seizures depends solely on neurochemical factors. This is not to exclude the important contributions of the quantity and duration of alcohol abuse in the causation of withdrawal seizures. Rather, the important point to stress is that a host of other factors can also determine the likelihood of an alcoholic to have seizures during withdrawal. These factors include the individual's genetic makeup, seizure threshold, health status, malnutrition, polydrug abuse, histories of epilepsy, and prior alcohol withdrawal seizures and trauma.

Despite difficulties in data interpretation outlined above, some of the neurochemical changes associated with ethanol withdrawal are similar to those postulated to be involved in the mechanisms of epileptic seizures. Strong similarities are found in changes involving Ca^{++} and the GABA-BZD-Cl⁻ ionophore complex, while fewer correlations can be found in alterations involving Ad, opiates, 5-HT, and ACh. These correlations suggest but do not prove a possible role of one or more of these systems in withdrawal seizures. The availability of specially bred strains of mice which differ in severity of alcohol withdrawal seizures (Kosobud and Crabbe, 1986) and rodents that differ in the susceptibility to epileptic seizures, as well as various experimental models of epilepsy, are particularly useful in testing the hypothesis that the neurochemical systems mentioned in this chapter are involved in alcohol withdrawal seizures.

ACKNOWLEDGMENTS

The authors thank Darlene Spino, Michelle Spino, and Carol Tixier for skillful typing and Donna L. Schanley for proofreading.

REFERENCES

Abbasakoor, A., Beanlands, D. S., and MacLeod, S. M. (1976). Electrocardiographic changes during ethanol withdrawal. *Ann. N.Y. Acad. Sci. 173*:364–370.

Adams, J. H., Graham, D. I., Murray, L. S., and Scott, G. (1982). Diffuse axonal injury due to nonmissle head injury in humans: An analysis of 45 cases. *Ann. Neurol. 12*:557–563.

Adinoff, B., Majchrowicz, E., Martin, P. R., and Linnoila, M. (1986). The benzodiazepine antagonist Ro15-1788 does not antagonize the ethanol withdrawal syndrome. *Biol. Psychiatr. 21*:643–649.

Airaksinen, M. M., and Peura, P. (1987). Mechanisms of alcohol withdrawal syndrome. *Med. Biol. 65*:105–112.

Alexander, C. S. (1968). The concept of alcoholic myocardiopathy. *Med. Clin. North Am. 52*:1183–1191.

Altura, B. M., Altura, B. T., and Gebrewold, A. (1983). Alcohol-induced spasms of cerebral blood vessels: Relation to cerebrovascular accidents and sudden death. *Science 220*:331–333.

Alves, W. M., and Jane, J. A. (1985). Mild brain injury: Damage and outcome. In *Central Nervous System Trauma Status Report–1985*, D. P. Becker and J. T. Povlishock (Eds.). National Institutes of Health, Washington, D.C., pp. 255-270.

Ault, B., and Wang, C. M. (1986). Adenosine inhibits epileptiform activity arising in hippocampal area CA3. *Br. J. Pharmacol. 87*:695–703.

Bagdy, G., and Arato, M. (1987). Serum dopamine-β-hydroxylase activity and alcohol withdrawal symptoms. *Drug Alcohol Depend. 19*:45–50.

Bajorek, J. G., Lee, R. J., and Lomax, P. (1984). Neuropeptides: A role as endogenous mediators or modulators of epileptic phenomena. *Ann. Neurol. (Suppl) 16*:S31–S38.

Balldin, J., Alling, C., Gottfries, C. G., Lindstedt, G., and Langestrom, G. (1985). Changes in dopamine receptor sensitivity in humans after heavy alcohol intake. *Psychopharmacology 86*:142–146.

Banki, C. M., and Molnar, G. (1981). Cerebrospinal fluid amine metabolites in delirium tremens. *Psychiatria Clin. 14*:167–177.

Barry, D. I., Kikvadze, I., Brundin, P., Bolwig, T. G., Bjorklund, A., and Lindvall, O. (1987). Grafted noradrenergic neurons suppress seizure development in kindling-induced epilepsy. *Proc. Nat. Acad. Sci. USA 84*:8712–8715.

Baumgartner, G. R., and Rowen, R. C. (1987). Clonidine vs. chlordiazepoxide in the management of acute alcohol withdrawal syndrome. *Arch. Intern. Med. 147*:1223–1226.

Berman, R. F., Lee, J. A., Olson, K. L., and Goldman, M. S. (1984). Effects of naloxone on ethanol dependence in rats. *Drug Alcohol Depend. 13*:245–254.

Blankenhorn, M. A. (1945). The diagnosis of beri beri heart disease. *Ann. Intern. Med. 23*:398–404.

Borg, S., Kvande, H., and Valverius, P. (1986). Clinical conditions and central dopamine metabolism in alcoholics during acute withdrawal under treatment with different pharmacological agents. *Psychopharmacology 88*:12–17.

Brambilla, F., Zarattini, F., Gianelli, A., Bianchi, M., and Painerai, A. (1988). Plasma opioids in alcoholics after acute alcohol consumption and withdrawal. *Acta Psychiatr. Scand. 77*:63–66.

Brennan, F. N., and Lyttle, J. A. (1987). Alcohol and seizures: A review. *J. R. Soc. Med. 80*:571–573.

Brigden, W., and Robinson, J. (1964). Alcoholic heart disease. *Br. Med. J. 5420*: 1277–1289.

Brown, M. E., Anton, R. F., Malcolm, R., and Ballenger, J. C. (1988). Alcohol detoxification and withdrawal seizures: Clinical support of a kindling hypothesis. *Biol. Psychiatr. 23*:507–514.

Buckingham, T. A., Kennedy, H. L., Goenjian, A. K., Vasilomanolakis, E. C., Shriver, K. K., Sprague, M. K., and Lyyski, D. (1985). Cardiac arrhythmias in a population admitted to an acute alcoholic detoxification center. *Am. Heart J. 110*:961–965.

Burley, E. S., and Ferrendelli, J. A. (1984). Regulatory effects of neurotransmitters on electroshock and pentylenetetrazol seizures. *Fed. Proc. 43*:2521–2524.

Burroughs, A. K., Morgan, M. Y., and Sherlock, S. (1985). Double-blind controlled trial of bromocriptine, chlordiazepoxide and chlormethiazole for alcohol withdrawal symptoms. *Alcohol Alcoholism 20*:263–271.

Caldecott-Hazard, S., and Engel, J. (1987). Limbic postictal events: Anatomical substrates and opioid receptor involvement. *Prog. Neuro-Psychopharmacol. Biol. Psychiatr. 11*:389–418.

Camerlingo, M., Franceschi, M., Bottacchi, E., Truci, G., Sferrazza-Papa, A., and Mamoli, A. (1986). Neuroendocrinological abnormalities in chronic alcoholic men after withdrawal. *Neuroendocrinol. Lett. 8*:123–127.

Camps, F. E. (Ed.) (1976). *Gradwohl's Legal Medicine*. Year Book Medical, Chicago.

Carlsson, C., and Haggendal, J. (1967). Arterial noradrenaline levels after ethanol withdrawal. *Lancet 2*:889.

Chan, A. W. K. (1985). Alcoholism and epilepsy. *Epilepsia 26*:323–333.

Chan, A. W. K., Schanley, D. L., Leong, F. W., and Casbeer, D. (1982). Dissociation of tolerance and physical dependence after ethanol/chloridazepoxide intake. *Pharmacol. Biochem. Behav. 17*:1239–1244.

Cicero, T. J. (1980). Alcohol self-administration, tolerance and withdrawal in humans and animals: Theoretical and methodological issues. In *Alcohol Tolerance and Dependence*, H. Rigter and J. C. Crabbe (Eds.). Elsevier/North Holland, New York, pp. 1–51.

Clemmesen, L., Lindvall, O., Hemmingsen, R., Ingvar, M., and Bolwig, T. G. (1985). Convulsive and non-convulsive ethanol withdrawal behaviour in rats with lesions of the noradrenergic locus coeruleus system. *Brain Res. 346*:164–167.

Coffman, J. A. and Petty, F. (1985). Plasma GABA levels in chronic alcoholics. *Am. J. Psychiatr. 142*:1204–1205.

Conway, N. (1968). Hemodynamic effects of ethyl alcohol in patients with coronary heart disease. *Br. Heart J. 30*:638–644.

Cooper, S. D., and Sellers, E. M. (1974). Serum dopamine hydroxylase activity in alcohol withdrawal. *Proc. Can. Fed. Biol. Soc. 17*:120.

Craig, D. R. (1984). Evidence for a role of neurotransmitters in the mechanism of topical convulsant models. *Fed. Proc. 43*:2525–2528.

Craig, J. R., Johnson, L., Lundberg, G. D., Tattler, D., Edmonson, H. A., and McGah, S. (1980). An autopsy survey of clinical and anatomic diagnoses associated with alcoholism. *Arch. Path. Lab. Med. 104*:452–455.

Culebras, A., Miller, M., Bertram, L., and Koch, J. (1987). Differential response of growth hormone, cortisol, and prolactin to seizures and to stress. *Epilepsia 28*:564–570.

Dar, M. S., and Wooles, W. R. (1984). Striatal and hypothalamic neurotransmitter changes during ethanol withdrawal in mice. *Alcohol 1*:453–458.

Dar, M. S., Mustafa, S. J., and Wooles, W. R. (1983). Possible role of adenosine in the CNS effects of ethanol. *Life Sci. 33*:1363–1374.

De Sarro, G. B., Meldrum, B. S., and Nistico, G. (1988). Anticonvulsant effects of some calcium entry blockers in DBA/2 mice. *Br. J. Pharmacol. 93*:247–256.

Diamond, I., Wrubel, B., Estrin, W., and Gordon, A. (1987). Basal and adenosine receptor-stimulated levels of cAMP are reduced in lymphocytes from alcoholic patients. *Proc. Nat. Acad. Sci. USA 84*:1413–1416.

Dick, P., Costa, C., Fayolle, K., Grandjean, M. E., Khoshbeen, A., and Tissot, R. (1984). DSIP in the treatment of withdrawal syndromes from alcohol and opiates. *Eur. Neurol. 23*:364–371.

Dolin, S., Little, H., Hudspith, M., Pagonis, C., and Littleton, J. (1987). Increased dihydropyridine-sensitive calcium channels in rat brain may underlie ethanol physical dependence. *Neuropharmacology 26*:275–279.

Engle, J., Jr. (1983). Functional localization of epileptogenic lesions. *Trends Neurosci. 6*:660–665.

Espir, M. L. E., and Rose, F. C. (1987). Alcohol, seizures and epilepsy. *J. R. Soc. Med. 80*:542–543.

Evans, W. (1964). Alcoholic myocardiopathy. *Prog. Cardiovasc. Dis. 7*:151–171.

Fadda, F., Mosca, E., Meloni, R., and Gessa, G. L. (1985). Suppression by pro-
gabide of ethanol withdrawal syndrome in rats. *Eur. J. Pharmacol. 109*:321–
325.

Falconer, M. A. (1974). Mesial temporal (Ammon's horn) sclerosis as a common
cause of epilepsy. Etiology, treatment, and prevention. *Lancet 2*:767–770.

Fariello, R. G. (1985). Biochemical approaches to seizure mechanisms: The
GABA and glutamate systems. In *The Epilepsies*, R. J. Porter and P. L. Morselli (Eds.). Butterworths, London, pp. 1–19.

Ferrendelli, J. A. (1983). Relationship between seizures and cyclic nucleotides in
the central nervous system. In *Advances in Neurology*, Vol. 34, *Status Epilepticus*, A. V. Delgado-Escueta, C. G., Wasterlain, D. M., Treiman, and R. J.
Porter (Eds.). Raven Press, New York, pp. 353–357.

Fisher, J., and Abrams, J. (1977). Life threatening ventricular tachyarrhythmias
in delirium tremens. *Arch. Intern. Med. 137*:1238–1241.

Fowler, N. O., Gueron, M., and Rowlands, D. T. (1961). Primary myocardial disease. *Circulation 23*:498–508.

Frederiksen, P., and Hed, R. (1945). Clinical studies in chronic alcoholism. *Acta
Med. Scand. 162*:203.

Freytag, E., and Lindenberg, R. (1964). 294 medicolegal autopsies in epileptics.
Arch. Pathol. 78:274–286.

Friedman, H. J. (1980). Assessment of physical dependence on and withdrawal
from ethanol in animals. In *Alcohol Tolerance and Dependence*, H. Rigter
and J. C. Crabbe (Eds.). Elsevier/North-Holland, New York, pp. 93–121.

Gale, K. (1985). Mechanisms of seizure control mediated by γ-aminobutyric
acid: Role of the substantia nigra. *Fed. Proc. 44*:2414–2424.

Goldstein, D. B. (1978). Animal studies of alcohol withdrawal reactions. In *Re-
search Advances in Alcohol and Drug Problems*, Vol. 4, Y. Israel, F. B. Glaser,
H. Kalant, R. E. Popham, W. Schmidt, and R. G. Smart (Eds.). Plenum, New
York, pp. 77–109.

Goldstein, D. B. (1986). The alcohol withdrawal syndrome. A view from the
laboratory. In *Recent Developments in Alcoholism*, Vol. 4, M. Galanter (Ed.).
Plenum, New York, pp. 231–240.

Gonzalez, L. P. (1985). Changes in physostigmine-induced hippocampal seizures
during ethanol withdrawal. *Brain Res. 335*:384–388.

Goodwin, D. W. (1987). Genetic influences in alcoholism. *Adv. Intern. Med. 32*:
283–298.

Gordon, A. S., Collier, K., and Diamond, I. (1986). Ethanol regulation of adenosine receptor-stimulated cAMP levels in a clonal neural cell line: An in vitro
model of cellular tolerance to ethanol. *Proc. Nat. Acad. Sci. USA 83*:2105–
2108.

Gorelick, D. A., and Wilkins, J. N. (1986). Special aspects of human alcohol
withdrawal. In *Recent Developments in Alcoholism*, Vol. 4, M. Galanter
(Ed.). Plenum, New York, pp. 283–305.

Gottlieb, L. D. (1988). The role of beta blockers in alcohol withdrawal syndrome. *Postgrad. Med. (Special No.)*:169–174.

Gould, L., Jaynal, F., Zahir, M., and Gomprecht, R. F. (1972). Effects of alcohol on the systolic time intervals. *Q. J. Stud. Alcohol 33*:451–463.

Grcevic, N. (1989). The concept of inner cerebral trauma. *Scand. J. Rehabil. Med. (Suppl.)*.

Green, A. R., Heal, D. J., and Vincent, N. D. (1987a). The effects of single and repeated electroconvulsive shock administration on the release of 5-hydroxytryptamine and noradrenaline from cortical slices of rat brain. *Br. J. Pharmacol. 92*:25–30.

Green, A. R., Metz, A., Minchin, M. C. W., and Vincent, N. D. (1987b). Inhibition of the rate of GABA synthesis in regions of rat brain following a convulsion. *Br. J. Pharmacol. 92*:5–11.

Green, A. R., Minchin, M. C. W., and Vincent, N. D. (1987c). Inhibition of GABA release from slices prepared from several brain regions of rats at various times following a convulsion. *Br. J. Pharmacol. 92*:13–18.

Gunnar, R. M., Sutton, G. C., Pietras, R. J., and Tobin, J. R. (1971). Alcoholic cardiomyopathy. *Disease-A-Month*, September: 1–30.

Hariton, C., Ciesielski, L., Cano, J. P., and Mandel, P. (1988). Studies on benzodiazepine receptor subtypes in a model of chronic spontaneous petit mal-like seizures. *Neurosci. Lett. 84*:97–102.

Harper, C. (1979). Wernicke's encephalopathy: A more common disease than realised. A neuropathological study of 51 cases. *J. Neurol. Neurosurg. Psychiatr. 42*:226–231.

Hatch, R. C., and Jernigan, A. D. (1988). Effect of intravenously-administered putative and potential antagonists of ethanol on sleep time in ethanol-narcotized mice. *Life Sci. 42*:11–19.

Hauser, W. A. (1988). Alcohol abuse and epilepsy, the frequency of the problem. *Epilepsia 29*:492.

Hawley, R. J., Major, L. F., Schulman, E. A., and Linnoila, M. (1985). Cerebrospinal fluid 3-methoxy-4-hydroxyphenylglycol and norepinephrine levels in alcohol withdrawal. *Arch. Gen. Psychiatr. 42*:1056–1062.

Heinemann, U., and Hamon, B. (1986). Calcium and epileptogenesis. *Exp. Brain Res. 65*:1–10.

Heinemann, U., Konnerth, A., Pumain, R., and Wadman, W. J. (1986). Extracellular calcium and potassium concentration changes in chronic epileptic brain tissue. In *Advances in Neurology*, Vol. 44, A. V. Delgado-Escueta, A. A. Ward, D. M. Woodbury, and R. J. Porter (Eds.). Raven Press, New York, pp. 641–661.

Hillbom, M. (1980). Occurrence of cerebral seizures provoked by alcohol abuse. *Epilepsia 21*:459–466.

Hinkle, L. E., Jr., Carver, S. T., and Stevens, M. (1969). The frequency of asymptomatic disturbances of cardiac rhythm and conduction in middle-aged men. *Am. J. Cardiol. 24*:629–650.

Hiss, R. G., and Lamb, L. E. (1962). Electrocardiographic findings in 122,043 individuals. *Circulation 25*:947–961.

Hoffman, P. L., and Tabakoff, B. (1985). Ethanol's action on brain biochemistry. In *Alcohol and the Brain. Chronic Effects*, R. E. Tarter and D. H. Van Thiel (Eds.). Plenum, New York, pp. 19–68.

Hruska, R. E. (1988). Effect of ethanol administration on striatal D_1 and D_2 dopamine receptors. *J. Neurochem. 50*:1929–1933.

Hudspith, M. J., Brennan, C. H., Charles, S., and Littleton, J. M. (1987). Dihydropyridine-sensitive Ca^{2+} channels and inositol phospholipid metabolism in ethanol physical dependence. *Ann. N.Y. Acad. Sci. 492*:156–170.

Hunt, W. A. (1985). *Alcohol and Biological Membranes*. Guilford Press, New York.

Jay, G. W., and Leestma, J. E. (1981). Sudden death in epilepsy. A comprehensive review of the literature and proposed mechanisms. *Acta Neurol. Scand. (Suppl. 82):63*:1–66.

Jobe, P. C., Dailey, J. W., and Reigel, C. E. (1986). Noradrenergic and serotonergic determinants of seizure susceptibility and severity in genetically epilepsy-prone rats. *Life Sci. 39*:775–782.

Johnson, R. (1985). Alcohol and fits. *Br. J. Addict. 80*:227–232.

Kajita, S., Ogawa, N., and Sato, M. (1987). Long-term increase in striatal thyrotropin-releasing hormone receptor binding caused by amygdaloid kindling. *Epilepsia 28*:228–233.

Kamphuis, W., Wadman, W. J., Buijs, R. M., and Lopes da Silva, F. H. (1986). Decrease in number of hippocampal gamma-aminobutyric acid (GABA) immunoreactive cells in the rat kindling model of epilepsy. *Exp. Brain Res. 64*: 491–495.

Killam, E. K., and Killam, K. F. (1984). Evidence for neurotransmitter abnormalities related to seizure activity in the epileptic baboon. *Fed. Proc. 43*: 2510–2515.

Koppi, S., Eberhardt, G., Haller, R., and Konig, P. (1987). Calcium-channel-blocking agent in the treatment of acute alcohol withdrawal—Caroverine versus meprobamate in a randomized double-blind study. *Neuropsychobiology 17*:49–52.

Kosobud, A., and Crabbe, J. C. (1986). Ethanol withdrawal in mice bred to be genetically prone or resistant to ethanol withdrawal seizures. *J. Pharmacol. Exp. Ther. 238*:170–177.

Kotlinska, J., and Langwinski, R. (1986). Audiogenic seizures during ethanol withdrawal can be blocked by a delta opioid agonist. *Drug Alcohol Depend. 18*:361–367.

Kotlinska, J., and Langwinski, R. (1987). Does the blockade of opioid receptors influence the development of ethanol dependence? *Alcohol Alcoholism 22*: 117–119.

Kraus, M. L., Gottlieb, L. D., Horwitz, R. I., and Auscher, M. (1985). Randomized clinical trial of atenolol in patients with alcohol withdrawal. *New. Engl. J. Med. 313*:905–909.

Laidlaw, J., and Richens, A. (1976). *A Textbook of Epilepsy*. Churchill-Livingstone, New York.

Laird, H. E., Dailey, J. W., and Jobe, P. C. (1984). Neurotransmitter abnormalities in genetically epileptic rodents. *Fed. Proc. 43*:2505–2509.

Lang, R. M., Borow, K. M., Neumann, A., and Feldman, T. (1985). Adverse cardiac effects of acute alcohol ingestion in young adults. *Ann. Intern. Med. 102*:742–747.

Laurie, W. (1971). Alcohol as a cause of sudden unexpected death. *Med. J. Aust. 1*:1224–1227.

Leestma, J. E. (Ed.) (1988). *Forensic Neuropathology*. Raven Press, New York.

Leestma, J. E., and Grcevic, N. (1988). Impact injuries to the brain and head. In *Forensic Neuropathology*, J. E. Leestma (Ed.). Raven Press, New York, pp. 184–253.

Leestma, J. E., Kalelkar, M. B., Teas, S. S., Jay, G. W., and Hughes, J. R. (1984). Sudden unexpected death associated with seizures: Analysis of 66 cases. *Epilepsia 25*:84–88.

Leestma, J. E., Walczak, T., Hughes, J. R., Kalelkar, M., and Teas, S. (1989). A prospective study on sudden unexpected death in epilepsy. *Ann. Neurol. 26*: 195–203.

Lindenberg, R., and Freytag, E. (1957). Morphology of cortical contusions. *Arch. Path. 63*:23–42.

Little, H. J., Taylor, S. C., Nutt, D. J., and Cowen, P. J. (1985). The benzodiazepine antagonist, Ro15-1788 does not decrease ethanol withdrawal convulsions in rats. *Eur. J. Pharmacol. 107*:375–377.

Little, H. J., Dolin, S. J., and Halsey, M. J. (1986). Calcium channel antagonists decrease the ethanol withdrawal syndrome. *Life Sci. 39*:2059–2063.

Little, R. E., and Gayle, J. L. (1980). Epilepsy and alcoholism. *Alcohol Health Res. World 5*:31–36.

Littleton, J. M. (1984). Biochemical pharmacology of ethanol tolerance and dependence. In *Pharmacological Treatment for Alcoholism*, G. Edwards and J. Littleton (Eds.). Methuen, New York, pp. 119–144.

Loscher, W., and Czuczwar, S. J. (1985). Evaluation of the 5-hydroxytryptamine receptor agonist 8-hydroxy-2-(Di-n-propylamino) tetralin in different rodent models of epilepsy. *Neurosci. Lett. 60*:201–206.

Loscher, W., and Schwark, W. S. (1987). Further evidence for abnormal GABAergic circuits in amygdala-kindled rats. *Brain Res. 420*:385–395.

Lynch, M. A., Archer, E. R., and Littleton, J. M. (1986). Increased sensitivity of transmitter release to calcium in ethanol tolerance. *Biochem. Pharmacol. 35*: 1207–1209.

Manhem, P., Nilsson, L. H., Moberg, A. L., Wadstein, J., and Hokfelt, B. (1985). Alcohol withdrawal: Effect of clonidine treatment on sympathetic activity, the renin-aldosterone system, and clinical symptoms. *Alcoholism 9*:238–243.

Marrosu, F., Del Zompo, M., and Corsini, G. U. (1983). The role of dopamine in human epilepsy: Effect of apomorphine. In *Epilepsy: An Update on Research and Therapy*, G. Nistico, R. Di Perri, and H. Meinardi (Eds.). Alan R. Liss, New York, pp. 95–104.

Masello, III W. (1984). Sudden death mechanisms in the alcoholic. *Medico Legal Bull.* (Richmond, Va.) September–October, 1–7.

Matsumoto, A., Kumagai, T., Takeuchi, T., Miyazaki, S., and Watanabe, K. (1987). Clinical effects of TRH for severe epilepsy in childhood: A comparative study with ACTH therapy. *Epilepsia 28*:49–55.

McCloy, R. B., Prancan, A. V., and Nakano, J. (1974). Effects of acetyldehyde on the systemic, pulmonary, and regional circulations. *Cardiovasc. Res. 8*: 216–226.

McNamara, J. O. (1984). Role of neurotransmitters in seizure mechanisms in the kindling model of epilepsy. *Fed. Proc. 43*:2516–2520.

Meldrum, B. S., and Corsellis, J. A. N. (1984). Epilepsy, In *Greenfield's Neuropathology*, 4th ed., J. H. Adams, J. A. N. Corsellis, and L. W. Duchen (Eds.). Wiley, New York, pp. 921–950.

Messing, R. O., Carpenter, C. L., Diamond, I., and Greenberg, D. A. (1986). Ethanol regulates calcium channels in clonal neural cells. *Proc. Nat. Acad. Sci. USA 83*:6213–6215.

Meyer, F. B., Anderson, R. E., Sundt, T. M., Yaksh, T. L., and Sharbrough, F. W. (1987). Suppression of pentylenetetrazole seizures by oral administration of dihydropyridine Ca^{2+} antagonist. *Epilepsia 28*:409–414.

Morin, A. M., and Wasterlain, C. G. (1983). Role of receptors for neurotransmitters in status epilepticus. In *Advances in Neurology*, Vol. 34, *Status Epilepticus*, A. V. Delgado-Escueta, C. G. Wasterlain, D. M. Treiman, and R. J. Porter (Eds.). Raven Press, New York, pp. 369–374.

Mucha, R. F., and Pinel, J. (1979). Increased susceptibility to kindled seizures in rats following a single injection of alcohol. *J. Stud. Alcohol 40*:258–271.

Nakano, J., and Prancan, A. V. (1972). Effects of adrenergic blockage on cardiovascular responses to ethanol and acetylaldehyde. *Arch. Int. Pharmacodyn. Ther. 196*:259–268.

Naranjo, C. A., and Sellers, E. M. (1986). Clinical assessment and pharmacotherapy of the alcohol withdrawal syndrome. In *Recent Developments in Alcoholism*, Vol. 4, M. Galanter (Ed.). Plenum, New York, pp. 265–281.

Nevins, M. A., and Lyon, L. J. (1972). Sudden death and metabolic derangement in alcoholism with malnutrition. *J. Med. Soc. N.J. 69*:155–157.

Nicoletti, F., Barbaccia, M. L., Iadarola, M. J., Pozzi, O., and Laird, H. E. (1986). Abnormality of α_1-adrenergic receptors in the frontal cortex of epileptic rats. *J. Neurochem. 46*:270–273.

Nutt, D., Glue, P., Molyneux, S., and Clark, E. (1988). α-2-Adrenoceptor function in alcohol withdrawal: A pilot study of the effects of IV clonidine in alcoholics and normals. *Alcoholism 12*:14–18.

Ogata, M., Mendelson, J. H., Mello, N. K., et al. (1971). Adrenal function and alcoholism: II. Catecholamines. *Pyschosom. Med. 33*:159–180.

Olsen, R. W., Wamsley, J. K., Lee, R. J., and Lomax, P. (1986). Benzodiazepine/barbiturate/GABA receptor-chloride ionophore complex in a genetic model for generalized epilepsy. In *Advances in Neurology*, Vol. 44, A. V. Delgado-Escueta, A. A. Ward, D. M. Woodbury, and R. J. Porter (Eds.). Raven Press, New York, pp. 365–378.

Ono, K., Mori, K., Baba, H., and Wada, J. A. (1987). A role of the striatum in premotor cortical seizure development. *Brain Res. 435*:84–90.

Parale, M. P., and Kulkarni, S. K. (1986). Studies with α_2-adrenoceptor agonists and alcohol abstinence syndrome in rats. *Pyshcopharmacology 88*:237–239.

Pilke, A., Partinen, M., and Kovanen, J. (1984). Status epilepticus and alcohol use: An analysis of 82 status epilepticus admissions. *Acta Neurol. Scand. 70*: 443–450.

Pinel, J. P. J. (1980). Alcohol withdrawal seizures: Implications for kindling. *Pharmacol. Biochem. Behav. (Suppl. 1) 13*:225–231.

Pitkanen, A., Saano, V., Hyvonen, K., Airaksinen, M. M., and Riekkinen, P. J. (1987). Decreased GABA, benzodiazepine and picrotoxin receptor binding in brains of rats after cobalt-induced epilepsy. *Epilepsia 28*:11–16.

Pohorecky, L. A., and Brick, J. (1988). Pharmacology of ethanol. *Pharmacol. Ther. 36*:335–427.

Polson, C. J., Gee, D. J., and Knight, B. (1985). *The Essentials of Forensic Medicine*, 4th ed. Pergamon, New York, p. 564.

Racine, R. J., and McIntyre, D. (1986). Mechanism of kindling: A current view. In *The Limbic System: Functional Organization and Clinical Disorders*, B. K. Doane and K. E. Livingston (Eds.). Raven Press, New York, pp. 109–121.

Richards, H. G. (1964). Sudden death due to fatty degeneration of the myocardium and liver. *Med. Sci. Law 4*:182.

Rosen, J. B., and Berman, R. F. (1987). Differential effects of adenosine analogs on amygdala, hippocampus, and caudate nucleus kindled seizures. *Epilepsia 28*:658–666.

Saito, T., Lee, J. M., Hoffman, P. L., and Tabakoff, B. (1987). Effects of chronic ethanol treatment on the β-adrenergic receptor-coupled adenylate cyclase system of mouse cerebral cortex. *J. Neurochem. 48*:1817–1822.

Sanders, M. G. (1970). Alcoholic cardiomyopathy: A critical review. *Q. J. Stud. Alcohol 31*:324–368.

Sandler, M., Glover, V., Elsworth, J. D., and Clow, A. (1984). Ethanol and endogenous ligands in humans. *Psychopharmacol. Bull. 27*:485–486.

Santori, E. M., and Collins, R. C. (1988). Effects of chronic control seizures on GABA and benzodiazepine receptors within seizure pathways. *Brain Res. 442*:261–269.

Sataline, L. (1973). Cardiac standstill simulating seizures. *J. Am. Med. Assoc. 225*:747.

Schmutz, M. (1987). Relevance of kindling and related processes to human epileptogenesis. *Prog. Neuro-Psychopharmacol. Biol. Psychiatr. 11*:505–525.

Scollo-Lavizzari, G. (1983). Epilepsy in alcoholics. *Hexagon (Roche), 6*:20–24.

Segel, L. D., Klausner, S. C., Gnadt, J. T. H., and Amsterdam, E. A. (1984). Alcohol and the heart. *Med. Clin. North Am. 68*:147–161.

Sereny, G. (1971). Effects of alcohol on the electrocardiogram. *Circulation 44*: 558.

Sherwin, A., Matthew, E., Blain, M., and Guevremont, D. (1986). Benzodiazepine receptor binding is not altered in human epileptogenic cortical foci. *Neurology 36*:1380–1382.

Sherwin, A. L., and Van Gelder, N. M. (1986). Amino acid and catecholamine markers of metabolic abnormalities in human focal epilepsy. In *Advances in Neurology*, Vol. 44, A. V. Delgado-Escueta, A. A. Ward, D. M. Woodbury, and R. J. Porter (Eds.). Raven Press, New York, pp. 1011-1032.

Shin, C., Pedersen, H. B., and McNamara, J. O. (1985). γ-Aminobutyric acid and benzodiazepine receptors in the kindling model of epilepsy: A quantitative radiohistochemical study. *J. Neurosci.* 5:2696-2701.

Smile, D. H. (1984). Acute alcohol withdrawal complicated by supraventricular tachycardia: Treatment with intravenous propranolol. *Ann. Emergency Med.* 13:53-55.

Suranyi-Cadotte, B., Lafaille, F., Dongier, M., Dumas, M., and Quirion, R. (1988). Decreased dentistry of peripheral benzodiazepine binding sites on platelets of currently drinking, but not abstinent alcoholics. *Neuropharmacology* 27:443-445.

Swann, A. C. (1987). (Na^+, K^+)-ATPase and noradrenergic function: Effects of chronic ethanol. *Eur. J. Pharmacol.* 134:145-153.

Syapin, P. J., and Alkana, R. L. (1988). Chronic ethanol exposure increases peripheral-type benzodiazepine receptors in brain. *Eur. J. Pharmacol.* 147: 101-109.

Tabakoff, B., and Hoffman, P. L. (1980). Alcohol and neurotransmitters. In *Alcohol Tolerance and Dependence*, H. Rigter and J. C. Crabbe (Eds.). Elsevier/North-Holland, New York, pp. 201-226.

Tabakoff, B., and Hoffman, P. (1983). Neurochemical aspects of tolerance to and physical dependence on alcohol. In *The Biology of Alcoholism*, Vol. 7, B. Kissin and H. Begleiter (Eds.). Plenum, New York, pp. 199-252.

Talbott, G. D. (1976). Primary alcoholic heart disease. *Ann. N.Y. Acad. Sci.* 173:237-242.

Talbott, G. D., and Gander, O. F. (1974). Convulsive seizures in the alcoholic: A clinical appraisal. *Maryland State Med. J.* 23:81-85.

Tamborska, E., and Marangos, P. J. (1986). Brain benzodiazepine binding sites in ethanol dependent and withdrawal states. *Life Sci.* 38:465-472.

Tartara, A., Manni, R., and Mazzella, G. (1983). Epileptic seizures and alcoholism. Clinical and pathogenetic aspects. *Acta Neurol. Belg.* 83:88-94.

Torvik, A., Lindboe, C. F., and Rogde, S. (1982). Brain lesions in alcoholics. A neuropathological study with clinical correlations. *J. Neurol. Sci.* 56:233-248.

Valverius, P., Hoffman, P. L., and Tabakoff, B. (1987). Effect on mouse cerebral cortical β-adrenergic receptors. *Mol. Pharmacol.* 32:217-222.

Vetter, W. R., Cohn, L. H., and Reichgott, M. (1967). Hypokalemia and electrocardiographic abnormalities during acute alcohol withdrawal. *Arch. Intern. Med.* 120:536-541.

Victor, M., and Brausch, C. (1967). The role of abstinence in the genesis of alcoholic epilepsy. *Epilepsia* 8:1-20.

Victor, M., and Laureno, R. (1978). Neurologic complications of alcohol abuse: Epidemiologic aspects. *Adv. Neurol.* 19:603-617.

Ward, A. A. (1969). The epileptic neurone: Chronic foci in animals and man. In *Basic Mechanisms in the Epilepsies*, H. H. Jasper, A. A. Ward, and A. Pope (Eds.). Churchill-Livingstone, London, pp. 263–277.

White, H. S., Chen, C. F., Kemp, J. W., and Woodbury, D. M. (1985). Effects of acute and chronic phenytoin on the electrolyte content and the activities of Na^+-, K^+-, Ca^{2+}-, Mg^{2+}-, and HCO_3^--ATPases and carbonic anhydrase of neonatal and adult rat cerebral cortex. *Epilepsia 26*:43–57.

Wilkins, A. J., Jenkins, W. J., and Steiner, J. A. (1983). Efficacy of clonidine in treatment of alcohol withdrawal state. *Psychopharmacology 81*:78–80.

Wilkins, J. N., and Gorelick, D. A. (1986). Clinical neuroendocrinology and neuropharmacology of alcohol withdrawal. In *Recent Developments in Alcoholism*, Vol. 4, M. Galanter (Ed.). Plenum, New York, pp. 241–263.

Wilson, D. E., Schreibman, P. H., Brewster, A. C., and Avky, R. A. (1970). The enhancement of alimentary lipemia by ethanol in man. *J. Lab. Clin. Med. 75*:264–274.

20
Glycoside-Induced Arrhythmias and Seizures

CLAIRE M. LATHERS*   *The Medical College of Pennsylvania, Eastern Pennsylvania Psychiatric Institute, Phildelphia, Pennsylvania*

I. INTRODUCTION

Digitalis-induced toxicity characteristically elicits unwanted cardiac arrhythmias that are primary ventricular in origin (Lathers, in press; Lathers et al., 1977, 1978, 1981, 1982). Central nervous system side effects, including headache, malaise, drowsiness, confusion, psychosis, changes in color vision, and/or convulsions may also occur with digitalis toxicity (Frankl et al., 1984a,b; Lathers and Roberts, 1980, 1986). As early as 1785 Whithering noted the possibility of the occurrence of epileptic seizures with the use of glycoside preparations. Others have also reported the occurrence of convulsions or myoclonic jerks (Fowler et al., 1964; McNamara et al., 1964; Potter et al., 1964; Shermann and Locke, 1960; Tettelbaum, 1931). Feuerstein and colleagues (1973) reported a case in which a 2.5 month old baby was admitted with infectious rhinopharyngitis with dyspnea. A congenital heart disease was detected. During treatment, a toxic dose of digitalis solution was accidentally administered. Eight hour later, respiratory pauses of short duration occurred. Twelve hours later the electrocardiogram displayed alternating phases of bigeminy and trigemy along with changes in the ST segment. Twenty-four hours after ingestion, intermittent, generalized, and asymmetric focal convulsions developed. The convulsions always developed during periods of apnea, beginning after the cardiac arrest and stopping before the return of spontaneous breathing movements (Figures 1 and 2). Not all periods of apnea were associated with motor phenomena. Four days after treatment with antibiotics, corticosteroids, adjustment of the electrolyte balance, intravenous feeding, oxygen, artificial respiration, Tris(trimethylol-

Current affiliation: FDA, Rockville, Maryland.

375

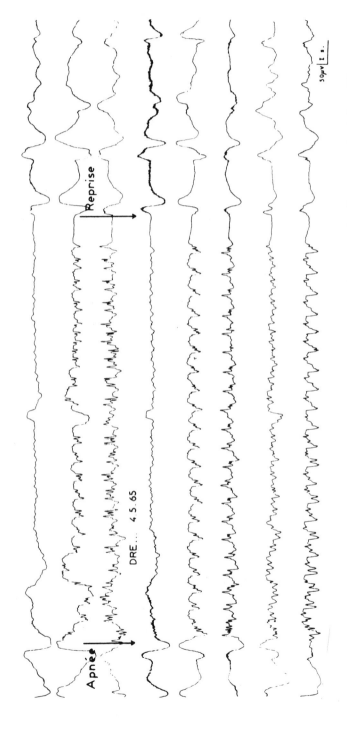

Figure 1 Short-duration apnea (17 seconds) associated with a generalized seizure. Note the disappearance of the artifacts, caused by spontaneous respiratory movements, when the spike discharges occur (respiratory rate between the apneas 28–30/minute). Speed 15 mm/sec. Calibration mark: 50 μV. [From Feuerstein et al. (1973), modified with permission.]

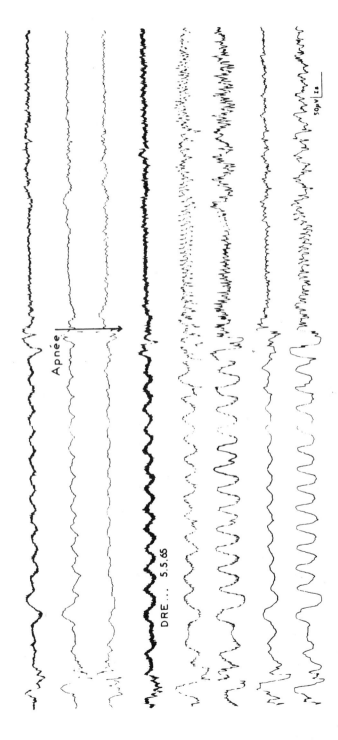

Figure 2 Beginning of apnea concomitant with a left hemisphere seizure. Respiratory arrest is shown by the disappearance of breathing movement artifacts. Speed: 15 mm/sec. Calibration mark: 50 μV. [From Feuerstein et al. (1973), modified with permission.]

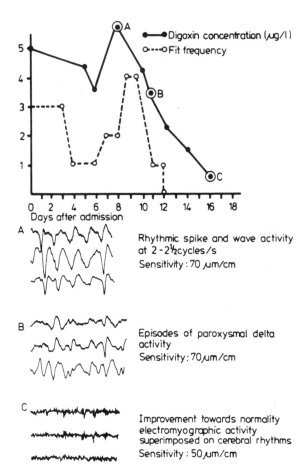

Figure 3 Profile of plasma digoxin concentration and frequency of observed daily fits with associated electroencephalographic appearances at 5–8 µg/L (A), 3–6 µ/L (B), and 0–7 µg/L (C). [From Kerr et al. (1982), reproduced with permission.]

aminomethane) solution, phenobarbital, and chloral hydrate enema, the general state of the child improved.

Digoxin toxicity is generally associated with plasma concentrations of 2–4 µg/L (Sarangi et al., 1980). Convulsions may complicate acute intoxication with nontherapeutic doses of digoxin; epileptiform activity may also be associated with the clinical symptoms of chronic digoxin toxicity. Kerr et al. (1982) reported the case of a 64-year-old female who presented with angina, atrial fibrillation, rheumatic valvular disease, and signs of digitalis toxicity, including bradycardia, xanthopsia, nausea, vomiting, and neurologic events characterized as a clouding of consciousness, total disorientation, lip-smacking, and coarse tremor of all limbs. The electroencephalographic abnormalities and epileptiform activity persisted while the plasma digoxin levels remained in the toxic range and resolved when the concentration fell to the therapeutic range (Figure 3).

II. THE EPILEPTOGENIC EFFECT OF OUABAIN

Digitalis glycosides have been demonstrated to induce seizures in man as well as in laboratory animals (Batterman and Gutner, 1948; Douglas et al., 1971; Feuerstein et al., 1973; Gold et al., 1947; Lebovitz, 1974; Oedley et al., 1969, Pedley et al., 1969). Ouabain, digoxin, gitalin, and squill glycosides produced convulsions in rats (Gold et al., 1947). Intracerebroventricular injection of ouabain produced convulsions in conscious mice (Doggett et al., 1970). Digitoxigenin, the aglycone of digitoxin, produced convulsions in cats (Chen et al., 1938), mice (Lage and Spratt, 1966), and rats (Butterbaugh and Spratt, 1970). Ouabain applied locally to the cerebral cortex elicits epileptic seizure patterns that appear at fairly regular intervals and are present for several hours (Bignami and Palladini, 1966). The application of a pledget soaked in a saline solution containing ouabain to the cortex of conscious rats provided a model of focal cortical epilepsy (Lewin, 1970). Of 22 rats, 15 manifested epileptiform discharges in the EEG at some time within the first 24 hours; 6 had observable focal seizures. Ouabain inhibits the sodium–potassium-dependent ATPase (Skou, 1965) and thus produces a decrease in membrane potential and an enhanced tendency to self-sustained seizure activity. Cellular uptake of potassium is associated with increased intracellular water; this leads to deterioration of glia and nerve cells. Ultimately, local brain edema with a characteristic spongioform state develops (Petsche and Seitelberger, 1967). Ouabain-induced seizures have been used to study neurophysiological events associated with seizures and as a model to test the efficacy of anticonvulsant agents.

Petsche et al. (1973) performed a craniotomy under local anesthesia in rabbits suspended in a hammock. Electrophysiologic recordings were made from several different cortical zones, including striata, parietal cortex, and precentral cortex, before and after the cortical application of ouabain (g-strophanthin). As depicted in Figure 4, ouabain initially produced a slow decrease in spontaneous EEG activity prior to the seizures. Generalized seizures started earlier with higher concentrations of ouabain. When concentrations of 10^{-3} M or greater were used, ouabain elicited seizures of hippocampal type, i.e., groups of spikes with a high repetition rate, sooner in the course of status epilepticus, which partially replaced the cortical seizures.

Petsche et al. (1973) also examined the phenomena within the cortex after administration of ouabain by using laminar microelectrodes. Electrophysiological

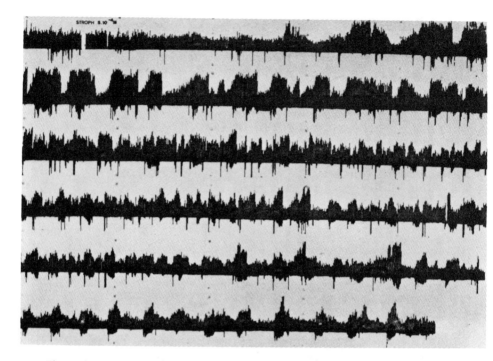

Figure 4 Integrated EEG activity precentral vs. striatal area (upward deflections) and motor seizure activity of head and right forelimb (downward deflections); low-speed recording (1 cm = 1 min). After application of ouabain $5-10^{-4}$ M, the spontaneous activity slowly decreases and a few voltage oscillations of several minutes duration appear before generalized seizures start (at first only in the EEG, later together with jerks). The status epilepticus was recorded for almost six hours in this experiment. [From Petsche et al. (1973), reproduced with permission.]

activity recorded from the deep layers beneath the zone of necrosis induced by ouabain did not decrease in voltage to the same extent as the surface activity. The seizures begin with flattening of the cortical surface EEG, which was accompanied by intracortical high-voltage fast activity and regularly discharging negative spikes, which gradually increased in amplitude and slowly involved adjacent regions. When the deeper activity decreased in frequency, the typical seizure pattern on EEG was recorded with the surface electrodes. The surface activity became more and more uniform over time, while the deeper intracortical activity retained its original character. The amount of higher frequencies on the surface EEG diminished, whereas the activity monitored within the deep cortical layers did not. As the duration of ouabain effect increased, there was decreased correlation between deep and surface activity. Progressive deterioration of the uppermost cortical layers occurred, related in extent and degree to the concentration of ouabain and to its duration of application. The decrease in voltage of the seizure activity was related to the number of neurons destroyed.

Petsche et al. (1973), as well as Scherrer and Calvet (1972) and Peronnet et al. (1972), concluded that the EEG recorded from the cortical surfaces was composed of several activities that originated at different cortical layers, reaching more or less up to the surface and even existing independently of each other. Petsche et al. (1973) hypothesized that if a close relationship between wave patterns at the surface and at deep intracortical layers occurred during seizures, then some synchronizing force existed in a vertical direction of the cortex. Petsche and Rappelsberger (1970) noted that the application of ouabain to the rabbit cortex was experimentally advantageous in that it caused constant irritation to one region of the cortex, giving rise to electrographic seizures which were constant in amplitude, duration, and interval and that the action of sequential anticonvulsant drugs given to one animal could be studied. Clonazepam reduced synchronization within the cortex both in the horizontal and in the vertical direction (Petsche, 1972). After clonazepam, most of the electrographic seizure activity decayed into a pattern of dispersed, locally circumscribed patterns in different layers and different regions of the cortex.

Bergman et al. (1970) used a preparation similar to that of Petsche et al. (1973) to study intracerebral connections. They reported that application of ouabain or digitoxin to the hypothalamus evoked seizure activity first in the hippocampus and subsequently in the subcortical and cortex regions. Implantations of the drugs into the hippocampus elicited epileptic discharges initially in the hypothalamus and then in other parts of the brain (Figure 5). Bergman and colleagues concluded that in the rabbit brain, both the lateral geniculate body and the caudate nucleus were linked to the contralateral hippocampus.

Pharmacologic stimulation of central dopaminergic receptors with dopamine agonists such as apomorphine reduces the intensity of bioelectrical and behavioral seizures (Meldrum et al., 1975), audiogenic seizures (Anlezark and Meldrum, 1975), and electroconvulsive shock seizures (Stull et al., 1973). The cause of certain drug-induced seizures has also been attributed to a depression of cerebral gamma-aminobutyric acid (GABA) concentration, particularly that resulting in inhibition of glutamic acid decarboxylase (GAD) activity (Abrahams and Wood, 1970; Gottesfeld and Elazar, 1975; Karlsson et al., 1974; Tapia et al., 1975; Wood and Petsche, 1975). Thus, Stach and Kacz (1977) hypothesized that dopamine and GABA receptor-stimulating agents given together might mutually potentiate their anticonvulsant activities. They administered ouabain via cortical applications to freely moving rabbits to elicit epileptiform activity. Combined treatment of dopamine and GABA receptor-stimulating agents exhibited a much

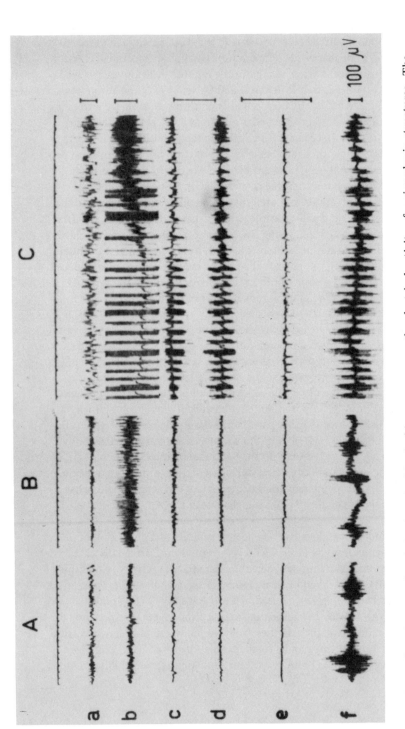

Figure 5 Influence of ouabain, deposited in the hippocampus, on the electrical activity of various brain structures. The rabbit received 5 μg of the drug into the posterior part of the right dorsal hippocampus. Recording from (a) right-left motor cortex; (b) left, and (c) right dorsal hippocampus; (d) right and (e) left thalamus; and (f) right hypothalamus. (A) Two minutes after application of ouabain; (B) after 20 minutes; (C) after 120 minutes. Time in seconds on top scale; vertical bars on right side indicate individual calibrations of 100 μV; the third bar belongs to records c and d. [From Bergman et al. (1970), reproduced with permission.]

better anticonvulsant action than any of the compounds alone. They concluded that the effectiveness of the inhibition of ouabain-induced seizures depends on simultaneous stimulation of dopamine and GABA receptors in the central nervous system. They noted that although drugs that stimulate GABA receptors seem to possess antiepileptic properties, they may simultaneously impair transmission in the dopaminergic system in the striatum. This action may be an unfavorable antiepileptic activity since compounds that impair dopaminergic transmission by specific blockade of dopamine receptors potentiate epileptiform activity, while dopaminergic stimulation inhibits it (Jobe et al., 1974; Vernadakis, 1972). Thus Stach and Kacz (1977) suggested that the addition of a dopamine receptor–stimulating agent will overcome the inhibitory effect of GABA-mimetic treatment on dopaminergic transmission, thus increasing the anticonvulsant action of GABA mimetics.

III. PROPOSED MECHANISMS OF GLYCOSIDE-INDUCED SEIZURES

A relationship has been proposed to exist between Na^+/K^+-ATPase activity and epilepsy. Donaldson et al. (1971) discussed data supporting this suggestion. First, ouabain inhibits Na^+/K^+-ATPase and elicits clonic tonic seizures. Divalent cations such as copper and zinc also inhibit the enzyme and elicit seizure activity. Intraventricular injection of ouabain, copper, and zinc greatly decreases the enzyme activity in the hippocampus and hypothalamus of rat brains. Donaldson et al. (1971) also reported that the decrease in enzyme activity in these brain areas is associated with an increase in total sodium content and in the Na^+/K^+ ratio during ouabain-induced seizures. Copper and zinc also increases brain regional sodium content and the Na^+/K^+ ratio. Chronic administration of phenytoin decreased the brain sodium content.

Donaldson et al. (1973) also reported that the regional distribution of ^{3}H-ouabain was very similar to the regional distribution of ^{3}H-GABA in rat brain. Earlier, Roberts and Kuriyama (1968) had suggested that altered brain level of GABA may be related to seizure susceptibility. Yessaian et al. (1971) proposed that GABA-related changes in rat brain tissue slices may be associated with changes in Na^+/K^+-ATPase activity at the level of the synaptosomal membrane.

Stone and Javid (1982) reported that phenytoin, phenobarbital, chlordiazepoxide, and valproic acid antagonized the seizures induced by the intracerebral injection of ouabain into mice. Phenobarbital, but not phenytoin, antagonized seizures induced by the intracerebral injection of pentylenetetrazol. It was concluded that phenytoin may be specific for seizures arising from a derangement of mechanisms involving the intracellular–extracellular sodium relationships. Ouabain-induced seizures would be included in this class since ouabain inhibits Na^+/K^+-ATPase, thereby depressing the activity of the sodium pump and thus

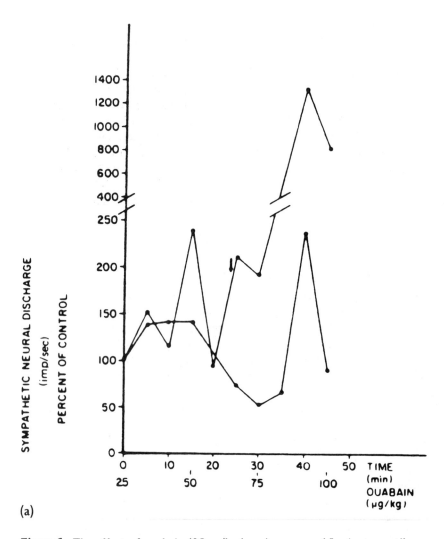

(a)

Figure 6 The effect of ouabain (25 μg/kg i.v. given every 15 minutes until death) on postganglionic cardiac sympathetic neural discharge (impulses/second, % of control). The data are graphed as a function of time (minutes).

inducing depolarization (Woodbury, 1980a,b). Electroconvulsive shock is also thought to produce seizures associated with an altered ionic relationship. Stone and Javid (1982) concluded that additional studies, designed to examine ionic changes associated with seizure activity, are needed.

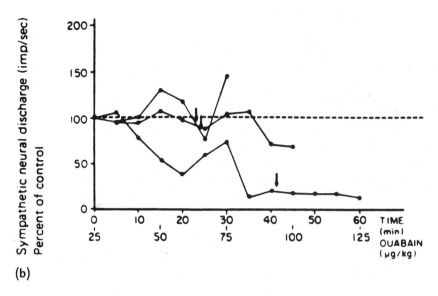

(b)

Figure 6 (continued) One postganglionic cardiac sympathetic nerve was monitored in three different animals (*a*) and three prostaglandic branches in one cat (*b*). The arrows indicate the development of arrhythmia. [From Lathers (1980), reproduced with permission.]

IV. NEURAL EFFECTS OF DIGITALIS GLYCOSIDES

Experiments in laboratory animals have demonstrated that alteration of neural activity occurs at many sites, including the brain stem cardiovascular and respiratory centers, spinal cord, autonomic ganglia, peripheral nerves, and autonomic nerve terminals (Basu-Ray et al., 1972a,b; Bircher et al., 1963; Frazer and Tillie, 1925; Gillis, 1969; Gillis et al., 1972; Konzett and Rothlin, 1952; Lathers, 1980; Lathers et al., 1977, 1978, 1981, 1982; Levitt et al., 1970; McLain, 1969; Melville and Shister, 1957; Perry and Reinert, 1954; Sohn et al., 1970; Ten Eick and Hoffman, 1969; Weaver et al., 1975, 1976). Lathers and colleagues (1977, 1978; Lathers, 1980) recorded in one postganglionic nerve in one cat (Figure 6a) or simultaneously from two or three postganglionic cardiac sympathetic nerves monitored in the same anesthetized cat (Figure 6b) and demonstrated that just prior to ouabain-induced arrhythmias, the neural discharge was elevated in some branches, depressed in some, and unaltered in others. This discharge was designeated nonuniform; the discharge was thought to be one mechanism contributing to the initiation of arrhythmias. The reader is also referred to Chapter 9 of this book for additional details of the neural action of glycosides.

Osterberg and Raines (1973) reported that the action of digitoxigenin, acetyl-strophanthidin, and ouabain on spinal synaptic processes in the cat represented a spectrum with decreasing order of lipid solubility and propensity to excite neural structures in the anesthetized cat. Digitoxigenin caused clonic and tonic convulsive movements; acetylstrophanthidin, only muscle twitching; and ouabain, no convulsive symptoms. Only digitoxigenin, in large doses, facilitated high-frequency transmission through the monosynaptic reflex pathway. All three enhanced posttetanic potentiations of the monosynaptic reflex pathway due to a reduced pretetanic spike amplitude rather than to an increase in poten-tiated responses. Unconditional responses of the monosynaptic reflex were de-pressed by all three; the exception was observed after large doses of digitoxigen, on which occasion the monosynaptic responses were highly variable, being either depressed or enhanced. Digitoxigenin and acetylstrophanthidin increased the poly-synaptic responses. When seizures were arrested, the postsynaptic activity was enhanced. Digitoxigenin and acetylstrophanthidin produced partial depolariza-tion of the intraspinal primary afferent nerve endings. It was concluded that these digitalis glycosides alter spinal cord synaptic reflex pathways in a manner that predisposes to convulsions and other central nervous system excitatory manifestations. Most importantly, it was noted that the increased variability of the ventral root monosynaptic reflex observed during convulsive dose of digi-toxigenin also occurs with pentylenetetrazol. It was therefore suggested that this mechanism may be responsible for moment-to-moment fluctuations in the back-ground activity produced by disorganization of the balance of facilitatory and inhibitory influences on motorneurons from internuncial cells (Lewin and Es-plin, 1961).

Lewin and Esplin (1961) reported that after administration of pentylenetetra-zol there was an enhancement of recurrent inhibition. Osterberg and Raines (1973) also found this effect at a time corresponding with convulsant activity in-duced by digitoxigenin. Glycosides enhance acetylcholine release from neuro-secretory endings in ganglia and in the neuromuscular junction (Birks, 1963). Os-terberg and Raines (1973) speculated that if digitoxigenin produced the same effect in the recurrent collateral terminals, enhanced acetylcholine release would be a potent stimulus to the Renshaw cells, resulting in an inhibition of this sys-tem. Alternatively, digitoxigenin could increase the transmitter output of inhibi-tory interneurons. Thus it appears that digitoxigenin has an action similar to that of pentylenetetrazol, and that both may share a common mechanism in the de-velopment and sustenance of seizure activity. Furthermore, both digitoxigenin and pentylenetetrazol (Boyd et al., 1966) reduce presynaptic inhibition, although it is more difficult to correlate the effects of drugs that increase or decrease presynaptic inhibition with seizure production (Osterberg and Raines, 1973).

V. NEURAL ACTIONS OF GLYCOSIDES AND PENTYLENETRAZOL AND THE OCCURRENCE OF CARDIAC ARRHYTHMIAS

It is of interest to note that epileptogenic activity elicited by both pentylenetetrazol and digitalis glycosides has been associated with the occurrence of cardiac arrhythmias (Lathers and Schraeder, 1982; Schraeder and Lathers, 1983). Thus it may well be that neurally induced arrhythmias associated with epileptogenic activity in persons with epilepsy place these individuals at risk for death in a sudden, unexpected manner. It would appear that the digitalis glycosides offer an alternative method to study the neural cardiac component of arrhythmias associated with epileptogenic activity in an animal model.

REFERENCES

Abrahams, D. E., and Wood, J. D. (1970). Hydrazide-induced seizures and cerebral levels of γ-aminobutyric acid: A re-evaluation. *J. Neurochem. 17*:1197–1204.

Anlezark, G. M., and Meldrum, B. S. (1975). Effects of apomorphine, ergocornine and piribedil on audiogenic seizures in DBA/2 mice. *Br. J. Pharmacol. 53*: 419–421.

Basu-Ray, B. N., Booker, W. M., Dutta, S. N., and Pradhan, S. N. (1972a). Effects of microinjection of ouabain into the hypothalamus in cats. *Br. J. Pharmacol. 45*:197–206.

Basu-Ray, B. N., Dutta, S. N., and Pradhan, S. N. (1972b). Effects of microinjections of ouabain into certain medullary areas in cats. *J. Pharmacol. Exp. Ther. 181*:357–361.

Batterman, R. C., and Gutner, L. B. (1948). Hitherto undescribed neurological manifestations of digitalis toxicity. *Am. Heart J. 36*:582–586.

Bergman, N. F., Costin, A., Chaimovitz, M., et al. (1970). Seizure activity evoked by implantation of ouabain and related drugs into cortical and subcortical regions of the rabbit brain. *Neuropharmacology 9*:441–449.

Bignami, A., and Palladini, G. (1966). Experimentally produced cerebral status spongiosus and continuous pseudorhythmic electroencephalographic discharges with a membrane-ATPase inhibitor in the rat. *Nature (Lond.) 209*: 413–414.

Bircher, R. P., Kanai, T., and Wang, S. C. (1963). Mechanisms of cardiac arrhythmias and blood pressure changes induced in dogs by pentylenetetrazol, picrotoxin, and deslanoside. *J. Pharmacol. Exp. Ther. 141*:6–14.

Birks, R. I. (1963). The role of sodium ions in the metabolism of acetylcholine. *Can. J. Biochem. Physiol. 41*:2573–2597.

Boyd, E. S., Merill, D. A., and Gardner, L. C. (1966). The effect of convulsant drugs on transmission through the cuneate nucleus. *J. Pharmacol. Exp. Therap. 154*:398–406.

Butterbaugh, G., and Spratt, J. (1970). Observations on the possible role of central mechanisms in acute digitoxigenin toxicity. *Toxicol. Appl. Pharmacol.* *17*:387-399.

Chen, K. K., Robbins, E. B., and Worth, H. (1938). The significance of the sugar component in the molecule of cardiac glycosides. *J. Am. Pharm. Assoc. 27*: 189-195.

Doggett, N. S., Spencer, P. S. J., and Turner, T. A. R. (1970). The pharmacological effects of ouabain administered intracerebrally to conscious mice. *Br. J. Pharmacol. 40*:138-139.

Donaldson, J., Minnich, J. L., Izumi, K., and Barbeau, A. (1973). Ouabain-induced seizures in rats: Relationship to brain monoamines. *Can. J. Biochem. 51*:198-203.

Donaldson, J., St-Pierre, T., and Minnich, J. (1971). Seizures in rats associated with divalent cation inhibition of Na^+/K^+-ATPase. *Can. J. Biochem. 49*: 1217-1224.

Douglas, E. F., White, P. T., and Nelson, J. W. (1971). Three per second spike wave in digitalis toxicity. *Arch. Neurol. 25*:373-375.

Feuerstein, J., Mantz, J. M., and Kurtz, D. (1973). EEG and massive digitalis intoxication. A case of epilepsy with respiratory manifestations and prolonged apnea. *Electroencephalogr. Clin. Neurophysiol. 34*:213-316.

Fowler, R. S., Rathl, L., and Keith, J. D. (1964). Accidental digitalis intoxication in children. *J. Pediatr. 64*:188-199.

Frankl, W., and Lathers, C. M. (1984a). Cardiogenic shock and low output syndrome. In *Cardiovascular Therapeutics in Clinical Practice*, W. Frankl, J. Roberts, and C. M. Lathers (Eds.). Wiley, New York, Chapter 4. pp. 175-196.

Frankl, W., Roberts, J., and Lathers, C. M. (1984b). Congestive heart failure. In *Cardiovascular Therapeutics in Clinical Practice*, W. Frankl, J. Roberts, and C. M. Lathers (Eds.). Wiley, New York, Chapter 3, pp. 115-174.

Frazer, D., and Tillie, R. (1925). In *Digitalis and Its Allies*, A. R. Chushny (Ed.). Longmans, Green, London, pp. 176-180.

Gillis, R. A. (1969). Cardiac sympathetic nerve activity: Changes induced by ouabain and propranolol. *Science 166*:508-510.

Gillis, R. A., Raines, A., Sohn, Y. J., Levitt, B., and Standoert, F. G. (1972). Neuroexcitatory effects of digitalis and their role in the development of cardiac arrhythmias. *J. Pharmacol. Exp. Ther. 183*:154-168.

Gold, H., Modell, W., Cattell, M., et al. (1947). Action of digitalis glycosides on the central nervous system with special reference to the convulsant action of red squill. *J. Pharmacol. Exp. Ther. 91*:15-30.

Gottesfeld, Z., and Elazar, A. (1975). GABA synthesis and uptake in penicillin focus. *Brain. Res. 84*:346-350.

Jobe, P. C., Stull, R. E., and Geiger, P. F. (1974). The relative significance of norepinephrine, dopamine, and 5-hydroxytryptamine in electroshock seizure in the rat. *Neuropharmacology 13*:961-968.

Karlsson, A., Fonnum, F., Malthe Strennsen, D., et al. (1974). Effect of the convulsive agent 3-mercaptopropionic acid on the level of GABA, other amino acids and glutamate decarboxylase in different regions of the rat brain. *Biochem. Pharmacol. 23*:3053-3061.

Kerr, D. J., Elliott, H. L., and Hillis, S. (1982). Epileptiform seizures and electroencephalographic abnormalities as manifestations of digoxin toxicity. *Br. Med. J. 284*:162–163.

Konzett, H., and Rothlin, E. (1952). Effect of cardioactivty glycosides on a sympathetic ganglion. *Arch. Int. Pharmacodyn. Ther. 89*:343–352.

Lage, G. L., and Spratt, J. L. (1966). Structure-activity correlation of the lethality and central effects of selected cardiac glycosides. *J. Pharmacol. Exp. Ther. 152*:501–508.

Lathers, C. M. (1980). Effect of timolol on prostaganglionic cardiac and preganglionic splanchnic sympathetic neural discharge associated with ouabain-induced arrhythmia. *Eur. J. Pharmacol. 64*:95–106.

Lathers, C. M. (in press). Digitalis glycosides. In *Textbook of Pharmacology*, A. M. Reynard and C. M. Smith (Eds.). W. B. Saunders, Philadelphia.

Lathers, C. M., and Roberts, J. (1980). Minireview: Digitalis cardiotoxicity revisited. *Life Sci. 27*:1713–1733.

Lathers, C. M., and Roberts, J. (1986). Digitalis glycosides. In *Pharmacology in Medicine: Principles and Practice. Textbook of Pharmacology* S. N. Pradham, R. P. Maickel, S. N. Dutta, and S. P. Press (Eds.). International, Maryland, pp. 555–571.

Lathers, C. M., and Schraeder, P. L. (1982). Autonomic dysfunction in epilepsy. Characterization of autonomic cardiac neural discharge associated with pentylenetetrazol-induced epileptogenic activity. *Epilepsia 23*:633–648.

Lathers, C. M., Roberts, J., and Kelliher, G. J. (1977). Correlation of ouabain-induced arrhythmia and nonuniformity in the histamine-evoked discharge of cardiac sympathetic nerves. *J. Pharmacol. Exp. Ther. 203*:467–479.

Lathers, C. M., Kellilher, G. J., Roberts, J., and Beasley, A. B. (1978). Nonuniform cardiac sympathetic nerve discharge: Mechanism for coronary occlusion and digitalis-induced arrhythmias. *Circulation 57*:1058–1065.

Lathers, C. M., Gerard-Ciminera, J. L., Baskin, S. I., Krusz, J. C., Kelliher, G. J., and Roberts, J. (1981). The action of reserpine, 6-hydroxydopamine, and bretylium on digitalis-induced cardiotoxicity. *Eur. J. Pharmacol. 76*:371–379.

Lathers, C. M., Gerard-Ciminera, J. L., Baskin, S. I., Krusz, J. C., Kelliher, G. J., Goldberg, P. B., and Roberts, J. (1982). Role of the adrenergic nerve terminal in digitalis-induced cardiac toxicity. A study of the effects of pharmacological and surgical denervation. *J. Cardiovasc. Pharmacol. 4*:91–98.

Lebovitz, R. M. (1974). Reactivity of penicillin-induced epileptogenic foci to selective blockade of membrane sodium-potassium ATPase via ouabain. *Exp. Neurol. 42*:647–660.

Levitt, B., Raines, A., Sohn, Y. J., Standaert, F. G., and Hirshfeld, J. W. (1970). The nervous system as a site of action for digitalis and antiarrhythmic drugs. *Mt. Sinai J. Med. 37*:227–240.

Lewin, E. (1970). Epileptogenic foci induced with ouabain. *Electroencephalogr. Clin. Neurophysiol. 29*:402–403.

Lewin, J., and Esplin, D. (1961). Analysis of the spinal excitatory action of pentylenetetrazol. *J. Pharmacol. Exp. Ther. 132*:245–250.

McLain, P. L. (1969). Effects of cardiac glycosides on spontaneous efferent activity in vagus and sympathetic nerves of cats. *Int. J. Neuropharmacol. 8*: 379-387.

McNamara, R. C., Brewer, E. A., and Ferry, G. R. (1964). Accidental poisoning of children with digitalis. *New Engl. J. Med. 251*:1106-1108.

Meldrum, B., Anlezark, G., and Trimble, M. (1975). Drugs modifying dopamin- ergic activity and behavior, the EEG and epilepsy in *Papio papio. Eur. J. Pharmacol. 32*:203-213.

Melville, K. I., and Shister, H. E. (1957). General systemic effects and electro- cardiographic changes following injections of digitalis glycosides into the lateral ventricle of the brain. *Am. Heart J. 53*:425-438.

Osterberg, R. E., and Raines, A. (1973). Changes in spinal cord neural mecha- nisms associated with digitalis administration. *J. Pharmacol. Exp. Ther. 187*: 246-259.

Pedley, T. A., Zuckerman, E. C., and Glaser, G. H. (1969). Epileptogenic effects of localized ventricular perfusion of ouabain on dorsal hippocampus. *Exp. Neurol. 25*:207-219.

Peronnet, F., Sindou, M., Laviron, A., et al. (1972). Human cortical electrogene- sis: Stratigraphy and spectral analysis. In *Synchronization of EEG Activity in Epilepsies*, H. Petsche and M. A. B. Brazier (Eds.). Springer, Vienna, pp. 235- 262.

Perry, W. L. M., and Reinert, H. (1954). The action of cardiac glycosides on autonomic ganglia. *Br. J. Pharmacol. 9*:324-328.

Petsche, H. (1972). Zum Nachweis des kortilalen Angriffspunktes des antikon- vulsiven benzodiazepinderivates Chlorazepam. *Z. EEG-EMG 3*:145-152.

Petsche, H., and Rappelsberger, P. (1970). A method to determine the efficiency of anti-epileptic drugs on experimental cortical seizures. *Electroencephalogr. Clin. Neurophysiol. 29*:316-318.

Petsche, H., and Seitelberger, F. (1967). Hirnelektrische Tatigkeit und Rinden- struktur. *Wein Klin. Wiss. 79*:492-496.

Petsche, H., Rappelsberger, P., Frey, Z., et al. (1973). The epileptogenic effects of ouabain (g-strophanthin): Its action on the EEG and cortical morphology. *Epilepsia 14*:243-260.

Potter, M., Vedrinne, J., Perrot, L., et al. (1964). In *L'intoxication Digitalique Massive*. Masson, Paris, p. 135.

Roberts, E., and Kuriyama, K. (1968). Biochemical-physiological correlation in studies of the gamma-aminobutyric acid system. *Brain Res. 8*:1-35.

Sarangi, A., Tripathy, N., Laii, D., Patnaik, B. C., and Swain, A. K. (1980). Study of serum digoxin status in digitoxicity by radioimmunoassay. *Am. Heart J. 28*:289-293.

Scherrer, J., and Calvet, J. (1972). Normal and epileptic synchronization at cor- tical level in animals. In *Synchronization of EEG Activity in Epilepsia*, H. Petsche and M. A. B. Brazier (Eds.). Springer, Vienna, pp. 112-132.

Schraeder, P. L., and Lathers, C. M. (1983). Cardiac neural discharge and epileptogenic activity in the cat: An animal model for unexplained sudden death. *Life Sci. 32*:1371–1382.

Shermann, J. L., and Locke, R. J. (1960). Transplacental neonatal digitalis intoxication. *Am. J. Cardiol. 6*:834–837.

Skou, J. C. (1965). Enzymatic basis for active transport of Na^+ and K^+ across cell membranes. *Physiol. Res. 45*:596–617.

Sohn, Y. J., Raines, A., and Levitt, B. (1970). Respiratory actions of the cardiac glycoside, ouabain. *Eur. J. Pharmacol. 12*:19–23.

Stach, R., and Kacz, D. (1977). Effect of combined dopaminergic and GABAergic stimulation on ouabain-induced epileptiform activity. *Epilepsia 18*: 417–423.

Stone, W. E., and Javid, M. J. (1982). Interactions of phenytoin with ouabain and other chemical convulsants. *Arch. Int. Pharmacokyn. 260*:28–35.

Stull, R. E., Jobe, P. C., Geiger, P. F., et al. (1973). Effects of dopamine receptor stimulation and blockade on Ro4-1284-induced enhancement of electroshock seizure. *J. Pharm. Pharmacol. 25*:842–844.

Tapia, R., Pasantes-Morales, H., Taborda, E., et al. (1975). Seizure susceptibility in the developing mouse and its relationship to glutamate decarboxylase and pyridoxal phosphate in brain. *J. Neurobiol. 6*:159–170.

Ten Eick, R. E., and Hoffman, B. F. (1969). The effect of digitalis on the excitability of autonomic nerves. *J. Pharmacol. Exp. Ther. 169*:95–108.

Tettlebaum, J. (1931). Troubles du rythme cardique provoques par l'intoxication digitalique massive du coeur humain normal. Thèse, Lyon.

Vernadakis, A. (1972). Spontaneous seizures in rat treated with chlorpromazine during postnatal development. *Experientia 28*:173–174.

Weaver, L. C., Akera, T., and Brody, T. M. (1975). Opposing responses in sympathetic nerve activity induced by central injections of ouabain. *J. Pharmacol. Exp. Ther. 195*:114–125.

Weaver, L. C., Akera, T., and Brody, T. M. (1976). Digoxin toxicity: Primary sites of drug action on the sympathetic nervous system. *J. Pharmacol. Exp. Ther. 197*:1–9.

Whithering, W. (1785). *An account of the foxglove and some of its medical use, with practical remarks on dropsy and other diseases*. Robinson, Birmingham. Reprinted in Cardiac Classics, C. V. Mosby, St. Louis, 1941.

Wood, J. D., and Petsche, S. J. (1975). The anticonvulsant action of GABA-elevating agents: A re-evaluation. *J. Neurochem, 25*:277–286.

Woodbury, D. M. (1980a). Convulsant drugs: Mechanism of action. In *Antiepileptic Drugs*, G. H. Glaser, J. K. Penry, and D. M. Woodbury (Eds.). Raven Press, New York, pp. 249–303.

Woodbury, D. M. (1980b). Phenytoin: Proposed mechanism of anticonvulsant action. In *Antiepileptic Drugs*, G. H. Glaser, J. K. Penry, and D. M. Woodbury (Eds.). Raven Press, New York, pp. 447–471.

Yessaian, N. H., Armenian, A. R., Kazarova, E. K., et al. (1971). On the involvement of inorganic ions in the effect of gamma-aminobutyric acid on brain serotonin and norepinephrine. *J. Neurochem. 18*: 307-321.

21

Cocaine-Induced Seizures, Arrhythmias, and Sudden Death

CLAIRE M. LATHERS,* MICHELLE M. SPINO, ISHA AGARWAL, and
LAURIE S. Y. TYAU   *The Medical College of Pennsylvania, Eastern
Pennsylvania Psychiatric Institute, Philadelphia, Pennsylvania*

WALLACE B. PICKWORTH   *Addiction Research Center, National Institute
on Drug Abuse, Baltimore, Maryland*

I. INTRODUCTION

The presence of coca leaves in the tombs of South American Indian mummies
suggests that cocaine was used as early as A.D. 600. The use of cocaine is becoming prevalent in modern society. Cregler and Mark (1986a) reviewed the
demographics of current cocaine users and found that approximately 22 million
to 30 million, or 1 out of every 10 Americans, have used cocaine at least once
and there are over 5 million chronic users of cocaine and another 5000 persons
trying it each day (Cregler and Mark, 1987). The fallacy that cocaine is a benign,
nonaddicting substance may be part of the reason for the alarming rise in abuse
(Cregler and Mark, 1986b). This increase is also attributed to the limited information published on the short- and long-term effects of cocaine. Published accounts of the action of cocaine on the systems of the body are fairly recent and
often controversial, consisting almost entirely of individual case reports (Fischman et al., 1976; Loveys, 1987; Pitts et al., 1987).

Although cocaine has been found to be a cardiotoxin, the pathogenesis of this
toxicity is not well defined (Cregler and Mark, 1987). Cocaine use has also been
linked to the occurrence of subarachnoid hemorrhage, hypertension, ventricular
arrhythmia, tachycardia, acute myocardial infarction, seizure, and sudden death
(Lichtenfeld et al., 1984; Nahas et al., 1985; Tazelaar et al., 1987; Young and

---

Current affiliation; FDA, Rockville, Maryland.
This chapter was written as an outside activity and does not reflect the views of the
Addiction Research Center, NIDA, or the U.S. Government.

Glauber, 1947). Persons with epilepsy have been shown to manifest autonomic dysfunctions similar to those manifest by cocaine users, including changes in blood pressure and heart rate and rhythm, phenomena that may be contributory to sudden unexpected death (Leestma, 1984; Penfield and Erickson, 1941; Phizackerly et al., 1954; Walsh et al., 1968). Thus one must ask whether the use of cocaine in individuals with epilepsy places these individuals at risk of dying in a sudden unexplained manner.

II. MECHANISMS OF ACTION OF COCAINE

Cocaine (Figure 1), extracted from the leaves of *Erythroxylon coca*, is a potent local anesthetic agent (Cregler and Mark, 1986a; Gould et al., 1985) possessing membrane-stabilizing effects at low plasma levels (Tazelaar et al., 1987). It is also a sympathomimetic agent at higher plasma concentrations (Benchimol et al., 1978; Duke, 1986).

Cocaine amplifies the effect of catecholamines by blocking the re-uptake at the synaptic junctions, causing a local excess of norepinephrine at the synaptic cleft. As a result of the excess of norepinephrine at the nerve terminal, there is a prolongation and potentiation of the activity of norepinephrine (Weiss, 1986). Norepinephrine is the primary neurotransmitter of the sympathetic nervous system. Excitation of the sympathetic nervous system produces physiological characteristics, such as mobilization of adrenal catecholamines, causing an increase in blood pressure, an increase in heart rate, dilatation of the pupils, a rise in blood sugar levels, vasoconstriction of vessels in the brain and muscles, tightening of the sphincters, and an elevation of body temperature. The intense peripheral vasoconstriction retards reabsorption. Drug effects include intense euphoria and elation, garrulousness, excitability, and irritability; with repeated administration paranoid ideation, delirium, and assaultiveness occur. Table 1 summarizes the

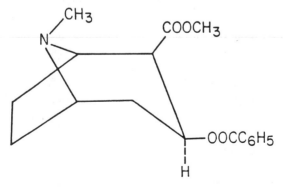

Figure 1   Structure of cocaine ($C_{17}H_{21}NO_4$).

Table 1 The Cocaine Reaction

Phase	Central nervous system	Cardiovascular system	Respiratory system
I: Early stimulation	Euphoria; stated feelings of "soaring," well being Elation, expansive good humor, laughing Mydriasis Talkative, garrulous Excited, flighty, emotionally unstable Restless, irritable; apprehensive; unable to sit still Stereotyped movements (such as "picking" or "stroking"), bruxism Nausea, vomiting, vertigo Sudden headache Cold sweats Tremor (nonintentional) Twitching of small muscles, especially of the face, fingers, and feet Tics, generalized Preconvulsive, tonic and clonic jerks Possible psychosis, hallucinations Core body temperature rises Verbalization of impending doom (precedes imminent total collapse)	Pulse varies at first, may immediately slow because of reflex vagal effect; will increase 30% to 50% above normal with system absorption of 25 mg of cocaine Blood pressure usually elevates 15% to 20% above normal with similar dosages as noted above Skin pallor caused by vasoconstriction Premature ventricular contractions	Increased respiratory rate and depth Dyspnea
II: Advanced stimulation	Unresponsive to voice; decreased responsiveness to all stimuli Increased deep tendon reflexes Generalized hyperreflexia Convulsions, tonic and clonic Status epilepticus Incontinence Malignant encephalopathy possible	Increased pulse and blood pressure; high output failure possible Blood pressure falls as ventricular dysrhythmias supervene and inefficient cardiac output results Pulse becomes rapid, weak, and irregular Peripheral, then central cyanosis	Gasping, rapid, or irregular respiration (Cheyne-Stokes)
III: Depressive	Flaccid paralysis of muscles Coma Pupils fixed and dilated Loss of reflexes Loss of vital support functions Paralysis of medullary brain center Exitus	Ventricular fibrillation Circulation failure Ashen gray cyanosis No palpable pulse Cardiac arrest Paralysis of medullary brain center Exitus	Agonal gasps Respiratory failure Gross pulmonary edema Paralysis of medullary brain center Exitus

actions of cocaine on the cardiovascular, respiratory, and central nervous system (Gay, 1982).

Cocaine as a hydrochloride salt is brought into the United States ranging up to 95% in its purity (Gay, 1982). The purity is decreased to 25–90% of its original state through the addition of diluents and adulterants such as procaine, lidocaine (Cregler and Mark, 1986b), caffeine, benzocaine, amphetamines, heroin, quinine, talc, and phencyclidine. All adulterants contribute to the toxicity of cocaine. Finally, it is combined with sugars such as mannitol, lactose, and glucose to attain a final volume and weight (Gay, 1982). The resulting cocaine product can be administered by various routes, including intravenous and subcutaneous injections, intranasal inhalation (snorting), and the current vogue of smoking a "free base" form of cocaine (crack). Free base smoking or intravenous injections of cocaine cause a euphoric or "rush" experience, which occurs within 45 seconds and is associated with a rapid increase in plasma cocaine concentrations. The effect lasts for approximately 20 minutes. In contrast, intranasal administration results in euphoria occurring within three to five minutes of administration and lasts for one to one and a half hours (Van Dyke and Byck, 1983). Regardless of the route of administration, accounts of cocaine-induced sudden death have become common.

III. COCAINE-INDUCED SUDDEN DEATH

Sudden death has been shown to be induced by cocaine (Amon et al., 1986; Estroff and Gold, 1986; Mittleman and Welti, 1987; Welti and Fishbain, 1985). Reports indicate 1.2 g to be a lethal dose; however, severe toxic effects have been reported with doses as low as 20 mg (Estroff and Gold, 1986). Because it is so sudden, medical personnel do not ordinarily witness cocaine-induced death; victims usually collapse and die before resuscitation efforts can begin.

Confusion or convulsions precede death induced by cocaine. Estroff and Gold (1986) reported seven cases of sudden death associated with the use of cocaine, in whom a state of excited delirium was the fatal symptom. The initial symptom was intense paranoia, followed by bizarre and violent behavior necessitating the use of force to restrain the patient. The unexpected outbursts of strength were associated with hyperthermia, which was thought to be due to a direct effect of cocaine on the central nervous system center for temperature regulation, and due to peripheral vasoconstriction, with resultant reduction in heat (Ritchie and Greene, 1980). Status epilepticus, respiratory paralysis, or cardiac arrhythmias genrally precede sudden death induced by cocaine. Abramowicz (1986) suggested that most sudden deaths associated with cocaine use are caused by seizures leading to anoxia. Recent clinical data have been correlated with pathological findings, generating several hypotheses which attempt to define forensically the pathological mechanisms of cocaine-induced sudden death.

A. Cocaine-Induced Changes in Mean Arterial Blood Pressure and Heart Rate

The circulatory effects of cocaine are believed to be of both central and peripherally induced vasoconstriction and cardioacceleration (Young and Glauber, 1947). Change in heart rate is a sensitive measure of cocaine-induced cardiovascular effect (Fischman et al., 1976). Cocaine results in dose-related changes in heart rate (Javiad et al., 1978), with small doses decreasing heart rate via central vagal action and moderate doses increasing heart rate via atrial and peripheral sympathetic stimulation (Benchimol et al., 1978). Extremely high intravenous

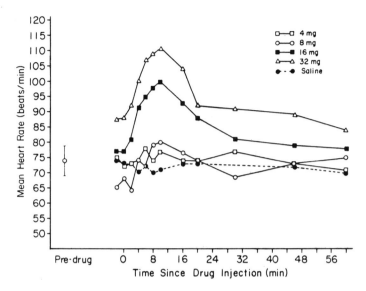

Figure 2 Mean heart rate as a function of the time after cocaine was injected.

doses have direct toxic effects on the heart and cause immediate death (Nanji and Filipenko, 1984; Young and Glauber, 1947). The duration of the cardiovascular action is dependent on the dose of cocaine. Fischman et al. (1976) showed that an increase in heart rate was evident after intravenous injections of varying doses of cocaine; the increase began 2–5 minutes after infusion, peaked at 10 minutes, and rapidly returned to baseline (Figure 2). Cocaine also increased blood pressure in a dose-related manner, but more variability is seen in this measure. In one study (Pitts et al., 1987) cocaine was administered intravenously and evoked a rapid, transient, dose-dependent rise in mean arterial pressures (Figure 3).

Jain et al. (1987) reported that the administration of cocaine (0.25 mg/kg i.v.) to anesthetized cats increased systolic and diastolic blood pressure by 33 ± 11 and 31 ± 7 mm Hg, respectively. The dose also enhanced the pressor responses to intravenous norepinephrine and to bilateral carotid occlusion. Doses of 0.5 and 1.0 mg/kg i.v. also caused an increase in blood pressure and responses to intravenous norepinephrine but did not increase the blood pressure response to bilateral carotid occlusion. Higher doses had no additive effect on the blood pressure, but rather slowed the heart rate, attenuated blood pressure responses to norepinephrine, prolonged the QRS duration, and decreased tidal volumes. All effects were increased after a dose of 4 mg/kg or greater of cocaine intravenously, with arrhythmias occurring with 4 and 8 mg/kg. Doses as low as 0.25

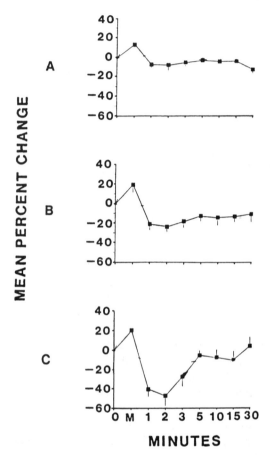

Figure 3   Time course for the cardiovascular and respiratory effects of three different doses of cocaine: 0.312, 1.25, and 5 mg/kg i.v. depicted in panels A (*N* = 6), B (*N* = 5), and C (*N* = 4), respectively. Ordinate scale is percentage of change and the abscissa scale is time in minutes. *M* = period during maximal pressor response. Squares represent mean value for the arterial pressure. Vertical lines represent standard error of the mean. All animals were anesthetized with pentobarbital (6.5 mg/kg i.p.). [Modified from Pitts (1987).]

mg/kg i.v. evoked substantial cardiovascular responses and lethal responses of apnea.

In another study, the administration of cocaine intravenously to conscious rats increased arterial blood pressure (Rockhold et al., 1987). The heart rate was elevated initially but subsequently was decreased. With the onset of cocaine-induced seizures a further elevation in heart rate and blood pressure occurred, ultimately progressing to cardiovascular collapse and death. Preliminary studies utilizing intravenous administration of cocaine to anesthetized dogs elicited a dose-dependent increase in blood pressure and heart rate and alterations in the S-T segment (Tackett and Jones, 1987). These changes were associated with elevated cerebrospinal fluid levels of norepinephrine and dopamine, findings which suggest a role for central catecholaminergic mechanisms in the cardiovascular actions of cocaine. Therefore, as cocaine raises the blood pressure and heart rate to excessively high levels, there is an increased risk of aneurism, arterovenous malformation, or stroke and/or hemorrhage from ruptures of cerebral arteries weakened by drug-related arteritis.

B. Cocaine-Induced Myocardial Ischemia, Infarction, Arrhythmia, and Cardiomyopathies

There has been a recent and dramatic increase of cardiac abnormalities among cocaine users (Duke, 1986; Wiener and Putnam, 1987; Wiener et al., 1986), which has raised questions concerning the effect of cocaine on the cardiovascular system. Indeed, cocaine is clearly cardiotoxic, being temporally linked to myocardial ischemia, arrhythmias, and many cardiomyopathies. Cocaine use in the presence of preexisting coronary artery disease may predispose the individual to the development of angina, arrhythmias, or myocardial infarction (Coleman et al., 1982; Young and Glauber, 1947). It is possible that a patient with hypercholesterolemia who is using cocaine may be further increasing the likelihood of coronary artery spasm (Rosendorff et al., 1981), leading to myocardial ischemia and necrosis.

Numerous cases of suspected cocaine-induced myocardial ischemias and infarctions have been reported (Isner et al., 1985, 1986; Kassowsky and Lyon, 1984; Mathias, 1986; Rod and Zucker, 1987; Rollingher et al., 1986; Schachne et al., 1984; Simpson and Edwards, 1986). Simpson and Edwards (1986) reported a case of a 21-year-old man with a history of recreational intravenous cocaine abuse who developed chest pain within one minute and cardiopulmonary collapse within one hour after injection of cocaine. Postmortem findings revealed severe coronary obstructive lesions and acute platelet thrombosis, with secondary chronic and acute myocardial ischemic lesions, focal endothelial injury, and platelet aggregations being observed. The author proposed that coronary artery spasm induced by cocaine caused the endothelial lesions and favored platelet adherence and aggregation. The chronic obstructions that were also found may have resulted from a similar mechanism. According to Weiss (1986), fixed coronary atherosclerotic lesions play a permissive role in the induction of coronary vasospasm. It has been proposed that the ability of both intrinsic atherosclerotic plaques and cocaine-induced norepinephrine uptake blockade increases local levels of catecholamine, producing coronary vasospasms. Furthermore, preexisting coronary artery disease sensitizes the vascular smooth muscle to norepinephrine-induced vasoconstriction, predisposing the cocaine user to life-threatening ischemia (Gould et al., 1985; Weiss, 1986). Also, with chronic cocaine abuse, the excessive accumulation of norepinephrine may prime the myocardium for a fatal arrhythmia (Tazelaar et al., 1987).

Cocaine increases the local concentrations of catecholamines from blocked adrenergic nerve endings to other cell receptors by inhibiting the neuronal uptake of norepinephrine. Thus the adrenergic response in susceptible organs is increased, leading to the development of catecholamine supersensitivity (Benchimol et al., 1978; Trendlenberg, 1968). Therefore, cocaine is capable of eliciting both an inhibitory and an excitatory response of sympathetically innervated structures to endogenous and exogenous catecholamines (Pitts et al., 1987). It has also been suggested that cocaine accentuates the action of norepinephrine on beta receptors in the heart (Nanji et al., 1984) by increasing the concentration of norepinephrine at the synaptic cleft. Beta stimulation increases automaticity, heart rate, and the conduction velocity of the His-Purkinje system and decreases atrioventricular nodal refractoriness (Tazelaar et al., 1987).

Tazelaar et al. (1987) characterized cocaine-induced pathophysiology in a postmortem study of 30 cocaine-related deaths. Morphologic characteristics of acute ischemia were observed in 93% of the cases. These involved the formation of myocardial contraction bands in association with polymorphonucleocytes in the initial 12–24 hours; they were replaced with lymphocytes by 24–48 hours. The formation of contraction bands and myocardial interstitial fibrosis may be one pathogenic mechanism for fatal arrhythmias. These contraction bands may also represent an anatomical route for reentrant mechanism, thus priming the heart for fatal arrhythmias. It is quite possible that arrhythmias may be generated by cocaine through a decrease in the refractoriness of the myocardial fibers, accumulation of excess norepinephrine, formation of contraction bands, and production of interstitial fibrosis.

Cocaine causes myocardial ischemia by direct and indirect actions (Vitullo et al., 1987). Direct effects are the stimulation of the sinoatrial node, with an increase in heart rate, contractility, and wall tension. Indirectly, the effects can be due to the sympathetic vasoconstriction of the peripheral smooth muscle vasculature. Arterial vasoconstriction leads to an increase in afterload and blood pressure, which, in turn, increases the work that the heart must pump against.

Both the direct and the indirect actions increase the oxygen consumption of the myocardium, with an ischemic event occurring when the demand for oxygen supersedes the supply (Tyau and Lathers, 1988).

Pasternack et al. (1985) reported three male patients in their middle to late thirties who were referred for coronary angiography after having angina pectoris and/or an acute myocardial infarction, coincident with an increase in the frequency of cocaine abuse. The onset of angina and acute myocardial infarctions may have been caused by a cocaine-induced potentiation of the activities of the central nervous system resulting in systemic hypertension and tachycardia. Isner et al. (1986) reported a temporal relationship between cocaine and cardiac sequelae in seven nonintravenous cocaine abusers. It was concluded that cocaine may precipitate fatal arrhythmias, myocarditis, acute infarctions, and possible sudden death in patients with either anatomically normal or abnormal coronary arteries. In these cases there was a temporal relationship between the administration of cocaine and the onset of a myocardial ischemia and/or infarction. Because of many other medical factors involved, it is difficult to discern the actual etiological mechanisms of the infarctions. However, in a case report by Howard et al. (1985), a young woman with normal coronary arteries, blood glucose, and lipid levels and no history of cardiovascular disease or smoking was admitted to the hospital for loss of consciousness and epigastric pain; five hours prior she had inhaled 1.5 g of cocaine. On admission, an ECG showed precordial ST segment elevation and a loss of R waves. On the day following admission, an echocardiography revealed akinesis and dyskinesis of the left ventricle apex and septum. In this healthy individual with no coronary risk factors or demonstrable coronary artery disease, infarction occurred. This finding suggests that cocaine-induced myocardial infarctions should be considered when examining individuals who may not appear to be vulnerable. The cardiovascular events produced through cocaine abuse can be seen to involve a range of pathological responses, including coronary vasospasm, arrhythmia, myocardial ischemia, infarction, and cardiomyopathies.

Therapeutic use of cocaine is not without risk. For example, Chiu et al. (1986) reported a patient who was anesthesized for a closed reduction of a nasal fracture by spraying 2 ml of 1% cocaine solution into the nasal airways. The patient complained of an acute onset of chest pain and shortness of breath. An electrocardiogram indicated ST-T wave changes in the precordial leads, suggestive of an acute coronary ischemic event. The rise in the MB creatine kinase fraction and reversed LDH isoenzyme fractional values were consistent with a small nontransmural myocardial infarction. The published accounts of cardiovascular events, myocardial infarction, and mortality related to cocaine use as described here are fairly recent and consist almost entirely of case reports (Loveys, 1987). Experimental research looking into the cardiovascular effects of cocaine is warranted.

C. Cocaine-Induced Changes in Postganglionic Cardiac Sympathetic Neural Function

Cocaine potentiates the ganglionic blocking action of norepinephrine (Christ et al., 1982). In the isolated hamster stellate ganglia preparation, cocaine exaggerated the inhibitory action of exogenously applied norepinephrine. In pithed rats, cocaine potentiated the pressor effect of norepinephrine more than it potentiated the pressor effect of sympathetic stimulation (Bayorh et al., 1983). Cocaine increased plasma norepinephrine levels and extended the inotropic and chronotropic responses to sympathetic neural stimulation in anesthetized dogs (Matsuda et al., 1980). These actions were attributed to the inhibition of the neuronal catecholamine uptake by cocaine (Matsuda, 1980). It is possible that cocaine-induced exaggeration of sympathetic discharge may enhance the arrhythmias experimentally caused by ouabain (Lathers et al., 1977), coronary occlusion (Lathers et al., 1978), and seizures (Lathers and Schraeder, 1982; Schraeder and Lathers, 1983). Experimental arrhythmias are hypothesized to be a useful model to study possible mechanisms of sudden death associated with myocardial infarctions (Lathers et al., 1986) and epilepsy (Lathers and Schraeder, 1987; Schraeder and Lathers, 1989). Consequently, any changes induced by cocaine in cardiac sympathetic neural discharge may well augment the development of arrhythmias and/or sudden death.

On the other hand, Dart et al. (1983) demonstrated that stimulation of postganglionic cardiac sympathetic nerves in a Langendorff rat-isolated heart preparation produced a stimulation frequency-dependent overflow of endogenous norepinephrine into the venous effluent with an increase in the heart rate. Cocaine significantly reduced the norepinephrine outflow while the heart rate continued to increase.

D. Central Actions of Cocaine

Many of the effects of cocaine result from actions in the central nervous system. Cocaine-induced euphoria, for example, was among the first effects described (Freud, 1884) and is the most well known central effect. Generalized convulsions, which often precede cocaine-induced death, unfortunately are less well known outside the medical community. It has been shown that seizures are a major determinant of cocaine-induced death (Catravas and Waters, 1981; Catravas et al., 1978). The common concomitants of generalized seizures, including hyperthermia, acidosis, increased blood pressure, cardiac arrhythmia, and hypoventilation, may be responsible for the lethality.

In animal studies, many of the effects of cocaine have been localized to limbic structures. For example, Castellani et al. (1983) found that cocaine initiated high-voltage spindles that began in the amygdala 5–25 seconds following the in-

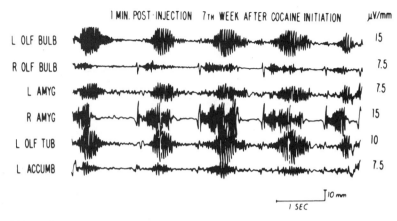

Figure 4 Electrographic amygdala–olfactory spindling and spike response to 5 mg/kg intravenous cocaine during preseizure behaviors.

jection of cocaine (Figure 4) and spread within seconds to other olfactory sites in synchronous bursts. Cocaine induced an increase in spindle frequency in the olfactory bulb and amygdala that was inhibited by atropine administration. Yasuda et al. (1984) reported that low concentrations of cocaine potentiated a norepinephrine-induced increase in spike amplitude of hippocampal splices. The authors concluded that the action was due to the inhibition of catecholamine uptake based on the observation that other inhibitors had the same effect.

Lesse and Collins (1979) found that cocaine increased the speed at which epileptiform discharge spread to the amygdala and hippocampus. They postulated that subconvulsive doses of cocaine have an excitatory effect on limbic structures, which increases their sensitivity to repetitive discharges from distant foci. Matsuzaki (1978) reported that chronic high doses of cocaine in the rhesus monkey engendered persistent behavioral depression, with cortical and limbic slowing of EEG. They concluded that it was the action of cocaine on limbic structures that played an important role in the persistence of these effects. Overall, the evidence indicates that cocaine enhances the propagation of limbic seizures. Since activity has been associated with cardiac arrhythmia (Lathers and Schraeder, 1982; Schraeder and Lathers, 1983), it is quite possible that cocaine-induced seizures could be a factor in the deaths of persons using the drug.

The cortical EEG effects of cocaine in humans were among the earliest documented effects of the drug (Berger, 1937). Cocaine increases power in the fast frequency (beta bands) of the resting EEG after subcutaneous, intravenous, or oral administration (Berger, 1937; Herning et al., 1985). Four-hour intravenous

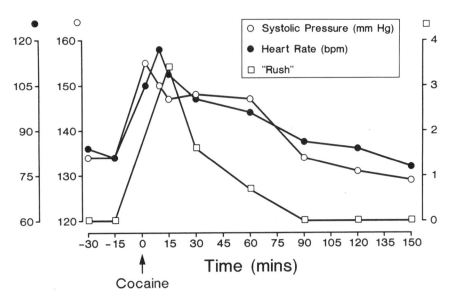

Figure 5   Effects of intravenous cocaine (60 mg) in seven drug-experienced volunteers. The high dose caused a transient "rush" (drug-induced euphoria) but
prolonged increases in blood pressure and heart rate.

infusions of high doses of cocaine in humans sustains the increase in EEG beta
power (Pickworth et al., 1986). The increase of power in the fast EEG frequency bands is ordinarily associated with increased attention, vigilance, or
arousal. Pickworth et al. (1986) measured subjective, cardiovascular, and EEG
effects of large (60 mg) intravenous doses of cocaine in human volunteers. Although the subjective report of "rush" lasted for only a few moments, the pressor effect and tachycardia persisted for up to 60 minutes (Figure 5). The rush, or
intense cocaine-induced euphoria, is the effect for which the drug is self-administered. It is quite probable that inadvertent overdosage may occur when subjects readminister cocaine at a time when the cardiovascular and central nervous
systems are at jeopardy.

In reviewing the effect of cocaine on the electrophysiology of the central
monoaminergic neurons, Pitts and Marwah (1986) found that intravenous cocaine activated cerebellar Purkinje neurons and inhibited serotonergic dorsal
raphe and noradrenergic locus coeruleus neurons. The authors concluded that
cocaine-induced increases in the mean arterial blood pressure were correlated
with changes in the discharge of the central neurons.

Pitts and Marwah (1987) also found that reserpine pretreatment diminished
the inhibitory effects of intravenous cocaine on neuronal discharges in the locus

coeruleus and dorsal raphe as well as the excitatory action of cocaine on the cerebellar Purkinje neurons. Thus, although stimulation of the inhibitory locus coeruleus afferent input to the cerebellar Purkinje neurons can reduce the activity of the Purkinje neurons via a beta-adrenoceptor mechanism, intravenous cocaine (1 mg/kg) did not precipitate the inhibitory actions of locus coeruleus stimulation on cerebellar Purkinje neurons. This dose of cocaine also did not potentiate the inhibitory effects of iontophoretically applied norepinephrine or GABA on cerebellar Purkinje neurons. Locus coeruleous neurons were inhibited by intravenous cocaine (1 mg/kg) in conscious animals paralyzed with gallamine. It was proposed that intravenous cocaine (1 mg/kg) reduced impulse flow in locus coeruleus neurons, possibly through an alpha$_2$ -autoreceptor mechanism, without augmenting the effect of norepinephrine at the level of the noradrenergic terminals impinging on postsynaptic cerebellar Purkinje neurons.

The action of cocaine on norepinephrine-containing locus coeruleus neurons was also evaluated in freely moving, unanesthetized cats (Trulson and Trulson, 1987). Cocaine elicited a dose-dependent reduction in the activity of the neurons, which was suppressed by a prior administration of an alpha$_2$ antagonist, piperoxane. Also, the activity of the locus coeruleus remained unchanged by the administration of the structurally related local anesthetic agent procaine. It was concluded that the local anesthetic actions of cocaine were not the inhibitory factor in its effect on the activity of norepinephrine-containing neurons. Nevertheless, as Yasuda et al. (1984) stated, "It is remarkable that its effects upon the electrophysiological activity of the brain remain virtually unknown." Whether cocaine-induced changes in the activity of central neurons contributes to sudden death remains to be determined.

E. Cocaine-Induced Seizures

Seizures have been shown to play an essential role in the pathophysiology of cocaine toxicity. A major determinant of lethality in cocaine-treated dogs was the presence of seizures (Catravas and Waters, 1981; Catravas et al., 1978). Cocaine infusions produced prolonged seizures that led to lactic acidosis and hyperthermia prior to death while cardiac output, systemic vascular resistance, respiration, and oxygenation were stable just prior to death. Seizures and death could have been prevented with pretreatment using diazepam, high-dose chlorpromazine, or neuromuscular blockade with pancuronium (Antelman et al., 1981; Fekete and Borsy, 1971). The use of diazepam is particularly important since it also counteracts the sympathomimetic action of cocaine on the heart. Treatment of acidosis alone did not prevent death, unless the animals were maintained in a hypothermic state.

Jonsson et al. (1983) reported one patient who, as a result of cocaine intoxication, showed combined metabolic and respiratory acidosis consequent to seizures and hypoventilation. Improved ventilation and the administration of bicarbonate reversed the hypotension and accelerated idioventricular rhythm to sinus rhythm. Blood pH increased from 6.33 to normal and the pCO_2 decreased from 70 to 46 mm Hg. Jonsson et al. concluded that respiratory arrest compounded the acidosis in patients intoxicated with cocaine and may have contributed significantly to their deaths. Acidosis has a particularly negative effect on myocardial contractility (Fabiato and Fabiato, 1978; Spivey et al., 1985) and acidosis can heighten the effects of catecholamines on the heart (Ford et al., 1968; Lathers et al., 1988; Spivey et al., 1986), and thereby contribute to the initiation of arrhythmias by cocaine.

Carbamazepine is an antiepileptic drug that seems to be particularly effective in treating limbic system seizures. In experimental studies, repeated high doses of cocaine produce a convulsive response classified as pharmacologic kindling. Weiss et al. (1987) reported that chronic carbamazepine administration inhibited the development of lidocaine- or cocaine-kindled seizures and lethality. Chronic, but not acute pretreatment with carbamazepine inhibited the high-dose cocaine seizures. It was suggested that carbamazepine may interact with local anesthetic mechanisms mediating the progressive development of seizures and that the effects of this antiepileptic drug at the level of the sodium channels should be further explored since both carbamazepine and the local anesthetics are believed to interact at this site. Investigation of the mechanism responsible for this effect should be undertaken, as it may prove clinically useful in preventing cocaine toxicity.

IV. TREATMENT OF COCAINE-INDUCED ARRHYTHMIAS AND SEIZURES

Treatment of cocaine toxicity must ultimately involve deconditioning therapy to reduce drug craving and drug-seeking behavior (Kumor et al., 1988). Tricyclic antidepressants, bromocriptine, amantadine, methylphenidate, and lithium may decrease cocaine self-medication. The hypertension and tachycardia that follow administration of cocaine are mediated by both alpha-adrenergic and beta-adrenergic receptors to induce vasoconstriction and an increase in heart rate and cardiac output, respectively (Olsen et al., 1983). One clinical management procedure of the adrenergic cocaine crisis involves the judicious use of intravenous propranolol, given in doses of 1 mg at one-minute intervals to a total of up to 6 mg (Gay, 1982). Although intervention calms the excitable patient and decreases tachyarrhythmias, the efficacy of propranolol is limited by its receptor sensitivity. It has been argued that although propranolol effectively blocks beta receptors to decrease heart rate, it leaves the alpha-adrenergic receptors unopposed (Olsen et al., 1983). Thus stimulation of the $alpha_1$-adrenergic receptors in the smooth muscle vasculature results in a worsening of vasoconstriction with resultant dangerous hypertension. Olsen et al. (1983) propose the use of phentolamine or nitroprusside to effect rapid vasodilatation. However, Gay (1983) argues that the nonselective alpha-adrenergic blockade properties of phentolamine may, in fact, further aggravate matters. Indeed, phentolamine will block alpha$_1$ postsynaptic receptors to decrease vasoconstriction, but it will also block alpha$_2$ presynaptic receptors. This blocks the normal regulatory control of the catecholamines, resulting in an increase in synthesis and output of norepinephrine, and may even spur a reflex sympathetic response to the heart. One agent recently used to treat cocaine toxicity is labetalol, which possesses both alpha- and beta-blocking capabilities. Thus the establishment of alpha blockade counters the cocaine-induced vasoconstriction and hypertension while the beta blockade decreases the tachyarrhythmias (Gay and Loper, 1988).

The use of chlorpromazine and haloperidol to calm the hyperkinetic state is contraindicated in the cocaine user as they can lower seizure threshold activity and cause cardiac arrhythmias and/or sudden death (Lathers and Lipka, 1986, 1987; Lipka and Lathers, 1987). Instead, effective means of quieting the stimulatory phase of cocaine intoxication is the use of diazepam, 15–20 mg orally every eight hours. Antelman et al. (1981) serendipitously found that amytriptiline, a tricyclic antidepressant, protected against sudden cardiac death due to cocaine intoxication in animals. Amytriptiline 10 mg/kg administered experimentally in animals one hour prior to intraperitoneal injection of cocaine (35 mg/kg) resulted in no protection against sudden death. However, 24-hour pretreatment with a single injection of amytriptiline markedly increased survival, while 10-day pretreatment conferred complete protection against sudden death. The mechanism of action, to date, has not been defined. However, pretreatment is not a useful tool in the management of clinical toxicity associated with cocaine use.

It has recently been suggested that Ca^{2+} channel blockers may be a useful antidote for cocaine toxicity (Duke, 1986; Mittleman and Welti, 1987; Trouve and Nahas, 1986). Ca^{2+} channel blockers inhibit the vasoconstrictive effects of norepinephrine by blocking the release of Ca^{2+} into the smooth muscle of the vasculature. Trouve and Nahas (1986) studied the cocaine antagonistic effects of nitrendepine, a Ca^{2+} channel blocker, in animals. Nitrendipine was selected for its lack of myocardial depressant activity and its ability to cause coronary vasodilatation. Nitrendipine, 1.46×10^{-3} mg/kg/min, was concomitantly administered with 2 mg/kg/min of cocaine and caused an inhibition of cocaine-induced tachycardia, pressor, and vasoconstriction. Nitrendipine also suppressed the cocaine-induced arrhythmias observed in control animals. In a comparative study, nitrendipine and propranolol were able to slow cocaine-induced tachycardia while nitrendepine alone increased coronary flow and pulse pressure. Nitrendipine

alone and in combination with propranolol decreased coronary flow and performance (Trouve and Nahas, 1986). In addition to its cardioprotective properties, nitrendipine appears to possess central activity. Nitrendipine prevented
motor tremors, convulsions, and seizures (Trouve and Nahas, 1986). It was concluded that the sympathomimetic properties of cocaine can be antagonized by
Ca^{2+} channel blockers. Ca^{2+} channel blockers may become the drugs of choice
for the treatment of cocaine intoxication.

V. USE OF COCAINE IN PERSONS WITH EPILEPSY

Since cocaine use has been reported to produce hypertension, ventricular arrhythmias, tachycardia, myocardial infarction, seizures, and sudden death
(Nahas et al., 1985; Tazelaar et al., 1987), and since persons with epilepsy have
been shown to manifest autonomic dysfunction, including changes in blood pressure, heart rate, and rhythm (Leestma et al., 1984; Penfield and Erickson, 1941;
Phizackerly et al., 1954; Walsh et al., 1968), one must raise the question of
whether the use of cocaine in individuals with epilepsy places them at risk of dying in a sudden, unexplained manner. Furthermore, dysfunction in the activity
of peripheral cardiac autonomic neural discharge contributes to the production
of cardiac arrhythmias (Gillis, 1969; Gillis et al., 1972; Lathers et al., 1974,
1977, 1978; Verrier and Lown, 1978; Weaver et al., 1976) and to sudden death
(Lown and Verrier, 1978). Lathers et al. (1977, 1978) and Lathers (1980) reported that nonuniform discharge in the cardiac postganglionic nerves, i.e.,
simultaneous increases and decreases in the various sympathetic branches innervating the myocardium, contributes to the production of arrhythmias by altering
ventricular automaticity and excitability in the manner reported by Han and
Moe (1964). Similar autonomic cardiac neural dysfunction was reported in association with arrhythmias and interictal and ictal discharges (Carnel et al.,
1985; Lathers and Schraeder, 1982, 1987; Lathers et al., 1984, 1987; Schraeder
and Lathers, 1983, 1988). Cocaine also modifies postganglionic cardiac sympathetic neural function, increasing the inotropic and chronotropic responses to
sympathetic neural stimulation (Matsuda et al., 1980). Thus it is possible that
the actions of cocaine and the autonomic cardiac neural dysfunction associated
with epileptogenic activity may combine to produce cardiac arrhythmias and, at
worst, sudden unexpected death. The question of whether cocaine use in the individual with epilepsy places the individual at risk for sudden death should be
examined.

VI. SUMMARY

This chapter has reviewed the incidence, characteristics, risk factors, and clinical
management of cocaine-induced toxicity. Cocaine causes death by actions on the

cardiovascular system, including cardiomyopathy, arrhythmia production, accelerated heart rate, and increased blood pressure. Seizures often accompany cocaine toxicity, leading to death. Cocaine is known to activate the EEG in humans, cause seizures in animals, and lower the seizure threshold. Patients with preexisting risk factors for cardiovascular pathology (high cholesterol, high blood pressure, cardiac arrhythmia, etc.) and those with epilepsy may be especially sensitive to cocaine-induced toxicity. Most research in animals suggests that cocaine-induced cardiovascular responses are due to enhanced noradrenergic response on the heart and arteriolar smooth muscles. While there is controversy surrounding the management of cocaine-induced toxicity, a symptomatic approach involves controlling the seizures with diazepam, the cardiovascular response with beta-adrenergic blockers or labetolol, a combined alpha- and beta-blocking agent, while correcting the systemic acidosis and hyperthermia. Use of the Ca^{2+} channel blockers may represent a new, more effective treatment. Finally, since both cocaine and epilepsy alone are associated with sudden unexpected death and since both are capable of modifying cardiac sympathetic neural discharge to produce changes in heart rate and rhythm, the question of whether the use of cocaine in the epileptic person places this individual at risk for sudden death must be raised.

REFERENCES

Abramowicz, M. (1986). "Crack." *Med. Lett. Drug Ther. 28*:69–70.

Amon, C. A., Tate, L. G., Wright, R. K., and Matusiak, W. (1986). Sudden death due to ingestion of cocaine. *J. Ann. Toxicol. 10*:217–218.

Antelman, M., Kocan, D., Rowland, N., De Giovanni, L., and Chiodo, L. A. (1981). Amitriptyline provides long-lasting immunization against sudden cardiac death from cocaine. *Eur. J. Pharmacol. 69*:119–120.

Bayorh, M. A., Zukowska-Grojec, Z., and Kopin, I. J. (1983). Effect of desipramine and cocaine on plasma norepinephrine and pressor responses to adrenergic stimulation in pithed rats. *J. Clin. Pharmacol. 23*:24–31.

Benchimol, A., Bartall, H., and Desser, K. (1978). Accelerated ventricular rhythm and cocaine abuse. *Ann. Intern. Med. 88*:519–520.

Berger, H. (1937). Hans Berger on the electroencephalogram of Man. *Arch. Psychiatr. Nervenk. 106*:577–584. Translated in P. Gloor (Eds.). *EEG Clin. Neurophysiol. Suppl. 28*, pp. 291–297.

Carnel, S. B., Schraeder, P. L., and Lathers, C. M. (1985). Effect of phenobarbital pretreatment on cardiac neural discharge and pentylenetetrazol-induced epileptogenic activity in the cat. *Pharmacology 30*:225–240.

Castellani, S., Ellinwood, E. H., Jr., Kilbey, M. M., et al. (1983). Cholinergic effects on arousal and cocaine-induced olfactory-amygdala spindling and seizures in cats. *Sociol. Behav. 31*:461–466.

Catravas, J. D., and Waters, I. W. (1981). Acute cocaine intoxication in the conscious dog: Studies on the mechanism of lethality. *J. Pharmacol. Exp. Ther. 217*:350–356.

Catravas, J. D., Waters, I. W., Walz, M. A., et al. (1978). Acute cocaine intoxication in the conscious dog: Pathophysiologic profile of acute lethality. *Arch. Int. Pharmacodyn. 235*:328–340.

Chiu, Y. C., Brecht, K., DasGupta, D. S., and Mhoon, E. (1986). Myocardial infarction with topical cocaine anesthesia for nasal surgery. *Arch. Otolaryngol. Head Neck Surg. 112*:988–990.

Christ, D., Curry, J., and Zitaglio, T. (1982). Potentiation of the ganglionic blocking action of norepinephrine by cocaine. *J. Pharmacol. Exp. Ther. 220*: 97–101.

Coleman, D. L., Ross, T. F., and Naughton, J. L. (1982). Myocardial ischemia and infarction related to recreational cocaine use. *West. J. Med. 136*:444–446.

Cregler, L. L., and Mark, H. (1986a). Medical complications of cocaine abuse. *New Engl. J. Med. 315*:1495–1500.

Cregler, L. L., and Mark, H. (1986b). Cardiovascular dangers of cocaine abuse. *Am. J. Cardiol. 57*:1185–1186.

Cregler, L. L., and Mark, H. (1987). Cocaine-induced myocardial ischemia. *Am. J. Med. 82*:388.

Dart, A. M., Dietz, R., Kubler, W., Schömig, A., and Strasser, R. (1983). Effects of cocaine and desipramine on the neurally evoked overflow of endogenous noradrenaline from the rat heart. *Br. J. Pharmacol. 79*:71–74.

Duke, M. (1986). Cocaine, myocardial infarction and arrhythmias—A review. *Conn. Med. 50*:440–442.

Estroff, T. W., and Gold, M. S. (1986). Medical and psychiatric complications of cocaine abuse with possible points of pharmacological treatment. In *Advances in Alcohol Substance Abuse*, Vol. 5. Haworth Press, New York, pp. 61–68.

Fabiato, A., and Fabiato, F. (1978). Effects of pH on the myofilaments and the sarcoplasmic reticulum of skinned cells from cardiac and skeletal muscle. *J. Physiol 276*:233–255.

Fekete, M., and Borsy, J. (1971). Chlorpromazine–cocaine antagonism: Its relation to changes of dopamine metabolism in the brain. *Eur. J. Pharmacol. 16*: 171–175.

Fischman, M. W., Schuster, C. R., Resnekov, L., et al. (1976). Cardiovascular and subjective effects of intravenous cocaine administration in humans. *Arch. Gen. Psych. 33*:983–989.

Freud, S. (1884). Oncoca. Centralblatt für die Gesammte Theupie (Wien) Vol. 2: 289–314. Reprinted in the Cocaine Papers (S. Edminster, trans.). Vienna Dunquin Press, 1963.

Ford, G. D., Cline, W. H., Jr., and Flemin, W. W. (1968). Influence of lactic acidosis on cardiovascular response to sympathomimetic amines. *Am. J. Physiol. 215*:1123–1129.

Gay, G. R. (1982). Clinical management of acute and chronic cocaine poisoning. *Ann. Emergency Med. 11*:562–572.

Gay, G. R. (1983). Letter to the editor: In response to management of cocaine poisoning. *Ann. Emergency Med. 10*:656–657.

Gay, G. R., and Loper, K. A. (1988). Control of cocaine-induced hypertension with labetalol. *Anesth. Analg. 67*:92.

Gillis, R. A. (1969). Cardiac sympathetic nerve activity: Changes induced by ouabain and propranolol. *Science 166*:508–510.

Gillis, R. A., Raines, A., Sohn, Y. L., Levitt, B., and Standaert, F. G. (1972). Neuroexcitatory effects of digitalis and their role in the development of cardiac arrhythmias. *J. Pharmacol. Exp. Ther. 183*:154–168.

Gould, L., Gopalaswamy, C., Patel, C., and Betzu, R. (1985). Cocaine-induced myocardial infarction. *N.Y. State J. Med.*, November, pp. 660–661.

Han, J., and Moe, G. K. (1964). Nonuniform recovery of excitability in ventricular muscle. *Circ. Res. 14*:44–60.

Herning, R. I., Jones, R. T., Hooker et al. (1985). Cocaine increases EEG beta: A replication and extension of Hans Berger's historic experiments. *EEG Clin. Neurophysiol. 60*:470–477.

Howard, R. E., Hueter, D. C., and Davis, G. J. (1985). Acute myocardial infarction following cocaine abuse in a young woman with normal coronary arteries. *J. Am. Med. Assoc. 254*:95–96.

Isner, J. M., Estes, N. A. M., Thompson, P. D., Mark, et al. (1985). Cardiac consequences of cocaine: Premature myocardial infarction, ventricular tachyarrhythmia, myocarditis, and sudden death. *Circulation (Suppl. 3)72*:414.

Isner, J. M., Estes, N. A. M., Thompson, P. D., et al. (1986). Acute cardial events temporally related to cocaine abuse. *New Engl. J. Med. 315*:1438–1443.

Jain, R., Gatti, P. J., Visner, M., Albrecht, K. G., Moront, M. G., Rackley, C. E., and Gillis, R. A. (1987). Effects of cocaine on cardiorespiratory function and on cardiovascular responses produced by bilateral carotid occlusion and IV norepinephrine. *Fed. Proc. 46*:402.

Javiad, J. I., Fishman, M. W., Schuster, C. R., et al. (1978). Cocaine plasma concentration: Relation to physiological and subjective effects in humans. *Science 202*:227–228.

Jonsson, S., O'Meara, M., and Young, J. B. (1983). Acute cocaine poisoning. *Am. J. Med. 75*:1061–1064.

Kassowsky, W. A., and Lyon, A. F. (1984). Cocaine and acute myocardial infarction. A probable connection. *Chest 5*:729–731.

Lathers, C. M. (1980). Effect of timolol on postganglionic cardiac and preganglionic splanchnic sympathetic neural discharge associated with ouabain-induced arrhythmia. *Eur. J. Pharmacol. 64*:95–106.

Lathers, C. M., and Lipka, L. J. (1986). Chlorpromazine: Cardiac arrhythmogenicity in the cat. *Life Sci. 38*:521–538.

Lathers, C. M., and Lipka, L. J. (1987). Cardiac arrhythmia, sudden death and psychoactive agents. *J. Clin. Pharmacol. 27*:1–14.

Lathers, C. M., and Schraeder, P. L. (1982). Autonomic dysfunction in epilepsy. Characterization of autonomic cardiac neural discharge associated with pentylenetetrazol-induced epileptogenic activity. *Epilepsia 23*:633-648.

Lathers, C. M., Tumer, N., Schoffstall, J. M. (1989). The effect of different routes of sodium bicarbonate administration on plasma catecholamines, pH, and blood pressure during cardiac arrest in pigs. *Resuscitation 18*: 59-74.

Lathers, C. M., and Schraeder, P. L. (1987). Review of autonomic dysfunction, cardiac arrhythmias, and epileptogenic activity. *J. Clin. Pharmacol. 27*:346-356. .

Lathers, C. M., Roberts, J., and Kelliher, G. J. (1974). Relationship between the effect of ouabain on arrhythmia and interspike intervals (ISI) of cardiac accelerator nerves. *Pharmacologist 16*:201.

Lathers, C. M., Roberts, J., and Kelliher, G. J. (1977). Correlation of ouabain-induced arrhythmia and nonuniformity in the histamine-evoked discharge of cardiac sympathetic nerves. *J. Pharmacol. Exp. Ther. 203*:467-479.

Lathers, C. M., Kelliher, G. J., Roberts, J., and Beasley, A. B. (1978). Nonuniform cardiac sympathetic nerve discharge: Mechanism for coronary occlusion and digitalis-induced arrhythmia. *Circulation 57*:1058-1065.

Lathers, C. M., Spivey, W. H., Suter, L. E., Lerner, J. P., Turner, N., and Levin, R. M. (1986). The effect of acute and chronic administration of timolol on cardiac sympathetic neural discharge, arrhythmias, and beta receptor density associated with coronary occlusion in the cat. *Life Sci. 39*:2121-2141.

Lathers, C. M., Schraeder, P. L., and Cornel, S. B. (1984). Neural mechanisms in cardiac arrhythmias associated with epileptogenic activity: The effects of phenobarbital. *Life Sciences 34*:1919-1936.

Lathers, C. M., Schraeder, P. L., and Weiner, F. L. (1987). Synchronization of cardiac autonomic neural discharge with epileptogenic activity: The lockstep phenomenon. *Electroencephalogr. Clin. Neurophysiol. 67*:247-259.

Lathers, C. M., Spivey, W. H., and Tumer, N. (1988). The effect of timolol given five minutes post coronary occlusion on plasma catecholamines. *J. Clin. Pharmacol. 28*:289-299.

Lathers, C. M., Tumer, N., Schoffstall, J. M. (1989). The effect of different routes of sodium bicarbonate administration on plasma catecholemines, pH, and blood pressure during cardiac arrest in pigs. *Resuscitation 18*:59-74.

Leestma, J. E., Kalelkar, M. G., Teas, S. S., Jay, G. W., and Hughes, J. R. (1984). Sudden unexpected death associated with seizures: Analysis of 66 cases. *Epilepsia 25*:84-88.

Lesse, H., and Collins, J. P. (1979). Effects of cocaine on propagation of limbic seizure activity. *Pharmacol. Biochem. Behav. 11*:689-694.

Lichtenfeld, P. J., Rubin, D. B., and Feldman, R. S. (1984). Subarachnoid hemorrhage precipitated by cocaine snorting. *Arch. Neurol. 41*:223-224.

Lipka, L. J., and Lathers, C. M. (1987). Psychoactive agents, seizure production, and sudden death in epilepsy. *J. Clin. Pharmacol. 27*:169-183.

Loveys, B. J. (1987). Physiologic effects of cocaine with particular reference to the cardiovascular system. *Heart Lung 16*:175-181.

Lown, B., and Verrier, R. L. (1978). Neural factors and sudden death. In *Perspectives in Cardiovascular Research*, Vol. 2, *Neural Mechanisms in Cardiac Arrhythmias*, P. J. Schwartz, A. M. Brown, A. Malliani, and A. Zanchetti (Eds.). Raven Press, New York, pp. 87-98.

Mathias, D. W. (1986). Cocaine associated myocardial ischemia. *Am. J. Med. 81*:675-678.

Matsuda, Y., Masuda, Y., Blattberg, B., and Levy, M. N. (1980). The effects of cocaine, chlorpheniramine and tripelennamine on the cardiac responses to sympathetic nerve stimulation. *Eur. J. Pharmacol. 63*:25-33.

Matsuzaki, M. (1978). Alteration in pattern of EEG activities and convulsant effect of cocaine following chronic administration in the rhesus monkey. *EEG Clin. Neurophysiol. 45*:1-15.

Mittleman, R. E., and Welti, C. V. (1987). Cocaine and sudden "natural" death. *J. Forensic Sci. 32*:11-19.

Nahas, G., Trouve, R., Demus, J. F., and von Sitbon, M. (1985). A calcium-channel blocker as antidote to the cardiac effects of cocaine intoxication. *New Engl. J. Med. 313*:519-520.

Nanji, A. A., and Filipenko, J. D. (1984). Asystole and ventricular fibrillation associated with cocaine intoxication. *Chest 85*:132-133.

Olsen, K., Benowitz, N., and Pentel, P. (1983). Management of cocaine poisoning. *Ann. Emergency Med. 10*:655-656.

Pasternack, P. F., Colvin, S. B., and Baumann, F. G. (1985). Cocaine-induced angina pectoris and acute myocardial infarction in patients younger than 40 years. *Am. J. Cardiol. 55*:847.

Penfield, W., and Erickson, T. C. (1941). *Epilepsy and Cerebral Localizations.* Thomas, Springfield, Ill., pp. 320-362.

Phizackerly, P. J. R., Poole, E. W., and Whitty, C. W. M. (1954). Sinoauricular heart block as an epileptic manifestation: A case report. *Epilepsia 3*:89-91.

Pickworth, W. B., Herning, R. I., Kumor, K., and Sherer, M. (1986). Spontaneous EEG during chronic cocaine infusion. *Pharmacologist 28*:236.

Pitts, D. K., and Marwah, J. (1986). Electrophysiological effects of cocaine on central monoaminergic neurons. *Eur. J. Pharmacol. 131*:95-98.

Pitts, D. K., and Marwah, J. (1987). Cocaine inhibits central monoaminergic neurons and activates cerebellar Purkinje neurons. *Fed. Proc. 46*:400.

Pitts, D. K., Udom, C. E., and Marwah, J. (1987). Cardiovascular effects of cocaine in anesthetized and conscious rats. *Life Sci. 40*:1099-1111.

Ritchie, J. M., and Greene, N. M. (1980). Local anesthetics. In *The Pharmacological Basis of Therapeutics*, L. S. Goodman and A. Gilman (Eds.). Macmillan, New York, pp. 302-321.

Roberts, D. C. S., Corcoran, M. E., and Fibiger, H. C. (1977). On the role of ascending catecholaminergic systems in intravenous self-administration of cocaine. *Pharmacol. Biochem. Behav. 6*:615-620.

Rockhold, R. W., Hoskins, B., and Ho, I. K. (1987). Spontaneously hypertensive rats are resistant to convulsive and lethal actions of cocaine. *Fed. Proc. 46*: 402.

Rod, J. L., and Zucker, R. P. (1987). Acute myocardial infarction shortly after cocaine inhalation. *Am. J. Cardiol. 59*:161.

Rollingher, I. M., Belzberg, A. S., and MacDonald, I. L. (1986). Cocaine-induced myocardial infarction. *Can. Med. Assoc. 135*:45-46.

Rosendorff, C., Hoffman, J. T. E., Verrier, E. D., Rouleau, J., and Boerboom, L. E. (1981). Cholesterol potentiates the coronary artery response to norepinephrine in anesthetized and conscious dogs. *Circ. Res. 48*:320-329.

Schachne, J. S., Roberts, B. H., and Thompson, P. D. (1984). Coronary-artery spasm and myocardial infarction associated with cocaine use. *New Engl. J. Med.* *310*:1665–1666.

Schraeder, P. L., and Lathers, C. M. (1983). Cardiac neural discharge and epileptogenic activity in the cat: An animal model for unexplained sudden death. *Life Sci.* *32*:1371–1382.

Schraeder, P. L., and Lathers, C. M. (1989). Paroxysmal cardiovascular dysfunction and epileptogenic activity. *Epilepsy Res.* *3*:55–62.

Simpson, R. W., and Edwards, W. D. (1986). Pathogenesis of cocaine-induced ischemic heart disease. *Arch. Pathol. Lab. Med.* *110*:479–484.

Spivey, W. H., Lathers, C. M., Malone, D. R., Unger, H. D., Blat, S., McNamara, R. M., Schroffstall, J., and Turner, N. (1985). A comparison of intraosseous, central and peripheral routes of sodium bicarbonate administration during CPR in pigs. *Arch. Pathol. Lab. Med.* *14*:1135–1139.

Tackett, R. L., and Jones, L. F. (1987). Central catecholaminergic changes and cardiovascular responses following acute administration of cocaine. *Pharmacologist 29*:159.

Tazelaar, H. D., Karch, S. B., Stephens, B. G., and Billingham, M. E. (1987). Cocaine and the heart. *Hum. Pathol. 18*:195–199.

Trendelenburg, U. (1968). The effect of cocaine on the pacemaker of isolated guinea-pig atria. *J. Pharmacol. Exp. Ther. 161*:222–231.

Trouve, R., and Nahas, G. (1986). Nitrendipine: An antidote to cardiac and lethal toxicity of cocaine. *Proc. Soc. Exp. Biol. Med. 183*:392–397.

Trulson, T. J., and Trulson, M. E. (1987). Cocaine suppresses the activity of noradrenergic locus coeruleus neurons in freely moving cats. *Pharmacologist 29*: 159.

Tyau, L. S. Y., and Lathers, C. M. (1988). Cocaine-induced myocardial ischemia, infarction, and arrhythmias: A review of possible mechanisms causing sudden death. *FASEB J. 2*:A1518.

Van Dyke, C., and Byck, R. (1983). Cocaine use in man. *Adv. Subst. Abuse 3*: 1–24.

Verrier, R. L., and Lown, B. (1978). Sympathetic–parasympathetic interactions and ventricular electrical stability. In *Perspectives in Cardiovascular Research*, Vol. 2, *Neural Mechanisms in Cardiac Arrhythmias*, P. J. Schwarz, A. M. Brown, A. Malliani, and A. Zanchetti (Eds.). Raven Press, New York. pp. 75–85.

Vitullo, J. C., Lakios-Cherpas, C., and Khairallah, P. A. (1987). Effects of intra-aortic injection of cocaine hydrochloride on rat electrocardiograms. *Fed. Proc. 46*:1143.

Walsh, G., Masland, W., and Goldenshon, E. (1968). Paroxysmal cerebral discharge associated with paroxysmal atrial tachycardia. *Electroencephalogr. Clin. Neurophysiol. 24*:187.

Weaver, L. C., Akera, T., and Brody, T. M. (1976). Digoxin toxicity: Primary sites of drug action on the sympathetic nervous system. *J. Pharmacol. Exp. Ther. 197*:1–9.

Weiss, R. J. (1986). Recurrent myocardial infarction caused by cocaine abuse. *Am. Heart J. 111*:793.

Weiss, S. R. B., Costello, M., Woodward, R., et al. (1987). Chronic carbamazepine inhibits the development of cocaine-kindled seizures. *Abstr. Soc. Neurosci. 13*:950.

Welti, C. V., and Fishbain, D. A. (1985). Cocaine-induced psychosis and sudden death in recreational cocaine users. *J. Forensic Sci. 30*:873–880.

Wiener, M. D., and Putnam, C. (1987). Pain in the chest in a user of cocaine. *J. Am. Med. Assoc. 258*:2087–2088.

Wiener, R. S., Lockhart, J. T., and Schwartz, R. G. (1986). Dilated cardiomyopathy and cocaine abuse: Report of two cases. *Am. J. Med. 81*:699–701.

Wilkerson, R. D. (1987). Yohimbine pretreatment enhances the cardiovascular actions of cocaine in anesthetized dogs. *Fed. Proc. 46*:1143.

Yasuda, R. P., Zahniser, N. R., and Dunwiddie, T. V. (1984). Electrophysiological effects of cocaine in the rat hippocampus in vitro. *Neurosci. Lett. 45*: 199–204.

Young, D., and Glauber, J. J. (1947). Electrocardiographic changes resulting from acute cocaine intoxication. *Am. Heart J. 34*:272–279.

22

Stress, Arrhythmias, and Seizures

WALLACE B. PICKWORTH   *Addiction Research Center, National Institute on Drug Abuse, Baltimore, Maryland*

JUDY GERARD-CIMINERA   *Warminster General Hospital, Warminster, and Holy Redeemer Hospital, Meadowbrook, Pennsylvania*

CLAIRE M. LATHERS*   *The Medical College of Pennsylvania, Eastern Pennsylvania Psychiatric Institute, Phildelphia, Pennsylvania*

I. INTRODUCTION

About a million deaths in the United States are attributed to cardiac causes each year; approximately half are sudden deaths (Kuller et al., 1987; Moss, 1980). The relationship between emotional stress and sudden death is an important area of study because of the widespread occurrence of sudden death and the persistence of theories that causally link emotion to sudden death. Folklore is replete with accounts of individuals who died in the throes of fear, anger, or grief. The Bible recounts the tale of Ananias, who was charged by Peter as having "lied not to man but to God" and then fell to the ground dead. His wife Sapphira met a similar fate when told that those who had buried her husband were at the door and planning to "carry thee out" (Acts 5:1-11).

Although anecdotes circulate among physicians about patients who died during times of emotional stress, few case reports appear in the medical literature. The literature emphasizes the importance of coronary thrombus and coronary artery disease as causative factors in the production of fatal arrhythmias, but these factors often are not documented. In the majority of cases of sudden death, fresh lesions indicative of myocardial infarction or coronary thrombosis are absent (Gomez and Gomez, 1984; Warness and Robert, 1984). If the anec-

---

Current affiliation: FDA, Rockville, Maryland.

This chapter was written as an outside activity and does not reflect the views of the Addiction Research Center, NIDA, or the U.S. Government.

dotes are true and psychological factors are responsible for sudden death, the population at risk and the pathopsychologic mechanisms involved must be understood. Perhaps timely pharmacologic or psychotherapeutic intervention will prevent sudden death in "at-risk" groups.

II. TYPES OF EMOTIONAL STRESS THAT PRECEDE SUDDEN DEATH

Engel (1971) categorized 170 reports of sudden death for their precipitating situations. Situations that preceded sudden death included (1) illness or death of a close person; (2) acute grief; (3) threat of loss of a close person; (4) mourning or anniversary of a death; (5) the loss of status or self-esteem; (6) personal danger or the threat of injury; (7) relief from danger; and (8) reunion, triumph, or happy ending. Engle observed common denominators among situations which preceded sudden death in his subjects and others. The precipitating event was one that was impossible for the victim to ignore whether it was abrupt, unexpected, or dramatic or because of its intensity, irreversibility, or persistence. The individual experienced overwhelming excitement in a situation over which he had no control.

Similarly, stress (usually exterme anger) occurred in a high percentage of patients immediately preceding their arrhythmia (Verrier and Hagestad, 1985). The stressful episode generally preceded the onset of arrhythmia by one hour (Engel, 1971; Lown, 1982; Verrier and Hagestad, 1985). So-called trigger patients had less coronary artery disease than those patients without psychological precipitants (Lown, 1982). Sudden cardiac death has been causally linked with Monday return to work, social isolation, and educational level (Rabkin et al., 1980; Ruberman et al., 1984; Weinblatt et al., 1978). Theorell and Rahe (1975) reported that life changes, such as new employment, often peaked during the year prior to death in patients with coronary heart disease. The two cases that follow illustrate typical scenarios.

Olsson and Rehnqvist (1982) discussed the case of 70-year-old man who had two previous myocardial infarctions. After his second myocardial infarction, he was enrolled in a double-blind trial with placebo/metoprolol. The patient was placed on a Holter monitor. During the time of a recording he noted that his wallet with several important papers was missing. He phoned the hospital where he thought he had left his wallet. During the phone call, he did not complain of chest pain but was very excited. Suddenly he sighed and nothing more was heard; his wife later found him dead on the floor. The monitor showed the patient had developed sinus tachycardia with self-limiting bursts of ventricular activity. Ventricular tachycardia was initiated by premature ventricular contractions, which degenerated into ventricular fibrillation and asystole. On autopsy, there was no evidence of recent myocardial infarction or acute coronary occlusion.

Engel (1971) related the case of a 70-year-old woman who arrived in the emergency room accompanying her younger sister, who was pronounced dead on arrival. The older sister collapsed and died the instant she heard of the younger sister's death. An ECG showed atrioventricular dissociation and left bundle branch block had preceded ventricular fibrillation.

III. THE ROLE OF A HIGHER CENTER IN INDUCING CARDIAC ARRHYTHMIAS

Central nervous system disease causes abnormalities of the electrocardiogram such as long T waves and prolongation of the Q-T interval (Abildskov, 1975). This finding supports the concept that central nervous system activity influences the electrical activity of the heart. Direct evidence linking brain activity and cardiac arrhythmias was obtained from experiments in anesthetized animals (Lown and Verrier, 1976; Lown et al., 1973). Electrical stimulation of the frontal lobe, orbital cortex, hidden motor areas, anterior temporal lobe, insula, and cingulate gyrus caused changes in heart rate and blood pressure as well as the induction of atrial and ventricular extrasystoles. Arrhythmias were more readily produced by stimulation of subcortical areas, with stimulation of the posterior hypothalamus causing profound hypertension and occasional extrasystoles (Lown et al., 1977). In normal hearts ventricular fibrillation did not follow such stimulation. However, when myocardial ischemia produced by ligation of the coronary arteries preceded hypothalamic stimulation, ventricular fibrillation occurred in 62.5% of dogs tested. Lathers and colleagues (Kraras et al., 1987; Lathers and Lipka, 1987; Lathers and Schraeder, 1982, 1987; Lathers et al., 1984, 1987, 1988; Lipka and Lathers, 1987, O'Rourke and Lathers, Chapter 15, this book; Schraeder and Lathers, 1983, 1989; Stauffer et al., 1989) proposed explanations for the interaction between electrophysiological discharges in the brain and the concomitant occurrence of cardiac arrhythmias in association with interictal and ictal cerebral discharges.

Skinner and Reed (1981) tested whether blockade of a pathway from the frontal cortex through the posterior hypothalamus to the brain stem prevents the occurrence of ventricular fibrillation in ischemic stressed pigs. Stimulation of this frontocortical–brain stem pathway previously had been shown to elicit ventricular arrhythmias (Skinner et al., 1975). Skinner and Reed found that cryogenic blockade delayed or prevented ventricular fibrillation. These results indicate that a central neural projection to the heart must be intact for myocardial ischemia to precipitate ventricular fibrillation in stressed animals. This study and those by Lown described earlier clearly indicate that electrical stimulation of the central nervous system can evoke diverse arrhythmias, including ventricular fibrillation. However, electrical stimulation of the nervous system in an unasthetized animal is only an experimental model to study the effects of brain activity in the induction of arrhythmias. Studies of the ventricular response to psychological stress in humans are needed to delineate the causal relationship between the higher centers and sudden death by ventricular fibrillation.

IV. THE ROLE OF ELECTRICAL INSTABILITY OF THE MYOCARDIUM

Lown et al. (1977) reviewed the literature dealing with neural and psychological mechanisms and their influence on sudden death. Their conclusions indicate that sudden death is not the culmination of advanced coronary artery disease. Rather, it is generally the result of ventricular fibrillation which is reversible and unlikely to recur once reversed. Their hypothesis is that certain hearts are electrically unstable in association with ischemic heart disease, and that neural factors can alter the excitable properties of the myocardium. This alteration evoked by neural impulses from the brain may trigger ectopic activity in the normal heart and ventricular fibrillation in the electrically unstable heart. Moss (1980) also concluded that although many patients who die of sudden coronary death have underlying coronary artery disease, the event appears to be an electrical one, perhaps associated with myocardial ischemia, and not the results of acute coronary thrombosis. A vulnerable period exists in the cardiac cycle which coincides with the apex of the T wave on the electrocardiogram; during this time an electrical stimulus may cause repetitive extrasystoles leading to ventricular fibrillation. The repetitive extrasystole has been used as an electrophysiological endpoint for studying the effects of psychological stress on cardiac vulnerability (Lown and Verrier, 1976; Matta et al., 1976b; Verrier and Lown, 1982). This model correlates well with findings in patients who suffered sudden cardiac death while undergoing Holter monitoring. In these patients, increasing incidences of PVCs, increased ventricular couplets, and runs of ventricular tachycardia preceded ventricular fibrillation and cardiac arrest (Panidis and Morganroth, 1985; Savage et al., 1987). During acute experimentally induced myocardial infarction in dogs, the threshold for repetitive extrasystoles is reduced but still remains higher than the threshold for a single response (ectopic beat). The vulnerable period during which stimulation would cause extrasystoles was lengthened following experimental coronary occlusion in dogs. Electrical instability is considered present when a stimulus of just threshold levels can initiate repetitive electrical activity (Lown and Verrier, 1976).

Lown and his associates (Corbalan et al., 1974; DeSilva et al., 1978; Lown et al., 1973; Matta et al., 1976a,b) used the threshold of the ventricular vulnerable period for provoking repetitive extrasystoles as a measure of the susceptibility to ventricular fibrillation. Dogs exposed to electric shock had a significantly lower threshold when restrained in a sling than when in their familiar cage. The threshold-lowering effect was greater before the dogs had been acclimated to the sling apparatus. Administration of a cardioselective beta blocker prior to the stress situation ablated the response. Animals that underwent occlusion of the left anterior descending artery were permitted to recover and were then reexposed to the sling apparatus. This resulted in ventricular arrhythmias, including ventricular tachycardia, which did not occur when the animals were in their familiar cages. The arrhythmogenic responses to the sling apparatus lessened over several days, suggesting that the psychophysiological effects required a myocardium which was electrically unstable, such as that which occurs during or after myocardial ischemia.

Johansson et al. (1974) examined the effects of stress in pigs, a species whose cardiovascular system is considered to be comparable to that of humans. Healthy pigs were exposed to "restraint stress" during which they were subjected to electric shock while immobilized with succinylcholine. Severe cardiopathy occurred in all 23 experimental pigs and sudden death occurred in 13%. ECG changes included T wave inversion, arrhythmias, and transitory elevation of S-T segments. The most frequent arrhythmia was ventricular tachycardia, although there were two cases of sinus arrest with bradycardia and five cases of sinus bradycardia, two of which terminated in ventricular standstill and death. Histopathology showed fragmentation, granulation, and necrosis of cardiac cells, which had occurred within 24-48 hours after stress was induced. These findings are similar to those of animals dying in stress situations such as captivity (Dismdale, 1977) and of human patients who have died suddenly (Dimsdale et al., 1987; Eliot and Beull, 1985; Eliot et al., 1977).

V. THE PERIPHERAL AUTONOMIC NERVOUS SYSTEM AND CENTRALLY INDUCED ARRHYTHMIAS

Earlier studies suggested that sympathetic pathways leading from the hypothalamus to the heart were implicated in the genesis of ventricular arrhythmias. The mammalian heart is richly innervated by the autonomic nervous system (Gomez and Gomez, 1984). Levels of circulating catecholamines have been shown to rise during exposure to an adverse environment and to vary directly with changes in ventricular vulnerability (Verrier and Hagestad, 1985; Verrier and Lown, 1982). Susceptibility to ventricular ectopy associated with cortical and subcortical stimulation was blocked by cardiac sympathectomy or beta-adrenergic blockade (Lown and Verrier, 1976). However, bilateral vagotomy did not influence the arrhythmogenic effect of central nervous system stimulation, indicating that the parasympathetic system was not involved. Increased vagus nerve activity, whether by electrical or pharmacological means, appeared to exert a protective effect against ventricular fibrillation under circumstances (thoracotomy, sympa-

thetic nerve stimulation, or catecholamine infusion) in which sympathetic tone
is increased (DeSilva et al., 1978; Verrier and Hagestad, 1985). Hypothalamic
efferent neurons stimulate secretion of catecholamines from the adrenal medulla
via the splanchnic nerves (Khalsa, 1985). However, since removing the adrenal
glands did not ablate the response to brain stimulation, adrenal catecholamines
are not the primary mechanism of this brain-heart linkage (Lown, 1979).

   Lown and DeSilva studied patients with advanced grades of ventricular arrythmias when stressed by mental arithmetic, reading from colored cards, and re-
counting emotionally charged experiences (Lown, 1987; Lown and DeSilva,
1978). Stress significantly increased the frequency of ventricular ectopic activity. Similarly, Tavazzi et al. (1986) reported arrhythmias in postinfarction patients performing mental arithmetic. Autonomic reflex testing, including carotid
massage and evocation of the dive reflex, did not provoke an increase in ectopic
activity (Lown, 1987; Lown and DeSilva, 1978). Lown and DeSilva concluded
that passive stimulation of the autonomic systems through tilt maneuvers, carotid massage, valsalva, etc., was not sufficient to induce arrhythmia. A higher
neural mediator was likely required to provide the type of neural traffic that dis-
organizes cardiac rhythm. Although increased sympathetic tone is likely to be
the pathway, the peripheral autonomic system appears not to exert a decisive
role without the higher neural input.

   If emotional factors predispose to ventricular arrhythmias by increasing sympathetic tone, the diminution of sympathetic activity should decrease the incidence of sudden death. This assumption was supported by the finding that the
administration of a beta blocker abolished the decrease in threshold for ventricular fibrillation in dogs suffering myocardial ischemia (Matta et al., 1976a,b).
Likewise, activities such as sleep and meditation, which reduce sympathetic
tone, decrease ventricular arrhythmias (Brodsky et al., 1987; DeSilva, 1982;
Lown et al., 1975, 1980).

   Recent clinical literature has shown that the use of beta blockade following
myocardial infarction decreases the occurrence of sudden death (Ahlmark and
Saetre, 1976; Green et al., 1975; Wilhelmsson et al., 1974). The major effect of
beta-blocking agents on survival after myocardial infarction appears to be during
the first six months of therapy (Podrid, 1985). Even after three years, stress-
induced ventricular arrhythmias were less frequently observed in patients on
beta blockers when compared to placebo (Olsson et al., 1986), although discontinuation of treatment was not associated with any serious arrhythmias during
mental stress. Brodsky et al. (1987) studied patients with structurally normal
hearts who had been referred for evaluation of ventricular tachycardia and who
reported having experienced marked psychological stress. He demonstrated a
marked reduction in both arrhythmias and symptoms after beta-blocker therapy
was initiated. Beta blockade has not proven invariable effective in reduction of

stress-related arrhythmias, as shown by Lown's observation that sleep suppresses ventricular arrhythmias that could not be controlled by beta blockade (Lown et al., 1975; Verrier and Hagestad, 1985).

The long QT syndrome, in which prolongation of the Q-T interval appears to be associated with the development of serious cardiac arrhythmias and sudden deth (Zipes et al., 1987), provides a naturally occurring human model that can be used to study the effect of beta blockade. The evidence for neural influence in this syndrome comes from the observation that it may occur in association with neurological diseases (Abildskov, 1975). Wolf (1987) showed an association between prolonged Q-T interval and patients with significant emotional depression. Further, the evidence for the role of the sympathetic system stems from the observation that syncopal attacks, which are felt to be nonsustained attacks of ventricular fibrillation, can be triggered by intense emotions and exertion, and that the observed T wave abnormalities noted prior to syncope can be reproduced by asymmetric stellate ganglion stimulation (Verrier and Hagestad, 1985). Increased catecholamine levels have been shown in patients with prolonged QT syndrome and mitral valve prolapse (Wolf, 1987). Beta blockade or stellectomy is capable of reducing the Q-T interval and decreasing recurrent attacks (Abildskov, 1975; Verrier and Hagestad, 1985).

Taggart et al. (1973) studied the effect of beta blockade on the frequency of arrhythmia induced during public speaking. In untreated subjects, tachycardia, ectopic beats ($>$ 6/min) J-point depression, and ischemic S-T depression occurred. After oxprenolol, both the tachycardia and ECG changes were suppressed. Plasma catecholamines increased in both the treated and the untreated groups. These data support the concept that sympathetic innervation of the heart mediates stress-induced arrhythmia.

Morphine is commonly used to suppress anxiety and pain during the early phases of cardiac ischemia, a time when ventricular fibrillation often occurs. Restraining animals in an aversive environment reduced the threshold to repetitive ventricular response to electrical stimulation of the heart. Pretreatment with morphine diminished the restraint-induced increase in vulnerability by 50% (DeSilva et al., 1978). DeSilva and colleagues postulated that morphine protects the heart by increasing vagal tone and by sedative action which decreases sympathetic outflow. Other studies have shown that increasing efferent vagal tone, with phenylephrine, terminated sustained ventricular tachycardia (Lown, 1987; Zipes et al., 1987). The effect is indirect and mediated by a muscarinic inhibition of sympathetic activity. When sympathetic tone is low as a result of beta blockade, vagal stimulation no longer alters the vulnerability or threshold to ventricular fibrillation (DeSilva et al., 1978).

Reflex vagal inhibition of the heart has been postulated as a mechanism for sudden cardiac death using the dive reflex as a model. A dive reflex includes a

vagally mediated slowing of the heart during exposure of the face to cold. De-
Silva's (1982) search of the literature failed to reveal any electrocardiographic-
ally documented deaths attributed to this reflex, although there are reports of
short periods of asystole, heart block, and ventricular arrhythmias. Although
vagal stimulation alone does not have a significant effect on the threshold to
ventricular fibrillation, it attenuated the increased vulnerability produced by the
sympathetic stimulation (Zipes et al., 1987). The sympathetic–parasympathetic
interactions occur both at the prejunctional and postjunctional levels. Prejunc-
tionally, the acetylcholine released at the vagal endings diminishes the release of
norepinephrine from the neighboring sympathetic terminals. Postjunctionally,
acetylcholine and norepinephrine interact with receptors on the cardiac cell
membranes.

VI. PATIENT MANAGEMENT TO REDUCE RISK
OF SUDDEN DEATH

Eliot and Forker (1976) suggested the following methods for the management
and relief of excessive prolonged emotional stress: (1) establishing priorities;
(2) identifying objective, realistic, and obtainable goals; (3) attempting behavior
modification of type A personality; (4) reducing the frequency of stressful life-
change events; (5) using the daily technique of relaxation response; (6) practic-
ing aerobic physical exercise; and (7) engaging in group therapy. These methods
are to be used concurrently with beta-adrenergic blockade with propranolol to
blunt the pathophysiological effects of sympathetic stimulation to the heart.
Eliot and Forker further suggested that the physician identify patients who may
be in a state of invisible entrapment and help them to find personally acceptable
options. The patient who has already undergone a life change, such as the death
of a spouse, should be counseled that only a certain number of life changes can
be safely handled in a reasonable period of time and another change (in job or
location) could reasonably be postponed. Relaxation techniques were suggested
to diminish excessive sympathetic system input.

Beta-adrenergic blockade represents a medical option for the reduction of
sympathetic tone. Long-term therapy with timolol and propranolol decrease sudden cardiac death and mortality from all causes in postinfarction patients (Frishman et al., 1985). Beta blockers also reduced the incidence of sudden death in
patients with long QT syndrome (Schwartz et al., 1987).

A surgical option available to patients at risk for sudden death is high thoracic left sympathectomy or left stellectomy (Schwartz et al., 1987). This operation was recommended for patients who have long QT syndrome unresponsive
to a full-dose beta-blockade. The surgery may also benefit postinfarction patients who are not eligible for beta-blocker therapy.

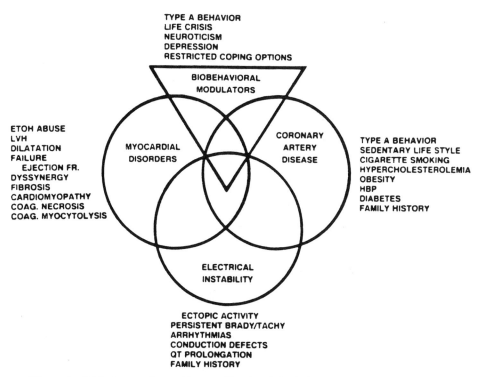

Figure 1 Risk factors for sudden cardiac death include coronary artery disease, electrical instability, and myocardial disorders. Each risk factor is associated with a number of causes; biobehavioral modulators influence the interaction and expression of the risk factors. [Adapted from Eliot and Buell (1985).]

A. Risk Factors for Sudden Death

Some of the risk factors for sudden cardiac deaths are illustrated in Figure 1 (Eliot and Buell, 1985). Figure 2 depicts the pathophysiological pathways involved in sudden cardiac death. The first of the three interconnected circles represents myocardial damage and vulnerability affected through ischemia, inflammation, or necrosis; this process has generally occurred on a long-term basis before the final event. The second circle represents electrical instability and diminished threshold to the ventricular ectopic activity, which culminates in sudden death. Neuroendocrine activation is represented in the third circle. Neuroendocrine arousals are capable of creating myocardial damage as well as independently inducing malignant rhythmic disturbances. Approximately 20% of resuscitated victims of sudden death have no structural heart disease (Reich et al.,

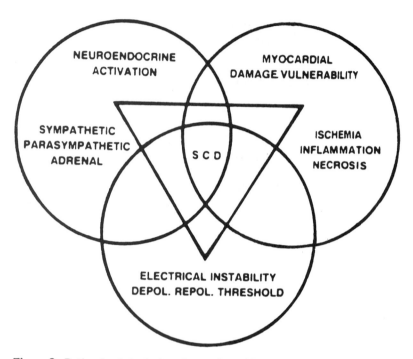

Figure 2   Pathophysiological pathways in sudden cardiac death involve myocardial damage/vulnerability, neuroendocrine factors, and electrical instability.
[Adapted from Eliot and Buell (1985).]

(1981). In these cases, arrhythmias may be precipitated exclusively by physiological stress.

    Figure 3 depicts the interactions between psychological variables and myo-
cardial electrical instability. When the heart is electrically stable (left of Figure
3) neither psychological state nor trigger can provoke ventricular fibrillation
(VF). However, in the presence of electrical instability (extreme right of Figure
3), no psychological trigger is required to induce ventricular fibrillation. In the
intermediate zone an interplay of these factors determines the predisposition to
ventricular fibrillation. Thus lesser magnitude of stimuli induce ventricular fibrillation with increased psychological state or with a greater degree of myocardial
electrical instability.

B.   Stress in Persons with Epilepsy

High levels of stress, when extended for long periods, cause harmful effect in
humans (Selye, 1956). An association between high levels of stress and the oc-

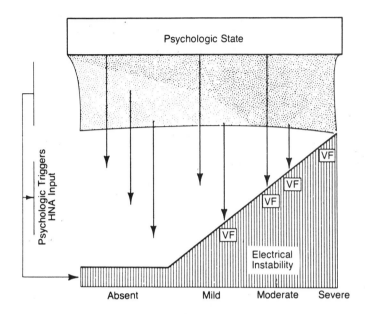

Figure 3 Interaction between psychological variables and myocardial electrical instability. Ventricular fibrillation (VF) is not likely to occur when electrical instability is low even in the presence of psychological triggers (at left) but it may occur in the absence of triggers if electrical instability is severe (at right); with intermediate levels psychological triggers and electrical instability interact to determine the predisposition. [Adapted from Lown et al. (1980).]

currence of seizures has been reported (Ames, 1982; Berlin and Yeager, 1951; Feldman and Paul, 1976; Gottschalk, 1953); an increase in seizures in 7 of 12 patients with epilepsy occurred when the daily stress level was high (Tempkin and Davis, 1984). Stress convulsions have been defined as seizures in persons who have not previously had unprovoked epileptic attacks and who, during the period immediately prior to the attack, were exposed to stressful stimuli such as emotional stress or intellectual or somatic overexertion (Mogens and Mogens, 1974). Friss and Lund (1974) reviewed records of 1250 patients with convulsive disorders; 37 patients had disorders that were defined as stress convulsions. One of the following diagnoses was reported for each of the 37 patients: symptomatic epilepsy, idiopathic epilepsy, suspected epilepsy, convulsions, or stress convulsions. The majority of patients were 20-50 years old and the occurrence of stress convulsions in men was twice as frequent as that in women. Of the 37 patients, 4 had been observed for 1-2 years, 21 for 2-4 years, and 12 for 5-12

Table 1   Seizure-Provoking Factors

Factor	Admission attack ($N = 37$)	Previous provoked attacks ($N = 11$)	Later provoked attacks ($N = 11$)
Lack of sleep	29	9	7
Emotional stress	15	7	7
Somatic stress (overexertion)	16	5	7
Intellectual stress	9	3	1
Abuse of alcohol	11	5	1
Abuse of drugs	2	1	1

Reproduced with permission from Friis and Lund: *Arch. Neurol. 31*: 158, 1974.

years, with a mean observation time of 5 years. A follow-up investigation was done in 36 patients; 1 had died of bronchopneumonia during the observation period. In addition, 27 children (< 20 years old) of 16 of the patients were interviewed. The follow-up examinations revealed that lack of sleep was the primary stress factor; emotional stress was the second most common (Table 1). Of the 37 patients, 1 had died, 2 of 36 developed unprovoked convulsions, and 10 experienced recurrence of stress convulsions. A familial disposition to epilepsy was not detected. Families of subjects exhibited increased incidences of febrile convulsions. One child had paroxysmal changes on the EEG only during photostimulation. Successful management involved avoidance of the provoking factors; further, anticonvulsant drugs did not appear to prevent recurrence (Table 2).

In a recent study, Snyder (1986) reviewed the literature of stress in persons with epilepsy and extracted 20 stressors. Six nurses working in epilepsy clinics or on inpatient epilepsy units evaluated the stressors and designated those that were appropriate; they were asked to add relevant stress factors that had been omitted from the list. The final list contains 22 stressors (Table 3). Patients with epilepsy then ranked the frequency of the stressor in their lives on a 5-point Likert scale, with almost always = 5 and never = 1; the right-hand column in Table 3 shows the results of this ranking. Table 4 gives a demographic analysis of the patients who participated. Scores did not differ significantly for the clinical sites, age groups, length of seizures, types of seizures, or frequency of seizures. Snyder (1986) concluded that the inventory list was easily administered and enabled the physician and patient to identify stressors. Most of the top stress factors related to uncertainty and to lack of control. The fear of having a seizure was a major stressor, even though the majority of patients had seizures infrequently.

Table 2 Relationship Between Prognosis and Treatment

Prognosis		Treatment				
Frequency of attacks after admission attack	No. of patients	No. of patients	Diphenyl-hydantoin	Pheno-barbital	Diphenyl-hydantoin + phenobarbital	No Treatment No. of patients
Free from attacks	24	14	12	2	0	10
1 provoked attack	8	4	3	0	1	4
> 1 provoked attack	2	0	0	0	0	2
1 unprovoked attack	—	—	—	—	—	—
> 1 unprovoked attack	1	1	0	0	1	0
> 1 unprovoked - > 1 provoked attack	1	1	1	0	0	0
Not examined (dead)	1	1	0	0	1	0

Reproduced with permission from Friis and Lund: *Arch. Neurol. 31*: 158, 1974.

Table 3   Rank Ordering and Means of Items On the Stressor Inventory

Rank	Stressor	Mean
1.	Need to take medications regularly	3.54
2.	Uncertainty about when a seizure will occur	2.78
3.	Increasing memory loss	2.74
4.	Inability to get driver's license	2.71
5.	Others not understanding epilepsy	2.65
6.	Lack of control over situation	2.61
7.	Limitation on type of activities	2.58
8.	Loss of driver's license	2.51
9.	Frustration with medicine not working	2.42
10.	Frustration that others assume you're not competent	2.38
11.	Side effects of medications	2.31
12.	Difficulty getting insurance	2.27
13.	Inability to "just like others"	2.26
14.	Overprotectiveness of family friends	2.22
15.	Dependency on others	2.18
16.	Fear of injuring self	2.13
17.	Cost of medications	2.08
18.	Being restricted in use of alcohol	2.04
19.	Fear about having children as they may have epilepsy	1.86
20.	Fear about sexual activity and marriage	1.80
21.	Rejection by others	1.79
22.	Fear others will find out about epilepsy	1.75

Reproduced with permission from *J. Neuroscience Nursing* April 1986, 72.

Table 4   Demographic Variables of Sample

Gender	
Males	74%
Females	36%
Age	
18–25	21.5%
26–35	30.8%
36–45	13.1%
46–55	15.9%
56–65	15.9%
Duration of Seizures	
1–5 years	19.6%
6–10 years	16.8%
Over 10 years	61.7%

Reproduced with permission from *J. Neuro-science Nursing* April 1986, 72.

Moffett and Scott (1984) compared the addition of a small dose of lorazepam with the addition of placebo to the preexisting anticonvulsant regime of 24 patients with drug-resistant epilepsy. Many epileptic patients complain that stress precipitates seizures. Lorazepam possesses both anticonvulsant and anxiolytic properties. Pretreatment assessment included a questionnaire to determine whether stress precipitated the subjects' seizures and whether they regarded themselves as tense. Interviews, visual analogue scales, and the Middlesex Hospital Questionnaire (Crown and Crisp, 1974) were given to determine problems with sleep, depression, or the presence of neurotic symptoms using a double-blind crossover design without a washout period between the lorazepam (1 mg) and placebo. Lorazepam reduced the seizure frequency, improved sleep, and led to a general improvement in the patients' sense of well-being. The benefits were most often seen in patients with seizures of focal origin.

Stewart and Bartucci (1986) reported a case associating posttraumatic stress disorder with partial complex seizures. A 33-year-old white male with a three-month history of increasingly frequent nightmares was admitted to the hospital one night after breaking a window with his fist. The patient was a Vietnam combat veteran who complained of irritability, anxiety, difficulty with interpersonal skills, feelings of survivor guilt, and frequent nightmares, often accompanied with motor activity. The history and physical revealed no psychotic symptoms, history of seizure, or recent substance abuse. He was admitted and maintained on alprazolam, a drug he had been taking for the prior six months. The nightmares with motor activity continued in the hospital. Because an EEG revealed independent bilateral temporal epileptiform sharp waves, carbamazepine was added to the medication regimen. Within two days of obtaining a therapeutic serum level, the nightmares stopped. Stewart and Bartucci (1986) remarked that although the dream content was based on the Vietnam experience, the positive response to carbamazepine implied an association with temporal lobe seizure activity. The prevalence of posttraumatic stress disorder among Vietnam veterans seems to be higher than initially suggested (Friedman, 1981). Recurrent disturbing nightmares are frequently reported in these patients (Ziarnowski and Broida, 1984). Thus it is important when treating an apparent posttraumatic stress disorder to consider the possibility of temporal lobe epilepsy with recurrent dreams and nightmares (Epstein, 1964; Epstein and Hill, 1966).

Numerous hypotheses have been proposed to explain why high levels of stress may precipitate seizures. The amygdala and the hippocampus are involved in emotions and both areas have a low seizure threshold. One explanation proposes that hyperventilation occurs with anxiety and the associated increases in blood pH may initiate a seizure. Increased epinephrine secretion and hypoglycemia caused by stress may precipitate seizures (Liberson, 1951; Revitch, 1955). Anxiety may ultimately result in immobilization and interference with socialization and work by initially taxing the individual's energy level, leaving subadequate energy for activities such as social interaction. Indeed, Dodrill et al. (1980) suggested that psychosocial difficulties interfere with the well-being of persons with epilepsy as much as the seizure disorder itself. The final section of this chapter addresses the neuroendocrine changes associated with the production of stress and/or cardiac arrhythmias.

VII. CORTICOTROPIN-RELEASING FACTOR

Acute or chronic stress has been shown to have cardiovascular consequences that may lead to sudden death. Chronic stress facilitates the development of hypertension, and stress management techniques are commonly recommended in the treatment of this disorder. Centrally originating neurogenic factors account for some of the dysfunctional cardiovascular consequences of epilepsy. A recently identified brain peptide, corticotropin-releasing factor (CRF), may be involved in stress-induced pathophysiology.

Corticotropin-releasing factor is a 41-amino acid peptide that was first isolated from ovine hypothalamic tissue (Vale et al., 1981). The amino acid sequences for rat (Rivier et al., 1983) and human (Shibihara et al., 1983) are identical but they differ from ovine CRF by seven amino acid residues. The discovery of CRF was the culminating event in a series of experiments beginning with the observation that stress causes an enlargement of the adrenal cortex (Selye, 1956). A number of studies have since demonstrated that stressful events increase the release of ACTH from the anterior pituitary. Harris (1948) reviewed evidence that the release of ACTH was controlled by a hypothalamic hormone, CRF, which reaches the pituitary through a portal blood supply. It was formerly thought that CRF was the major if not the only regulator of ACTH release from the pituitary. Recent evidence suggests that ACTH can be released and regulated by catecholamines, vasopressin, and vasoactive intestinal peptide, whereas corticosteroids and somatostatin inhibit ACTH release (Axelrod and Reisine, 1984). Thus brain peptides modulate ACTH release, which in turn increases plasma catecholamines and glucocorticoids, which are the humoral hallmarks of stress.

The mechanism responsible for the ACTH-induced increases in catecholamines and glucocorticoids were recently reviewed (Axelrod and Reisine, 1984; Valentino and Foote, 1986). ACTH stimulates the synthesis and release of corticosteroids from the adrenal cortex, which in turn inhibits further release of ACTH from the pituitary. Glucocorticoids enhance the synthesis of norepinephrine and epinephrine in the adrenal medulla by stimulating dopamine beta-hydroxylase and phenethanolamine-N-methyltransferase. Stress-induced adrenal catecholamine release is further regulated by presynaptic sympathetic neural activity. The emerging picture seems to suggest that increased sympathetic activity stimulates the rate-limiting enzymes of catecholamine synthesis, i.e., tyrosine hydroxylase and dopamine-beta-hydroxylase (Axelrod and Reisine, 1984).

Although a variety of stressors increase urinary catecholamine concentration (Bloom et al., 1963) as a general index of stress, plasma catecholamine levels are more precise measures of stress-induced activation of the sympathetic medullary system. Plasma norepinephrine levels generally indicate sympathetic nervous system activation, whereas plasma levels of epinephrine measure adrenal catecholamine secretion (Axelrod and Reisine, 1984). Plasma ratios of epinephrine to norepinephrine appear to depend on the nature of the precipitating stressor. For example, changes in posture increase norepinephrine levels twofold or threefold but have negligible effects on epinephrine (Lake et al., 1976). On the other hand, public speaking increased plasma norepinephrine levels by 50% but levels of epinephrine went up 100% (Dimsdale and Moss, 1980). Preexisting personality appears to be an important variable in the catecholamine response to stressful situations. When harassed, coronary-prone (type A) individuals showed greater increase in plasma catecholamines than non–coronary-prone subjects (type B) (Glass et al., 1980). In depressed subjects, the basal levels of plasma catecholamines were higher than basal levels in nondepressed subjects. These differences were attributed to the increased anxiety in the former subjects (Louis et al., 1975).

From these studies, it appears that stress increases plasma catecholamines through ACTH-mediated adrenal release, which is also partially regulated by CRF. Furthermore, the final levels of plasma catecholamines and the cardiovascular consequences of their changes depend on the stressor and the preexisting pathology of the individual. Victims of sudden death or those at risk may be especially sensitive to stressors or the increased catecholamines that attend them. In this at-risk population, the arrhythmogenic potential of the catecholamines might be increased as a result of previous treatment or as a consequence of existing conditions such as epilepsy, depression, or thyroid syndrome (Lathers and Lipka, 1987).

In addition to its role in the regulation of ACTH release, emerging evidence suggests that CRF may act as a neurotransmitter at widely distributed brain regions. CRF activity at several of these regions has been proposed to involve neural systems that could play a role in the pathogenesis of sudden death. Cummings et al. (1983) reported CRF immunoreactivity in the rat brain hypothalamus (paraventricular and anterior hypothalamic nuclei). CRF in this region could be involved in the regulation of ACTH release. Other hypothalamic and brain nuclei containing CRF immunoreactive neurons include bed nucleus of stria terminalis, amygdala, dorsal raphe, locus coeruleus (LC), external cuneate nucleus, and the medullary reticular formation. The widespread distribution of CRF-containing neurons was confirmed in studies by Swanson et al. (1983) and

Olschowka et al. (1982). Specific high-affinity binding sites for iodinated analogues of CRF delineated by DeSouza (1987) and DeSouza et al. (1985) in the
rat include neocortex, olfactory bulb, median eminence, several cranial nerve
nuclei, cerebellar nuclei, and cortex. Areas of moderate binding include olfactory tubercle, caudate-putamen, claustrum, nucleus accumbens, medullary reticular formation, and spinal cord. The authors concluded that CRF binding sites
are widely distributed and correspond with pharmacological sites of action of
CRF.

  Drug treatment can alter the CRF binding sites. Chronic atropine administration increased CRF binding in rat cortex but not in other brain regions (De-
Souza and Battaglia, 1986). Furthermore, CRF immunoreactivity is decreased
but CRF binding sites are increased in Alzheimer's disease (DeSouza et al.,
1986). These studies indicate that disease and drug therapy may influence CRF
activity.

  The extrahypothalamic location of CRF-containing neurons has led to suggestions that the neuropeptide may act directly as a neurotransmitter in regions
which are neuroanatomically associated with the stress response. For example,
CRF and CRF receptors have been identified in basal forebrain and brain stem
nuclei which participate in the autonomic concomitants of stress. CRF in the
spinal cord (Merchenthaler et al., 1983; Schipper et al., 1983) and in limbic
structures (Swanson et al., 1983) may be involved in the emotional and cogni-
tive consequences of stress, while the localization of the peptide in the cerebral
cortex could be a factor in the behavioral responses ordinarily associated with
stress.

  A direct neurotransmitter function for CRF is supported by studies showing
the autonomic, metabolic, and gastric effects of CRF are independent of ACTH
release. Brown et al. (1982a,b) and Fisher et al. (1982) reported that intracerebroventricular (i.c.v.) CRF injections increased plasma glucose, epinephrine
and norepinephrine, blood pressure, and heart rate. Gastric acid secretion is
decreased by i.c.v. CRF administration (Tache et al., 1983) in hypophysectomized and adrenalectomized animals and in animals pretreated with CRF anti-
serum. However, ganglionic blockade with chlorisondamine attenuated these
effects.

  These studies suggest that CRF acts centrally to increase sympathetic and
decrease parasympathetic tone during times of stress. This conclusion was
strengthened by studies where the levels of availability of CRF was diminished
prior to stress with dexamethasone (to decrease CRF release) or CRF antagonist alpha-helical CRF9-41. In these experiments, the stress-induced increase in
plasma catecholamines was diminished presumably by antagonizing the direct
neuronal actions of CRF (Brown et al., 1983, 1984). There is an extensive literature supporting the proposal that neurons emanating from the LC are involved

in the stress response (Valentino and Foote, 1986). The LC is the largest norepinephrine cell group in the brain and its neurons project to all levels of the neuraxis including the spinal cord, cerebellum, paleocortex, and neocortex (Swanson and Hartman, 1976). The structures innervated by the LC involved in autonomic cardiovascular function include hypothalamus, nucleus of tractus solitarius, dorsal motor nucleus of the vagus, and nucleus of the dorsal raphe (Valentine and Foote, 1986). Furthermore, nearly all of the norepinephrine in the cortex and hippocampus is of LC origin. The LC also projects to the paraventricular nucleus of the hypothalamus, the site of CRF-containing neurons (Sawchenko and Swanson, 1982). Since neurons containing CRF have been found in the LC, there is the possibility of reciprocal innervation and feedback control (Valentine and Foote, 1986).

The effects of LC stimulation and the characteristics of the noradrenergic LC fibers are consistent with the concept that the LC plays a physiological role in stress. The relationship between LC activity and blood pressure can be dissociated. Clonidine or CRF administration can change blood pressure without concomitant changes in LC firing. Conversely CRF increased LC firing without changing blood pressure (Valentino et al., 1986). The effects of electrical stimulation of the LC is mimicked by the direct application of norepinephrine on the target cells (Foote et al., 1983). The usual consequence is an enhancement of synaptically evoked responses in the target neurons, which may or may not accompany changes in the spontaneous activity of the neurons (Foote et al., 1983). Locus coeruleus-induced enhancement of the effects of other transmitters or of norepinephrine has been observed in neocortex, hippocampus cerebellum, and spinal cord (Valentino and Foote, 1986).

Neurons in the LC fire at rates which are determined by the behavioral state of the animal. In the anesthetized rat, LC fires at a slow (1-5 Hz) regular rate (Foote et al., 1980, 1983), which is increased by noxious stimuli (Aston-Jones and Bloom, 1981) but unaffected by other stimuli (Valentino and Foote, 1986). In the unanesthetized animal, the rate of LC firing depends on the state of arousal. Firing rate is maximal while attending to novel environmental stimuli; is diminished during consumptive behaviors such as eating, grooming, and slow-wave sleep; and is nearly absent during REM sleep (Aston-Jones and Bloom, 1981; Foote et al., 1980). In general, the characteristics of LC firing suggest that the nucleus is activated when the animal is vigilant and aroused by environmental stimuli. Further, LC activation enhances synaptic activity throughout the neuroaxis, which might amplify diverse behavioral responses to external stimuli. It is proposed that these activities enable the organism to effectively cope with threatening or noxious external stimuli (Valentino and Foote, 1986).

Another line of evidence implicates the interaction of LC and CRF under conditions of stress. It has been discovered that stressful stimuli which increase

LC firing, such as hemorrhage (Elam et al., 1984; Svenson and Thoren, 1979), electric shock, or hypercapnia (Elam et al., 1981), also increase ACTH release. On the other hand, stressors that do not increase LC firing, such as blood volume loading (Plotsky, 1985), decrease ACTH release. Since ACTH release is controlled by CRF activity, a parallel exists between LC activity and ACTH and CRF release.

A. Behavioral Effects of Corticotropin-Releasing Factor

Britton et al. (1982, 1985) reported that i.c.v. CRF caused dose-related increases in grooming and decreases in rearing, food approach, and food consumption. These behaviors were characteristic of stressed animals. The effects of CRF are diametrically opposite to those of anxyiolytics and differ from effects of ACTH administration. Sutton et al. (1982) found intracerebroventricular but not peripheral administration of CRF enhanced locomotor activity in rats. The effects were dose dependent, centrally mediated, and apparently not due to ACTH or beta-endophin release. In an operant conflict test in rats, CRF decreased punished and unpunished responding, with the former effect being reversed by a full benzodiazepine antagonist (Britton et al., 1988). However, the benzodiazepine partial agonist (Ro 15-1788) did not reverse the CRF-induced locomotor activation. The authors concluded that CRF is a stress-enhancing anxiogenic compound that is partially sensitive to benzodiazepine blockade. Opiate receptors may also be involved because naloxone prevented the pressor, tachycardia, and increased locomotion induced by i.c.v. administration of ACTH and CRF (Saunders and Thornhill, 1986). Behavioral stimulation and decreases in eating and grooming induced by CRF were localized to the paraventricular hypothalamus but not to other hypothalamic areas (Krahn et al., 1988).

B. Electrophysiological Effects of Corticotropin-Releasing Factor

Ehlers et al. (1983), studied the effect of intracerebroventricularly administered CRF on electrical activity in rats. They found that low doses of CRF caused EEG changes suggestive of arousal (cortical desynchrony and hippocampal theta). Higher doses caused electrographic and behavioral seizures similar to those caused by amygdala kindling. The larger doses of CRF increased locomotion and grooming, exaggerated the startle response, and increased urination and defecation. After one to three hours, paroxysmal EEG spiking was observed in the amygdala and then spread to the hippocampus and cortex. Behavioral evidence of seizures included myoclonic jaw movement, forelimb clonus, and loss of consciousness. On the day following the CRF administration, brief electrical stimulation of the amygdala caused similar behavioral convulsions. Ehlers et al. proposed that the EEG effects were due to a direct action of CRF on limbic structures. They distinguished the CRF-induced activity from the seizure activity caused by opioid peptides. Opioid peptides caused seizures that are brief, have a short latency, are limited to limbic sites, and are not associated with behavioral convulsions (Frenk et al., 1978; Henriksen et al., 1978; Urca et al., 1977). The separation of CRF action from that of the opiate peptides is especially important in light of evidence that CRF releases beta-endorphin from the pituitary (Young et al., 1986). The use of ovine CRF by Ehlers et al. (1983) may have been an important methodological choice. Studies by Marrosu et al. (1987) indicate that rat CRF and ovine CRF cause EEG and behavioral activation at low doses but the seizure activity of rat CRF was limited to the hippocampus and no myoclonic movements occurred.

Siggins et al. (1985) reviewed the electrophysiological actions of CRF in three types of studies. CRF usually caused EEG activation and, at higher doses, spiking and seizure activity. In single-unit studies, CRF ordinarily causes region-selective stimulation (LC, cortex, hypothalamus) or depression (thalamus, septum). In hippocampal slice preparations, application of CRF increases spontaneous firing and reduced after hyperpolarizations—which make cells more likely to fire. The literature implies that CRF plays a role in the central nervous system response to stress. This concept is supported by the local and direct effects of CRF on diverse neural tissue thought to be responsible for the electrophysiological, behavioral, and autonomic response to stress.

In addition to direct excitatory effects of CRF on neural structures, the CRF-induced release of ACTH and the subsequent increase in corticosteroids may lead to seizures. ACTH and corticosteroids have been reported to increase suscepibility to seizures in animal models (Ehlers and Killam, 1979) and humans (Gastaut, 1961). Although a number of other brain peptides (endorphins, beta-lipotropin, MSH) may be involved in this relationship, the evidence reviewed favors a dominant role for CRF. The peptide is clearly associated with ACTH regulation, which is known to be disrupted during stress. CRF is widely distributed through the brain. Its localization in the LC is of special interest because this nucleus controls many of the autonomic and behavioral responses to environmental stimuli. Furthermore, CRF acts directly on limbic structures, causing seizures which spread to cortical areas and lead to clonic convulsions.

VIII. SUMMARY

In this chapter, we have reviewed evidence that stress can be a factor associated with arrhythmias, seizures, and sudden death. Clinical studies suggest that sudden death is usually caused by ventricular fibrillation, which is precipitated by hemodynamic or neural mechanism. In patients at risk, stress-induced alterations in neural input to the heart can cause fatal arrhythmias. While these arrhythmias

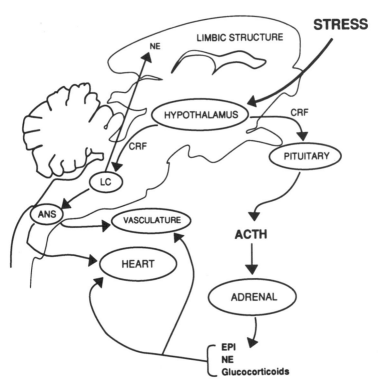

Figure 4 Summary of the effects of stress on CRF release and subsequent seizure and myocardial arrhythmias leading to sudden death. Stress-induced release of CRF stimulates ACTH release and enhances adrenal output of epinephrine and norepinephrine. CRF also stimulates the locus coeruleus (LC) causing norepinephrine release onto brain areas that control autonomic function (ANS) and seizure threshold in limbic areas. The combined neurogenic and endocrine effects and their sequela are thought to lead to sudden death.

may be a consequence of a thromboembolytic episode, they can occur following stress in patients without preexisting coronary artery disease. Although the mechanism by which stress can cause arrhythmia and seizures is unknown, it is proposed that CRF may be involved. Exogenous administration of CRF mimics stress-induced changes in operant behavior in animal tests, and the effects of CRF are inhibited by benzodiazepine anxiolytics. CRF is released in response to stress, lowers seizure threshold, and, through actions on the locus coeruleus, affects autonomic centers responsible for regulation of the heart. While stress is known to release other brain peptides including beta-endorphin, beta-lipotropin, and somatostatin, it is proposed that it is the action of CRF which mediates the mechanisms responsible for sudden death (Figure 4).

REFERENCES

Abildskov, J. (1975). The nervous system and cardiac arrhythmias. *Circulation (Suppl. 3) 51,52*:116–119.

Ahlmark, G., and Saetre, H. (1976). Longterm treatment with beta-blockers after myocardial infarction. *Eur. J. Clin. Pharm. 10*:77–83.

Ames, F. (1982). The evoked epilepsies. *S. Afr. Med. J. 61*:661–662.

Aston-Jones, G., and Bloom, F. E. (1981). Norepinephrine-containing locus coeruleus neurons in behaving rats exhibit pronounced responses to non-noxious environmental stimuli. *J. Neurosci. 1*:887–900.

Axelrod, J., and Reisine, T. D. (1984). Stress hormones: Their interaction and regulation. *Science 224*:452–459.

Berlin, I., and Yeager, C. (1951). Correlation of epileptic seizures, electroencephalograms, and emotional state. *Am. J. Dis. Child. 81*:644–670.

Bloom, G., Von Euler, U., and Frakenhaeuser, M. (1963). Catecholamine excretion and personality traits in paratroop trainees. *Acta Physiol. Scand. 58*: 77–89.

Britton, D. R., Koob, G. F., Rivier, J., and Vale, W. (1982). Intraventricular corticotropin-releasing factor enhances behavioral effects of novelty. *Life Sci. 31*:363–367.

Britton, K. T., Morgan, J., Rivier, J., Vale, W., and Koob, G. F. (1985). Chlordiazepoxide attenuates response suppression induced by corticotropin-releasing factor in the conflict test. *Psychopharmacology 86*:170–174.

Britton, K. T., Lee, G., and Koob, G. F. (1988). Corticotropin releasing factor and amphetamine exaggerate partial agonist properties of benzodiazepine antagonist R O 15-1788 in the conflict test. *Psychopharmacology 94*:306–311.

Brodsky, M., Sato, D., Iseri, L., Wolff, L., and Allen, B. (1987). Ventricular tachyarrhythmia associated with psychological stress: The role of the sympathetic nervous system. *J. Am. Med. Assoc. 257*:2064–2067.

Brown, M. R., Fisher, L. A., Rivier, J., Spiess, J., Rivier, C., and Vale, W. (1982a). Corticotropin-releasing factor: Effects on the sympathetic nervous system and oxygen consumption. *Life Sci. 30*:207–210.

Brown, M. R., Fisher, L. A., Spiess, J., Rivier, C., Rivier, J., and Vale, W. (1982b). Corticotropin-releasing factor: Actions on the sympathetic nervous system and metabolism. *Endocrinology 111*:928–931.

Brown, M. R., Fisher, L. A., and Vale, W. W. (1983). Sympathetic nervous system and adreno-cortical interactions. *Soc. Neurosci. Abstr. 9*:931.

Brown, M. R., Fisher, L. A., Vale, W. W., and Rivier, J. E. (1984). Corticotropin releasing factor: The role in central nervous system regulation of the adrenal medulla. *Soc. Neurosci. Abstr. 10*:1117.

Corbalan, R., Verrier, R., and Lown, B. (1974). Psychological stress and ventricular arrhythmias during myocardial infarction in the conscious dog. *Am. J. Cardiol. 34*:692–696.

Crown, S., and Crisp, A. H. (1974). The Middlesex Hospital Questionnaire clinical research. In *Psychological Medicine and Psychopharmacology*, P. Pichot (Ed.). Karger, Basel, pp. 111–124.

Cummings, S., Elde, R., Ells, J., and Lindall, A. (1983). Corticotropin-releasing factor immunoreactivity is widely distributed within the central nervous system of the rat: An immunohistochemical study. *J. Neurosci. 3*:1355–1368.

DeSilva, R. (1982). Central nervous system risk factors for sudden cardiac death. *Ann. N.Y. Acad. Sci. 382*:143–161.

DeSilva, R., Verrier, R., and Lown, B. (1978). The effect of psychological stress and vagal stimulation with morphine on vulnerability to ventricular fibrillation in the conscious dog. *Am. Heart J. 95*:197–203.

DeSouza, E. B. (1987). Corticotropin-releasing factor receptors in the rat central nervous system: Characterization and regional distribution. *J. Neurosci. 7*: 88–100.

DeSouza, E. B., and Battaglia, G. (1986). Increased corticotropin-releasing factor receptors in rat cerebral cortex following chronic atropine treatment. *Brain Res. 397*:401–404.

DeSouza, E. B., Insel, T. R., Perrin, M. H., Rivier, J., Vale, W. W., and Kuhar, M. J. (1985). Corticotropin-releasing factor receptors are widely distributed within the rat central nervous system: An autoradiographic study. *J. Neurosci. 5*:3189–3203.

DeSouza, E. B., Whitehouse, P. J., Kuhar, M. J., Price, D. L., and Vale, W. W. (1986). Reciprocal changes in corticotropin-releasing factor (CRF)-like immunoreactivity and CRF receptors in cerebral cortex of Alzheimer's disease. *Nature 319*:593–595.

Dimsdale, J. E. (1977). Emotional causes of sudden death. *Am. J. Psychiatr. 134*:1361–1366.

Dimsdale, J. E., and Moss, J. (1980). Plasma catecholamines in stress and exercise. *J. Am. Med. Assoc. 243*:340–342.

Dimsdale, J. E., Ruberman, W., et al. (1987). Task force 1: Sudden cardiac death: Stress and cardiac arrhythmias. *Circulation (Suppl. 1) 76*:I198–I201.

Dodrill, C., Batzel, L., Quiessen, H., and Temkin, N. (1980). An objective method for the assessment of psychological and social problems among epileptics. *Epilepsia 21*:123–135.

Ehlers, C. L., and Killam, E. K. (1979). The influence of cortisone on EEG and seizure activity in the baboon *Papio papio*. *Electroencephalogr. Clin. Neurophysiol. 47*:404–410.

Ehlers, C. L., Henriksen, S. J., Wang, M., Rivier, J., Vale, W., and Bloom, F. E. (1983). Corticotropin releasing factor produces increases in brain excitability and convulsive seizures in rats. *Brain Res. 278*:332–336.

Elam, M., Yao, T., Thoren, P., and Svensson, T. H. (1981). Hypercapnia and hypoxia: Chemoreceptor-mediated control of locus coeruleus and splanchnic sympathetic nerves. *Brain Res. 222*:373–381.

Elam, M., Yao, T., Svensson, T. H., and Thoren, P. (1984). Regulation of locus coeruleus neurons and splanchnic, sympathetic nerves by cardiovascular afferents. *Brain Res. 290*:281-287.

Eliot, R. S., and Buell, J. C. (1985). Role of emotions and stress in the genesis of sudden death. *J. Am. Coll. Cardiol. 5*:95B-98B.

Eliot, R. S., and Forker, A. (1976). Emotional stress and cardiac disease. *J. Am. Med. Assoc. 236*:2325-2326.

Eliot, R. S., Clayton, F. C., Pieper, G. M., and Todd, G. L. (1977). Influence of environmental stress on pathogenesis of sudden cardiac death. *Fed. Proc. 36*: 1719-1724.

Engel, G. (1971). Sudden and rapid death during psychological stress. *Ann. Intern. Med. 74*:771-782.

Epstein, A. W. (1964). Recurrent dreams: Their relationship to temporal lobe seizures. *Arch. Gen. Psychiatr. 10*:49-54.

Epstein, A. W., and Hill, W. (1966). Ictal phenomena during REM sleep of a temporal lobe epileptic. *Arch. Neurol. 15*:367-375.

Feldman, R. G., and Paul, N. L. (1976). Identity of emotional triggers in epilepsy. *J. Nerv. Ment. Dis. 162*:345-353.

Feldman, R., Ricks, N., and Orren, M. (1983). Behavioral methods of seizure control. In *Epilepsy*, T. Browne and R. Feldman (Eds.). Little, Brown, Boston, pp. 269-279.

Fisher, L. A., Rivier, J., Rivier, C., Spiess, J., Vale, W. W., and Brown, M. R. (1982). Corticotropin-releasing factor (CRF): Central effects on mean arterial blood pressure and heart rate in rats. *Endocrinology 110*:2222-2224.

Foote, S. L., Aston-Jones, G., and Bloom, F. E. (1980). Impulse activity of locus coeruleus neurons in awake rats and monkeys is a function of sensory stimulation and arousal. *Proc. Nat. Acad. Sci. USA 77*:3033-3037.

Foote, S. L., Bloom, F. E., and Aston-Jones, G. (1983). Nucleus locus coeruleus: New evidence of anatomical and physiological specificity. *Physiol. Rev. 63*: 844-914.

Frenk, H., Urca, G., and Liebeskind, J. C. (1978). Epileptic properties of leucine- and methionine-enkephalin: Comparison with morphine and reversibility by naloxone. *Brain Res. 147*:327-337.

Friedman, M. J. (1981). Post-Vietnam syndrome: Recognition and management. *Psychosomatics 22*:931-943.

Frishman, W., Laifer, L., and Furberg, C. (1985). Beta-adrenergic blockers in the prevention of sudden death. *Cardiovasc. Clin. 15*:249-264.

Friss, M. L., and Lund, M. (1974). Stress convulsions. *Arch. Neurol. 31*:155-159.

Gastaut, H. (1961). Introduction to ACTH, adrenocortical hormones and juvenile epilepsy. *Epilepsia 2*:343-344.

Glass, D. C., Krakoff, L. R., Contrada, R., Hilton, W. F., Kehoe, K., Mannucci, E. G., Collins, C., Snow, B., and Elting, E. (1980). Effect of harassment and competition upon cardiovascular and plasma catecholamine responses in type A and type B individuals. *Psychophysiology 17*:453-463.

Gomez, G., and Gomez, E. (1984). Sudden death: Biopsychosocial factors. *Heart Lung 13*:389–393.

Gottschalk, L. (1953). Effects of intensive psychotherapy on epileptic children. *Arch. Neurol. Psychiatr. 70*:361.

Green, K., et al. (1975). Improvement in prognosis of myocardial infarction by long term beta-adrenoceptor blockade using practolol. *Br. Med. J. 3*:735–740.

Harris, G. W. (1948). Neural control of pituitary gland. *Physiol. Rev. 23*:139–179.

Henriksen, S. J., Bloom, F. E., Ling, N., and Guillemin, R. (1978). β-Endorphin induces nonconvulsive limbic seizures. *Proc. Nat. Acad. Sci. USA 75*: 5221–5225.

Johansson, G., Jonsson, L., Lannek, N., Bloomgren, L., Lindberg, P., and Poupa, O. (1974). Severe stress-cardiopathy in pigs. *Am. Heart J. 87*:451–457.

Khalsa, D. (1985). Stress-related illness: Where the evidence stands. *Postgrad. Med. 78*:217–221.

Krahn, D. D., Gosnell, B. A., Levine, A. S., and Morley, J. E. (1988). Behavioral effects of corticotropin-releasing factor: Localization and characterization of central effects. *Brain Res. 443*:63–69.

Kraras, C. M., Tumer, N., and Lathers, C. M. (1987). The role of neuropeptides in the production of epileptogenic activity and autonomic dysfunction: Origin of arrhythmia and sudden death in the epileptic patient. *Med. Hypothesis 23*:19–31.

Kuller, L., Talbott, E., and Robinson, C. (1987). Environmental and psychosocial determinates of sudden death. *Circulation (Suppl. 1) 76*:I177–I185.

Lake, C. R., Ziegler, M. G., and Kopin, I. J. (1976). Use of plasma norepinephrine for evaluation of sympathetic neuronal function in man. *Life Sci. 18*: 1315–1326.

Lathers, C. M., and Lipka, L. J. (1987). Cardiac arrhythmia, sudden death, and psychoactive agents. *J. Clin. Pharmacol. 27*:1–14.

Lathers, C. M., and Schraeder, P. L. (1982). Autonomic dysfunction in epilepsy. Characterization of autonomic cardiac neural discharge associated with pentylenetetrazole-induced epileptogenic activity. *Epilepsia 23*:633–648.

Lathers, C. M., and Schraeder, P. L. (1987). Review of autonomic dysfunction, cardiac arrhythmias and epileptogenic activity. *J. Clin. Pharmacol. 27*:346–356.

Lathers, C. M., Schraeder, P. L., and Carnel, S. B. (1984). Neural mechanism in cardiac arrhythmias associated with epipetogenic activity: The effect of phenobarbital. *Life Sci. 34*:1919–1936.

Lathers, C. M., Schraeder, P. L., and Weiner, F. L. (1987). Synchronization of cardiac autonomic neural discharge with epileptogenic activity: The lock step phenomenon. *Electroencephalogr. Clin. Neurophysiol. 67*:247–259.

Lathers, C. M., Tumer, N., and Kraras, C. M. (1988). The effect of intracerebroventricular D-Ala^2-methionine enkephalinamide and naloxone on cardiovascular parameters in the cat. *Life Sci. 43*:2287–2298.

Liberson, W. (1951). Emotional and psychological factors in epilepsy. *Am. J. Psychiatr.* *112*:91.

Lipka, L. J., and Lathers, C. M. (1987). Psychoactive agents, seizure production, and sudden death in epilepsy. *J. Clin. Pharmacol.* *27*:169–183.

Louis, W. J., Doyle, A. E., and Anavekar, S. N. (1975). Plasma noradrenaline concentration and blood pressure in essential hypertension, pheochromocytoma and depression. *Clin. Sci. Mol. Med. (Suppl. 2) 48*:239–242.

Lown, B. (1979). Sudden cardiac death: The major challenge confronting contemporary cardiology. *Am. J. Cardiol.* *43*:313–328.

Lown, B. (1982). Mental stress, arrhythmias, and sudden death. *Am. J. Med. 72*: 177–179.

Lown, B. (1987). Sudden cardiac death: Biobehavioral perspective. *Circulation (Suppl. 1): 76*:I186–I196.

Lown, B., and DeSilva, R. (1978). Role of psychological stress and autonomic nervous system changes in provocation of ventricular premature complexes. *Am. J. Cardiol. 41*:979–985.

Lown, B., and Verrier, R. (1976). Neural activity and ventricular fibrillation. *New Engl. J. Med. 294*:1165–1170.

Lown, B., Verrier, R., and Corbalan, R. (1973). Psychological stress and the threshold for repetitive ventricular response. *Science 182*:834–836.

Lown, B., Calvert, A., Armington, R., and Ryan, M. (1975). Monitoring for serious arrhythmias and high risk of sudden cardiac death. *Circulation (Suppl. 3) 51,52*:III189–III198.

Lown, B., Verrier, R., and Rabinowitz, S. (1977). Neural and psychologic mechanisms and the problem of sudden cardiac death. *Am. J. Cardiol. 39*:890–902.

Lown, B., DeSilva, R. A., Reich, P., and Murawski, B. J. (1980). Psychophysiologic factors in sudden cardiac death. *Am. J. Psychiatr. 137*:1325–1335.

Marrosu, F., Mereu, G., Fratta, W., Carcanoiu, P., Camarri, F., and Gessa, G. L. (1987). Different epileptogenic activities of murine and ovine corticotropin-releasing factor. *Brain Res. 408*:394–398.

Matta, R., Lawler, J., and Lown, B. (1976a). Ventricular electrical instability in the conscious dog. *Am. J. Cardiol. 38*:594–598.

Matta, R., Verrier, R., and Lown, B. (1976b). Repetitive extrasystole as an index of vulnerability to ventricular fibrillation. *Am. J. Physiol. 230*:1469–1473.

Merchenthaler, I., Vigh, S., Petrusz, P., and Schally, A. V. (1983). The paraventriculo-infundibular corticotropin-releasing factor (CRF) pathway as revealed by immunocytochemistry in long-term hypophysectomized or adrenalectomized rats. *Regul. Pept. 5*:295–305.

Moffett, A., and Scott, D. F. (1984). Stress and epilepsy: The value of a benzodiazepine-lorazepam. *J. Neurol. Neurosurg. Psychiatr. 47*:165–167.

Mogens, L. F., and Mogens, L. (1974). Stress convulsions. *Arch. Neurol. 31*:155–159.

Moss, A. (1980). Prediction and prevention of sudden cardiac death. *Ann. Rev. Med. 31*:1–14.

Olschowka, J. A., O'Donohue, T. L., Mueller, G. P., and Jacobowitz, D. M. (1982). The distribution of corticotropin-releasing factor-like immunoreactive neurons in rat brain. *Peptides 3*:995-1015.

Olsson, G., and Rehnqvist, N. (1982). Sudden death preceded by psychological stress. *Acta Med. Scand. 212*:437-441.

Olsson, G., Hjemdahl, P., and Rehnqvist, N. (1986). Cardiovascular reactivity to mental stress during gradual withdrawal of chronic postinfarction treatment with metoprolol. *Eur. Heart J. 7*:765-772.

Panidis, I., and Morganroth, J. (1985). Initiating events of sudden cardiac death. *Cardiovasc. Clin. 15*:81-92.

Plotsky, P. M. (1985). Hypophyseotropic regulation of adenohypophyseal adrenocorticotropin secretion. *Fed. Proc. 44*:207-214.

Podrid, P. (1985). The role of antiarrhythmic drugs in prevention of sudden cardiac death. *Cardiovasc. Clin. 15*:265-286.

Rabkin, S., Matthewson, F., and Tate, R. (1980). Chronobiology of cardiac sudden death in men. *J. Am. Med. Assoc. 244*:1357-1358.

Reich, P., DeSilva, R. A., Lown, B., and Murawski, B. J. (1981). Acute psychological disturbance preceding life-threatening ventricular arrhythmias. *J. Am. Med. Assoc. 246*:233-235.

Revitch, E. (1955). Psychiatric aspects of epilepsy. *J. Med. Soc. N.J. 52*:634.

Rivier, J., Spiess, J., and Vale, W. (1983). Characterization of rat hypothalamic corticotropin-releasing factor. *Proc. Nat. Acad. Sci. USA 80*:4851-4855.

Ruberman, W., Weinblatt, E., Goldberg, J., and Chaudhary, B. (1984). Psychosocial influences of mortality after myocardial infarction. *New Engl. J. Med. 311*:552-559.

Saunders, W. S., and Thornhill, J. A. (1986). Pressor, tachycardic and behavioral excitatory responses in conscious rats following ICV administration of ACTH and CRF are blocked by naloxone pretreatment. *Peptides 7*:597-601.

Savage, H. R., Kissane, J. Q., Becher, E. L., Maddocks, W. Q., Murtaugh, J. T., and Dizadji, H. (1987). Analysis of ambulatory electrocardiograms in 14 patients who experienced sudden cardiac death during monitoring. *Clin. Cardiol. 10*:621-632.

Sawchenko, P. E., and Swanson, L. W. (1982). The organization of noradrenergic pathways from the brainstem to the paraventricular and supraoptic nuclei in the rat. *Brain Res. Rev. 4*:285-325.

Schipper, J., Steinbusch, H. W. M., Vermes, I., and Tilders, F. J. H. (1983). Mapping of CRF-immunoreactive nerve fibers in the medulla oblongata and spinal cord of the rat. *Brain Res. 267*:145-150.

Schraeder, P. L., and Lathers, C. M. (1983). Cardiac neural discharge and epileptogenic activity in the cat: An animal model for unexplained sudden death. *Life Sci. 32*:1371-1382.

Schraeder, P. L., and Lathers, C. M. (1989). Paroxysmal cardiovascular dysfunction and epileptogenic activity. *Epilepsy Res. 3*:55-62.

Schwartz, P., Randall, W., et al. (1987). Task force 4: Sudden cardiac death: Nonpharmacological interventions. *Circulation (Suppl. 1): 76*:I215-I219.

Selye, H. (1956). *The Stress of Life*. McGraw-Hill, New York.

Shibihara, S., Morimoto, Y., Furutani, Y., Notake, M., Takahashi, H., Shimizu, S. Horikawa, S., and Numa, S. (1983). Isolation and sequence analysis of human corticotropin-releasing factor precursor gene. *EMBO J.* 2:775–779.

Siggins, G. R., Gruol, P., Aldenhoff, J., and Pittman, Q. (1985). Electrophysiological actions of corticotropin-releasing factor in the central nervous system. *Fed. Proc.* 44:237–242.

Skinner, J. E., and Reed, J. C. (1981). Blockade of frontocortical–brain stem pathway prevents ventricular fibrillation of ischemic heart. *Am. J. Physiol.* 240 *(Heart Circ. Physiol. 9)*:H156–163.

Skinner, J. E., Lie, J. T., and Entman, M. L. (1975). Modification of ventricular fibrillation latency following coronary artery occlusion in the conscious pig: The effects of psychologic stress and beta-adrenergic blockage. *Circulation 51*: 656–667.

Snyder, M. (1986). Stressor inventory for persons with epilepsy. *J. Neurosci. Nurs.* 18:71–73.

Stauffer, A. Z., Dodd-o, J., and Lathers, C. M. (1989). The relationship of the lockstep phenomenon and precipitous changes in mean arterial blood pressure. *Electroencephalogr. Clin. Neurophysiol.* 72:340–345.

Stewart, J. T., Bartucci, R. J. (1986). Posttraumatic stress disorder and partial complex seizures. *Am. J. Psychiatr.* 143:113–114.

Sutton, R. E., Koob, G. F., Le Moal, M., Rivier, J., and Vale, W. (1982). Corticotropin releasing factor produces behavioural activation in rats. *Nature 297*: 331–333.

Svensson, T. H., and Thoren, P. (1979). Brain noradrenergic neurons in the locus coeruleus: Inhibition by blood volume load through vagal afferents. *Brain Res.* 172:174–178.

Swanson, L. W., and Hartman, B. K. (1976). The central adrenergic system. An immunofluorescence study of the location of cell bodies and their efferent connections in the rat utilizing dopamine β hydroxylase as a marker. *J. Comp. Neurol.* 163:467–506.

Swanson, L. W., Sawchenko, P. E., Rivier, J., and Vale, W. W. (1983). Organization of ovine corticotropin-releasing factor immunoreactive cells and fibers in the rat brain: An immunohistochemical study. *Neuroendocrinology 36*:165–186.

Tache, Y., Goto, Y., Gunion, M. W., Vale, W., Rivier, J., and Brown, M. (1983). Inhibition of gastric acid secretion in rats by intracerebral injection of corticotropin-releasing factor. *Science 222*:935–937.

Taggart, P., Carruthers, M., and Somerville, W. (1973). Electrocardiogram, plasma catecholamines and lipids and their modification by oxyprenolol when speaking before an audience. *Lancet 2*:341–346.

Tavazzi, L., Zotti, A., and Rondanelli, R. (1986). The role of psychologic stress in the genesis of lethal arrhythmias in patients with coronary artery disease. *Eur. Heart J. (Suppl. A)* 7:99–106.

Temkin, N., and Davis, G. (1984). Stress as a risk factor for seizures among adults with epilepsy. *Epilepsia 25*:450–456.

Theorell, T., and Rahe, C. R. (1975). Life change events, ballistocardiography and coronary death. *J. Hum. Stress. 1*:18–24.

Urca, G., Frenk, H., Libeskind, J. C., and Taylor, A. N. (1977). Morphine and enkephalin: Analgesic and epileptic properties. *Science 197*:83–86.

Vale, W., Spiess, J., Rivier, C., and Rivier, J. (1981). Characterization of a 41-residue ovine hypothalamic peptide that stimulates secretion of corticotropin and β-endorphin. *Science 213*:1394–1397.

Valentino, R. J., and Foote, S. L. (1986). Brain noradrenergic neurons, corticotropin-releasing factor, and stress. In *Neural and Endocrine Peptides and Receptors*, T. W. Moody (Ed.). Plenum, New York, pp. 101–120.

Valentino, R. J., and Foote, S. L. (1987). Corticotropin-releasing factor disrupts sensory responses of brain noradrenergic neurons. *Neuroendocrinology 45*: 28–36.

Valentino, R. J., Martin, D. L., and Suzuki, M. (1986). Dissociation of locus coeruleus activity and blood pressure. *Neuropharmacology 25*:603–610.

Verrier, R., and Hagestad, E. (1985). Role of the autonomic nervous system in sudden death. *Cardiovasc. Clin. 15*:41–63.

Verrier, R., and Lown, B. (1982). Experimental studies of psychological factors in sudden cardiac death. *Acta Med. Scand (Suppl.) 660*:57–68.

Warness, C., and Robert, W. (1984). Sudden coronary death: Comparison of patients with coronary thrombus to those without coronary thrombus at necropsy. *Am. J. Cardiol. 54*:1206–1211.

Weinblatt, E., Ruberman, W., Goldberg, J. D., Frank, C. W., Shapiro, S., and Chaudhary, B. S. (1978). Relation of education of sudden death after myocardial infarction. *New Engl. J. Med. 299*:60–65.

Wilhelmsson, C., Vedin, J. A., Wilhelmsson, L., Tibblin, G., and Werko, L. (1974). Reduction of sudden death after myocardial infarction by treatment with alprenolol. *Lancet 2*:1157–1160.

Wolf, S. (1987). Behavioral aspects of cardiac arrhythmia and sudden death. *Circulation (Suppl. 1) 76*:I174–I176.

Young, E. A., Lewis, J., and Akil, H. (1986). The preferential release of beta-endorphin from the anterior pituitary lobe by corticotropin releasing factor (CRF). *Peptides 7*:603–607.

Ziarnowski, A. P., and Broida, D. C. (1984). Therapeutic implications of the nightmares of Vietnam combat veterans. *VA Pract. 1*:63–68.

Zipes, D., et al. (1987). Task force 2: Sudden cardiac death: Neural-cardiac interventions. *Circulation (Suppl. 1) 76*:I202–I207.

23
Psychoactive Agents, Epilepsy, Arrhythmia, and Sudden Death

CLAIRE M. LATHERS* *The Medical College of Pennsylvania, Eastern Pennsylvania Psychiatric Institute, Philadelphia, Pennsylvania*

JAN E. LEESTMA *Chicago Neurosurgical Center, Columbus Hospital, Chicago, Illinois*

I. INTRODUCTION

Not long after the introduction of chlorpromazine (Thorazine) and other phenothiazine drugs for the management of psychotic patients, reports began to appear which suggested that these revolutionary drugs might be responsible for the phenomenon of sudden unexpected deaths in patients receiving them. One of the first of these (Ayd, 1956) involved the death of an agitated schizophrenic, being medicated with more than 2000 mg/day of chlorpromazine, who collapsed and died. Many reports followed during the 1960s in which individuals taking one or more phenothiazine derivatives (of which at that time there were more than a dozen) suddenly collapsed and died or were found dead (Caffey et al., 1966; Hollister and Kosek, 1965; Kelly et al., 1963; Reinert and Hermann, 1960; Wendkos and Clay, 1965). In most of these cases, autopsy examination failed to reveal an obvious cause of death. In some it appeared that the individuals suffered fatal aspiration of gastric contents, apparently without distress or obvious premonitory signs. In some cases of collapse, attempts were made to resuscitate the individuals and it was noted that cardiac arrhythmias and cardiac standstill were present and/or there was profound hypotension and shock (Graupner et al., 1964; Kelly et al., 1963). A controversy developed over the role of this important group of drugs in these sudden deaths. To some degree this controversy continues.

In an attempt to survey the issue Leestma and Koenig in 1968 reviewed all known reported cases of apparent sudden death in psychiatric patients in which phenothiazine tranquilizing drugs were alleged to play a role. A synopsis of these

---

Current affiliation: FDA, Rockville, Maryland.

Table 1   Data Relating to 58 Psychiatric Patients Who Died Suddenly and Unexpectedly

		Probable anatomic cause of death				Circumstances of death			
Age group[a]	No. of patients[a]	Cardiac	Aspiration	None	Other	Collapse death	Found dead or dying	Unexpected death	Other
15–24	3	0	2	1	0	3	0	0	0
25–34	17	0	2	15	0	7	6	3	1
35–44	17	1	2	14	0	5	9	2	1
45–54	15	1	2	11	1	6	4	3	2
55–64	3	0	1	2	0	1	1	1	0
65+	3	0	0	3	0	2	1	0	0
Total	58	2	9	46	1	24	21	9	4

[a]The study involved 40 men and 18 women with a mean age of 41 years.
Source: Leestma and Koenig (1968), reproduced with permission.

cases can be found in Table 1. It is apparent that over half the deaths occurred in persons of 40 years of age or younger, that no anatomic cause of death could be determined in the majority, but that aspiration was the cause of death in about 16% (9/58) of the cases and some degree of cardiac pathology was found in 3.4% (2/58). The onset of symptoms preceding the fatal event appeared to be sudden and often catastrophic. Chlorpromazine was the most common phenothiazine tranquilizer being taken, closely followed by thioridazine. It appeared that the number of cases in which thioridazine was involved was overrepresented, since at the time this drug was relatively new and the numbers of persons taking it were only a fraction of those taking the more prevalent and popular chlorpromazine. About half the cases could be considered to be taking "extreme" (Baldessarini, 1985) doses of one or more phenothiazines at the time of death and another 25% were taking maximal or near maximal "usual" (Baldessarini, 1985) doses of one or more phenothiazines.

An additional seven cases, reported by Plachta (1965) and reviewed by Leestma and Koenig (1968), did not have a great deal of information concerning drugs taken or their dosage. These cases were reported to have died because of sudden aspiration of gastric contents, apparently because pharyngeal guarding reflexes were absent or weakened by the tranquilizing medication. While little has been made of this observation, one of us (JEL) regularly observed cases of this type in the autopsy population of a large custodial psychiatric institution over a six-year period between 1973 and 1979. These cases are perplexing since

While Receiving Phenothiazine Drugs

		Phenothiazine-drugs at time of death					
Chlor-promazine	Trifluo-dazine	Chlor promazine and thiori-perazine	Trifluo perazine	Pro mazine	Prochlor-perazine	Other	Unknown
2	1	0	0	0	0	0	0
7	4	4	0	0	0	1	1
7	3	1	4	1	1	2	1
3	7	0	1	0	2	1	1
2	0	1	0	0	0	0	0
2	1	0	0	0	0	0	0
23	16	6	5	1	3	4	3

the victim, apprently without warning, collapses at the dining table or in the ward room. Resuscitation attempts usually were fruitless. At autopsy, massive aspiration was found. The clinical picture is very similar to the well-known "cafe coronary." The basis for this curious phenomenon was discussed by Plachta (1965), von Brauchitsch and May (1968), and more recently by Solomon (1977), who regards it as a drug-induced bulbar palsy–like syndrome.

Since the review (Leestma and Koenig, 1968) a number of reports and reviews on phenothiazine-associated sudden death have appeared in the literature (Alexander and Nino, 1969; Brown and Kocsis, 1984; Craig and Lin, 1982; Guillan et al., 1970; Laposata et al., 1988; Liberatore and Robinson, 1984; Moore and Book, 1970; Solomon, 1977; Swett, 1975; Wakasugi et al., 1986; Warnes and Ananth, 1971; Yang and Guillan, 1979; Zugibe, 1980). Although the proposed mechanism of death in these patients is most commonly thought due to an arrhythmogenic effect on the heart (discussed in detail later), hypotensive effects and the effect on pharyngeal guarding reflexes are still considered possible mechanisms of death, especially when high doses of phenothiazines are employed, often in the highly agitated psychotic individual. The possibility that these various, often fatal, complications of phenothiazine therapy are dose related or related to other conditions such as extreme stress and agitation have not fully been elucidated. Several aspects of these questions will be discussed in this chapter.

Some recent reports of sudden death in psychiatric patients, presumably on phenothiazines, invoke another mechanistic possibility for the deaths, so-called lethal catatonia. The reviews of Goodson and Litkenhous (1976) and of Peele and von Loetzen (1973) summarize the essence of the arguments. There are still those who allege no role of phenothiazines in such sudden deaths in psychotic individuals since there is a literature which reports that there has been no increase in sudden deaths in hospitalized psychotic patients from the days before phenothiazines existed (Brill and Patton, 1962; Hollister, 1957; Hussar, 1962). There are opposing views, however (Richardson et al., 1966; Swett and Shader, 1977; Ungvari, 1980).

Perhaps part of the etiological controversy, which was not addressed during the 1960s and is no longer practicable to analyze in the United States, is the complicating factor that a significant and probably unknown number of hospitalized psychiatric patients cited in the older literature and still used for comparison purposes also were epileptics (Hollister and Kosek, 1957; Wardell, 1957; Zielinski, 1974). Changes in demographics, philosophy, and patterns of therapy as well as societal changes make such comparisons unreliable.

Another complicating factor was, and is, that some phenothiazine-medicated individuals collapsed with a "seizure" or agonal event that might have represented a nonepileptic event such as spontaneous aspiration of gastric contents, apparently without warning, perhaps owing to some loss or suppression of the pharyngeal guarding reflexes as an effect of phenothiazine administration (Leestma and Koenig, 1968; Plachta, 1965; Solomon, 1977).

The phenomenon of sudden unexpected death in the general population and in the epileptic population is reviewed in Chapter 5. Many of the same issues and aspects apply to the phenomenon of sudden and unexpected death in a nonepileptic psychiatric patient. To repeat the essence of these aspects: most sudden deaths are thought, because of their suddenness, to be due to some malfunction of the heart, great vessels, or pulmonary tree (Kuller, 1966; Kuller et al., 1967) and can occur in apparently normal or mentally ill individuals, regardless of age (Hollister and Kosek, 1965; Jefferson, 1975; Kelly et al., 1963; Lathers and Lipka, 1987; Leestma, 1988; Simpson et al., 1988; Wendkos, 1979). It is also well known that autopsy diagnosis of functional disorders of the heart is very nearly impossible except by inference and circumstantial observations. The fact that there are many cardiovascular and neural effects of phenothiazines and related compounds that could affect cardiovascular function to produce a suddenly fatal outcome, alone or in combination with other factors, has led to considerable attention to these drugs in relation to sudden death. The added complication that some of the phenothiazines lower the seizure threshold and/or cause seizures by themselves provides further opportunities for thought regarding the phenomenon of sudden death in epileptics and the possible interaction of multiple events in its pathogenesis.

This chapter will discuss the clinical risks and side effects, including the initiation of cardiac arrhythmias and seizure activity, associated with the administration of psychoactive agents to epileptic persons. Experimental studies defining the effects of these drugs in models of epilepsy will be presented. Clinical findings obtained from patients taking psychoactive agents and dying in a sudden manner will be presented and, finally, guidelines for the management of the epileptic patient who requires a psychoactive drug will be discussed.

II. ARRHYTHMIAS ASSOCIATED WITH THE USE OF PSYCHOACTIVE AGENTS

Although psychoactive agents may initiate cardiac arrhythmias, they have been demonstrated to exhibit an antiarrhythmic action when arrhythmias were induced by succinylcholine in rabbits and adrenaline in guinea pigs (Courvoiser et al., 1953) and against acetylcholine-induced atrial fibrillation and ether-induced ventricular arrhythmias (Arora and Madan, 1956; Lathers et al., 1987; Melville, 1958). The antiarrhythmic action of chlorpromazine has been attributed to its action in the central nervous system, to quinidine or antiadrenaline properties, and to a local anesthetic action on myocardial cell membranes (Arora, 1979; Lathers and Lipka, 1986). Other psychoactive agents, including promazine, promethazine, perphenazine, trifluoperazine, levopromazine, prochlorperazine, thioridazine, chlorprothixene, droperidol, reserpine, imipramine, amitriptyline, desipramine, and nortriptyline have also been shown to possess antiarrhythmic properties (Arora, 1956; Baum et al., 1971; Giardina, 1984; Giardina et al., 1979; Gould et al., 1985; Koishnanarao and Achari, 1972; Landmark, 1970; Reynolds et al., 1969; Shamsi et al., 1971; Singh and Sharma, 1970; Somberg et al., 1984; Szekeres and Papp, 1971). In spite of these antiarrhythmic actions, relatively large doses of psychoactive agents have been reported to cause sudden death in primates (Domino, 1983, 1985; Domino and Kovacic, 1984). Therapeutic and toxic levels have initiated ventricular arrhythmias and sudden death in humans (Burgess et al., 1979; Byck, 1975; Coull et al., 1970a,b; Fowler et al., 1976; Hollister and Kosek, 1965; Jefferson, 1975; Kelly et al., 1963; Langou et al., 1980; Leestma and Koenig, 1968; Lipscomb, 1980; Reid and Harrower, 1984; Williams and Sherter, 1971).

Since sudden death associated with psychoactive drug use has often been ascribed to cardiac arrhythmia (Crawley and Kolodner, 1981; Leestma and Koenig, 1968), the cardiac electrophysiological changes initiated by these drugs have been studied (Axelsson and Aspenstrom, 1982; Lathers and Lipka, 1987; Nasrallah, 1978). Men ranging in age from 23 to 41 years and undergoing treatment with phenothiazines developed cardiovascular electrophysiological abnormalities reflected by changes in the electrocardiogram (ECG) (Alexander and Nino,

452   Lathers and Leestma

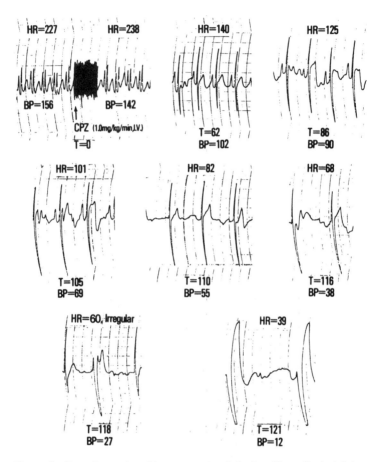

Figure 1   Data from the chlorpromazine infusion (1 mg/kg/min) in one anesthetized cat. Heart rate (HR) in beats/min, blood pressure (BP) mmHg and lead
II ECG are shown as functions of time (T) in minutes. The paper speed was 25
mm/sec except for the time period indicated by the arrow at time 0; here the
paper speed was 0.25 mm/sec. The chlorpromazine infusion (CPZ; 1 mg/kg/min)
was begun at time T = 0. Reproduced with permission from Lathers and Lipka:
Life Sciences 38:521–538, 1986.

1969). Chlorpromazine use has produced ventricular and atrial tachycardia, bigeminal rhythm, premature atrial beats, varying degrees of heart block, and ventricular fibrillation (Tri and Combs, 1975). Although the incidence of fatal
arrhythmias in patients taking chlorpromazine is small, alterations in the ECG,
including T wave changes, ST segment depression, and PQ and QT_c interval

prolongation, have been reported in up to 50% of patients (Huston and Bell, 1966). A prolonged QT interval is an ominous sign because of its association with a polymorphous ventricular tachycardia exhibiting the specific configuration known as torsade de pointe.

The administration of chlorpromazine to anesthetized cats produced arrhythmias and death (Figure 1; Lathers and Lipka, 1986). Tricyclic antidepressants induce T wave flattening and tachycardia (Byck, 1975). Toxic doses of imipramine induce T wave changes, prolonged QT_c intervals, depression of the ST segment, QRS widening, and supraventricular and ventricular tachyarrhythmias in experimental animals and in humans (Aronson and Serlick, 1977; Bianchetti et al., 1977; Langslet, 1969, 1970; Surawicz and Lasseter, 1970). Ventricular arrhythmias occurred in 14% of patients hospitalized for tricyclic antidepressant overdose who had prolonged QRS complexes (≥ 0.01 second) (Boehnert and Lovejoy, 1985). This study suggested that QRS prolongation is a better index for the prediction of ventricular arrhythmia than are serum drug levels. Even at therapeutic antidepressant concentrations, however, ECG changes such as prolonged P-R interval, QRS complex duration, and QT_c interval have occurred (Bigger et al., 1977). Desipramine induced consistent prolongation of intracardiac conduction in physically healthy young patients (Rudorfer and Young, 1980).

A. The Autonomic Nervous System, Arrhythmias, and Psychoactive Agents

Psychoactive agents do act on the autonomic nervous system to modify cardiac function. Jakobsen et al. (1984) reported that patients treated with tricyclic antidepressants for three weeks or more have reduced heart rate variation, induced by shortening of the R-R interval consequent to complex reflex mechanism. The heart rate variation is primarily influenced by respiratory changes and is referred to as sinus arrhythmia (Angelone and Coulter, 1964); the efferent portion of the reflex pathway is vagal. Normally, heart rate variation is abolished by cutting the autonomic vagus nerve or by treating with atropine; sympathetic blockade has no effect. Jakobsen and coworkers (1984) concluded that the direct anticholinergic effect of the tricyclic antidepressants is most probably responsible for the reduction in the heart rate variation.

The importance of a prolonged QT interval is related in many instances to the underlying autonomic nervous system balance (Surawicz and Knoebel, 1984). Psychoactive agents may induce a prolonged QT interval and ventricular tachycardias designated as torsade de pointe; thus it is important to consider the role of the autonomic nervous system in the production of arrhythmia by these drugs.

Alteration of the activity of the autonomic nervous system will produce arrhythmia (Gillis et al., 1979; Lathers and Roberts, 1980; Lathers et al., 1977,

1978, 1985; Levitt et al., 1976; Malliani et al., 1980; Roberts and Kelliher, 1973; Roberts et al., 1976; Schwartz et al., 1978), and psychoactive agents alter the functioning of the autonomic nervous system (Carpenter et al., 1982; Chai and Wang, 1966; Guzman-Harty et al., 1985; Hockman and Livingston, 1971; Kiem and Sigg, 1973; Raisfeld, 1972; Schallek and Zabransky, 1966; Sherif et al., 1958; Sigg and Sigg, 1969; Sigg et al., 1971).

Sigg and Sigg (1969) examined the effect of chlorpromazine and diazepam on preganglionic nerve activity in the cervical sympathetic splanchnic and vagal nerves which was evoked by hypothalamic stimulation. Both of these agents reduced the evoked impulse traffic in the sympathetic fibers but had little effect on the traffic in the vagal fibers. In 1971, Sigg et al. reported that after electrical stimulation of the hypothalamus, diazepam selectively attenuated the vasopressor response, whereas pentobarbital had a depressant effect on several autonomic parameters. Chlorpromazine, in addition to possessing an alpha-adrenergic blocking action, also decreased sympathetic outflow. It was concluded that the central sympathetic system is not homogeneous and may be selectively affected by different psychoactive agents.

Intravenous (i.v.) imipramine slowed atrial and ventricular conduction, depressed ventricular excitability, and inhibited atrioventricular (AV) conduction in the pentobarbital-anesthetized dog, effects that could be conducive to the production of imipramine-induced arrhythmia (Baum et al., 1971). Cairncross and Gershon (1962) reported that low doses of imipramine (0.5-2.5 mg/kg i.v.) did not produce any effect on the ECG of normotensive, pentobarbital-anesthetized dogs; a larger dose (5 mg/kg i.v.) produced extrasystoles, whereas 8 mg/kg caused ST segment depression, QRS broadening, and T wave abnormalities. Amitriptyline increased heart rate, left ventricular end-diastolic pressure, and the PR and QT intervals, the QRS complex, and the ST segments in anesthetized dogs (Fiedler et al., 1985b). Blood pressure, left ventricular pressure, and left ventricular dp/dt fell. Similar effects were obtained in conscious dogs. The occurrence of sustained ventricular arrhythmia induced by amitriptyline was increased by chromonar, an antianginal drug, suggesting that chromonar may be an effective therapy for amitriptyline-induced arrhythmia associated with cardiovascular collapse. The infusion of imipramine into rats or dogs elicited hypotension, bradycardia, intraventricular conduction delay, tachyrhythmia, and AV block. Chromonar, but not dipyridamole, protected the animals against heart failure (Fiedler et al., 1985a). Ventricular arrhythmias induced in dogs by amitriptyline were decreased by the administration of either lidocaine or sodium bicarbonate. Lidocaine action was transient and associated with a decreased blood pressure. Sodium bicarbonate induced reversal of arrhythmias for a longer time (Nattel and Mittleman, 1984).

After six weeks of oral imipramine 15 mg/day, the mean arrhythmogenic dose of epinephrine was increased in anesthetized dogs (Spiss et al., 1984). Imipramine treatment did not modify the alpha-adrenergic responsiveness induced by a dose of phenylephrine that caused a 75% increase in the mean arterial blood pressure; the dose of isoproterenol that increased the heart rate by 75% was also not changed. It was concluded that chronic imipramine dosing alters neither the arrhythmogenicity of epinephrine nor the adrenergic response to phenylephrine because compensatory mechanisms at the sympathetic nerve terminal reverse the initial hyperresponsiveness toward normal.

B. Effect of Psychoactive Agents on Autonomically Influenced Arrhythmias Induced by Digitalis

The interaction of psychoactive agents with the autonomic nervous system has been defined using models of arrhythmias that are influenced by the autonomic nervous system, i.e., those elicited by digitalis glycosides. Anesthetized cats were pretreated with chlorpromazine (5, 10, 20, 30, 40, or 60 mg/kg i.v.) and then administered ouabain (2 μg/kg/min i.v.) (Lathers and Lipka, 1986). There was no significant effect by the doses of chlorpromazine upon the dosages of ouabain that induced premature ventricular contractions, ventricular tachycardia, and death. It was concluded that these doses of chlorpromazine could be considered neither arrhythmogenic nor antiarrhythmic in the ouabain model.

In another study, Wilkerson (1978) infused ouabain at 2 μg/kg/min until death in anesthetized dogs and found that imipramine pretreatment at a dose of 3 mg/kg i.v. increased the dose of ouabain necessary to produce premature ventricular contractions, ventricular tachycardia, and ventricular fibrillation. When given alone, these doses of imipramine did not produce changes in the ECG. Desipramine (2.4 ± 0.4 mg/kg) converted ventricular arrhythmias produced by ouabain (66 ± 1.5 μg/kg i.v.) to a normal sinus rhythm. Basu Ray et al. (1977) reported that desipramine reduced the arrhythmogenic dose of ouabain but did not affect the lethal dose of ouabain; they concluded that the cardiotoxic effect of this agent is a result of its action on the sympathetic nervous system. Desmethylimipramine reduced the arrhythmogenic dose of ouabain but did not alter the fatal dose of this glycoside. Attree et al. (1972) found that stressed rats administered 40 mg/kg imipramine intraperitoneally (i.p.) required less digoxin to develop cardiac arrest. Chronic imipramine or desipramine (10 mg/kg/day for 14 days) significantly decreased the amount of digoxin required to produce cardiotoxicity. Acutely administered desipramine (20 or 40 mg/kg i.p) decreased the dose of digoxin necessary to produce cardiac arrest in rats.

The induction of ventricular extrasystoles in anesthetized, artificially respired dogs by the intravenous injection of lanatoside C (20 μg/kg at 10-minute intervals) was suppressed by a dose of 16.45 ± 1.23 mg/kg i.v. chlordiazepoxide infused at a rate of 0.5 mg/kg/min (Kuruvilla and Stephen, 1984). A stable ventricular arrhythmia of one-minute duration was induced by the administration of deslanoside (25 μg/kg i.v., 15 minutes) and was successively reverted to a normal sinus rhythm when chlordiazepoxide (10-15 min i.v.) was administered in increments given at approximately 45-second intervals in 9 of 12 cats (Gillis et al., 1974). This exact protocol was also employed (Pearl et al., 1978) with the addition of diazepam dissolved in propylene glycol. Conversion to normal sinus rhythm was observed in only two cats, whereas more serious rhythm changes were observed in three. Gascon (1977) also found that diazepam (5-150 mg/kg/day) resulted in a greater incidence of cardiac arrhythmias. Employing the ouabain infusion model in the dog, Brissette and Gascon (1978) found that oral diazepam pretreatment (0.25-25.00 mg/kg/day for 25 days), decreased the time to ouabain-induced arrhythmia and death.

Taken collectively, all of the foregoing studies indicate that there are differences in arrhythmogenicity among psychoactive agents, as digitalis-induced toxicity was increased by some agents, decreased by others, and not modified by still others. These diverse observations suggest the existence of differences in the actions of the various digitalis glycosides on the autonomic nervous system (Caldwell et al., 1978; Cook et al., 1982; Lathers and Roberts, 1985; Pace et al., 1974). The fact that chlordiazepoxide (Gillis et al., 1974) but not diazepam protected the majority of cats against digitalis-induced ventricular arrhythmia (Brissette and Gascon, 1978; Pearl et al., 1978) suggests that differences in solvents may be an alternative explanation. Chlordiazepoxide is water soluble, whereas diazepam is insoluble in water but soluble in aqueous vehicles containing propylene glycol. The increased potency of benzodiazepines dissolved in propylene glycol can be ascribed to either the increased solubility of the drugs or to a synergistic pharmacologic activity of the solvent (Crankshaw and Raper, 1971; Pearl et al., 1978).

C. Role of Adrenal Medullary Catecholamines in the Production of Arrhythmia by Psychoactive Agents

Adrenal catecholamine release, regulated in part by the autonomic nervous system, may cause arrhythmia (Ceremuzynski et al., 1969; Kelliher et al., 1975). Ouabain modifies cardiac neural discharge (Lathers et al., 1977, 1978) and releases catecholamines from the adrenal medulla and induced arrhythmia (Banks, 1967; Nadeau and DeChamplain, 1973). Desipramine, imipramine, trifluoperazine, and chlorpromazine reduce catecholamine secretion from the perfused rat adrenal gland; secretion was induced by the injection of acetylcholine, excess potassium ions, or by stimulation of the splanchnic nerves. The release of norepinephrine elicited by postganglionic sympathetic nerve stimulation in the perfused salivary gland was enhanced by lower concentrations of desipramine (0.3-30.0 μM); higher concentrations (100 μM) decreased the secretion of catecholamines. Leestma and Koenig (1968) hypothesized that the sudden unexplained death of a patient taking phenothiazines may be related to the increase in sympathetic neural discharge and release of adrenal medullary catecholamines induced by stress, since abnormally high blood norepinephrine levels (> 7 $\mu g/L$) have been reported in schizophrenic patients receiving large doses of chlorpromazine (Carlsson et al., 1966). A biphasic response to chlorpromazine, characterized by an accelerated rate of release of epinephrine from rabbit adrenal medulla at phenothiazine concentrations of approximately 10^{-4} M and an inhibition of release at lower concentrations of drug, has been reported by Weil-Malherbe (1965).

Bilateral adrenal ligation decreased the dose of chlorpromazine necessary to produce arrhythmia and death in the anesthetized cat (Lathers and Lipka, 1986). Thus not only did the adrenal catecholamines not appear to contribute to chlorpromazine-induced arrhythmia, but the bilateral ligation appeared to be deleterious when combined with the use of chlorpromazine. Bilateral adrenal ligation also failed to protect against thioridazine-induced arrhythmias in the cat (Lathers et al., 1986). Both chlorpromazine and thioridazine depressed blood pressure without producing the reflex tachycardia normally observed with hypotension, suggesting that these agents may be interfering with a baroreceptor reflex arc.

D. Role of the Central Nervous System in the Cardiac Actions of Psychoactive Agents

The central nervous system plays a major role in the production of cardiac arrhythmias via cardiac sympathetic outflow. The infusion of thioridazine into cats with spinal cords sectioned at the atlanto-occipital junction did not modify the dose that produced arrhythmia or death when compared with animals with intact spinal cords (Lathers et al., 1986), suggesting that the central sympathetic component above Cl does not play a significant role in acute thioridazine-induced arrhythmia. The thioridazine-induced arrhythmia is therefore attributable primarily to a direct myocardial effect.

Chlorpromazine, trifluoperazine, or haloperidol injected into the cerebral ventricles of unanesthetized cats induced emotional behavior such as restlessness, meowing, rage, attack, defense, fighting with paws, and biting; autonomic changes such as tachypnea, dyspnea, panting, salivation, defecation, urination, mydriasis, licking, and vomiting; and motor effects such as ataxia, motor weakness, and adynamia (Brieslin et al., 1985). The autonomic effects occurred inconsistently and were of low intensity.

Since the psychoactive agents produce their mood-altering effects by acting in the central nervous system (Snyder et al., 1974), studies have examined whether these agents also act centrally to alter cardiovascular control. Chlorpromazine administered into the cerebral ventricles in dogs produced hypotension, bradycardia, an inverted, lowered, or biphasic T wave, and single ventricular extrasystoles or salvos of two or three ventricular extrasystoles (Tangri and Bhargava, 1960; Weinberg and Haley, 1956). Chlorpromazine (up to 27 mg/kg i.v.) response to electrical stimulation of the medullary vasomotor center in the recipient dogs in the cross-perfused dog model, but neither arrhythmia nor death occurred. In addition, the blood pressure of the recipient dogs did not change significantly with chlorpormazine administration to donor dogs, whereas 8 of the 10 donor dogs developed hypotension (Wang et al., 1964). Although these data suggest that the inhibition of the pressor response produced by chlorpromazine is centrally mediated and that the hypotension is not necessarily centrally mediated, when chlorpromazine was injected intraventricularly in anesthetized respired cats, hypotension did not occur without significant changes in heart rate or arrhythmias (Lipka and Lathers, 1985). It was concluded that the hypotension induced by the peripheral administration of chlorpromazine is probably a result of a supraspinal action of chlorpromazine.

Signs of central nervous system toxicity and cardiotoxicity of amitriptyline were common in awake dogs during infusion into the cephalic vein (Nattel et al., 1984). These included barking, salivation, and vomiting in the earlier stages of the infusion, frequently followed by sedation. Five of the six dogs exhibited a seizurelike rhythmic motor activity in their limbs, which occurred immediately before the onset of arrhythmias in two dogs, long before the development of arrhythmia in three animals. The signs of central nervous system toxicity were not observed in dogs that were anesthetized. Heart rate, QRS duration, and AH and HV intervals were increased by amitriptyline. Ventricular tachyarrhythmias of varying duration occurred after the development of a marked degree of QRS prolongation. Sodium bicarbonate rapidly reversed this arrhythmia, perhaps as a result of alkalinization or of changes in serum sodium concentrations.

E. Link Between Sudden Unexplained Death and Psychoactive Agents

Turbott and Cairns (1984) reviewed the controversial nature of the link between sudden unexplained death and neuroleptic medication. There is general agreement that neuroleptics may cause cardiac arrhythmias, but neither the existence of a plausible mechanism nor case reports of sudden death establish a casual relationship. They also note that most case reports describe sudden death in young, healthy individuals, whereas many patients taking neuroleptics are in an older age group, more likely to be characterized by coronary artery disease. In the latter group, the sudden death may be a result of a convergence of factors rather than a single cause. These assertions cannot be dismissed but it should be remembered that sudden unexpected death is not limited by any means to the young (Haerem, 1978; Kuller, 1966). That neuroleptic drug use is not limited to the aged, and attempting a distinction on these bases would not seem called for. Brown and Kocsis (1984) recently summarized the controversy about whether any relationship exists between use of antipsychotic drugs and the causes for the sudden death of patients treated with antipsychotics. They listed rapid vascular collapse, drug-induced seizures, mucus plugs in asthmatic individuals, asphyxia caused by aspirated food, pulmonary neuroembolization, and arrhythmias as possible causes of death. In addition, they stressed that to minimize the number of sudden deaths in patients taking antipsychotics, careful consideration of any predisposing medical conditions, avoidance of potentially dangerous drug combinations such as phenothiazines with tricyclic antidepressants, and monitoring of vital signs, cardiac function, and respiration during the course of therapy must be performed.

Data obtained in both humans (Axelrod and Reisine, 1984; Rabkin et al., 1980; Ruberman et al., 1984; Weinblatt et al., 1978) and animals suggest that stress may lead to changes in myocardial function and sudden death. Stress can be either acute or chronic and its role in sudden death is indirect. A detailed discussion of the role of stress in sudden death in epileptic persons may be found in Chapter 2 and 22 in this book and in the recently published reviews by Lipka and Lathers (1987) and Simpson et al. (1989).

III. THE PRODUCTION OF SEIZURES BY PSYCHOACTIVE AGENTS

A. Phenothiazines

In addition to cardiac arrhythmia production, the phenothiazines may induce clinical seizures (Anton-Stephens, 1953; Kline and Angst, 1978; Logothetis, 1967; Lomas et al., 1955; Simpson et al., 1981). Leestma and Koenig (1968) reported several cases of sudden death associated with seizures in patients maintained on phenothiazines. In another study chlorpromazine induced seizures in 1 out of 453 patients administered the agent, while prochlorperazine induced repeated seizures in 1 out of 1214 patients without previous histories of epilepsy (Jick et al., 1972). Thus the overall frequency of seizures associated with phenothiazine administration appears to be low, with Logothetis (1967) suggesting that the incidence of convulsions is between 0.3 and 5%.

One study examined the clinical problems of seizure production associated with neuroleptic drug administration by comparing psychiatric patients who developed seizures while taking either antipsychotic or antidepressant agents with a control group who had been similarly managed but had not developed seizures (Toone and Fenton, 1977). Patients who experienced seizures were more commonly firstborn children who often had a history of perinatal brain damage, suggesting that firstborn children more often had traumatic deliveries and thus had a greater risk of brain damage than subsequent children. Furthermore, during the week prior to the seizure, there had been a significant increase in the number of new drugs introduced in the treatment regimen and/or an increase in dosage of drugs previously prescribed in those patients who developed seizures. For example, chlorpromazine was either introduced or the dose increased 24 hours to 7 days before the development of a seizure.

Only 10 of 1528 hospitalized psychiatric patients developed seizures over the course of 4 1/2 years (Logothetis, 1967), with 9 having generalized tonic clonic and 1 having a focal motor seizure. All 10 patients with convulsions were taking phenothiazines, which appeared to be the immediate precipitating cause of the seizures in 1.2% among the 859 patients on these drugs. Convulsions were not observed in the 669 patients not receiving phenothiazines. Among patients receiving large therapeutic doses the incidence of seizures increased to 9%; for those receiving low to moderate doses the incidence decreased to 0.5%. Seizures generally occurred at the onset of drug therapy or after a sudden increase in the dose. Patients with organic brain disease appeared more susceptible to convulsions than did patients without organic brain disease.

Logothetis (1967) found that the electroencephalograms (EEGs) of the patient who developed seizures differed from their EEGs before phenothiazine treatment, with slower frequencies, increased amplitude of background activity, and irregular theta and/or delta activity occurring. Nevertheless, the alterations in the background EEG activity of patients who developed convulsions did not differ from those of patients taking phenothiazines who did not develop seizures. Phenothiazine-induced changes in the EEG disappeared over a few days to two months after the agents had been discontinued. In general, chlorpromazine produces a slowing of the EEG pattern, an increase in theta and delta waves, and more frequent occurrence of burst activity and spiking (Baldessarini, 1985; Itil and Soldatos, 1980). Increased voltage and an enhanced tendency toward synchronization defined as a decrease in the variability of frequencies have been reported. Chlorpromazine may also produce an increase in alpha waveforms if the predrug EEG shows little alpha activity, or a decrease in the occurrence of alpha waves if the predrug EEG contains predominantly alpha activity (Kiloh et al., 1980b).

Chlorpromazine has also been found to alter abnormal EEG rhythms. In 20 hospitalized psychiatric patients, chlorpromazine normalized the slightly abnormal EEG of 1 patient and did not produce any effect on the abnormal EEG of another patient (Jorgensen and Wulff, 1958). A slightly abnormal EEG was defined by the presence of more than 15% of 6-7/second wave activity. Chlorpromazine enhanced already abnormal EEGs of two other patients by inducing 2-6/second spike–wave activity. Before chlorpromazine, photic stimulation did not evoke paroxysmal EEG changes; during drug treatment, photic stimulation produced paroxysmal changes in 3 of 20 patients. In another study, chlorpromazine was found to produce more enhancement of abnormalities in EEG activity in a group of elderly patients with organic brain syndrome than in a control group of elderly patients (Swain and Litteral, 1960).

Chlorpromazine-induced alteration of the EEG has been used diagnostically: 50 mg i.m. activated the EEG of 17 of 28 patients who had focal epilepsy (Stewart, 1957), and 100 i.v. has been used to diagnose focal irritative activity (Simons, 1958). The optimum safe dose of chlorpromazine is 50 mg i.v. over a period of five minutes (Kilow et al., 1980a).

Phenothiazines exhibit both anticonvulsant and convulsant properties in in vivo animal preparations. Tedeschi et al. (1958) defined the minimal electroshock seizure threshold in mice as the minimum current needed to produce facial, lower jaw, and/or forelimb clonus without loss of upright posture. They found that chlorpromazine (9-18 mg/kg p.o.) produced a decrease in the threshold and thus acted as a convulsant; doses of 4.5 and 27 mg/kg p.o. did not produce any changes in the threshold. Prochlorpromazine and trifluoperazine did not decrease the seizure threshold in mice at any of the doses tested. Tedeschi et al. (1958) indicated that there had been no prior reports in the literature of clinical seizures associated with the administration of prochlorpromazine or trifluoperazine. However, since that time, cases of seizures associated with prochlorperazine and trifluoperazine were reported (Jick et al., 1972; Toone and Fenton, 1977). Chen et al. (1968) found the extensor seizure threshold model in mice, i.e., the minimum current necessary to elicit clonic hindlimb extension, to be useful in the study of the effects of chlorpromazine on seizure threshold. Chlorpromazine produced a decrease in extensor seizure threshold in mice at low doses ($<$ 10 mg/kg i.p.), while an increase in the threshold occurred at higher doses ($>$ 40 mg/kg i.p.). Thus chlorpromazine exhibited dose-related anticonvulsant and convulsant properties.

Using the cortical alumina gel model of epilepsy, Morrell and Baker (1961) found frequent clinical seizures both in the control and guinea pigs treated with chlorpromazine (10 mg/kg p.o.). In the control group the seizures were usually focal, whereas after chlorpromazine the seizures were bilaterally symmetric and myoclonic. Often these myoclonic seizures were not associated with an electrographic seizure pattern at the cortical level, allowing speculation that primarily subcortical pathways were involved in the seizure production. In another study, chlorpromazine potentiated spike–wave responses elicited by direct thalamic stimulation, again suggesting subcortical pathways were involved in seizure production (Perot and Jasper, quoted in Morrell and Baker, 1961).

In *Papio papio*, a species of baboon in which seizure activity is produced in response to flashing light in 60% of the population, three of six animals that either were insensitive or exhibited attenuated response to light flashing became responsive to the light flashing and exhibited maximal seizure activity after the administration of chlorpromazine (Killam et al., 1967). Sensitivity lasted for three to five days, presumably a result of the long half-life of chlorpromazine. Thus in the majority of animal models examined, chlorpromazine at low doses enhances seizure susceptibility.

Phenothiazines also alter the seizure threshold of in vitro models. In the isolated, perfused rat brain an increase in amplitude and slowing in frequency of the EEG occurred after the addition of either promazine or monodesmethylpromazine. Grouped spikes, characterized by high amplitude and sudden ascension from background activity, were observed after administration of promazine and indicated the induction of seizure activity. The monodesmethyl metabolite of promazine produced grouped sharp waves characterized by slower sharp wave potentials. Both of these waveforms expressed a tendency toward neuronal synchronization.

The effect of psychoactive agents on potassium- and penicillin-induced interictal spike activity in isolated perfused guinea pig hippocampal slices has also been examined (Oliver et al., 1982). Chlorpromazine (50 ng/ml) produced an increase of 30% in neuronal firing compared with no drug; concentrations of 100–400 ng/ml inhibited the firing rate. Thioridazine (50 ng/ml) induced a 23% increase in neuronal discharge; 200 ng/ml produced a 33% increase; and after 400 ng/ml there was virtually no increase. Fluphenazine did not produce any significant effect at 20 ng/ml; 50 ng/ml produced a 12.5% increase; and 200 ng/ml induced an increase of 31%. The dose–response curves for chlorpromazine and thioridazine implicated a maximum potential for seizure production at concentrations that may be less than therapeutic, suggesting that patients would be at increased risk when first given the drug or upon drug withdrawal. Furthermore, these data parallel the in vivo data obtained with chlorpromazine discussed earlier. Thus chlorpromazine enhanced seizure susceptibility at low concentrations and inhibited this susceptibility at higher concentrations in both in vivo and in vitro models.

B. Butyrophenones

Butyrophenones exhibit a variable and unpredictable action on seizure activity (Kline and Angst, 1978; Remick and Fine, 1979). Haloperidol has been reported to induce a psychomotor status–like episode (Kaminer and Munitz, 1984). Low doses of haloperidol (< 10 mg/kg i.p.) produced a slight lowering of the extensor seizure threshold in mice, whereas higher doses (20 mg/kg i.p.) increased the threshold (Morell and Baker, 1961). In the photosensitive baboon, haloperidol (0.6–1.2 mg/kg i.v.) increased the incidence of spontaneous EEG spikes and waves and enhanced paroxysmal EEG activity concomitant with light stimulation (Meldrum et al., 1975).

In potassium- and penicillin-treated guinea pig hippocampal slices, haloperidol (10 ng/ml) produced a 29% increase in neuronal discharge; 50 ng/ml produced a 35% increase; 100 ng/ml, a 56% increase; and 200 ng/ml, a 50% increase (Oliver et al., 1982). Since the therapeutic range of this agent in patients is from 5 to 50 ng/ml, and since large doses in patients have not been associated with an unusual incidence of seizures (Aubree and Lader, 1980), it was concluded that the plateau in effect seen with haloperidol experimentally paralleled the low incidence of clinical seizures.

C. Non-MAOI Antidepressant Agents

Tricyclic antidepressant agents also may lower seizure threshold. Imipramine produced seizures in up to 4% of patients administered the agent during early clinical trials (Leyberg and Denmark, 1959). Imipramine induced myoclonus in 1 of 29 patients treated (Brooke and Weatherly, 1959). Ayd (1959) reported an additional case of imipramine-associated convulsions in 1 of 100 patients. A total of 35 convulsions have been reported in patients administered amitriptyline, an agent that in 1979 accounted for 34.2% of the prescriptions for antidepressants (Edwards, 1979). Betts et al. (1979) reported seizure activity in seven patients administered amitriptyline, five of whom had neither familial nor personal histories of epilepsy. Introduction of this agent or increasing the dose was associated with the development of clinical seizures. In nine patients, all with predisposing factors, seizures developed soon after the start of management of depression with tricyclic agents, including amitriptyline, imipramine, or protriptyline (Dallos and Heathfield, 1969). The administration of imipramine or amitriptyline to depressed patients was associated with an overall incidence of seizures of approximately 1%. Factors predisposing to seizure production included a personal or family history of epilepsy and a baseline epileptiform EEG (Lowry and Dunner, 1980).

There exist a few scattered reports of convulsions following administration of the tetracyclic mianserin (Tyrer et al., 1979) as well as the tricyclic agent viloxazine (Edwards, 1977; Edwards and Glen-Bott, 1984). The incidence of convulsions with mianserin (Edwards and Glen-Bott, 1984), the unicyclic bupropion (Peck et al., 1983), with bicyclic zimelidine, and the tricyclic maprotiline (Edwards, 1979) is reported to be as great as or greater than that associated with the established tricyclic antidepressants (Trimble, 1984). There may be differences among these newer agents; for example, Crome and Newman (1977) reported fewer instances of convulsions associated with mianserin toxicity than with maprotiline. Although a disproportionately large number of convulsions have been reported in association with maprotiline administration, early controlled clinical trials with this drug revealed a low incidence of seizures (17 cases out of more than 26,000 patients) (Trimble, 1985). It was suggested that seizures occurring in patients within a week of starting maprotiline therapy may be associated with predisposing conditions, such as a past history of epilepsy or drug addiction. Seizures occurring with this group of drugs after the first week of therapy may be due to the administration of large doses.

Some of these agents are less frequently associated with seizures than are the tricyclic antidepressant agents. A tetrahydroisoquinoline, nomifensine, has been associated with a single clinical case of seizure production (Gillman and Sandyk, 1984). No significant differences were found in the seizure frequency of 12 depressed patients for the four weeks before nomifensine (25 mg tid) treatment compared to the four weeks of treatment (Trimble, 1984). The administration of doxepin (5-400 mg/day) in patients with epilepsy improved seizure control in 15 patients, increased the seizure incidence in 2, and resulted in no change in 2 (Ojemann et al., 1983). Viloxazine appears to be less epileptogenic than tricyclic antidepressants and may have minimal convulsive properties (Brion, 1975; Edwards and Glen-Bott, 1984; Magnus, 1975; Pichot et al., 1975).

D. Seizure Production Association with Non-MAOI Antidepressant Toxicity

Self-administered overdoses of antidepressant agents have been increasing in frequency. Starkey and Lawson (1980) noted that 20% of patients hospitalized because of overdoses had ingested an antidepressant agent, with grand mal convulsions seen in 40%. In another study Kathol and Henn (1983) found that nearly half of the adult overdoses resulting in admission to a medical intensive care unit resulted from tricyclic antidepressant administration. Flechter et al. (1983) describe convulsions occurring with toxic doses of dibenzepine (14.4 g), chlorimipramine (2.5 g), and maprotiline (200 mg/day). Crome and Newman (1977) reported that 7 of 36 adults who developed maprotiline poisoning had convulsions. Parker and Laymeyer (1984) describe one case of maprotiline toxicity in which cardiac arrhythmia accompanied major motor seizures. Boehnert and Lovejoy (1985) reported that seizures occurred in 34% of patients hospitalized for tricyclic antidepressant overdose who manifested prolonged QRS complexes (≥ 0.015), suggesting that QRS prolongation is a better predictor of seizures and ventricular arrhythmia than serum tricyclic levels.

Numerous case reports of accidental antidepressant toxicity in children also exist. One of five children with maprotiline toxicity had repeated convulsions after ingestion of 525 mg (Crome and Newman, 1977). Pulst and Lombroso (1983) described a 13-year-old boy who developed seizures after an overdose of approximately 1000 mg of imipramine. Steel et al. (1967) reported that convulsions were characteristic of severe poisoning with imipramine or amitriptyline in children. Of 60 children with overdoses on tricyclic agents, 6 who had ingested amitriptyline and 2 who had ingested imipramine developed seizures (Goel and Shanks, 1974). Many children come in contact with these antidepressant agents because they or their siblings had nocturnal enuresis.

Reports of seizures associated with antidepressants used in the management of behavior disorders in children have also appeared. Brown et al. (1973) noted three cases of seizures associated with the use of imipramine (150-225 mg/day) for treatment of hyperactive behavior disorders. All three patients had organic brain disorders but none had a prior history of convulsions. Other cases of seizures have been associated with the use of imipramine for childhood autism and schizophrenia (Campbell et al., 1971; Petti and Campbell, 1975).

E. The Effect of Non-MAOI Antidepressants on the Human EEG

The EEG changes attributed to the tricyclic antidepressants are similar to changes produced by the phenothiazines (Baldessarini, 1985). These agents also have a tendency to potentiate epileptiform discharges. Imipramine increased hypersynchronization on the EEG, administering high doses of imipramine to patients whose spontaneous EEGs are irritated prior to drug administration (Delay and Deniker, 1959).

Like the phenothiazines, the tricyclic antidepressants may be used in the diagnosis of epilepsy (Kiloh et al., 1961). The administration of imipramine (75 mg i.v.) to 24 depressed patients without epilepsy and 36 patients with the disorder resulted in differing amounts of EEG activation in half of the patients with epilepsy with no change in those without epilepsy. Greater activation was found in those whose EEGs showed "epileptiform features" before the administration of imipramine. Similar alterations in the EEG occurred with amitriptyline (30 mg i.v.) over a period of five minutes (Davison, 1965). Mianserin and maprotiline administration in depressed patients did not show any changes in the frequency of alpha, beta, and theta bandwidths before and at the end of four weeks of treatment with the latter drug (Sedgwick and Edwards, 1983). The EEGs of the mianserin-treated group did show a slight increase in beta frequency over control.

Seizures induced in experimental animals have also been employed to examine the risk of epilepsy induction in patients administered tricyclic antidepressants. In general, the convulsive properties of these agents appear to be dose related. Thus, just as tricyclic antidepressants have been reported to produce anticonvulsant (Fromm et al., 1972; Pineda and Russell, 1974) and convulsant (Greenblatt et al., 1976; Richens et al., 1983; Trimble, 1978, 1980; Vernier, 1961) effects clinically, these agents also increase or decrease seizure thresholds in experimental animals, depending on the drug dosages examined. Subcutaneous (s.c.) administration of imipramine at low doses (10-30 mg/kg) raised both the maximal electroshock and pentylenetetrazol seizure thresholds in mice (Sigg, 1959). In nonanesthetized rabbits imipramine, amitriptyline, and desmethylamitriptyline increased the cortical afterdischarge threshold by over 100%, indicating a reduction in cortical excitability to convulsive electrical stimulation (Stille and Sayers, 1964). The demethylated metabolite of imipramine, desipramine, did not alter the threshold. Although these data suggested that imipramine, amitriptyline, and desmethylamitriptyline had anticonvulsant effects, the experimental method used evaluated generalized cortical seizure thresholds rather than limbic seizure thresholds. In addition, toxic doses (20 mg/kg i.v.) of imipramine, amitriptyline, or desmethylamitriptyline produced seizure activity that appeared to originate in the hippocampus. Thus it was suggested that these three agents may produce seizures via the limbic system and that, if tested by a different method, they would prove to be convulsant in nature.

At low doses, imipramine (17.5-25.0 mg/kg i.p.) blocked maximal electroshock seizures in mice but did not affect pentylenetetrazol seizures (Lange et al., 1976). At higher doses, imipramine induced clonic seizures in mice. In cats, imipramine (2.5-15.0 mg/kg i.v.) decreased the frequency of seizure discharge, shortened the afterdischarge duration, and increased afterdischarge threshold in both the penicillin and estrogen epilepsy models in the cat. In doses greater than 20 mg/kg i.v., imipramine exacerbated electrically and chemically induced convulsions and also induced spontaneous seizures. These studies correlated with dose-related anticonvulsant and convulsant properties of the tricyclic antidepressants which are seen clinically.

Steiner and Himwich (1963) found that the intravenous administration of a series of psychoactive agents to rabbits indicated that agents with an imipramine-like structure and known antidepressant action produced "EEG seizures" in nearly all animals. Desipramine was an exception, with only one of five rabbits developing convulsive activity. The induction of seizures was associated with high doses. Van Meter et al. (1959) found that high doses of imipramine (30-50 mg/kg i.v.) in rabbits produced an increase in amplitude and a decrease in the background frequency of the EEG. Monophasic and biphasic spikes occurred in recordings obtained from the amygdala and the hippocampus. High doses of amitriptiline, desipramine, and imipramine (25-50 mg/kg i.p.) produced convulsions in unanesthetized cats (Wallach et al., 1969). A lower dose of imipramine (0.5 mg/kg i.v.) produced cortical synchronization as well as desynchronization of hippocampal activity (Dasberg and Feldman, 1968). With higher doses, sleep spindles were observed; after doses above 4.0 mg/kg the electrocorticogram becam slow and irregular. Recordings from the amygdala revealed single spikes and sharp waves. Single spikes and sharp waves were observed in hippocampal recordings at doses of 8 mg/kg and higher. The arousal threshold, as assessed by electrically stimulating the midbrain reticular formation, was elevated by imi-pramine in a dose-dependent manner. Imipramine in doses greater than 4 mg/kg did not produce arousal. Thus the effects of these agents on seizure production appear to be dose dependent.

Intravenous doses of 10 or 20 mg/kg of chlorimipramine or imipramine not-ably depressed the convulsive threshold and induced seizures in all photosensi-tive baboons in which they were administered (Trimble et al., 1977). This find-ing appears to parallel the epileptogenic potential of these agents observed clin-ically.

In one in vitro study, imipramine increased the amplitude of the EEG activity and the slow-wave activity in the isolated perfused rat brain when compared with control perfusions without drug. Grouped spikes were elicited. However, the EEG waves produced by desipramine were not significantly different from the EEG of the control perfusion without drug. Thus in this preparation imipra-mine was distinguishable from its monodemethylated metabolite, desipramine.

In mice, oral viloxazine (10–30 mg/kg) protected against seizures produced either electrically or by pentylenetetrazol (Mallion et al., 1972). The same doses also protected against electrically induced seizures in the rat. Viloxazine (2.6 mg/kg i.v.) protected against photically induced seizures in *P. papio* one to two hours after drug administration (Meldrum et al., 1982). Maprotiline (10 mg/kg) or nomifensine (10 or 20 mg/kg i.v.) did not alter the seizure threshold (Trimble, 1984). Viloxazine exhibited anticonvulsant properties when used in the maximal electroshock test in mice and rats (Meldrum et al., 1982) and protected against pentylenetetrazol and 3-mercaptopropionic acid–induced convulsions and against seizure production in audiogenic mice (Miller and Wheatley, 1978). A frequency analysis of the EEG after administration of nomifensine, viloxazine, or bupropion to rats showed EEG arousal to be blocked by pimozide, a dopa-mine antagonist. After either acute intravenous or chronic oral administration of viloxazine, signs of epileptogenic activity were not noted on the electrocorti-cogram of the cat encephalae isole preparation (Neal and Bradley, 1978, 1979). In conscious rats, viloxazine produced desynchronization of the EEG (Mallion et al., 1972). In nonanesthetized rabbits, amitriptyline and imipramine were found to be equipotent in their production of the first convulsion, whereas mal-protiline was less potent and mianserin was least potent of the agents examined (Hughes and Radman, 1978). Koella et al. (1979) found differences in the EEG patterns of seizure activity in cats administered maprotiline when compared with imipramine, chlorimipramine, and amitriptyline. Although all four agents did evoke signs of epileptiform abnormalities, the EEG pattern of the period after maprotiline-induced seizures suggested that this agent might be less likely to sustain convulsive activity than the other three.

An examination of the effects of antidepressants on potassium- and penicillin-induced rhythmic interictal spiking in isolated, perfused guinea pig hippocampal slices revealed an increase in spike activity with imipramine, nortriptyline, maprotiline, and desipramine in decreasing order of potency (Luchins et al., 1984). Both nomifensine and doxepin enhanced spike discharges at lower concentrations but depressed activity after higher concentrations. Increasing concentratins of proptriptyline and trimipramine decreased the frequency of spike discharge; mianserin and viloxazine had a minimal effect at any concentration. In summary, the results obtained in this model paralleled the epileptogenic properties of these agents noted in humans. The data obtained with nomifensine, however, do not appear to be predictive, as use of this agent has been associated only rarely with clinical seizures (Gillman and Sandyk, 1984).

F. Mechanism by Which Psychoactive Agents Produce Seizure Activity

It has been hypothesized that the dopamine-blocking properties of the major tranquilizers render the patient susceptible to convulsions (Trimble, 1977). Dopamine agonists partially or completely block photically induced epilepsy in baboons; dopamine-blocking agents enhance spike and wave EEG activity and increase susceptibility to seizures in this model (Meldrum et al., 1975).

Many of the non-MAOI antidepressant agents have been shown to inhibit serotonin re-uptake at the synaptic cleft (Tang and Seeman, 1980). Thus enhanced serotonin concentration at the nerve terminal has been examined as a possible mechanism of seizure production. Holinger and Klawans (1976) and Burks et al. (1974) hypothesized that increased concentrations of serotonin at striatal interneuron sites produce the myoclonic jerks observed with seizures associated with tricyclic antidepressants. Westheimer and Klawans (1974) showed that a serotonin precursor , 5-hydroxytryptophan (5-HTP), produced myoclonic seizures when administered to guinea pigs. Subthreshold doses of 5-HTP in combination with imipramine (35 mg/kg) produced myoclonic seizures; administration of either agent individually at these doses did not. Antagonists of acetylcholine, norepinephrine, and dopamine did not block these seizures but methysergide did. Thus it was concluded that imipramine may be acting through serotonergic mechanisms to produce myoclonic seizures. When the photosensitive baboon was used as the animal model, 5-HTP (10–35 mg/kg i.p.) decreased EEG and motor responses to photic stimulation (Wada et al., 1972). Two days after administration of a tryptophan hydroxylase inhibitor, parachlorophenylalanine (pCPA), myoclonic responses to photic stimulation were enhanced. It was concluded that serotonergic mechanisms may be important in the photomyoclonic syndrome in this species.

It has also been hypothesized that mechanisms other than an enhanced serotonin concentration are responsible for seizure production by non-MAOI antidepressant agents. Trimble et al. (1977) suggested that enhanced serotonin tone may protect against seizure production since 5-HTP protected against the enhancement of convulsive responses to photic stimulation produced by chlorimipramine or imipramine in baboons. The effects of these agents on other neurotransmitters have also been hypothesized to alter seizure production. The anticholinergic action of some agents has been postulated to produce seizures (Flechter et al., 1983). Furthermore, since dopamine agonists have been found to increase seizure thresholds (Meldrum et al., 1975), it has been hypothesized that the dopaminergic agonist property that monifensine possesses may make this agent less likely to induce convulsions (Trimble, 1984). To date there is no clear experimental evidence to suggest the mechanism whereby non-MAOI antidepressant agents lower the seizure threshold.

IV. RECOMMENDATIONS FOR THE CLINICAL USE OF ANTIDEPRESSANTS AND NEUROLEPTICS

In general, patients with normal predrug EEGs who are without organic brain disease and do not have a history of epilepsy can be considered to be nearly free of risk from seizures during treatment with major tranquilizers or antidepressant agents. Sudden alterations of dose should be avoided, and the patient should be monitored for clinical seizures during the initial portion of treatment with these drugs (Itil and Saldatos, 1980). In patients with symptoms or a history of organic brain disease or epilepsy, management should be done cautiously, even if abnormalities are not seen on the EEG. Relevant clinical tests should be done before the onset of therapy. Agents with a high association of seizure production should be avoided if possible. Drugs with less convulsive potential should be substituted for those with greater epilepsy-induction potential. The dose of antidepressant or tranquilizer should be increased slowly until the desired serum levels are achieved (Remick and Fine, 1979; Robertson and Trimble, 1983).

Seizures that develop in persons with a history of epilepsy who have also been given psychoactive drugs should be controlled with concomitant administration of antiepileptic medication. In general, the dosage of antiepileptic drugs must be adjusted when there is simultaneous administration of psychoactive drugs (Itil and Soldatos, 1980). Pharmacologic interactions between anticonvulsant and psychoactive agents must be considered, since patients receiving anticonvulsants often have lower serum antidepressant levels. Hepatic enzyme induction by antiepileptic drugs may be the cause of this phenomenon (Richens et al., 1983). Tricyclic agents appear to have varying effects on anticonvulsant serum levels in that nortriptyline, viloxazine, and imipramine have been noted to increase serum phenytoin levels (Perucca and Richens, 1977).

In general, the psychoactive agents are more likely to induce negative reactions and EEG slowing in the aged (Hamilton, 1966; Thompson et al., 1983a,b).

The use of antipsychotic agents in elderly patients with known seizure disorders must be undertaken very cautiously (Popkin et al., 1982). The initial doses should be no more than one-third of that prescribed for younger patients (Zisook and Finkel, 1982). In the elderly, elimination half-lives may be increased to 80 hours. Thus careful monitoring for signs of adverse effects should be done (Lowry and Dunner, 1980).

The clinical manifestations of neurotoxicity associated with psychoactive drug administration may differ depending on the age of the patient. Van Sweden (1984) reported that the few clinical seizures occurring in a given patient population did so during the first week of dosing in patients less than 50 years of age who were administered combinations of drugs, including aminoalkylphenothiazines and tricyclic depressants. The early signs of neuroleptic neurotoxicity included stupor and myoclonic jerking. In the elderly, signs of neurotoxicity developed within several days of initiation of drug administration. In these patients, however, an alteration in the state of consciousness predominated. Additionally, changes in EEG pattern differed depending on the age of the patient. In patients less than 50 years old the EEG showed cerebral hypofunction and irritation and indicated dysfunction at the level of the brain stem reticular system within a few days after the start of drug administration. Diffuse slow-wave activity, with a desynchronized low-voltage pattern and signs of irritation, appered most often in the frontocentral regions with bilateral and irregular paroxysms. Late-onset EEG changes occurred after several weeks of treatment, often with use of more sedating agents. In elderly patients, periodic sharp transient discharges were noted, particularly on EEGs of patients treated with aminoalkylphenothiazines.

V. SUMMARY

The major tranquilizers and the antidepressant agents have been associated with clinical seizures. The incidence of such seizures is generally low when therapeutic doses are used; the use of large doses has been associated with many cases of convulsions. In animal models of epilepsy, phenothiazines are convulsant at lower doses, whereas higher doses are anticonvulsant. In contrast, antidepressants are anticonvulsant at low and convulsant at high doses. The mechanism by which these agents alter the seizure threshold is unknown. When treating patients with epilepsy who also have psychiatric problems, drugs of lower seizure production potential should be substituted for those with greater potential.

Sudden death in epileptic persons has been attributed most frequently to autonomic dysfunction and cardiac arrhythmias. The contribution of stress in sudden death production in these individuals must be evaluated (see Chapter 22, this book). Additionally, some psychoactive agents have been associated with sudden death and/or initiation of arrhythmias and seizures. Since there is the possibility that the factors involved in the production of sudden death may be additive (Lipka and Lathers, 1987), the administration of a psychoactive agent to an epileptic patient should be approached with caution. Pharmacological agents that do not alter cardiac rhythm or seizure threshold should be used if a psychoactive agent is required to manage psychiatric problems in the patient with epilepsy.

ACKNOWLEDGMENTS

The authors would like to thank Darline Spino for typing the manuscript.

REFERENCES

Alexander, S., and Nino, A. (1969). Cardiovascular complications in young patients taking psychotropic drugs. A preliminary report. *Am. Heart J. 78*: 757-769.

Angelone, A., and Coulter, N. A. (1964). Respirator sinus arrhythmia. A frequency dependent phenomenon. *J. Appl. Physiol. 19*:479-482.

Anton-Stephens, D. (1953). Preliminary observations on the psychiatric uses of chlorpromazine (Largactil). *J. Ment. Sci. 100*:543-557.

Aronson, C. E., and Serlick, E. R. (1977). Effects of chlorpromazine on the isolated perfused rat heart. *Toxicol. Appl. Pharmacol. 39*:157-176.

Arora, R. B., and Madan, B. R. (1979). Antiarrhythmia action of minor and major tranquilizers. *Pharm. Ther. 4*:633.

Attree, T., Sawyer, P., and Turnbull, M. J. (1972). Interaction between digoxin and tricyclic antidepressants in the rat. *Eur. J. Pharmacol. 19*:294-296.

Aubree, J. C., and Lader, M. H. (1980). High and very high dosage antipsychotics: A critical review. *J. Clin. Psychiatr. 41*:341-350.

Axelsson, R. and Aspenstrom, G. (1982). Electrocardiographic changes and serum concentrations in thioridazine-treated patients. *J. Clin. Psych. 43*: 332-335.

Ayd, F. J. (1959). Tofranil therapy for depressed states. *J. Neuropsychiatry 1*: 35-38.

Ayd, F. J. (1956). Fatal hyperpyrexia during chlorpromazine therapy. *J. Clin. Exp. Psych. 17*:189-192.

Baldessarini, R. J. (1985). Drugs and the treatment of psychiatric disorders. In *Goodman and Gilman's The Pharmacological Basis of Therapeutics*, 7th ed., A. G. Gilman, L. S. Goodman, T. W. Rall, amd F. Murad (Eds.). Macmillan, New York, pp. 387-445.

Banks, P. (1967). The effect of ouabain on the secretion of catecholamines and on the intracellular concentration of potassium. *J. Physiol. (Lond.) 193*: 631-637.

Basu Ray, B. N., Dutta, S. N., and Booker, W. M. (1977). Effects of lithium chloride, desmethylimipramine and cocaine on the cardiovascular actions of ouabain in dogs with or without carotid and aortic baroreceptor reflexes. *Arch. Int. Pharmacodyn. Ther. 228*:99–107.

Baum, T., Shropshire, A. T., Rowles, G., et al. (1971). Antidepressants and cardiac conduction: Iprindole and imipramine. *Eur. J. Pharmacol. 13*:287–291.

Baum, T., Eckfeld, D. K., Shropshire, A. T., et al. (1971). Observations on models used for evaluation of antiarrhythmic drugs. *Arch. Int. Pharmacodyn. Ther. 193*:149.

Beleslin, D. B., Jovanovic-Micic, D., Japundzic, N., et al. (1985). Behavioral, autonomic and motor effects of neuroleptic drugs in cats: Motor impairment and aggression. *Brain. Res. Bull. 15*:353–356.

Betts, W.C., Johnston, F. S., Jr., and Patt, M. J. (1979). An effective pallaitive treatment for phenothiazine-induced tardive dyskinesia. *NC Med. J. 40*:286. 286.

Bianchetti, G., Bonacloisi, A., Chiodorol, A., et al. (1977). Plasma concentrations and cardiotoxic effects of desipramine and protriptyline in the cat. *Br. J. Pharmacol. 60*:11–19.

Bigger, J. T., Giardina, E. G. V., Peterl, J. M., et al. (1977). Cardiac arrhythmic effect of imipramine hydrochloride. *New Engl. J. Med. 296*:206–208.

Boehnert, M. T., and Lovejoy, F. H. (1985). Value of the QRS duration versus the serum drug level in predicting seizures and ventricular arrhythmia after an acute overdose of tricyclic antidepressants. *New Engl. J. Med. 313*:474–479.

Brill, H., and Patton, R. E. (1962). Clinical-statistical analysis of population changes in New York State mental hospitals since introduction of psychotropic drugs. *Am. J. Psychiatr. 119*:20–35.

Brion, S. (1975). Open studies with viloxazine (Vivalan). *J. Intern. Med. Res. (Suppl. 3)*:87–91.

Brissette, Y., and Gascon, A. L. (1978). Increase in cardiac toxicity of ouabain in dogs after repetitive treatment with diazepam. *Toxicol. Appl. Pharmacol. 44*:127–135.

Brooke, G., and Weatherly, J. R. C. (1959). Imipramine. *Lancet 2*:568–569.

Brown, D., Winsberg, B. G., Bialer, I., et al. (1973). Imipramine therapy and seizures: Three children treated for hyperactive behavior disorders. *Am. J. Psychiatr. 130*:210–212.

Brown, R. P., and Kocsis, J. H. (1984). Sudden death and antipsychotic drugs. *Hosp. Comm. Psychiatr. 35*:486–491.

Burgess, K. R., Kefferis, R. W., and Stevenson, K. F. (1979). Fatal thioridazine cardiotoxicity. *Med. J. Aust. 2*:177–178.

Burks, J. S., Walker, J. E., Rumack, B. H., et al. (1974). Tricyclic antidepressant poisoning: Reversal of coma, choreoathetosis, and myoclonus by physostigmine. *J. Am. Med. Assoc. 230*:1405–1407.

Byck, R. (1975). Drugs and the treatment of psychiatric disorders. In *The Pharmacological Basis of Therapeutics*, 5th ed., L. S. Goodman and A. Gilman (Eds.). Macmillan, New York.

Caffey, E. M., et al. (1966). Antipsychotic, antianxiety and antidepressant drugs. Medical Bulletin MB-11. Veterans Administration, Washington, D.C., p. 11.

Cairncross, K. D., and Gershon, S. (1962). A pharmacological basis for the cardiovascular complications of imipramine. *Eur. J. Pharmacol. 13*:287–291.

Caldwell, R. W., Puryear, S. K., and Nash, C. B. (1978). Interaction of sympathetic nervous system in cardiac toxicity of digoxin or aminosugar cardiac glycosides. *Proceedings of the Seventh International Congress for Pharmacology, Paris*, p. 914.

Campbell, M., Fish, B., Shapiro, T., et al. (1971). Imipramine in preschool autistic and schizophrenic children. *J. Autism Childh. Schizophrenia 1*:267–282.

Carlsson, C., Dencker, S. J., Grimby, G., et al. (1966). Noradrenaline in blood-plasma and urine during chlorpromazine treatment. *Lancet 1*:1208.

Carpenter, P., Gobel, F. L., and Husing, D. J. (1982). Desipramine cardiac toxicity. *Minn. Med. 65*:231–234.

Ceremuzynski, L., Staszewska-Barczak, J., and Herbaczynska-Cedr, K. (1969). Cardiac rhythm disturbances and the release of catecholamines after acute coronary occlusion in dogs. *Cardiovasc. Res. 3*:190–197.

Chai, C. Y., and Wang, S. C. (1966). Cardiovascular actions of diazepam in the cat. *J. Pharmacol. Exp. Ther. 154*:271–280.

Chen, G., Ensor, C. R., and Bohner, B. (1968). Studies of drug effects on electrically induced extensor seizures and clinical implications. *Arch. Int. Pharmacodyn. 172*:183–218.

Cook, L. S., Caldwell, R. W., Nash, C. B., et al. (1982). Adrenergic and cholinergic mechanisms in digitalis inotropy. *J. Pharmacol. Exp. Ther. 223*:761–765.

Coull, D. C., Crooks, J., Dingwall-Fordyce, K., et al. (1970a). A method of monitoring drugs adverse reaction. II: Amitryptiline and cardiac disease. *Eur. J. Clin. Pharmacol. 3*:51–55.

Coull, D. C., Crooks, J., Dingwall-Fordyce, K., et al. (1970b). Amitriptyline and cardiac disease. *Lancet 2*:590–591.

Courvoiser, S., Fournel, J., Ducrot, R., et al. (1953). Properties pharmacodynamiques des chlor-e-(dimethylamine-3′)-propyl-10-phenothiazine. *Arch. Int. Pharmacodyn. Ther. 92*:305.

Craig, T. J., and Lin, S. P. (1982). Sudden death and neuroleptics. *Psychopharm. Bull. 18*:2.

Crankshaw, D. P., and Raper, C. (1971). The effect of solvents on the potency of chlordiazepoxide, diazepam, medazepam, and nitrazepam. *J. Pharm. Pharmacol. 23*:313–321.

Crawley, I. S., and Kolodner, R. M. (1981). The effects of psychotropic drugs on the heart. In *Clinical Essays on the Heart*, J. W. Hurst (Ed.). McGraw-Hill, New York, pp. 285–311.

Crome, P., and Newman, B. (1977). Poisoning with maprotiline and mianserin. *Br. Med. J. 2*:260 (abstract).

Dallos, V., and Heathfield, K. (1969). Iatrogenic epilepsy due to antidepressant drugs. *Br. Med. J. 4*:80–82.

Dasberg, H., Feldman, S. (1968). Effect of imipramine, physostigmine and amphetamine on the electrical activity of the brain in the cat. *Psychopharma-cologia 13*:129-139.

Davison, K. (1965). EEG activation after intravenous amitriptyline. *Electroen-cephalogr. Clin. Neurophysiol. 19*:298-300.

Delay, J., and Deniker, P. (1959). Efficacy of Tofranil in the treatment of various types of depression: A comparison with other antidepressant drugs. *Can. Psychiatr. Assoc. J. 4*:S100-S112.

Domino, E. F. (1983). Sudden death, acute and chronic extrapyramidal syndromes including tardive dyskinesia and self-mutilation induced by fluphenazine and haloperidol in monkeys. *Soc. Neurosci. Abs. 9*.

Domino, E. F. (1985). Sudden death and neuroleptic medication in subhuman primates. *Am. J. Psychiatr. 142*:145.

Domino, E. F., and Kovacic, B. (1984). Monkey models of tardive dyskinesia. In *Catecholamines: Neuropharmacology and Central Nervous System – The Therapeutic Aspect*. Alan R. Liss, New York.

Doyle, J. T. (1976). Mechanisms and prevention of sudden death. *Med. Conc. Cardiovasc. Dis. 45*:111-116.

Edwards, J. G., and Glenn-Bott, M. (1983). Mianserin and convulsive seizures. *Br. J. Clin. Pharmacol. 15 (Suppl.)*:299-311.

Edwards, J. G., and Glenn-Bott, M. (1984). Does viloxazine have epileptogenic properties? *J. Neurol. Neurosurg. Psychiatr. 47*:960-964.

Edwards, J. C. (1977). Convulsive seizures and viloxazine. *Br. Med. J. 2*:96-97.

Edwards, J. G. (1979). Antidepressants and convulsions. *Lancet 2*:1368-1369.

Fiedler, V. B., Gobel, H., and Nitz, R. E. (1985a). Cardioprotective effects of carbocromen in awake and anesthetized dogs with amitriptyline poisoning. *J. Cardiovasc. Pharmacol. 7*:666-672.

Fiedler, V. B., Kettenback, B., Gobel, H., et al. (1985b). Treatment of haemodynamic and electrocardiographic side-effects resulting from imipramine toxicity in rats and dogs. *Naunyn Schmiedebergs Arch. Pharmacol. 330*:155-161.

Flechter, S., Rabey, J. M., Regev, I., et al. (1983). Convulsive attacks due to antidepressant drug overdoses: Case reports and discussion. *Gen. Hosp. Psychiatr. 5*:217-221.

Fowler, N. O., McCall, D., Chou, T. C., Holmes, J. C., and Hanenson, I. B. (1976). Electrocardiographic changes and cardiac arrhythmias in patients receiving psychotropic drugs. *Am. J. Cardiol. 37*:223-230.

Freytag, E., and Lindenberg, R. (1964). 294 medicolegal autopsies in epileptics. *Arch. Pathol. 78*:274-286.

Fromm, G. H., Amores, C. Y., and Thies, W. (1972). Imipramine in epilepsy. *Arch. Neurol. 27*:198-204.

Gascon, A. L. (1977). Effect of acute stress and ouabain administration on adrenal catecholamine content and cardiac function of rats pretreated with diazepam. *Can. J. Physiol. Pharmacol. 55*:65-71.

Giardina, E. G. (1984). Cardiac and antiarrhythmic effects of imipramine in patients with ventricular arrhythmias. *Biomed. Pharmacother. 38*:128-130.

Giardina, E. G., Bigger, J. T., Glassman, A. H., et al. (1979). The electrocardiographic and antiarrhythmic effects of imipramine hydrochloride at therapeutic plasma concentrations. *Circulation 60*:1045.

Gillis, R. A., Thibodeauz, H., and Barr, L. (1974). Antiarrhythmic properties of chlordiazepoxide. *Circulation 49*:272–282.

Gillis, R. A., Quest, J. A., and Diaz Souza, J. (1979). The role of the nervous system in the cardiovascular effects of digitalis. *Pharmacol. Ref. 31*:19–97.

Gillman, M. A., and Sandyk, R. (1984). Nomifensine exacerbates depression and seizures in epileptic patients. *Neurology 34*:1620–1621.

Goel, K. M., and Shanks, R. A. (1974). Amitriptyline and imipramine poisoning in children. *Br. Med. J. 4*:261–263.

Goldney, R. D., Spoence, N. D., and Bowes, J. A. (1986). The safe use of high dose neuroleptics in a psychiatric intensive care unit. *Aust. N.Z. J. Psychiatr. 20*:370–375.

Goodson, W. H., Jr., and Litkenhous, E. E., Jr. (1976). Sudden unexplained death in a psychiatric patient taking thioridazine. *South. Med. J. 69*:311–315, 320.

Gould, R. J., Steeg, C. N., Eastwood, A. B., et al. (1985). Potentially fatal cardiac dysrhythmia and hyperkalemia periodic paralysis. *Neurology 35*:128–130.

Graupner, K. I., Murphree, O. D., and Meduna, L. J. (1964). Electrocardiographic changes associated with the use of thioridazine. *J. Neuropsychiatr. 5*:344–350.

Greenblatt, D. J., Shader, R. I., and Lofgren, S. (1976). Rational psychopharmacology for patients with medical diseases. *Ann. Rev. Med. 27*:407–420.

Guillan, R. A., Zelman, S., Reinert, R. E., and Smalley, R. L. (1970). Electron microscopy. Sudden death in patients under phenothiazine therapy: Study of three cases. *J. Kans. Med. Soc. 71*:213–218.

Guzman-Harty, M., Tjioe, S. A., and O'Neill, J. J. (1985). Effects of chlorpromazine and its dihydroxy metabolite on calcium movement and electrical activity in the superior cervical ganglia. *Arch. Toxicol. 56*:272–278.

Haerem, J. W. (1978). Sudden, unexpected coronary death. The occurrence of platelet aggregates in the epicardial and myocardial vessels of man. *Acta Pathol. Microbiol. Scand. (Suppl. 265)*:1–47.

Hamilton, L. D. (1966). Aged brain and phenothiazines. *Geriatrics 21*:131–138.

Hirsch, C. S., and Martin, D. L. (1971). Unexpected death in young epileptics. *Neurology 21*:682–690.

Hockman, C. H., and Livingston, K. E. (1971). Inhibition of reflex vagal bradycardia by diazepam. *Neuropharmacology 10*:307–314.

Holinger, P. C., and Klawans, H. L. (1976). Reversal of tricyclic-overdosage-induced central anticholinergic syndrome of physostigmine. *Am. J. Psychiatr. 133*:1018–1022.

Hollister, L. E. (1957). Unexpected asphyxial death and tranquilizing agents. *J. Psychiatr. 114*:366–367.

Hollister, L. H., and Kosek, J. C. (1965). Sudden death during treatment with phenothiazine derivatives. *J. Am. Med. Assoc. 192*:1035–1038.

Horowitz, L. N., and Morganroth, J. A. (1982). Can we prevent sudden cardiac death? *Am. J. Cardiol. 50*:535–538.

Hughes, I. E., and Radman, S. (1978). Relative toxicity of amitriptyline, imipramine, maprotiline and mianserin after intravenous infusion in conscious rabbits. *Br. J. Clin. Pharmacol. (Suppl. 1) 5*:19S–20S.

Hussar, A. E. (1962). Effect of tranquilizers on medical morbidity and mortality in a mental hospital. *J. Am. Med. Assoc. 179*:682–686.

Huston, J. R., and Bell, G. E. (1966). The effect of thioridazine hydrochloride and chlorpromazine on the electrocardiogram. *J. Am. Med. Assoc. 198*:134–138.

Itil, T. M., and Soldatos, C. (1980). Epileptogenic side effects of psychotropic drugs. Practical recommendations. *J. Am. Med. Assoc. 244*:1460–1463.

Itil, T. M., Polvan, N., and Hsu, W. (1972). Clinical and EEG effects of GB-94, a tetracyclic antidepressant: EEG model in discovery of a new psychotropic drug. *Curr. Ther. Res. 14*:395–413.

Jakobsen, J., Hauksson, P., and Veslergaard, P. (1984). Heart rate variation in patients treated with antidepressants. An index of anticholinergic effects? *Psychopharmacology 84*:544–548.

Jay, G. W., and Leestma, J. E. (1981). Sudden death in epilepsy: A comprehensive review of the literature and proposed mechanisms. *Acta Neurol Scand. (Suppl. 82)*:1–66.

Jefferson, J. W. (1975). A review of the cardiovascular effects and toxicity of tricyclic antidepressants. *Psychosom. Med. 37*:160–179.

Jick, H., Slone, D., Shapiro, S., et al. (1972). Drug-induced convulsions. Report from Boston collaborative drug surveillance program. *Lancet 2*:677–679.

Jorgensen, R. S., and Wulff, M. H. (1958). The effect of orally administered chlorpromazine on the electroencephalogram of man. *Electroencephalogr. Clin. Neurophysiol. 10*:325–329.

Kaminer, Y., and Munitz, H. (1984). Case report: Psychomotor status-like episodes under haloperidol treatment. *Br. J. Psychiatr. 145*:87–90.

Kannel, W. B., Doyle, J. T., McNamara, P. M., et al. (1975). Precursors of sudden coronary death. Factors related to the incidence of sudden death. *Circulation 51*:606–613.

Kannel, W. B., and Thomas, H. E. (1982). Sudden coronary death: The Framingham study. In *Annals of the New York Academy of Science*, Vol. 382, *Sudden Coronary Death*, H. M. Greenberg and E. M. Dwyer (Eds.). New York Academy of Science, New York.

Kathol, R. G., and Henn, F. A. (1983). The most common agent used in potentially lethal overdose. *J. Nerv. Ment. Dis. 171*:250–252.

Keilson, M. J., Hauser, W. A., Magrill, J. P., et al. (1987). EEG abnormalities in patients with epilepsy. *Neurology 37*:1624–1626.

Kelliher, G. J., Widmer, C., and Roberts, J. (1975). Influence of the adrenal medulla on cardiac rhythm disturbances following acute coronary artery occlusion. In *Recent Advances in Studies on Cardiac Structure and Metabo-*

lism, Vol. 10, *The Metabolism of Contraction*, P. Roy and G. Rona (Eds.). University Park Press, Baltimore, pp. 387–4ʋ0.

Kelly, H. G., Fay, J. E., and Laverty, S. G. (1963). Thioridazine hydrochloride (Mellaril): Its effect on the electrocardiogram and a report of two fatalities with electrocardiographic abnormalities. *Can. Med. Assoc. J. 89*:546–554.

Kiem, K. L., and Sigg, E. B. (1973). Vagally mediated cardiac reflexes and their modulation by diazepam and pentobarbital. *Neuropharmacology 12*:319–325.

Killam, K. F., Killam, E. K., and Naquet, R. (1967). An animal model of light sensitive epilepsy. *Electroencephalogr. Clin. Neurophysiol. 22*:497–513.

Kiloh, L. G., Davison, K., and Osselton, J. W. (1961). An electroencephalographic study of the analeptic effects of imipramine. *Electroencephalogr. Clin. Neurophysiol. 13*:216–223.

Kiloh, L. G., McComas, A. J., and Osselton, J. W. (1980a). Epilepsy. In *Clinical Electroencephalography*, 3rd ed., L. G. Kiloh, A. J. McComas, and J. W. Osselton (Eds.), Butterworth, London, pp. 71-108.

Kiloh, L. G., McComas, A. J., and Osselton, J. W. (1980b). Psychiatry. In *Clinical Electroencephalography*, 3rd ed. L. G. Kiloh, A. J. McComas, and J. W. Osselton (Eds.). Butterworths, London, pp. 168–200.

Kline, N. A., and Angst, J. (1978). Side effects of psychotropic drugs. *Psychiatr. Ann. 5*:441–458.

Koella, W. P., Glatt, A., Klebs, K., et al. (1979). Epileptic phenomena induced in the cat by the antidepressants maprotiline, imipramine, clomipramine, and amitriptyline. *Biol. Psychiatr. 14*:485–497.

Koishnanarao, K., and Achari, G. (1972). Antiarrhythmic action of two new phenothiazine derivatives. *J. India Med. Assoc. 98*:1.

Kuller, L. (1966). Sudden and unexpected non-traumatic deaths in adults: Review of epidemiological and clinical studies. *J. Chron. Dis. 19*:1165–1192.

Kuller, L., Lilienfeld, A., and Fisher, R. (1966). Sudden and unexpected death in young adults. *J. Am. Med. Assoc. 198*:248–252.

Kuller, L., Lilienfeld, A., and Fisher, R. (1967). An epidemiological study of sudden and unexpected death in adults. *Medicine 46*:341–361.

Kuruvilla, A., and Stephen, P. M. (1984). Effect of chlordiazepoxide on experimentally induced centrogenic arrhythmias in anesthetized dogs. *Indian J. Exp. Biol. 22*:653–656.

Lamy, P. P. (1980). Psychopharmacologic drugs. In *Prescribing for the Elderly*, P. P. Lamy (Ed.). PSG Publishing Co., Littleton, Mass, pp. 501–591.

Landmark, K. (1970). Changes in excitability of rat atria caused by phenothiazine derivatives. *Acta Pharm. Toxicol. (Suppl. 1) 28*:59.

Lange, S. C., Julien, R. M., and Fowler, G. W. (1976). Biphasic effects of imipramine in experimental models of epilepsy. *Epilepsia 17*:183–196.

Langou, R. A., Van Dyke, C., Tahan, S. R., et al. (1980). Cardiovascular manifestations of tricyclic antidepressant overdose. *Am. Heart J. 100*: 458-464.

Langslet, A. (1969). Changes in coronary flow and ECG in the isolated perfused rat heart induced by phenothiazine drugs. *Acta Pharmacol. Toxicol. 27*: 183–192.

Langslet, A. (1970). ECG-changes induced by phenothiazine drugs in the anesthetized rat. *Acta Pharmacol. Toxicol. 28*:258-264.

Laposata, E. A., Hale, P., and Poklis, A. (1988). Evaluation of sudden death in psychiatric patients with special reference to phenothiazine therapy: Forensic pathology. *J. Forensic Sci. 33*:432-440.

Lathers, C. M., and Lipka, L. J. (1986). Chlorpromazine: Cardiac arrhythmogenicity in the cat. *Life Sci. 38*:521-538.

Lathers, C. M., and Lipka, L. J. (1987). Cardiac arrhythmia, sudden death, and psychoactive agents. *J. Clin. Pharmacol. 27*:1-14.

Lathers, C. M., and Roberts, J. (1980). Minireview: Digitalis cardiotoxicity revisited. *Life Sci. 27*:1713-1733.

Lathers, C. M., and Roberts, J. (1985). Are the sympathetic neural effects of digoxin and quinidine involved in their action on cardiac rhythm? *J. Cardiovasc. Pharmacol. 7*:350-360.

Lathers, C. M., and Schraeder, P. L. (1983). Autonomic dysfunction, cardiac arrhythmias, and epileptogenic activity. Unexpected, unexplained death in epileptic persons. Presented at the Epilepsy International Symposium and American Epilepsy Society Meeting 15:14.

Lathers, C. M., Roberts, J., and Kelliher, G. J. (1977). Correlation of ouabain-induced arrhythmia and nonuniformity in the histamine-evoked discharge of cardiac sympathetic nerves. *J. Pharmacol. Exp. Ther. 203*:467-479.

Lathers, C. M., Kelliher, G. J., Roberts, J., and Beasley, A. B. (1978). Nonuniform cardiac sympathetic nerve discharge: Mechanism for coronary occlusion and digitalis-induced arrhythmia. *Circulation 57*:1058-1065.

Lathers, C. M., Lipka, L. J., and Klions, H. A. (1985). Controversies in the actions of digitalis substances: Are all digitalis derivatives alike? *J. Clin. Pharmacol. 25*:501-506.

Lathers, C. M., Flax, R. F., and Lipka, L. J. (1986). The effect of C_1 spinal cord transection or bilateral adrenal vein ligation on thioridazine-induced arrhythmia and death in the cat. *J. Clin. Pharmacol. 26*:515-523.

Leestma, J. E. (1988). Forensic neuropathology. Raven Press, New York.

Leestma, J. E., and Koenig, K. L. (1968). Sudden death and phenothiazines: A current controversy. *Arch. Gen. Psychiatr. 18*:137-148.

Leestma, J. E., Kalelkar, M. B., Teas, S. S., Jay, G. W., and Hughes, J. R. (1984). Sudden unexpected death associated with seizures: Analysis of 66 cases. *Epilepsia 25*:84-88.

Levitt, B., Cagin, N. A., Somberg, J. C., et al. (1976). Neural basis for the genesis and control of digitalis arrhythmias. *Cardiology 61*:50-60.

Leyberg, J. T., and Denmark, J. C. (1959). The treatment of depressive states with imipramine hydrochloride (Tofranil). *J. Ment. Sci. 105*:1123-1126.

Liberatore, M. A., and Robinson, D. S. (1984). Torsade de pointe: A mechanism for sudden death associated with neuroleptic drug therapy? *J. Clin. Psychopharmacol. 4*:143-146.

Lipka, L. J., and Lathers, C. M. (1985). Cardiovascular effects of intracerebroventricular administration of chlorpromazine in the cat. *J. Clin. Pharmacol. 25*:462 (abstract).

Lipka, L. J., and Lathers, C. M. (1987). Psychoactive agents, seizure production, and sudden death in epilepsy. *J. Clin. Pharmacol. 27*:169–183.

Lipscomb, P. A. (1980). Cardiovascular side effects of phenothiazines and tricyclic antidepressants. A review with precautionary measures. *Postgrad. Med. 67*:189–196.

Logothetis, J. (1967). Spontaneous epileptic seizures and electroencephalographic changes in the course of phenothiazine therapy. *Neurology 17*:869–877.

Lomas, J., Boardman, R. H., and Marlowe, M. (1955). Complications of chlorpromazine therapy in 800 mental-hospital patients. *Lancet 1*:1144–1147.

Lowry, M. R., and Dunner, F. J. (1980). Seizures during tricyclic therapy. *Am. J. Psychiatr. 137*:1461–1462.

Luchins, D. J., Oliver, A. P., and Wyatt, R. J. (1984). Seizures with antidepressants: An in vitro technique to assess relative risk. *Epilepsia 25*:25–32.

Magnus, R. V. (1975). A placebo controlled trial of viloxazine with and without tranquilizers in depressive illness. *J. Intern. Med. Res. 3*:207–213.

Malliani, A., Schwartz, P. J., and Zanchetti, A. (1980). Neural mechanisms in life-threatening arrhythmias. *Am. Heart. J. 100*:705–715.

Mallion, K. B., Todd, A. H., Turner, R. W., et al. (1972). 2-(2-Ethoxyphenoxymethyl) tetrahydro-1,4-oxazine hydrochloride, a potential psychotropic agent. *Nature 238*:157–158.

Meldrum, B., Anlezark, G., and Trimble, M. (1975). Drugs modifying dopaminergic activity and behavior, the EEG and epilepsy in *Papio papio. Eur. J. Pharmacol. 32*:203–213.

Meldrum, B. S., Anlezark, G. M., Adam, H. K., et al. (1982). Anticonvulsant and proconvulsant properties of viloxazine hydrochloride: Pharmacological and pharmacokinetic studies in rodents and the epileptic baboon. *Psychopharmacology 76*:212–217.

Melville, K. L. (1958). Studies on the cardiovascular action of chlorpromazine. I. Antiadrenergic and antifibrillatory actions. *Arch. Int. Pharmacodyn. Ther. 115*:278.

Miller, A. A., and Wheatley, P. L. (1978). Effects of some newer antidepressants on the EEG of the conscious rat. *Abstracts of the International Congress of Pharmacology, Paris*, p. 346.

Moore, M. T., and Book, M. H. (1970). Sudden death in phenothiazine therapy. A clinicopathologic study of 12 cases. *Psychiatr. Q. 44*:389–402.

Morrell, F., and Baker, L. (1961). Effects of drugs on secondary epileptogenic lesions. *Neurology 11*:651–664.

Nadeau, R., and DeChamplain, J. (1973). Comparative effects of 6-hydroxydopamine and reserpine on ouabain toxicity in the rat. *Life Sci.* 1753–1761.

Nasrallah, H. A. (1978). Factors influencing phenothiazine-induced ECG changes. *Am. J. Psychiatr. 135*:118–119.

Nattel, S., and Mitterman, M. (1984). Treatment of ventricular tachyarrhythmias resulting from amitriptyline toxicity in dogs. *J. Pharmacol. Exp. Ther. 231*:430–435.

Nattel, S., Keable, H., and Sasynuik, B. I. (1984). Experimental amitriptyline intoxication: Electrophysiologic manifestations and management. *J. Cardiovasc. Pharmacol. 6*:83–89.

Neal, H., and Bradley, P. B. (1978). Electrophysiological studies with a new antidepressant drug: Comparison of the effects of viloxazine HCl (ICI 58,834) with three tricyclic antidepressants in the encephale isole. *Neuropharmacology 17*:835–849.

Neal, H., and Bradley, P. B. (1979). Electrocortical changes in the encephale isole cat following chronic treatment with antidepressant drugs. *Neuropharmacology 18*:611–615.

Ojemann, L. M., Friel, P. N., Trejo, W. J., et al. (1983). Effect of doxepin on seizure frequency in depressed epileptic patients. *Neurology 33*:646–648.

Oliver, A. P., Luchins, D. J., and Wyatt, R. J. (1982). Neuroleptic-induced seizures. *Arch. Gen. Psycyiatr. 39*:206–209.

Pace, D. G., Quest, J. A., and Gillis, R. A. (1974). The effect of the vagus nerve on the bradycardia and ventricular arrhythmias induced by digitoxin and digoxin. *Eur. J. Pharmacol. 28*:288–293.

Parker, J., and Laymeyer, H. (1984). Maprotiline poisoning: A case of cardiotoxicity and myoclonic seizures. *J. Clin. Psychiatr. 45*:312–314.

Pearl, D. S., Quest, J. A., and Gillis, R. A. (1978). Effect of diazepam on digitalis-induced ventricular arrhythmias in the cat. *Toxicol. Appl. Pharmacol. 44*:643–652.

Peck, A. W., Stern, W. C., and Watkinson, C. (1983). Incidence of seizures during treatment with tricyclic antidepressant drugs and bupropion. *J. Clin. Psychiatr. (Sec. 2) 44*:197–210.

Peele, R., and von Loetzen, I. S. (1973). Phenothiazine deaths: A critical review. *Am. J. Psychiatr. 130*:306–309.

Perucca, E., and Richens, A. (1977). Interaction between phenytoin and imipramine. *Br. J. Clin. Pharmacol. 4*:485–486.

Petti, T. A., and Campbell, M. (1975). Imipramine and seizures. *Am. J. Psychiatr. 132*:538–540.

Pichot, P., Guelfi, J., and Dreyfus, J. F. (1975). A controlled multicentre therapeutic trial of viloxazine (Vivalan). *J. Intern. Med. Res. (Suppl. 3) 3*:80–86.

Pineda, M. R., and Russell, S. C. (1974). The use of tricyclic antidepressant in epilepsy. *Dis. Nerv. Syst. 35*:322–323.

Plachta, A. (1965). Asphyxia relatively inherent to tranquilization: Review of the literature and report of seven cases. *Arch. Gen. Psychiatr. 12*:152–158.

Popkin, M. K., Hall, R. C. W., and Gradner, E. R. (1982). Clinical use of antipsychotics in the elderly: Considerations for optimal technique. In *Geriatric Psychopharmacology: Optimal Technique*, A. J. Levenson (Ed.). Springfield, Ill., Thomas, pp. 39–58.

Pulst, S. M., and Lombroso, C. T. (1983). External ophthalmoplegia, alpha and spindle coma in imipramine overdose. Case report and review of the literature. *Ann. Neurol. 14*:587–590.

Rabkin, J. G. (1980). Stressful life events and schizophrenia. A review of the research literature. *Psychol. Bull. 87*:408–425.

Raisfeld, I. H. (1972). Cardiovascular complications of antidepressant therapy: Interactions at the adrenergic neuron. *Am. Heart. J. 83*:129–133.

Reid, W., and Harrower, A. D. B. (1984). Cardiac arrest after apparent recovery from an overdose of chlorpromazine. *Br. Med. J. 228*:1880.

Reinert, R. E., and Hermann, C. G. (1960). Unexplained deaths during chlorpromazine therapy. *J. Nerv. Ment. Dis. 131*:435–442.

Remick, P. A., and Fine, S. H. (1979). Antipsychotic drugs and seizures. *J. Clin. Psychiatr. 40*:78–80.

Reynolds, A. K., and Horne, M. L. (1969). Studies on the cardiotoxicity of ouabain. *Can. J. Phys. Pharm. 47*:165.

Richardson, H. L., Graupner, K. I., and Richardson, M. E. (1966). Intramyocardial lesions in patients dying suddenly and unexpectedly. *J. Am. Med. Assoc. 195*:254–260.

Richens, A., Nawishy, S., and Trimble, M. (1983). Antidepressant drugs, convulsions and epilepsy. *Br. J. Clin. Pharmacol. 15 (Suppl.)*: 295–298.

Roberts, J., and Kelliher, G. J. (1973). Adrenergic innervation of the heart as a site for the genesis and control of arrhythmia. Recent advances in studies on cardiac structure and metabolism. In *Myocardial Metabolism*, N. S. Dhalla (Eds.). University Park Press, Baltimore, pp. 357–366.

Roberts, J., Kelliher, G. J., and Lathers, C. M. (1976). Role of adrenergic influences in digitalis-induced ventricular arrhythmia. *Life Sci. 18*:665–678.

Robertson, M. M., and Trimble, M. R. (1983). Depressive illness in patients with epilepsy: A review. *Epilepsia (Suppl. 2) 24*:S109–S116.

Rudorfer, M. V., and Young, R. C. (1980). Desipramine: Cardiovascular effects and plasma levels. *Am. J. Psychiatr. 137*:984–986.

Schallek, W., and Zabransky, F. (1966). Effects of psychotropic drugs on pressor responses to central and peripheral stimulation in cat. *Arch. Int. Pharmacodyn. Ther. 161*:126–131.

Schwartz, P. J., Brown, A. M., Malliani, A., and Zanchettia, A. (Eds.) (1978). *Neural Mechanisms in Cardiac Arrhythmias*, Vol. 2. Raven Press, New York.

Sedgwick, E. M., and Edwards, J. G. (1983). Mianserin, maprotiline and the electroencephalogram. *Br. J. Clin. Pharmacol. 15 (Suppl)*:255–259.

Shamsi, M. A., Kulshrestha, V. K., Dhawan, K. N., et al. (1971). Correlation of chemical structure of phenothiazines with their coronary dilator and antiarrhythmic activities. *Jpn. J. Pharmacol. 21*:747.

Sherif, M. A. F., Chata, M. K., and Madkour, M. K. (1958). Action of chlorpromazine on autonomic ganglia. *Arch. Int. Pharmacodyn. Ther. 115*:269–277.

Sigg, E. B. (1959). Pharmacological studies with Tofranil. *Can. Psychiatr. Assoc. J. 4*:S75–S85.

Sigg, E. B., and Sigg, T. D. (1969). Hypothalamic stimulation of preganglionic autonomic activity and its modification by chlorpromazine, diazepam, and pentobarbital. *Int. J. Neuropharmacol. 8*:567–572.

Sigg, E. B., Keim, K. L., and Kepner, K. (1971). Selective effect of diazepam on certain central sympathetic components. *Neuropharmacology 10*:621–629.

Simons, A. J. R. (1958). EEG-activation by means of chlorpromazine. *Electro-encephalogr. Clin. Neurophysiol. 10*:356–357.

Simpson, G. M., Jefferson, J. W., Perez-Cruet, J., and Davis, J. (1989). Sudden death in psychiatric patients: Role of neuroleptic drugs, *APA Task Force on Sudden Death*. American Psychiatric Press, Washington, D.C. In press.

Simpson, G. M., Pi, E. H., and Sramek, J. J. (1981). Adverse effects of antipsy-chotic agents. *Drugs 21*:138–151.

Singh, K., and Sharma, V. N. (1970). Clinical construction and drug action of *N*-substituted phenothiazines in ventricular ectopic tachycardia. *Jpn. J. Pharmacol. 20*:173.

Snyder, S. H., Banerjee, S. P., Yamamura, H. I., et al. (1974). Drugs, neurotrans-mitters, and schizophrenia. *Science 184*:1243–1253.

Solomon, K. (1977). Phenothiazine-induced bulbar palsy-like syndrome and sud-den death. *Am. J. Psychiatr. 134*:308–311.

Somberg, J. C., Butler, B., Rorres, V., et al. (1984). Antiarrhythmic action of bethanidine. *Am. J. Cardiol. 54*:343–346.

Spiss, C. K., Smith, C. M., and Maze, M. (1984). Halothane-epinephrine arrhyth-mias and adrenergic responsiveness after chronic imipramine administration in dogs. *Anesth. Analog. 63*:825–828.

Starkey, I. R., and Lawson, A. A. H. (1980). Poisoning with tricyclic and related antidepressants—A ten year review. *Q. J. Med. 49*:33–49.

Steel, C. M., O'Duffy, J., and Brown, S. S. (1967). Clinical effects and treatment of imipramine and amitryptiline poisoning in children. *Br. Med. J. 3*:663–667.

Steiner, W. G., and Himwich, H. E. (1963). Effects of antidepressant drugs on limbic structures of rabbit. *J. Nerv. Ment. Dis. 137*:277–284.

Stewart, L. F. (1957). Chlorpromazine: Use to activate electroencephalographic seizure patterns. *Electroencephalogr. Clin. Neurophysiol. 9*:427–440.

Stille, G., and Sayers, A. (1964). The effect of antidepressant drugs on the con-vulsive excitability of brain structures. *Int. J. Neuropharmacol. 3*:605–609.

Surawicz, B., and Knoebel, S. B. (1984). Good, bad or indifferent? *J. Am. Coll. Cardiol. 4*:398–411.

Surawicz, B., and Lasseter, K. C. (1970). Effect of drugs on the electrocardio-gram. *Prog. Cardiovasc. Dis. 13*:26–54.

Swain, J. M., and Litteral, E. B. (1960). Prolonged effect of chlorpromazine: EEG findings in a senile group. *J. Nerv. Ment. Dis. 131*:550–553.

Swett, C. (1975). Cardiac side effects and sudden death among psychiatric in-patients. *Psychopharm. Bull. 11*:16–17.

Swett, G. P., and Shader, R. I. (1977). Cardiac side effects and sudden death in hospitalized psychiatric patients. *Dis. Nerv. Syst. 38*:69.

Szekeres, L., and Papp, J. G. (1971). *Experimental Cardiac Arrhythmia and Anti-Arrhythmic Drugs*. Akademiai Kaido, Budapest.

Tang, W. W., and Seeman, P. (1980). Effect of antidepressant drugs on seroton-ergic and adrenergic receptors. *Naunyn Schmiedebergs Arch. Pharmacol. 311*:255–261.

Tangri, K. K., and Bhargava, K. P. (1960). The central hypotensive action of 1-hydrazinophthalazine (C-5968). *Arch. Int. Pharmacodyn. Ther. 125*:331–342.

Tedeschi, D. H., Benigni, J. P., Elder, C. J., et al. (1958). Effects of various phenothiazines on minimal electroshock seizure threshold and spontaneous motor activity of mice. *J. Pharmacol. Exp. Ther. 123*:35-38.

Terrence, D. F., Jr., Wisotskey, H. M., and Perper, J. A. (1975). Unexpected, unexplained death in epileptic patients. *Neurology 25*:594-598.

Thompson, T. L., Moran, M. G., and Niles, A. S. (1983a). Psychotropic drug use in the elderly. I. *New Engl. J. Med. 308*:134-138.

Thompson, T. L., Moran, M. G., and Niles, A. S. (1983b). Psychotropic drug use in the elderly. II. *New Engl. J. Med. 308*:194-199.

Toone, B. K. and Fenton, G. W. (1977). Epileptic seizures induced by psychotropic drugs. *Psychol. Med. 7*:265-270.

Tri, T. B., and Combs, D. T. (1975). Phenothiazine induced ventricular tachycardia. *West. J. Med. 123*:412-416.

Trimble, M. (1977). The relationship between epilepsy and schizophrenia: A biochemical hypothesis. *Biol. Psychiatry 12*:299-304.

Trimble, M. R. (1978). Non-monoamine oxidase inhibitor antidepressants and epilepsy: A review. *Epilepsia 19*:241-250.

Trimble, M. R. (1980). New antidepressant drugs and the seizure threshold. *Neuropharmacology 19*:1227-1228.

Trimble, M. R. (1984). Epilepsy, antidepressants, and the role of nomifensine. *J. Clin. Psychiatr. (Sec. 2) 45*:39-42.

Trimble, M., Anlezark, G., and Meldrum, B. (1977). Seizure activity in photosensitive baboons following antidepressant drugs and the role of serotonergic mechanisms. *Psychopharmacology 51*:159-164.

Turbott, J., and Cairns, F. J. (1984). Sudden death and neuroleptic medication. *Am. J. Psychiatr. 141*:919-920.

Tyrer, P., Steinberg, B., and Watson, B. (1979). Possible epileptogenic effect of mianserin. *Lancet 2*:798-799.

Ungvari, G. (1980). Neuroleptic related sudden death: Proven or a mere hypothesis. *Pharmakopsychiatry 13*:29.

Van Meter, W. G., Owens, H. F., and Himwich, H. E. (1959). Effects of Tofranil, an antidepressant drug on electrical potentials of rabbit brain. *Can. Psychiatr. Assoc. J. 4*:S113-S119.

Van Sweden, B. (1984). Neuroleptic neurotoxicity: Electroclinical aspects. *Acta Neurol. Scand. 69*:137-146.

Vernier, V. G. (1961). The pharmacology of antidepressant agents. *Dis. Nerv. Syst. 22*:7-13.

von Brauchitsch, H., and May, W. (1968). Deaths from aspiration and asphyxiation in a mental hospital. *Arch. Gen. Psychiatr. 18*:129-136.

Wada, J. A., Balzamo, E., Meldrum, B. S., et al. (1972). Behavioral and electrographic effects of *L*-5-hydroxytryptophan and *D, L*-parachlorophenylalanine on epileptic senegalese baboon (*Papio papio*). *Electroencephalogr. Clin. Neurophysiol. 33*:520-526.

Wakasugi, C., Nishi, K., and Yamada, M. (1986). Sudden death in a patient taking neuroleptics. *Am. J. Forensic Med. Pathol. 7*:165-166.

Wallach, M. B., Winters, W. D., Mandell, J., et al. (1969). A correlation of EEG, reticular multiple unit activity and gross behavior following various antidepressant agents in the cat. IV. *Electroencephalogr. Clin. Neurophysiol. 27*: 563–573.

Wang, H. H., Kanai, T., Markee, S., et al. (1964). Effects of reserpine and chlorpromazine on the vasomotor center in the medulla oblongata of the dog. *J. Pharmacol. Exp. Ther. 144*:186–195.

Wardell, D. W. (1957). Untoward reactions to tranquilizing drugs. *Am. J. Psychiatr. 113*:745.

Warnes, H., and Ananth, J. V. (1971). Complications of psychotropic medications in high dosage. *Psychiatr. Q. 45*:87–91.

Weil-Malherbe, H. (1965). The biphasic effect of phenothiazines on the release of adrenaline from adrenomedullary granules and its dependence on pH. In *Pharmacology of Cholinergic and Adrenergic Transmission*, G. B. Koelle, W. W. Douglas, A. Carlssan, and Z. Trcka (Eds.). Macmillan, New York, pp. 235–239.

Weinberg, S. J., and Haley, T. J. (1956). Effect of chlorpromazine on cardiac arrhythmias induced by intracerebral injection of tryptamine-strophanthidin. *Arch. Int. Pharmacodyn. Ther. 105*:209–220.

Wendkos, M. H. (1979). Psychotropic agents. In *Sudden Death and Psychiatric Illness*, Vol. 15, SP Medical & Scientific Books, New York, pp. 281–316.

Wendkos, M. H., and Clay, R. W. (1965). Unusual hospitalized schizophrenic patients. *J. Am. Geriatr. Soc. 13*:622–671.

Westheimer, R., and Klawans, H. L. (1974). The role of serotonin in the pathophysiology of myoclonic seizures associated with acute imipramine toxicity. *Neurology 24*:1175–1177.

Wilensky, A. J., Leal, L. W., Dudley, D. L., et al. (1981). Characteristics of psychotropic drug use in the epilepsy center population. *Epilepsia 22*:247 (abstract).

Wilkerson, R. D. (1978). Antiarrhythmic effects of tricyclic antidepressant drugs in ouabain-induced arrhythmias in the dog. *J. Pharmacol. Exp. Ther. 206*: 666–674.

Williams, R. B., Jr., and Sherter, C. (1971). Cardiac complications of tricyclic antidepressant therapy. *Ann. Intern. Med. 74*:395–398.

Yang, C. P. and Guillan, R. A. (1979). Sudden death syndrome. Reports of 16 pages on high doses of phenothiazine. *J. Kan. Med. Soc. 80*:547–563.

Zielinski, J. J. (1974). Epilepsy and mortality rate and cause of death. *Epilepsia 15*:191–201.

Zisook, S., and Finkel, S. I. (1982). Tricyclic antidepressant medication in later life. In *Geriatric Psychopharmacology*, A. J. Levenson (Ed.). Thomas, Springfield, Ill., pp. 86–97.

Zugibe, F. T. (1980). Sudden death related to the use of psychotropic drugs. *Legal Med.*:75–90.

24

Antiepileptic Activity of Beta-Blocking Agents

CLAIRE M. LATHERS*, KAM F. JIM†, and WILLIAM H. SPIVEY *The Medical College of Pennsylvania, Eastern Pennsylvania Psychiatric Institute, Philadelphia, Pennsylvania*

CLAIRE KAHN,‡ KATHLEEN DOLCE,‡ and WILLIAM D. MATTHEWS‡ *Smith Kline & French Laboratories, Upper Merion (Kahn), King of Prussia (Dolce), and Swedeland (Matthews), Pennsylvania*

I. INTRODUCTION

The etiology of unexplained sudden death in epilepsy is unknown but autonomic dysfunction is a frequently presented hypothesis (Hirsch and Martin, 1971; Leestma et al., 1984). Autonomic neural dysfunction contributes to the development of cardiac arrhythmias (Gillis, 1969; Lathers et al., 1977, 1978; Randall et al., 1978) and sudden death (Lown and Verrier, 1978). Stimulation of the sympathetic ventrolateral cardiac nerve produces tachyarrhythmias (Randall et al., 1978). Sympathetic neural imbalance, or "neural nonuniformity," is defined to exist when neural activity is recorded simultaneously from two or three postganglionic cardiac sympathetic nerves in the same cat and increases and/or decreases in activity develop (Lathers et al., 1977, 1978). The neural discharge is associated with arrhythmias; it is hypothesized that the nonuniform neural discharge induced nonuniform changes in excitability and conduction in the heart, producing arrhythmia, as reported by Han and Moe (1964).

Autonomic sympathetic and parasympathetic cardiac neural dysfunction and cardiovascular abnormalities, e.g., changes in blood pressure, heart rate, and rhythm, as well as alterations in cardiac depolarization and repolarization, are associated with interictal and ictal spike activity induced by pentylenetetrazol (PTZ) (Carnel et al., 1985; Lathers and Schraeder, 1982; Lathers et al., 1984,

Current affiliation:
*FDA, Rockville, Maryland
†Wyeth-Ayerst Research, Philadelphia, Pennsylvania.
‡Smithkline Beecham Pharmaceuticals, Swedeland, Pennsylvania.

1985; Schraeder and Lathers, 1983). The major action of PTZ is thought to be
mediated via the central nervous system and not by direct stimulation of the
peripheral systems (Toman and Davis, 1949). Furthermore, Gremels (1931) and
Hildebrandt (1937), quoted by Hahn (1960), concluded that PTZ did not exert
a positive inotropic action on the heart. Thus the cardiovascular changes observed using the PTZ model of epilepsy in our study appear to be due to autonomic dysfunction associated with epileptiform activity rather than to a direct action of PTZ on the heart and peripheral vascular system. To exclude the possibility that the autonomic dysfunction observed with the epileptiform activity in
our previous studies was due to the peripheral effects of PTZ, we examined the
action of intracerebroventricularly (i.c.v.) administered PTZ to induce epileptiform activity and autonomic dysfunction. It was hypothesized that if the autonomic dysfunction, including the development of arrhythmias, also occurred in
humans, it might contribute to sudden unexplained death of epileptic patients.

    This study examined whether the beta-blocking agent timolol, given centrally
and then peripherally, would eliminate the cardiac arrhythmias, epileptiform activity, and changes in the blood pressure and heart rate induced by PTZ intracerebroventricularly administered to anesthetized cats. To further examine the
potential anticonvulsant action of beta-blocking agents in a different animal
model, the action of propranolol on epileptogenic activity induced by intravenously (i.v.) administered PTZ in anesthetized pigs was studied.

II. METHOD

A. Seizure Studies in Anesthetized Cats

Twenty-four cats of either sex, weighing from 2.5 to 3.4 kg, were used. Animals
were anesthetized with alpha-chloralose (80 mg/kg i.v.) and cannulated as described by Lathers and Schraeder (1982). Cats were positioned in a stereotaxic
apparatus. Coordinates A+0.5, HD+8.5, and RL+4 (Snider and Niemer, 1970),
were used to locate the cannula through a burr hole at a 90° angle. Pentylenetetrazol (10 or 20 mg) was dissolved in 50 μl saline and injected by using a 26G
spinal needle placed into the left lateral ventricle. The electrocorticogram
(ECoG) was monitored using silver ball electrodes placed on the surface of the
sigmoid gyri unilaterally after a bifrontal craniectomy and dural resection. A
recording electrode was inserted into the right hippocampus (A+7; HD-6.0 and
RL+11.8) using a concentric bipolar electrode.

    Four experimental groups of cats were examined. In the first, only 10 mg
i.c.v PTZ was administered (N = 8 cats). In the second, PTZ 10 and/or 20 mg
i.c.v. was administered and followed by timolol 10, 100, 500 μg/kg i.c.v. and 1,
5, 10, and/or 20 mg/kg i.v. (N = 6 cats). Doses were given at 5-minute intervals.
In the third group, the pharmacological agent (D-Ala[5]) methionine-enkephalin-
amide or prostaglandin E_2 was administered i.c.v. prior to the administration of
PTZ and timolol (N = 7). In the fourth group (N = 3 cats), the same doses of

timolol were administered at different time intervals, i.e., one cat received timolol every 10 minutes and a second cat received timolol every 15 minutes after
the administration of PTZ. In the third cat, timolol doses were given every 15
minutes but no PTZ was administered.

A one-factor repeated-measures analysis of variance (ANOVA) was performed
to determine whether changes in the mean arterial blood pressure and heart rate
after the i.c.v. injection of PTZ ($N = 8$ cats) were significantly different from the
control.

To verify that it would be appropriate to combine the data obtained in the
experimental cats receiving other pharmacological agents prior to the administration of PTZ and timolol with those cats receiving only PTZ and timolol, a two-
factor ANOVA with repeated measures on time and nonrepeated measures on
group was used to analyze the effects of time course, group membership, and the
interaction of these two variables on blood pressure and heart rate, separately.
The time course reflects the effect over time of PTZ and timolol on blood pressure or heart rate.

To determine whether the PTZ–timolol actions on heart rate and blood pressure varied from the actions of only PTZ, a two-way ANOVA was done in which
the independent variables were the presence or absence of timolol and the time
course. Simple effect tests and Tukey-HSD (Honestly Significantly Different)
post-hoc tests were used where appropriate.

For the 13 cats receiving PTZ and timolol, the ECoG data for the left and
right cortex and for the hippocampus were analyzed separately by dividing the
number of episodes of epileptiform activity into categories of $\leq$ 10-second and
$>$ 10-second duration. For each cat, the mean numbers of episodes for the two
durations were calculated for the control and for each dose of PTZ and timolol.
Means were calculated by combining the ECoG data from all cats. To determine
if there were any statistically significant differences among the means, data were
analyzed by a Friedman rank analysis of variance followed by a Bonferroni-
corrected Wilcoxon post-hoc tests. The following time points were analyzed:
control; PTZ 10 mg and 20 mg; and timilol 10 μg, 100 μg, 500 μg, and 1 mg/kg.

B. Seizure Studies in Anesthetized Pigs

Domestic swine weighing 13–20 kg were anesthetized with ketamine (20 mg/kg
i.v.) and alpha-chloralose (80 mg/kg i.v.). Animals were prepared as described by
Spivey et al. (1987). After a 10-minute equilibration period, seizure activity was
induced by PTZ (100 mg/kg i.v.). Sixty seconds following the onset of epileptogenic activity, the animals were treated with no drug (control group) or propranolol 2.5 mg/kg i.v. Seizure activity was monitored for 20 minutes.

Plasma levels of propranolol were determined by withdrawing blood samples
(8 ml) at 1, 2, 5, 10, 15, and 20 minutes after propranolol. The samples were
centrifuged at 1000 g for 5 minutes and the plasma (3 ml) was stored frozen at
–20 degrees centigrade. The concentrations of propranolol in plasma were deter-

mined by a modification of the method of Albani et al. (1982). The procedure involves reverse-phase high-pressure liquid chromatographic (HPLC) resolution with fluorometric detection of propranolol and an internal standard, carvedilol 1-(4-carbazolyloxy)-3-[2-(2-methoxyphenoxy)ethylamino]-2-propranol.

III. RESULTS

A. Data Obtained in Anesthetized Cats

A one-factor repeated-measures ANOVA revealed that the increase in the control blood pressure of 103 ± 13 mm Hg to 149 ± 13 mm Hg 3 minutes after PTZ i.c.v. was significant, whereas the mean heart rate increase from 159 ± 17 to 162 ± 10 bpm 3 minutes after PTZ and to 175 ± 14 bpm 15 minutes after PTZ was not significant. The PTZ-induced increase in blood pressure and heart rate preceded the initiation of epileptiform activity in the majority of these cats (Table 1). This trend was also observed in the 13 cats receiving PTZ and then timolol (Table 2). During the occurrence of PTZ-induced epileptiform activity, premature ventricular contractions with a duration of three to eight minutes were observed in three of the eight cats.

Data obtained from one cat are illustrated in Figure 1. In panel A (control) the cerebral activity present was that associated with the induction of anesthesia. With the i.c.v. administration of 10 mg PTZ (panel B), there was induction of epileptiform activity, a slight increase in blood pressure, and a slight decrease in

Table 1 Sequence in Which Incidence of the Epileptiform Activity and an Increase in Mean Arterial Blood Pressure and Heart Rate Occurred after I.C.V. Pentylenetetrazol[a]

Preceded[b]	Same time	Proceeded[c]	No change
BP[d] 5	0	2	0
HR[d] 5	0	1	1
BP[e] 11	1	1	0
HR[e] 12	0	1	0

[a]Incidence indicates the number of cats of the 13 studied.
[b]Preceded indicates that the increase in blood pressure or heart rate occurred before the onset of epileptiform activity elicited by PTZ.
[c]Proceeded indicates that the increase in blood pressure or heart rate occurred after the onset of epileptiform activity elicited by PTZ.
[d]Seven cats receiving only PTZ; the ECoG activity was not recorded in the eighth cat.
[e]Thirteen cats receiving PTZ and timolol.

Table 2 Incidence of the Sequence in Which Suppression of I.C.V. Pentylenetetrazol-Induced Epileptiform Activity and a Decrease in Mean Arterial Blood Pressure and Heart Rate Occurred After Timolol[a]

	Partial suppression compared to control			Total suppression compared to control				Total suppression compared to mean of previous 5-minute interval			
	Preceded[b]	Same	Proceeded[c]	Preceded	Same	Proceeded	No change	Preceded	Same	Proceeded	No change
BP	1	0	12	11	0	1	1	7	0	4	2
HR	0	0	13	12	0	0	1	2	1	6d	5d

[a]Incidence indicates the number of cats of the 13 studied.
[b]Preceded indicates that the decrease in blood pressure or heart rate occurred before the partial or total suppression of epileptiform activity.
[c]Proceeded indicates that the decrease in blood pressure or heart rate occurred after the partial or total suppression of epileptiform activity.
[d]Includes same cat, hippocampus no change; both left and right cortex proceeded total suppression of epileptogenic activity.

489

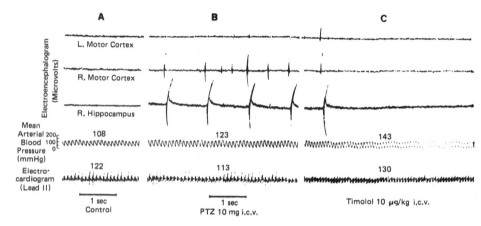

Figure 1 Effect of timolol on the electrocorticogram and cardiovascular parameters associated with i.c.v. pentylenetetrazol-induced epileptiform activity in one
cat. Represented in all three panels are electrocorticograms from the left and
right motor cortex and right hippocampus, as well as mean arterial blood pressure, and electrocardiogram from top to bottom, respectively. Reproduced with
permission from Lathers et al., *Epilepsy Res. 4*:42–54, 1989.

heart rate. When timolol (10 μg/kg i.c.v.) was administered (panel C), the epileptiform activity was diminished, although the blood pressure and heart rate
values were still elevated above control.

The i.c.v. administration of PTZ increased both the mean arterial blood pressure and the heart rate in six cats receiving only PTZ and timolol; no other pharmacological agents were administered (data not shown). When timolol was given
to the six cats after the administration of PTZ, the mean arterial blood pressure
and heart rate values began to decrease. Similar data were obtained when PTZ
and timolol were administered to cats that had previously received other agents
(N = 7 cats). In the cats receiving other pharmacological agents prior to the administration of PTZ, the blood pressure, heart rate, and ECoG activity had returned to baseline values prior to the administration to PTZ. No significant effect of previous drugs or interaction between previous drug and time was found.
The lack of a significant effect indicated that the two groups of animals responded the same ways to the drug injections over time and permitted combination of the two groups for purposes of analysis (N = 13 cats; Figure 2). Thus the
administration of PTZ increased both mean arterial blood pressure and heart
rate. When timolol was given intracerebroventricularly, the mean arterial blood
pressure and heart rate values began to decrease. In the two-way ANOVA, both
main effects and the interaction were significant for the heart rate. A comparison of the two experimental groups (PTZ i.c.v. and PTZ–timolol, N = 13 cats)

at each experimental time showed that the timolol group was lower in the control period, sharply rising to a nonsignificant difference after the second dose of PTZ and after the first and second doses of timolol. At higher doses of timolol, the timolol group was consistently significantly lower in heart rate than the group receiving only PTZ. Experimental times within groups, done as separate one-way repeated-measures ANOVAs, due to the different variances, showed no significant difference across time in the heart rate for the cats receiving no timolol and a sharp rise followed by a fall (Tukey–HSD) in the cats receiving PTZ and increasing doses of timolol.

The two-way ANOVA revealed that the group main effects on blood pressure were not significant. The time effect and the interactions were significant. When the experimental groups were compared at each experimental time, no differences were found until the two highest doses of timolol. The data in the control group were steady at the time equivalent to that when timolol would have been administered to the animals in the experimental group, while the timolol group exhibited a rapid fall in blood pressure. Consequently, the latter group was significantly lower. Experimental times within each group showed no significant effect of time course on blood pressure in those cats receiving only PTZ, while in the cats receiving both PTZ and timolol, the PTZ increased the blood pressure and timolol reversed the effect of PTZ.

In the two cats receiving the same doses of timolol at time intervals other than 5 minutes (i.e., 10 or 15 minutes), timolol suppressed the epileptogenic discharges and decreased the blood pressure and heart rate. In the one cat in which all doses of timolol were given every 15 minutes but no epileptogenic activity occurred since PTZ was not given, both the heart rate and blood pressure values were decreased, but the magnitude of the decrease was much less than that observed in the cats dosed with PTZ.

Although PTZ induced both interictal and ictal epileptiform discharges in all cats, most epileptiform activity exhibited durations of ≤ 10 seconds, i.e., interictal and brief ictal activity (Table 3 and Figure 3). The dashed curve in Figure 3 depicts the epileptiform activity with a duration of ≤ 10 seconds obtained in the left cortex of the cats receiving only PTZ and no timolol. The mean number of episodes of epileptiform activity remained approximately the same for the 45-minute period, the time equivalent to the entire experimental duration in the cats receiving both PTZ and increasing doses of timolol. The mean number of episodes of epileptiform activity lasting ≤ 10 seconds for the other three brain areas depicted in Figure 3 decreased with increasing doses of timolol. Timolol produced this decrease even though most cats in this group received two doses of PTZ, i.e., 10 and 20 mg.

In all 13 cats receiving timolol after PTZ, the timolol partially suppressed the epileptiform activity evident in the left and right cortices and in the hippocampus

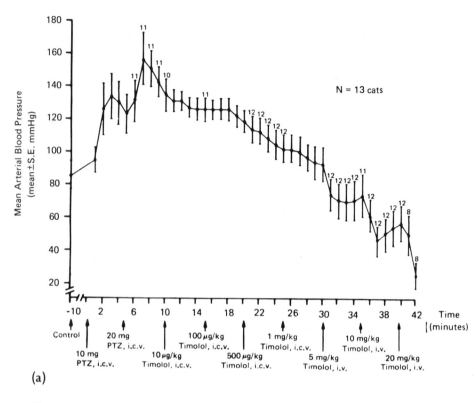

(a)

Figure 2   The effect of timolol on mean arterial blood pressure and heart rate changes induced by pentylenetetrazol-administered intracerebroventricularly in 13 cats. In the upper graph the mean arterial blood pressure is graphed as a func-

after the first dose of 10 μg. The mean times to partial suppression for the left and right cortices and for the hippocampus were 36 ± 11, 33 ± 11, and 50 ± 15 seconds, respectively, after 10 μg timolol. In 12 of the 13 cats, the time to partial suppression was the same for all three brain areas. In one cat, epileptiform activity was suppressed 27 seconds earlier in the left and right cortices when compared to the hippocampus. Higher doses of timolol, ranging from 1 to 20 mg, were required to induce a total suppression of the epileptiform activity. Table 4 indicates the number of cats in which a given dose of timolol induced total suppression of epileptiform activity. Using the time of administration of the first dose of timolol 10 μg as zero, the mean times to total suppression of epileptiform activity in the left and right cortices and the hippocampus were 26 ± 2, 26 ± 2, and 27 ± 2 min, respectively. In six cats, the time to total sup-

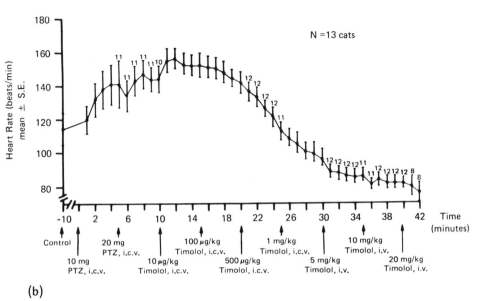

(b)

Figure 2 (continued)   tion of time. The lower graph depicts the mean heart rate. The arrows along the abscissa indicate the administration of PTZ i.c.v. and timolol i.c.v. or i.v. Reproduced with permission from Lathers et al., *Epilepsy Res. 4*:42–54, 1989.

Table 3   Mean Duration of Episodes of Epileptogenic Activity Lasting > 10 Seconds (seconds/minute; mean ± S.E.)

Experimental groups	Left cortex	Right cortex	Right hippocampus
Control[a]	0	0	0
PTZ, 10 mg i.c.v.	0	0	1.21 ± 1.21[b]
PTZ, 20 mg i.c.v.	0.31 ± 0.31[b]	0.54 ± 0.54[b]	1.00 ± 0.65
Timolol, 10 μg/kg i.c.v.	0.50 ± 0.50[b]	0.45 ± 0.45[b]	5.51 ± 4.63
Timolol, 100 μg/kg i.c.v.	0	0	4.22 ± 4.22[b]
Timolol, 500 μg/kg i.c.v.	0	0	0
Timolol, 1 mg/kg i.c.v.	0	0	4.62 ± 4.62[b]
Timolol, 5 mg/kg i.v.	0	0	0.89 ± 0.89[b]
Timolol, 10 mg/kg i.v.	0	0	0

[a]Defined as the mean ± S.E. for the 13 cats in which a mean 10-minute control period was obtained.
[b]Mean ± S.E. was calculated by averaging 12 zeros and 1 number, resulting in an S.E. value that is the same as the mean. Reproduced with permission from Lathers et al., *Epilepsy Res. 4*:42–54, 1989.

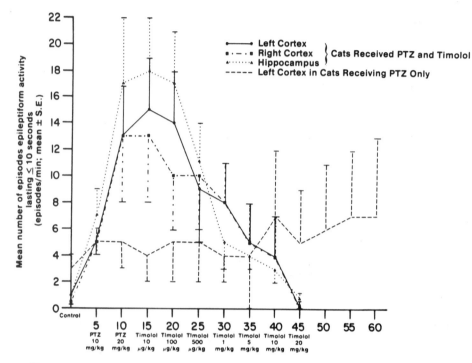

Figure 3 Epileptiform activity with a duration of ≤ 10 seconds obtained in cats treated with pentylenetetrazol and timolol. For purposes of comparison, data obtained in cats receiving only pentylenetetrazol are shown for the comparable experimental duration. The control values obtained in the cats receiving both pentylenetetrazol and timolol are means obtained in the 10-minute period prior to the first dose of pentylenetetrazol. Reproduced with permission from Lathers et al., *Epilepsy Res. 4*:42–54, 1989.

Table 4 Number of Cats and Dose of Timolol Inducing Total Suppression of Epileptiform Activity[a]

	Number of cats			
Doses of timolol (mg)	1	5	10	20
Left cortex	2	3	1	6
Right cortex	2	3	1	5
Hippocampus	2	2	2	7

[a]Epileptiform activity was not induced by PTZ in the left and right cortex of one cat and in the right cortex of a second animal.

pression of epileptiform activity was the same in only three brain regions. In six of the other seven cats, the dose of timolol producing total suppression of epileptiform activity was the same for all three brain areas; the times to suppression varied by only a few seconds. In one cat the epileptiform activity was suppressed in the left and right cortices at a dose of 5 mg timolol, while a dose of 10 mg was required to elicit total suppression in the hippocampus. The administration of timolol decreased the duration of all types of epileptiform activity, i.e., prolonged ictal (> 10 seconds), brief ictal, and interictal (Table 3).

The Friedman ANOVAs were significant ($p \leq 0.0001$) for all three areas of the brain. The Wilcoxon post-hoc tests revealed the expected PTZ-induced increase in epileptiform activity from control. In the 10 cats receiving 20 mg PTZ, this dose was not different from control (for any of the three areas) even though the means were higher than for 10 mg PTZ. In fact, none of the Bonferroni-corrected Wilcoxon tests were significant between 20 mg PTZ and any other dose, for any area. The first dose of timolol elicited slightly (not significant) higher rates of prolonged and brief ictal and interictal activity than 20 mg PTZ, after which a steady decrease in epileptiform activity occurred, becoming significant (one-tailed) by the dose of 1 mg/kg i.c.v. timolol. This trend occurred in all three areas of the brain. None of the Friedman ANOVAs or duration above 10 seconds approached significance; this was anticipated since many subjects had no prolonged ictal episodes at any dose.

Table 2 indicates the sequence in which the mean arterial blood pressure and heart rate were depressed by timolol in relation to the time when timolol partially or totally suppressed the epileptiform activity. In 12 of 13 cats the epileptiform activity was partially suppressed prior to the fall in mean arterial blood pressure, i.e., the fall in this parameter followed partial suppression induced by 10 μg timolol. The heart rate decreased in all 13 cats after the epileptiform activity was partially suppressed by this dose of timolol. In almost all of the cats the decrease in the mean arterial blood pressure and heart rate preceded total suppression of epileptogenic activity when the cardiovascular parameters were compared to control values. When mean arterial blood pressure and heart rate values at the time of total suppression of epileptogenic activity were compared to blood pressure and heart rate values in the preceding 5-minute interval, in most cats (7/13) the blood pressure decreased prior to total suppression of the epileptiform activity by timolol. However, the decrease in the mean heart rate followed total suppression of epileptogenic activity in six cats. In five cats the heart rate did not change immediately before or after the occurrence of total suppression of epileptiform activity.

B. Data Obtained in Anesthetized Pigs

A transient increase (16.3–50.0%) in the mean arterial blood pressure occurred following the PTZ administration. The elevated blood pressure gradually de-

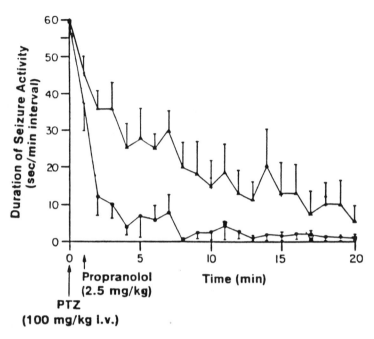

Figure 4   The effect of intravenous propranolol (2.5 mg/kg) on seizure activity
induced by PTZ (100 mg/kg i.v.) in pigs (*N* = 5-6). PTZ was given to induce seizure activity. Propranolol was administered 60 seconds after the onset of seizure
activity. The seizure activity at time zero was determined from the seizure duration of 0-1-minute interval. A significant suppression of seizure activity was observed at one minute following propranolol administration. Modified and reproduced with permission from Lathers et al., *Epilepsia 30*:473-479, 1989.

clined to the basal level within 10 minutes following PTZ. Intravenously administered propranolol significantly reduced this transient pressor response and returned the elevated blood pressure to the basal level at 2 minutes following drug
infusion (Figure 4). There was no significant change in the basal heart rate following PTZ administration. However, a marked bradycardia was observed at 1
minute after i.v. propranolol administration. Propranolol produced a maximal
decrease of 32-38% in the basal heart rate; the bradycardia persisted throughout
the experiment (Figure 5). Epileptogenic activity induced by PTZ was associated
with the occurrence of premature ventricular contractions in some pigs, similar
to those observed in anesthetized cats when administered PTZ. Figure 4 illustrates the duration of seizure activity elicited by PTZ over an experimental
period of 20 minutes. The seizure activity was continuous from *t* = 0 to 1 minute

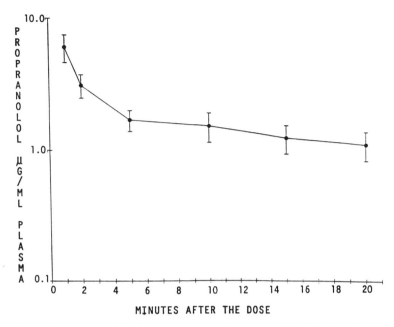

Figure 5 Propranolol plasma concentrations versus time in pigs administered propranolol 2.5 mg/kg i.v. Values are means ± deviation ($N = 6$).

for both groups. Intravenous propranolol produced a significant reduction in the duration of seizure activity one minute following drug infusion; the seizure durations (second per minute interval) were 36.3 ± 4.8 and 12.3 ± 5.1 for the control and i.v. groups, respectively. Animals treated with i.v. propranolol had reduced duration of seizure activity throughout the entire experiment when compared to the control animals.

Plasma propranolol concentrations were determined from 1 minute to 20 minutes after the intravenous administration of 2.5 mg/kg. After a rapid fall from 6.04 ± 1.43 μg/ml at minute 1 to 1.69 ± 0.31 μg/ml at minute 5, a steady decline in plasma concentration was observed out to 20 minutes, with a mean half-life of 23.3 ± 4.8 minutes (Figure 5). The brevity of the experiment precluded the determination of further kinetic parameters.

IV. DISCUSSION

Previous studies have shown that pentylenetetrazol administered intravenously induced epileptiform activity associated with cardiac arrhythmias and changes in the mean arterial blood pressure and heart rate (Carnel et al., 1985; Lathers and Schraeder, 1982; Lathers et al., 1984; Schraeder and Lathers, 1983). The present study demonstrated that the central administration of pentylenetetrazol produced similar effects within seconds of its intracerebroventricular injection. These data support the conclusion that the intravenous administration of pentylenetetrazol has little direct effect on the heart in eliciting cardiac arrhythmias, and that such arrhythmias are associated with the epileptiform discharges induced by PTZ.

The central administration of timolol decreased mean arterial blood pressure and heart rate. In another study, timolol administered intravenously to anesthetized cats also decreased the mean arterial blood pressure and heart rate (Lathers, 1980) and exhibited an antiarrhythmic action against ouabain-induced arrhythmias. Lathers et al. (1986) demonstrated that chronic oral dosing with timolol for one or two weeks increased the time, although not significantly, to arrhythmia induced by acute permanent occlusion of the left anterior descending coronary artery. In the present study, increasing doses of timolol administered intracerebroventricularly and intravenously not only significantly decreased the elevation of mean arterial blood pressure and heart rate but also decreased and subsequently abolished the incidence of cardiac arrhythmias associated with the epileptiform activity.

Epileptiform activity elicited in the present study with a duration less than or equal to 10 seconds includes both interictal and brief ictal discharges. Pentylenetetrazol-induced bilateral interictal spike activity is indicative of increased cortical excitability often evident in the EEG records of epileptic individuals. Pentylenetetrazol-induced generalized asynchronous clonic movements followed by a tonic convulsion in which limb movements are flexion followed by extension are analogous to the brief ictal discharges. Motor activity characterized by forelimb clonus is analogous to the prolonged ictal activity, i.e., duration greater than 10 seconds. In the animal model employing the cat and intracerebroventricular injection of pentylenetetrazol, most of the epileptiform activity elicited was interictal and/or brief ictal activity. It has been hypothesized that the cardiac arrhythmias associated with interictal activity could be one potential mechanism for sudden unexplained death in epileptic persons (Carnel et al., 1985; Lathers and Schraeder, 1982; Lathers et al., 1984; Schraeder and Lathers, 1983). That timolol either partially or totally abolishes the epileptiform activity in the shorter duration category suggests that it may be a useful therapeutic agent to suppress the interictal discharges associated with cardiac arrhythmias.

The administration of PTZ elicited epileptiform activity that was followed by increases in blood pressure, heart rate, and cardiac arrhythmias. Exactly how these changes develop is unknown but this laboratory (Kraras et al., 1987; Suter and Lathers, 1984) has proposed a possible mechanism to explain how epileptogenic activity and autonomic dysfunction may occur in epileptic patients, resulting in fatal cardiovascular changes. PTZ, trauma, inhibition of prostaglandin transport across the blood-brain barrier, or altered synthesis or metabolism of central enkephalins may lead to increased central levels of PGE_2 and/or enkephalins. The consequence of this is thought to be inhibition of central GABA release, epileptogenic activity, increased blood pressure and heart rate, increased sympathetic and parasympathetic central neural outflow, impaired or imbalanced cardiac sympathetic and parasympathetic discharge, and a resultant arrhythmia and/or death. In the present study, the central i.c.v. administration of timolol partially suppressed the epileptiform activity and subsequently decreased the blood pressure and heart rate values elevated by PTZ. It may be that timolol is interfering with the central actions of PGE_2 or enkephalins to reverse their known capabilities to induce epileptiform activity (see Chapter 18, this book). Additional experimental studies are required to verify this suggestion. Additional mechanisms to explain the anticonvulsant and antiarrhythmic actions of timolol are discussed later.

It has been theorized that pharmacologic agents capable of suppressing epileptiform activity and the sympathetic component of cardiac arrhythmias may be the best regimens to prevent interictal activity and the associated cardiac arrhythmias that may contribute to the production of sudden unexplained death in the epileptic person (Carnel et al., 1985; Lathers and Schraeder, 1982; Lathers et al., 1984; Schraeder and Lathers, 1983). The data obtained in the present study indicate that in the experimental setting the pharmacologic agent timolol possesses components of both of these capabilities. Blockade of cardiac $beta_1$ receptors, a cardiac neurodepressant effect, and/or membrane depressant actions of beta-blocking agents are thought to contribute to the antiarrhythmic action of beta-blocking agents (Lathers and Spivey, 1987). PTZ has been used to induce seizure activity in humans (Franz, 1980; Van Buren, 1958); study seizure mechanisms (Faingold and Berry, 1973; Krall et al., 1978; Langeluddeke, 1936; Swinyard, 1972); examine autonomic dysfunction associated with epileptogenic activity (Lathers and Schraeder, 1982; Onuma, 1957; Orihara, 1952; Schraeder and Lathers, 1983; Van Buren, 1958; Van Buren and Ajmone-Marsan, 1960); and screen anticonvulsant agents (Carnel et al., 1985; Faingold and Berry, 1973; Lathers et al., 1984). Since it is accepted that PTZ is a convulsive model and that many drugs capable of suppressing the PTZ-induced epileptiform activity are anticonvulsant agents, the results of this study suggest that timolol exhibited an anticonvulsant action. Although the data indicate that timolol can reverse the effects of PTZ on the brain, this does not necessarily mean that timolol has intrinsic "anticonvulsant" properties separate from an ability to reverse the effects of PTZ. To answer this question, additional studies must be done to determine whether timolol will protect against seizures induced in other experimental models of epilepsy. In particular, it would be important to evaluate the capability of timolol to suppress interictal discharges and cardiac arrhythmias elicited in other in vivo experimental models not involving PTZ. If timolol also suppresses both the interictal discharges and the arrhythmias in these experimental models, this would provide additional evidence to support the possibility that timolol may be an effective agent to use in epileptic patients to prevent sudden unexplained death.

The concept that beta-blocking agents may possess anticonvulsant action is not new (Bose et al., 1963; Conway et al., 1978; Papanicolaou et al., 1982). The studies of Dashputra et al. (1985), Jaeger et al. (1979), Murmann et al. (1966), and Tocco et al. (1980) demonstrated that propranolol possesses anticonvulsant actions. Mueller and Dunwiddie (1983) showed that timolol selectively blocked the proconvulsant activity of 2-fluoro-norepinephrine and 1-isoproterenol in in vitro hippocampal slice preparations superfused with penicillin and elevated levels of potassium. Louis et al. (1982) reported that propranolol or timolol (0.25 μg/kg i.c.v.) produced an anticonvulsant action when pentylenetetrazol was used to induce convulsions in rats. The anticonvulsant action of timolol reported here for the data obtained in swine is similar to the anticonvulsant action of diazepam when employed in the same experimental model (Lathers et al., 1987; Spivey et al., 1987).

The anticonvulsant action of beta-blocking agents is commonly ascribed to a membrane-stabilizing effect, although exceptions have been reported (Lints and Nyquist-Battie, 1985). Other proposed anticonvulsant mechanisms include decreased central serotonergic (Conway et al., 1978) and monoamine oxidase activity (Bose et al., 1963). An additional possible antiepileptic mechanism of the beta-blocking agents may include beta-adrenoceptor blockade, especially beta$_2$ receptors in the central nervous system (Papanicolaou et al., 1982). Although norepinephrine is generally believed to be anticonvulsant, studies suggest that norepinephrine may exacerbate seizure activity via activation of beta receptors. The state of abnormal seizure susceptibility, but not severity, in genetically epilepsy-prone rats may be determined by norepinephrine deficits in the hypothalamus/thalamus (Dailey and Jobe, 1986). Both severity and susceptibility can be determined by norepinephrine deficits in the telencephalon, midbrain, and pons–medulla, while seizure severity but not susceptibility may be determined by norepinephrine abnormalities in the cerebellum. Noradrenergic effects may not be uniform throughout the hippocampus; thus selective activation of alpha or beta receptors by norepinephrine in the brain areas such as the hippocampus might produce either anticonvulsant- or proconvulsant effects, respectively (Mueller and Dunwiddie, 1983). Beta-blocking agents can increase norepinephrine concentration in cerebral spinal fluid (Tackett et al., 1981) and potentiate the effects of exogenously administered norepinephrine on vas deferens contraction (Patil et al., 1968). If a similar action occurred in this study, the establishment of beta blockade with timolol would increase the central norepinephrine concentration. The increased norepinephrine activity at the central postsynaptic alpha$_1$ receptor sites may account for the anticonvulsant effects of beta-blocking agents (Goldman et al., 1987). Thus the protective mechanism for timolol against seizures induced by pentylenetetrazol may be due to a selective blockade of seizure-inducing beta receptors, allowing available norepinephrine to stimulate the central alpha$_1$ receptors that exert an anticonvulsant action.

In addition to the possibility that the central alpha$_1$ receptors may be involved in the anticonvulsant action of beta-blocking agents, the role of central postsynaptic alpha$_2$ receptors must be evaluated. Activation of alpha$_2$ receptors decreases the excitability of CA1 pyramidal neurons (Mueller et al., 1982). Clonidine and 1-m-norepinephrine are more selective for alpha$_2$ than for alpha$_1$ receptors and inhibit epileptiform activity at low concentrations; the alpha$_1$ agonist 1-phenylephrine was ineffective at much higher concentrations. These data suggest that central postsynaptic alpha$_2$ receptors may play a greater role than the alpha$_1$ receptors in the anticonvulsant action of timolol observed in the present study. Definitive experiments will have to be done to confirm this possibility.

V. SUMMARY

The experiments in this study were designed to explore the ability of beta-blocking agents to suppress seizures induced by pentylenetetrazol in two species, the cat and the pig. Cats were anesthetized with alpha-chloralose and pentylenetetrazol (10–20 mg i.c.v.) was administered to elicit epileptiform activity, including both interictal and ictal discharges. Timolol 10, 100, 500 μg/kg i.c.v. and 1, 5, 10, and/or 20 mg/kg i.v. was then administered at five-minute intervals to determine whether it suppressed the epileptiform activity. Mean arterial blood pressure increased after the administration of pentylenetetrazol and was associated with the development of epileptiform activity. Heart rate also was increased after pentylenetetrazol. All doses of timolol caused a decrease in the blood pressure and heart rate elevated by pentylenetetrazol. The administration of timolol also suppressed the epileptiform activity. Similar findings were obtained in cats that received the same doses of timolol administered at different time intervals. The data indicate that the central administration of timolol reverses the epileptiform activity of pentylenetetrazol on the brain and suppresses the associated increases in blood pressure and heart rate.

Domestic swine (13–20 kg) were prepared for recordings of arterial blood pressure, ECG, and electrocortical activity. Seizure activity was induced by PTZ

(100 mg/kg i.v.). Sixty seconds after the onset of seizure activity, the animals received either no drug (control) or propranolol (2.5 mg/kg i.v.). A transient increase in the mean arterial blood pressure was observed following PTZ administration. Intravenous propranolol significantly suppressed the seizure duration (second per minute interval) at one minute following drug administration; seizure duration control, 36.3 ± 4.8; i.v. propranolol, 12.3 ± 5.1. Intravenous propranolol also produced a maximal decrease of 32-38% in the basal heart rate and reduced the transient increase in mean arterial blood pressure elicited by PTZ, with no significant effect on the basal mean arterial blood pressusre. Plasma propranolol levels were found to be 6.07 ± 1.43 μg/ml at 1 minute after administration, falling to 1.10 ± 0.27 μg/mg over the following 19 minutes of the experiment. The data demonstrate that propranolol possesses anticonvulsant activity against PTZ-induced seizures in both the pig and in the cat.

ACKNOWLEDGMENTS

The study was funded by a grant from the Epilepsy Foundation of America and from the Ben Franklin Partnership Fund, a program of the Commonwealth of Pennsylvania. The authors would like to thank Valerie Farris, Larry Pratt, and Michele Spino for technical help and also for typing the manuscript, and Dr. Edward Gracely for statistical analyses.

REFERENCES

Albani, F., Riva, R., and Baruzzi, A. (1982). Simple and rapid determination of propranolol and its active metabolite, 4-hydroxypropranolol, in human plasma by liquid chromatography with fluorescence detection. *J. Chromatogr.* 228:362–365.

Bose, B. C., Saifi, A. Q., and Sharma, S. (1963). Studies on anticonvulsant and antifibrillatory drugs. *Arch. Int. Pharmacodyn. 146*:106–113.

Carnel, S. B., Schraeder, P. L., and Lathers, C. M. (1985). Effect of phenobarbital pretreatment on cardiac neural discharge and pentylenetetrazol-induced epileptogenic activity in the cat. *Pharmacology 20*:225–240.

Conway, J., Greenwood, D. T., and Middlemiss, D. N. (1978). Central nervous actions of β-adrenoceptor antagonists. *Clin. Sci. Molec. Med. 54*:119–124.

Dailey, J. W., and Jobe, P. C. (1986). Indices of noradrenergic function in the central nervous system of seizure-naive genetically epilepsy-prone rats. *Epilepsy 27*:665–670.

Dashputra, P. G., Patki, V. P., and Hemnani, T. J. (1985). Antiepileptic action of beta-adrenergic blocking drugs: Pronethal and propranolol. *Mater. Med. Pol. 2*:88–92.

Faingold, C. L., and Berry, C. A. (1973). Quantitative evaluation of the pentylenetetrazol-anticonvulsant interaction on the EEG of the cat. *Eur. J. Pharmacol. 24*:381–388.

Franz, D. N. (1980). *The Pharmacological Basis of Therapeutics*. Macmillan, New York.

Gillis, R. A. (1969). Cardiac sympathetic nerve activity: Changes induced by ouabain and propranolol. *Science 166*:508–510.

Goldman, B. D., Stauffer, A. Z., and Lathers, C. M. (1987). Beta blocking agents and the prevention of sudden unexpected death in the epileptic person: Possible mechanisms. *Fed. Proc. 46*:705.

Gremels, H. (1931). Uber die Einwirkung einiger zentral-erregender Mittel auf Atmung und Kreislauf. *Arch. Exp. Pathol. Pharmacol. 162*:29–45.

Hahn, F. (1960). Analeptics. *Pharmacol. Rev. 12*:447–530.

Han, J., and Moe, G. K. (1964). Nonuniform recovery of excitability in ventricular muscle. *Circ. Res. 14*:44–60.

Hildebrandt, E. (1937). Pentamethylenetetrazol (Cardiazol). *Handb. Exp. Pharm. 5*:151–183.

Hirsch, C. S., and Martin, D. L. (1971). Unexpected death in young epileptics. *Neurology 21*:682–690.

Jaeger, V., Esplin, B., and Capek, R. (1979). The anticonvulsant effects of propranolol and beta-adrenergic blockade. *Experientia 35*:8081.

Krall, R. L., Perry, J. K., White, B. G., Kupferberg, H. J., and Swinyard, E. A. (1978). Antiepileptic drug development. II. Anticonvulsant drug screening. *Epilepsia 19*:409–428.

Kraras, C. M., Tumer, N., and Lathers, C. M. (1987). The role of enkephalins in the production of epileptogenic activity and autonomic dysfunction: Origin of arrhythmia and sudden death in the epileptic patient? *Med. Hypotheses 23*:19–31.

Langeluddeke, A. (1936). Die diagnostische Bedeutung experimentell erzeugter Krampfe. *Dsch. Med. Wehnschr. 62*:1588–1590.

Lathers, C. M. (1980). Effect of timolol on autonomic neural discharge associated with ouabain-induced arrhythmia. *Eur. J. Pharm. 64*:95–106.

Lathers, C. M., and Schraeder, P. L. (1982). Autonomic dysfunction in epilepsy: Characterization of autonomic cardiac neural discharge associated with pentylenetetrazol-induced epileptogenic activity. *Epilepsia 23*:633–647.

Lathers, C. M., and Spivey, W. H. (1987). The effect of timolol, metoprolol, and practolol on postganglionic cardiac neural discharge associated with acute coronary occlusion-induced arrhythmia. *J. Clin. Pharmacol. 27*:582–592.

Lathers, C. M., Stauffer, A. Z., Turner, N., Kraras, C. M., and Goldman, B. D. (1989). Anticonvulsant and antiarrhythmic actions of the beta blocking agent timolol. *Epilepsy Res. 4*:42–54.

Lathers, C. M., Roberts, J., and Kelliher, G. J. (1977). Correlation of ouabain-induced arrhythmia and nonuniformity in the histamine-evoked discharge of cardiac sympathetic nerves. *J. Pharmacol. Exp. Ther. 203*:467–479.

Lathers, C. M., Kelliher, G. J., Roberts, J., and Beasley, A. B. (1978). Nonuniform cardiac sympathetic nerve discharge. *Circulation 57*:1058–1064.

Lathers, C. M., Schraeder, P. L., and Carnel, S. B. (1984). Neural mechanisms in cardiac arrhythmias associated with epileptogenic activity: The effect of phenobarbital in the cat. *Life Sci. 34*:1919–1936.

Lathers, C. M., Tumer, N., and Kraras, C. M. (1985). Cardiovascular and epileptogenic effects of pentylenetetrazol administered intracerebroventricularly in cats. *Epilepsia 26*:520.

Lathers, C. M., Spivey, W. H., Suter, L. E., Lerner, J. P., Tumer, N., and Levin, R. M. (1986). The effect of acute and chronic administration of timolol on cardiac sympathetic neural discharge, arrhythmia, and beta adrenergic receptor density associated with coronary occlusion in the cat. *Life Sci. 39*:2121–2141.

Lathers, C. M., Jim, K., and Spivey, W. H. (1989). A comparison of intraosseous and intravenous routes of administration for antiseizure agents. *Epilepsia 30*: 472–479.

Leestma, J. E., Kalelkar, M. B., Teas, S. S., Jay, G. W., and Hughes, J. R. (1984). Sudden unexpected death associated with seizures: Analysis of 66 cases. *Epilepsia 1*:84–88.

Lints, C. E., and Nyquist-Battie, C. (1985). A possible role for beta-adrenergic receptors in the expression of audiogenic seizures. *Pharmacol. Biochem. Behav. 22*:711–716.

Louis, W. J., Papanicolaou, J., Summers, R. J., and Vajda, F. J. E. (1982). Role of central beta adrenoceptors in the control of pentylenetetrazol-induced convulsions in rats. *Br. J. Pharmacol. 75*:441–446.

Lown, B., and Verrier, R. L. (1978). Neural factors and sudden death. In *Perspectives in Cardiovascular Research*, Vol. 2, *Neural Mechanisms in Cardiac Arrhythmias*, P. J. Schwartz, A. M. Brown, A. Malliani, A. Zanchetti (Eds.). Raven Press, New York, pp. 87–88.

Mueller, A. L., and Dunwiddie, T. V. (1983). Anticonvulsant and proconvulsant actions of alpha- and beta-noradrenergic agonists on epileptiform activity in rat hippocampus *in vitro*. *Epilepsia 24*:57–64.

Mueller, A. L., Hoffer, B. J., and Dunwiddie, T. V. (1981). Noradrenergic responses in rat hippocampus: Evidence for mediation by alpha and beta receptors in the *in vitro* slice. *Brain Res. 214*:113–126.

Murmann, W., Almirante, L., and Saccani-Gueli, M. (1966). Central nervous system effects of four beta-adrenergic receptor blocking agents. *J. Pharm. Pharmacol. 18*:317–318.

Onuma, T. (1957). Relationships of the predisposition to convulsions with the action potentials of the autonomic nerves and the brain. II. Changes in action potential of the autonomic nerves and the brain under conditions for increasing the predisposition to convulsions. *Tohoku J. Exp. Med. 65*:121–129.

Orihara, O. (1952). Comparative observations of the action potential of autonomic nerve with EEG. *Tohoku J. Exp. Med. 57*:43–54.

Papanicolaou, J., Vajda, F. J., Summers, R. J., and Louis, W. J. (1982). Role of beta-adrenoreceptors in the anticonvulsant effect of propranolol on leptazol-induced convulsions in rats. *J. Pharm. Pharmacol. 34*:124–125.

Patil, P. N., Tye, A., May, C., Hetey, S., and Miyagi, S. (1968). Steric aspects of adrenergic drugs. XI. Interactions of dibenamine and beta adrenergic blockers. *J. Pharmacol. Exp. Ther. 163*:309–319.

Randall, W. C., Thomas, J. X., Euler, D. E., and Rozanski, G. J. (1978). Cardiac dysrhythmias associated with autonomic nervous system imbalance in the conscious dog. In *Perspectives in Cardiovascular Research*, Vol. 2, *Neural Mechanisms in Cardiac Arrhythmias*, P. J. Schwartz, A. M. Brown, A. Malliani, and A. Zanchetti (Eds.). Raven Press, New York, pp. 123-138.

Schraeder, P. L., and Lathers, C. M. (1983). Cardiac neural discharge and epileptogenic activity in the cat: An animal model for unexplained death. *Life Sci.* *32*:1371-1382.

Snider, R. S., and Neimer, W. T. (1970). *A Stereotaxic Atlas of the Brain*. University of Chicago Press, Chicago.

Spivey, W. H., Unger, H. D., Lathers, C. M., and McNamara, R. M. (1987). Intraosseous diazepam suppression of pentylenetetrazol-induced epileptogenic activity in pigs. *Ann. Emergency Med.* *16*:156-159.

Suter, L. E., and Lathers, C. M. (1984). Modulation of presynaptic gamma aminobutyric acid release by prostaglandin E_2: Explanation for epileptogenic activity and dysfunction in autonomic cardiac neural discharge leading to arrhythmias? *Med. Hypotheses 15*:15-30.

Swinyard, E. A. (1972). Assay of antiepileptic drug activity in experimental animals: Standard tests. In *Anticonvulsant Drugs, International Encyclopedia of Pharmacology and Therapeutics*. Pergamon Press, Oxford, Section 19.1:47-65.

Tackett, R. L., Webb, J. G., and Privitera, P. J. (1981). Cerebroventricular propranolol elevates cerebrospinal fluid norepinephrine and lowers blood pressure. *Science 213*:911-913.

Tocco, D. J., Clineschmidt, B. V., Duncan, A. E. W., Deluna, F. A., and Baer, J. R. (1980). Uptake of the beta-adrenergic blocking agents propranolol and timolol by rodent brains: Relationship to central pharmacological action. *J. Cardiovasc. Res. 2*:133-143.

Toman, J. E. P., and Davis, J. P. (1949). The effects of drugs upon the electrical activity of the brain. *Pharmacol. Rev. 1*:425-492.

Van Buren, J. M. (1958). Some autonomic concomitants of ictal autonomism. *Brain 81*:505-528.

Van Buren, J. M., and Ajmone-Marsan, C. (1960). Correlations of autonomic and EEG components in temporal lobe epilepsy. *Arch. Neurol. 3*:683-703.

Index

About the Editors

CLAIRE M. LATHERS is a Pharmacologist in the Division of Cardio-Renal Drug Products, Food and Drug Administration, Rockville, Maryland; a Universities Space Research Association Visiting Scientist working at the National Aeronautics and Space Administration, Houston, Texas; and a Visiting Scientist in the Department of Pharmacology of the Uniformed Services University of the Health Sciences, Bethesda, Maryland. Dr. Lathers was previously affiliated with the Medical College of Pennsylvania, Philadelphia, where she was an Associate Professor of Pharmacology. The author or coauthor of over 200 publications and a reviewer for several journals, she is a Regent to the Board of the American College of Clinical Pharmacology and a member of numerous professional societies including the American Society for Pharmacology and Experimental Therapeutics, American Federation for Clinical Research, Society for Experimental Biology and Medicine, Cardial Electrophysiological Group, and International Study Group for Research in Cardiac Metabolism. Dr. Lathers received the B.S. degree (1969) in pharmacy from Union University, Albany, College of Pharmacy, New York, and Ph.D. degree (1973) in pharmacology from the State University of New York at Buffalo, School of Medicine and Dentistry.

PAUL L. SCHRAEDER is Professor of Medicine and Neurology and Head of the Division of Neurology at the University of Medicine and Dentistry of New Jersey, Robert Wood Johnson Medical School, Camden. The author or coauthor of over 20 publications, he is a member of several professional organizations including the Professional Advisory Board of the Epilepsy Foundation of New Jersey, American Epilepsy Society, American EEG Society, American Academy of Neurology, and American Association for the Advancement of Science. Dr. Schraeder received the A.B. degree (1962) from Bucknell University, Lewisburg, Pennsylvania, and M.D. degree (1966) from Jefferson Medical College Philadelphia, Pennsylvania. He completed his residency in neurology at the University of Wisconsin.